NUTRITION AND FOOD CHOICES

KRISTEN W. McNUTT, Ph.D.

FASEB Congressional
Science Fellow for 1977–78

DAVID R. McNUTT, M.D., M.P.H.

Bureau of Health Manpower,
Health Resources Administration

Department of Health,
Education and Welfare

SCIENCE RESEARCH ASSOCIATES, INC.
Chicago, Palo Alto, Toronto, Henley-on-Thames, Sydney, Paris, Stuttgart
A Subsidiary of IBM

Acquisition Editors	Bob Bovenschulte
	Jerry Richardson
Project Editor	Gretchen Hargis
Designer/Illustrator	Barbara Ravizza
Medical Illustrator	Roger Myers
Technical Illustrator	Pat Rogondino
Compositor	York Graphic Services

Library of Congress Cataloging in Publication Data

McNutt, Kristen W
   Nutrition and food choices.

   Includes bibliographies and index.
   1. Nutrition. I. McNutt, David R., joint author.
II. Title
TX354.M26   641.1   77-13636
ISBN 0-574-20500-4

The opinions and conclusions expressed by the authors and their interpretations of data do not necessarily represent those of the Bureau of Health Manpower, Department of Health, Education and Welfare.

10 9 8 7 6 5 4 3 2 1

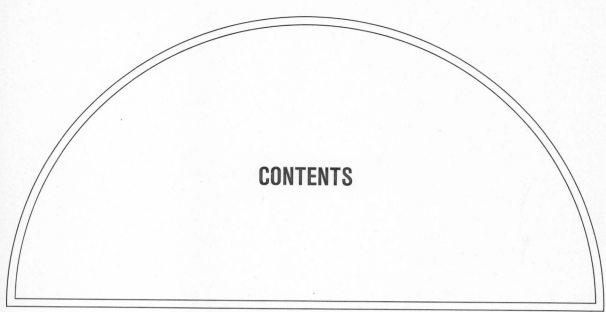

CONTENTS

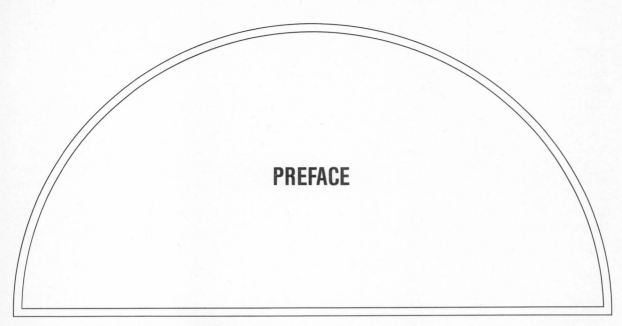

PREFACE

The basic objectives of *Nutrition and Food Choices* are to present current knowledge of the science of nutrition and to show how this science can be applied to guide an individual toward making appropriate food choices.

Nutrition and Food Choices uses terminology and explanations that can be comprehended by students who have not previously studied chemistry. A high-school basic science or biology course would be helpful background for Chapters 4, 6, and 7, but this preparation is not mandatory. Descriptive words and phrases are included as synonyms for technical vocabulary used by biochemists and physiologists. We make frequent use of analogies throughout the text, but especially in the first two sections. The key concepts printed at the top of each appropriate page are designed to help students remember the most important ideas presented and to reinforce information explained in greater detail within the text of that page.

The perspective of this book expands progressively from section to section. An overview of the fundamental concepts of nutrition is provided in the first two sections. Section I classifies the nutrients, describes their functions in the body, and lists the foods that supply (and do not supply) each nutrient.

Section II discusses how the energy and nutrients of food are rendered utilizable by the body. The physiological and metabolic roles of nutrients are explained, attention is given to how the nutrients function together to support health, and the importance of water is discussed.

The remainder of *Nutrition and Food Choices* applies and expands the principles presented in the first two sections. Teachers and students may choose from the following chapters those that are of greatest interest; not all of this material must be taught. Chapters may generally be covered independently and in whatever sequence is most useful for various course outlines. However, Chapter 8 (the first chapter in Section III) on food selection guides and Chapter 13 (the first chapter in Section IV) on nutrition surveys provide information necessary for fully appreciating the chapters that follow in each of these two sections.

Sections III and IV consider many different situations and conditions that influence the appropriateness of various food choices. Section III focuses on variables that determine which foods best fit the diet of an individual, regardless of that person's age or sex. These variables include body weight, activity level, snacking and meal patterns, financial means, and personal values. Section IV explains how nutrient needs vary throughout the lifespan. This information is integrated into a discussion of concurrent changes in physiological and psychosocial factors that influence the acceptability or appropriateness of foods for persons of different ages.

Section V discusses the role of food and nutrients in maintaining health and in preventing disease. Emphasis is given to developing thought processes that apply the science of nutrition to questions related to health. Discussions include topics such as development of scientific hypotheses, analysis of epidemiological data, similarity of manifestations of certain nutritional and non-nutritional disorders, dose-response correlations, toxicity calculations, dangers inherent in self-medication, benefit-risk evaluations, the significance of dietary risk factors associated with certain diseases, and the interrelationship between nutrition disorders and other diseases or conditions.

Section VI looks into the crystal ball. One chapter suggests how a person can continue to learn about nutrition without taking additional academic courses. The other touches upon how diets may change in the future and how the future of society will be affected by the success of efforts to resolve the world food problem and by the growth and application of nutrition knowledge.

The ultimate objective of *Nutrition and Food Choices* is not only that students master nutrition facts but also that they learn to ask critical questions about their own diets and about food-related issues. The significance of this objective is underscored by the current changes in the health delivery system of the United States (such as the increasing emphasis on consumer input into health planning and personal responsibility for health) and the growing interdependence between science and public policy. Both of these trends have important implications for nutrition education and indeed for all of health education. Nonscientists must be prepared to think analytically and scientists must be prepared to apply their knowledge to real life situations and problems. We hope that *Nutrition and Food Choices* proves to be a useful tool toward achieving these goals.

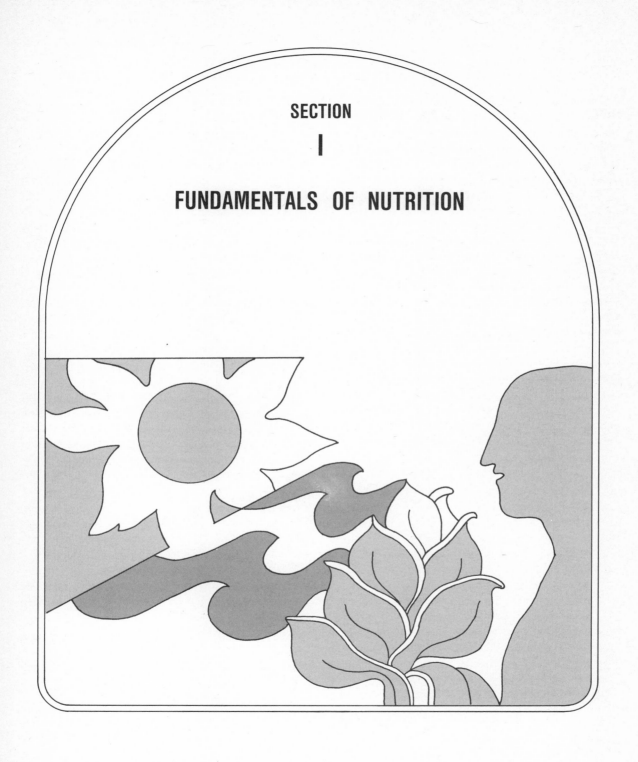

SECTION

I

FUNDAMENTALS OF NUTRITION

FUNDAMENTALS OF NUTRITION

Nutrition is the biological science that deals with the body's need for nutrients and how these nutrients function in the body to maintain health. Application of nutrition knowledge requires an appreciation of psychosocial factors that influence our diet selection patterns as well as an understanding of the nutrients required for health and the amounts of each nutrient provided by different types of food. Section I provides a foundation of nutrition information that is expanded and applied in the rest of the book.

CHAPTER 1 WHY WE EAT outlines the physiological reasons that food is needed by our bodies; points out some of the psychosocial factors that influence our diets; explains some of the benefits of good nutrition in combination with other sound health practices.

CHAPTER 2 WHAT WE EAT describes the macronutrients and micronutrients we need; tells which types of food are good or poor sources of each nutrient.

CHAPTER 3 WHY WE EAT WHAT WE EAT discusses the energy value of food and the energy needs of our bodies; explains the different functions of each macronutrient and micronutrient.

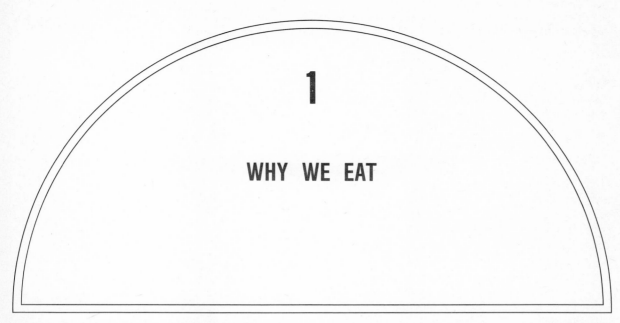

1

WHY WE EAT

Eating is such a fundamental part of our daily lives that there seems little reason to ask "Why do we eat?" But the response to this question is not as obvious as one might assume. Much of this book is devoted to answering this seemingly simple question.

Fundamentally, the science of nutrition deals with the physiological reasons for eating. Life in the human organism is dependent upon an adequate dietary supply of *nutrients*—proteins, carbohydrates, fats, water, vitamins, and minerals. These nutrients occur in myriad combinations as foods. In order for us to meet our physiological need for these nutrients, we must eat a proper combination of different types of foods.

Although nutrient composition of food is an important consideration, we eat for other reasons also. Factors such as personal preferences regarding taste, color, and texture affect food choices. Diet patterns are influenced by the way we live—such as our pace of life, our financial means, and the values of our family and our society. These psychosocial reasons for eating, which may seem peripheral to the discipline of nutrition, are actually the dominant factors (conscious or subconscious) that govern our patterns of food selection.

The purpose of this chapter is to highlight both the physiological and psychosocial reasons for eating. In the ultimate application of nutrition knowledge, we must not only understand the function of nutrients and become aware of the foods that supply these nutrients, but also adapt this basic knowledge to our individual patterns of eating and personal preferences for foods. Anyone who masters this information and puts it into practice will be able to select a diet that both meets individual nutrient needs and satisfies other criteria that determine diet patterns.

PHYSIOLOGICAL REASONS

Walking through the aisles of a grocery store, the shopper is confronted with thousands of foods, all differing in taste, cost, and appearance. Compared to the many different fruits, vegetables, meats, desserts, and other varieties of food, the types of nutrients found in food are small in number. There are six types or groups of nutrients: water, proteins, carbohydrates, lipids (fats), vitamins, and minerals.

Each of these nutrient groups, except water, contains several different nutrients. Important differences, both within and among these groups will be delineated in later chapters. The categorization that follows is a basic explanation of the general functions of nutrients.

Macronutrients and Micronutrients

The functions of each nutrient may be better understood if one appreciates the relative amounts of the different types of nutrients in the diet. Proteins, carbohydrates, lipids, and water together account for most of the weight of food. Vitamins and minerals, however, constitute less than 1 percent of the weight of the food we eat. These distinctions in weight between the *macronutrients* (proteins, carbohydrates, lipids, and water) and the *micronutrients* (vitamins and minerals) are related to differences in the physiological functions of each group.

Each nutrient within a group has many specific functions in the body. In most instances, several nutrients work together to sustain life-supporting tasks, such as building blood cells or conducting nerve impulses from the brain to the heart. These and the other functions of nutrients fall into one of three categories (Figure 1-1):

1. Providing energy to the body
2. Supporting the growth, maintenance, and repair of the body
3. Regulating the many reactions that occur within the body

Energy. The energy of food is bound up in the macronutrients—proteins, carbohydrates, and lipids. (Alcohol also provides energy, but it is not a dietary essential.) Several micronutrients—vitamins and minerals—are necessary for the release of this food energy and its utilization within the cells of the body.

The conversion of food energy to the energy necessary to support animal life is part of the flow of energy through the biosphere. In order to understand this conversion, we must know that energy

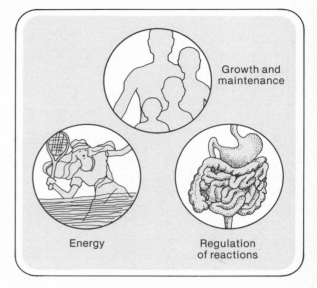

Figure 1–1. Functions of nutrients.

cannot be destroyed—it can only be transformed or converted from one energy state, or form, to another. For example, both the energy in the form of heat that maintains body temperature at 98.6°F (37°C) and the energy stored in chemical bonds that enables muscles to contract, originate in the rays of light emanating from the sun.

When light energy from the sun reaches plants on earth, it is transformed into chemical energy by *photosynthesis*, a process that involves the chlorophyll of green plants. These plants combine water obtained from the soil with carbon dioxide from the air to form oxygen and carbohydrate molecules (Figure 1-2). These molecules represent not only a stable way for plants to store the energy they receive from the sun; they also form the structural or building blocks of plants. When we eat plants, the stored energy is released and used to power activities within our bodies.

The food energy we eat is stored in the chemical bonds of carbohydrates, fats, and proteins in a manner similar to the storage of energy in coal or oil.

Our diets include large amounts of macronutrients (proteins, carbohydrates, lipids or fats, and water) and small amounts of micronutrients (vitamins and minerals).

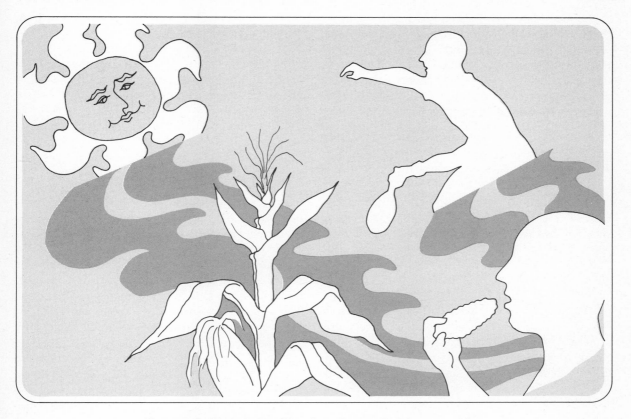

Figure 1–2. How energy flows from the sun to human muscles.

Table 1-1 compares the energy values of some food portions with corresponding portions of various types of fuels.

Food energy can be released as heat energy al-most instantaneously—a marshmallow falling into the fire or some cooking oil spattering onto the flame of a gas stove releases its energy just as a flaming log in a fireplace releases heat. In the

TABLE 1-1. The Energy in Food

Portions of Food	Calories	Energy Equivalents
Milk, 1 quart	634	Gasoline, $\frac{1}{3}$ cup
Beef, lean ground, 1 pound	812	Coal, $\frac{1}{4}$ pound
Root beer, 12 ounces	152	Natural gas, $\frac{1}{2}$ cubic foot

human body, however, food energy is released more slowly, as the chemical bonds of proteins, fats, and carbohydrates are broken and rearranged in a gradual, ordered series of reactions. Some food energy is released as heat, but most food energy is harnessed or captured in the formation of specialized, high-energy molecules that can later be used to power energy-requiring reactions throughout the body. If more food energy is consumed than is needed to maintain body temperature and body reactions, the excess energy is used to form body fat.

Growth and Maintenance. On a day-to-day basis it is difficult to appreciate the relationship between diet and body growth. Over a period of approximately eighteen years, however, this relationship is readily apparent. For example, a seven-pound baby will increase its body weight about fifteen fold if it is female and from twenty to twenty-five fold if it is male. This change, which is measurable on the bathroom scales, reflects the expansion of body tissues—bones grow longer; muscle girth expands; the volume of blood circulating through the heart, arteries, and veins increases; and skin grows to cover the larger person. These tissues and others are constructed solely from the nutrients of the food we eat.

The role of food in supporting growth is easier to visualize than the importance of diet in body maintenance. From the cradle to the grave, cells are constantly forming, maturing and dying throughout the body. For example, the need for haircuts, shaving, and manicures is due to the continuous synthesis and replacement of body cells. Peeling off a layer of dead skin after a sunburn or experiencing flaky, dry skin in cold weather are obvious manifestations of how cells die without threatening a person's life.

Cells in the liver, kidneys, intestines, thyroid, blood, and other tissues also have lifespans shorter than the lifespan of the entire body. When these cells break down, their constituents are either incorporated into new cells, broken down to produce energy, or excreted. Feces contain not only un-

digested food and bacteria, but also dead cells from the lining of the gastrointestinal tract, some breakdown products of blood, and cellular material excreted into the intestine by the liver. Urine normally contains dissolved minerals, vitamins, and other chemicals released from cells in the body, but few intact cells.

Food, therefore, must supply nutrients and energy not only for body growth, but also for replacing worn-out cells that are lost through normal processes or through excessive wear and tear.

Regulation of Reactions. The complexity and fine tuning of the numerous reactions constantly occurring within the human body are rarely appreciated by people outside the biological sciences. In order for your eyes to move across this page and for your brain to comprehend the words you read, hundreds of separate but integrated reactions occur. These reactions involve the muscles and retina of the eye, the optic nerve, and the brain. Even when you close your eyes and sit quietly, vital processes continue—the breaking down of macronutrients to release energy; the moving of molecules across membranes from one cell to another; the assembling of digested proteins, fats, and carbohydrates into biologically active components of the body. The reactions that occur within a fraction of a second are too numerous to count. The release of energy from one molecule of table sugar, for example, requires more than a hundred separate reactions.

Several important classes of chemical compounds regulate the physiological reactions in the body. *Hormones* are the master control molecules for maintaining the rate and direction of these reactions. Together with nerve tissues, they keep the body in tune with both its external and its internal environments. A class of proteins called *enzymes* facilitate specific steps in the reaction sequence. Certain vitamins and minerals, act as *cofactors* in the sequence of biological reactions by activating the enzyme that a particular reaction requires. If an enzyme or a cofactor essential to any one step in a process is missing, the entire sequence of reactions is slowed down or blocked. Deficiency of a vitamin or mineral cofactor, therefore, can have far-reaching effects upon the regulation of normal body functions. For example, synthesis of blood cells may be diminished, causing anemia; or the nervous system may not function properly, resulting in convulsions.

Integration of Functions

Although the functions of nutrients can be separated into the categories energy, growth and maintenance, and regulation of reactions, there are crucial interrelationships among these three basic functions: (Figure 1-3):

1. Energy release can occur only in the presence of regulatory enzymes and cofactors.
2. Growth, maintenance, and repair of the body are dependent upon an adequate supply of energy and of regulatory enzymes and cofactors.
3. The reactions that are regulated by enzymes and

cofactors are also dependent upon an adequate supply of energy; the ultimate purpose of these regulated reactions is the growth, maintenance, and repair of the body.

The interrelationship of nutrient functions is a concept woven through the chapters to follow. Although the academic explanations of these interactions fall within the disciplines of biochemistry and physiology, the general nutrition student, at this stage, should simply be aware that nutrients work together in the body to perform many functions. For example, the protein, calcium, and vitamin D in milk play many roles besides building bones and teeth; but these three nutrients cannot be used for building bones and teeth unless the diet also supplies enough of several other nutrients.

PSYCHOSOCIAL REASONS

A computer program based on food composition data and individual nutrient needs, which could rapidly print out a monthly cycle of nutritionally adequate meals, may sound like an easy solution to our nutrition problems. However, nutritive value is not the only consideration governing what we eat. Few people would be willing to follow a computer-generated diet and, for a number of reasons, many people would not be able to eat the recommended foods in the designated amounts according to the prescribed instructions.

Many psychosocial factors—some internal, some external—influence daily food selection patterns (Figure 1-4). Being aware of these factors that determine food choices is essential if we desire to change our patterns of selecting food. An appreciation of both the nutritional value of food and psychosocial reasons for eating enables a person to evaluate what is being gained or lost by altering the diet.

The nutrition information in the following chapters may reveal that your diet supplies too much or too little of certain types of nutrients. In some instances, changing your food intake to meet nutri-

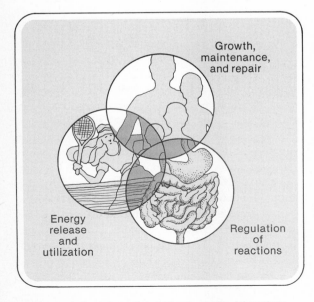

Figure 1-3. Integration of basic nutrient functions.

Biological reactions depend upon the presence of enzymes or cofactors—certain vitamins and minerals. Consumption of food (the source of nutrients) is greatly influenced by psychosocial factors.

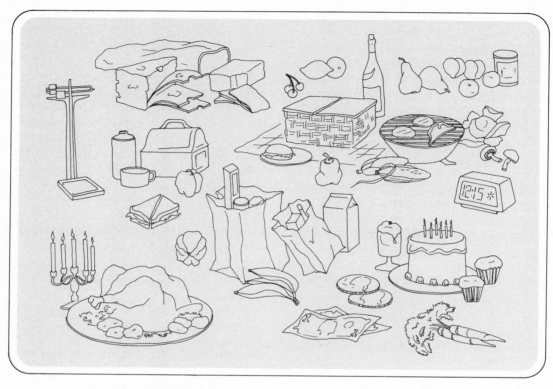

Figure 1–4. Food choices are determined by many psychosocial influences.

ent needs can be accomplished only through difficult adjustments—giving up things you like or making yourself eat foods you have never enjoyed. Most often, however, a person who recognizes the psychosocial or personal value of certain types of foods can learn to substitute for a nutritionally unwise food a food that is nutritionally more appropriate but that still satisfies personal reasons for eating.

Let's examine some of these psychosocial factors.

Availability

The primary criterion for whether one eats or does not eat is simply the availability of food. Civil disruptions and war have disastrous effects upon this factor. Production is curtailed, and transport to the marketplace of the few available commodities is often impossible. In a similar manner, food is not available to flood or snowstorm victms because roads and stores are closed.

The availability of food is also affected by the seasons. Inclement weather may drastically reduce crop yields; the limited supply of food that can be harvested is in such great demand that prices soar. The energy crunch is beginning to pose a similar threat to the availability of food. The lack of petroleum by-products from which fertilizers are made and the higher prices of energy used to harvest, transport, and process food may dramatically alter the price of the food and also affect the kinds of foods available to people all over the world.

The availability of food in grocery stores depends to a certain degree upon the preferences of the clientele. Many international items are not sold in some cities because of insufficient demand, and more expensive foods such as artichoke hearts and caviar are not stocked in the markets of low-income neighborhoods.

Factors closer to home also influence the availability of food. The elderly as well as people who do not own a car have limited access to food simply because they have difficulty carrying groceries home. Economic constraints may limit the amount and type of food an individual or family can afford, but financial security does not always enhance food availability. In families where both parents work, youngsters who prepare their own food may select diets that are inadequate in either quantity or quality. Access to food can also be indirectly affected by what a person wants to do with his or her money. Food must compete with other commodities in the budget—clothing, car, hobbies, cosmetics, housing, entertainment, a vacation, and so forth.

A person's lifestyle can impose limitations on the availability of food. The student who has only ten minutes to get to an afternoon job after a morning of classes has very little access to lunch. The executive who goes from a morning meeting in Boston to a two o'clock conference in New York gets no lunch on the commuter flight.

The list of factors affecting availability of food is not exhaustive. The important point is that if you realize that your diet can be improved, you should examine what foods are realistically available— when and where and why.

Social Reasons

Food is a part of almost every social gathering. The kind of gathering and other circumstances unrelated to nutrition often determine whether a food is considered appropriate or out-of-place. Popcorn is part of going to the movies, but is unacceptable at the opera. Barbecued spareribs are much too challenging for a formal dinner, but are suitable for a cookout. Watermelon balls may appear as a first course on a fancy menu, but a quarter melon is more enjoyable at a picnic.

The coffee break is perhaps the most common social use of food. Irrespective of what one drinks or eats, the coffee break serves many functions. For the desk worker, it is a chance to stretch one's legs; for people who have more active jobs, it is an opportunity to rest. The coffee break can also provide an opportunity to solicit an opinion or to get advice from a fellow worker or student. Although the food and/or beverages consumed at break time can improve the nutrient content of the total daily diet, this is rarely the purpose of the coffee break in American society.

The giving or receiving of food has greater social significance than simply eating at the same table with another person. Many people think twice before offering or accepting an invitation to dine with someone, because eating a meal together can affect the distance between people.

The social implications of exchanging food are similar throughout the world. The animal sacrifices of certain cultures and the food gifts exchanged among tribes in Africa and Polynesia may seem foreign to us, but the social reasons for these traditions are similar to those that determine food practices in the United States. For example, the work and cost involved in company meals are an expression of respect for the guest and for the friendship shared; delicacies not usually part of the daily diet are often reserved for this dinner. The food that we take to a bereaved family serves not only to ease the burden of meal preparation, but also to express sympathy. We use food also to communicate with our closest friends and loved ones. Gifts of candy or a favorite dessert may be part of patching up a quarrel—perhaps akin to appeasing the gods in more primitive societies.

The sensory qualities of food, our priorities and scheduling, and our emotions all affect both what we eat and when or if we eat.

Sensory Qualities

The sensory qualities of food—taste, odor, temperature, color, and texture—influence what we select to eat. Who would order hot coffee after a set of tennis or sip iced tea in front of the fireplace on a cold winter night? We feel that a firm banana is not yet ripe enough to eat, but we discard a mushy apple. Similarly, an odorless bowl of clam chowder or spaghetti has little appeal. Adults are often influenced by the appearance of food. For example, parsley, orange slices, or spiced apples may be used to decorate a plate rather than to provide basic nutrients. Children are also drawn to attractive foods, such as brightly colored breakfast cereals.

The person who recognizes the importance of the sensory qualities of food is better equipped to make nutritionally indicated dietary changes. The snacker who likes crunchy food but needs to cut down the amount of fat in the diet could substitute unbuttered popcorn for potato chips or peanuts. The overweight person with an unquenchable thirst for something cold could cut calories by reaching for unsweetened iced tea instead of soft drinks. The host or hostess who needs color to liven up a dinner plate would be doing a favor for overweight guests by serving carrots rather than sweet potatoes.

Lifestyle

Food selection and eating patterns are also greatly influenced by a person's schedule of activities. For example, breakfast options are affected by the means one chooses for getting the morning news. If you read the newspaper on the commuter train, you probably opt for coffee-to-go and a Danish. If you watch television at the breakfast table, many more food choices are feasible. The breakfast schedule also depends upon your priorities regarding time for sleeping, dressing, exercising, shaving, or putting on makeup. Breakfast foods, and therefore the nutrients consumed, are also affected by how many people are in the kitchen, helping or needing help in food preparation.

Frequency of eating is greatly influenced by the day's schedule and other activities. Jotting down the number of times you eat anything on a weekday and then comparing such a list to food consumption on a weekend reveals how strongly eating patterns are affected by where you are and by what else you are doing.

There are many other examples of priorities for eating versus priorities for other activities. The table-talker—who knows no age restriction—is a prime example. No doubt, among your friends there is one who dominates the group conversation and is always the last person to finish eating, or perhaps never finishes all the food on the plate. Some people skip meals because they have too much work (or play) or because they are more interested in these activities than in food.

Emotions

Eating patterns are closely related to one's mood or emotions. Part of this behavior may be physiological. Some nutritional deficiencies cause apathy and depression accompanied by a lack of appetite. Many other diseases, as well as drugs, can cause emotional changes that reduce incentive to eat or make food seem unappealing.

Psychological factors can trigger either an increase or a decrease in food consumption. Eating beyond one's physiological needs is one reaction pattern to emotionally disturbing experiences. Eating very little when upset or excited is another.

Rejection of food can symbolize emotions that are difficult to verbalize for some people. Adults, as well as children, express anger, alienation, or a plea for attention by refusing food. The overt action may be picking at the food on the plate or a stormy departure from the dinner table, but the message has little to do with the nutritional or other qualities of the meal.

Many other psychosocial reasons influence what we eat. Some of these are discussed further in Section III. It is important for each individual to identify the factors that determine his or her food choices.

BENEFITS OF GOOD NUTRITION

Most people in the United States today are well enough nourished that severe nutrient deficiency diseases such as *scurvy, pellagra,* and *rickets* are unlikely to occur. The rarity of these diseases among the general population tends to convey a feeling that all is well on the nutrition horizon. However, malnutrition does occur among Americans today, although its manifestations are subtle.

Evidence that the body is not adequately nourished usually appears first as an alteration in normal cellular reactions. Laboratory tests for nutritional status can detect such changes long before the entire body manifests the effects of poor food choices. Abnormalities detected in cellular function will eventually be mirrored in ill health if an appropriate diet is not adopted.

Good nutrition, like most sound health practices, rarely provides a person with immediate gratification. Some of the benefits of good nutrition and the reasons they are not readily perceived are discussed below.

Gradual, Cumulative Effects

Many of the benefits of good nutrition are the result of choosing foods wisely throughout a lifetime. The contribution of good nutrition to the attainment of optimal body proportion is spread over nearly two decades of childhood. Nutrition affects how tall a person becomes, but other factors such as heredity and the age at which growth spurts occur may also affect height. A direct correlation between diet and a person's height cannot therefore be easily perceived on an individual basis. This benefit of good nutrition becomes obvious, however, by comparing average heights of large groups of children whose diets have varied in quality.

The cumulative effects of nutrition also influence the health of adults. Nutrition can make a great difference in the physical condition of older people, and consequently in how active they can be during their later years.

Preventive Effects

Certain effects of good nutrition are hard to appreciate because they are preventive rather than curative. Healthy people who have good nutrition habits have little or no basis for linking the absence of disease with the quality of their diet.

Nutrition maintains one's resistance to infection. Good nutrition alone cannot always protect a person from disease; but, over a long time, a person will be sick less often if he or she is well nourished.

Knowing how to choose food wisely enables a person to maintain an ideal body weight. People who avoid becoming overweight are not as conscious, however, of the benefits of their good nutrition as obese people are aware of the disadvantages of being overweight.

Performance under Stress

Some of the benefits of good nutrition are not recognizable until the body is stressed. A less-than-optimal diet can provide sufficient nutrients to allow normal functioning of the body under ideal conditions. However, when the body is challenged by physiologically stressful conditions such as an infection or even physical exertion, marginal nutritional status (less than ideal but not severely deficient) becomes evident. In the case of an injury or an unexpected operation, if a person has failed to eat a balanced diet and to build up nutritional reserves with which to begin and sustain the reparative processes, then recovery may be prolonged and

11

Nutrition can determine physiological characteristics only within a person's genetic potential. To gain maximum benefit from good nutrition, a person must maintain other sound health practices.

TABLE 1-2. Indicators of Health and Factors Affecting Them

| Characteristic | Nutrition | | Other Factors |
	Good	Poor	
Height	Appropriate for age	Short for age	Genetics, posture
Weight	Appropriate for height	Overweight, underweight	Genetics, exercise, stress
Vision	Good	Impaired	Genetics, disease
Teeth	Few cavities	Many cavities	Genetics, fluoridation, brushing and flossing
Skin	Clear	Dry and scaly, oily	Genetics, weather, allergies, infection, trauma
Hair	Lustrous	Dry or oily	Genetics, hygiene
Fingernails	Strong	Cracked, split	Genetics, nervous behavior
Stamina	Capable of prolonged endurance	Easily worn out	Exercise, smoking habits
Susceptibility to infection	Resistant	Often sick	Stress, immunization, lack of rest, exposure to illness

the risk of complication may be increased. Pregnancy is also a physiological stress that requires maximal nutritional preparedness.

Nutrient reserves are necessary for the continuation of optimal physiological functioning should food intake be temporarily restricted. Exam week, for example, may wreak havoc with normal eating patterns, or an emotional crisis may cause a loss of appetite. The person who has chosen an appropriate diet prior to these stressful experiences is better prepared to meet these challenges.

Genetically Interrelated Effects

As Table 1-2 shows, many manifestations of nutritional status are greatly influenced by genetics. For instance, the maximal height to which a person can grow is genetically determined. Good nutrition cannot enable a person to grow taller than what is genetically possible. However, a person who is poorly nourished will fail to reach his or her height potential.

Appearance of the hair and skin, strength of fingernails, and oral health are other personal characteristics that are influenced by both genetics and nutritional status. Genetics determines what is physiologically possible; nutrition determines whether or not the potential is realized.

Interdependent Health Determinants

Almost all of the potential benefits of good nutrition will be negated if other sound health practices are neglected. Regardless of one's diet, a cavity-free mouth is rarely possible without good oral hygiene. Muscles become flabby and weak if a person never exercises. The risk of a heart attack is affected not only by obesity and certain diet patterns, but also by smoking and probably by inactivity, personality traits, and genetics. Resistance to certain infections requires immunization as well as adequate nutrition. Good nutrition alone cannot provide optimum health unless a person also respects other factors that influence how well the body functions.

STUDY QUESTIONS

1. List the macronutrients and the micronutrients that comprise your diet.

2. Name the three physiological reasons for eating.

3. Trace the flow of energy from the sun to the muscles of your legs.

4. Explain the role of macronutrients and micronutrients in supplying energy to the body.

5. What is the function of enzymes and cofactors?

6. In what ways is the consumption of food influenced by psychosocial factors?

7. What can be gained by understanding the psychosocial factors that influence food selection?

8. Name three factors that influence what you eat and when you eat.

9. Why is it difficult to recognize the consequences of poor nutrition?

10. What might happen to you that would make it advantageous to have good nutrient reserves? In other words, why are good nutrient reserves important?

11. How does a person's genetic potential interact with nutrition?

12. For your own body, which of the indicators of health in Table 1-2 are hampered by nonnutritional factors?

SUGGESTED READING

1. J. Mayer, "The American way of eating," *Family Health* 7(1975):30.

2. N. W. Jerome, "Flavor preferences and food patterns of selected U.S. and Caribbean Blacks," *Food Technology* 29(1975):46–51.

3. A. M. Brown, "British food habits," *Journal of Human Nutrition* 31(1977):41–44.

4. M. F. Futrell, L. T. Kilgore, and F. Windham, "Nutritional status of black preschool children in Mississippi: Influence of income, mother's education, and food programs," *Journal of the American Dietetic Association* 66(1975):22–27.

5. B. A. Cosper and L. M. Wakefield, "Food choices of women: Personal, attitudinal, and motivational factors," *Journal of the American Dietetic Association* 69(1976):152–54.

6. A. A. Hertzler and C. Owen, "Sociological study of food habits," *Journal of the American Dietetic Association* 69(1976):377–85.

7. J. J. Groen, "Psychocultural influences on nutritional behavior," *Nutrition* (London) 27(1973):393–403.

8. M. Mead, *Cultural Patterns and Technological Change* (chapter on nutrition). New York: New American Library, 1955.

9. M. E. Lowenberg, E. N. Todhunter, E. D. Wilson, J. R. Savage, and J. L. Lubawski, *Food and Man.* 2d ed. New York: John Wiley and Sons, 1974.

10. H. H. Gift, M. B. Washbon, and G. G. Harrison, *Nutrition, Behavior and Change.* Englewood Cliffs, N.J.: Prentice-Hall, Inc., 1976.

11. "The state of nutrition today," *FDA Consumer* 7(1973):13–17.

12. F. T. Hatch, "Interactions between nutrition and heredity in coronary heart disease," *American Journal of Clinical Nutrition* 27(1974):80–89.

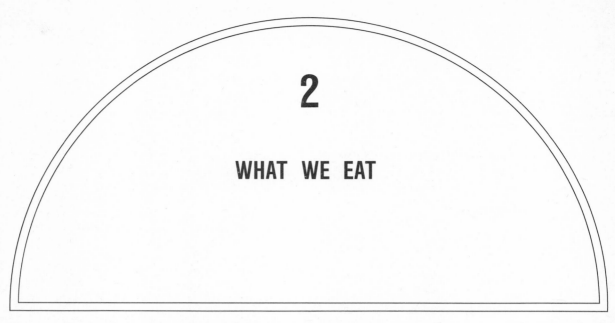

2

WHAT WE EAT

Almost everything we eat supplies the body with several nutrients, but the amount and the proportion of macronutrients and micronutrients in each food vary greatly. In order to select a total diet that will furnish the proper amount of each nutrient and thereby enable the body to function at its best, we must know what the nutrients are and how they are distributed in different foods.

DIET COMPOSITION

If all the solid food eaten during one day by an average adult were put in a half-gallon milk carton, the container would be about one-half to three-quarters full. If, after the bones were taken out, this mixture were transferred to a shallow dish and put in an oven at a temperature warm enough to evaporate the water without burning the food, the volume would be reduced eventually to about a pint. Heating this pint of residue in a laboratory oven at a much higher temperature would reduce the residue to about a teaspoonful.

This simple experiment tells us a great deal about the composition of the food we eat. A large percentage of our diet, excluding beverages, is water. Foods such as milk, tomatoes, and certain vegeta-

bles contain as much as 85 percent water; foods such as grains, flour, and cereal contain less than 15 percent water.

The pint or so of residue that remains after the water is evaporated comprises the carbohydrates, fats, proteins, vitamins, and minerals in the original sample of food. About one-half of the residue is carbohydrate; one-fourth, protein; and one-fourth, fat. Vitamins and minerals represent a minute fraction of the total mixture. The teaspoon of ash remaining after the macronutrients and vitamins are burned off comprises the diet's minerals, some of which can be destroyed by prolonged heating and elevated oven temperature.

THE MACRONUTRIENTS

Fat, protein, and *carbohydrate* are household words today; their use is not limited to the biochemist, nutritionist, or dietitian. These terms appear daily in newspaper columns, on food labels, and even in television advertisements for pet food and beer. Few people, however, know how a protein differs from a fat or a carbohydrate, and many of us have misconceptions about which foods contain each of these macronutrients. In this chapter, we shall lay the foundation for understanding why the body needs all three types of macronutrients (as explained in Chapter 3) by studying their chemical composition. Such information is the key to knowing why the protein of bread differs from that of beef, why the fat of butter differs from that of margarine, and why the carbohydrate of cereal differs from that of table sugar.

What Is a Carbohydrate?

The word *carbohydrate* tells us something about the composition of this nutrient. *Carbo-* stands for the chemical element *carbon*, commonly considered to be the basic building block of nature and the backbone element of all plant and animal life. A *hydrate* is a compound that contains water. In a carbohydrate, there is one atom of carbon (C) for every molecule of water (HOH). Each water unit exists as one hydrogen atom (H) and one hydroxyl group (OH), each linked, or *bonded*, to a carbon atom.

Simple Carbohydrates. Most simple food carbohydrates contain six pairs of carbon and water, and are called *hexoses*. A few of the simple carbohydrates we eat are *pentoses*—carbohydrates that contain five pairs of carbon and water. Both hexoses and pentoses are *monosaccharides*.

Structural representations of three hexoses (*glucose, galactose,* and *fructose*) are shown in Figure 2-1. We can see that their structures have certain similarities and differences—an observation that has nutritionally important corollaries. These three carbohydrates have the same energy value, but fructose tastes sweeter than glucose, which is slightly sweeter than galactose. With the help of vitamins, minerals, and enzymes, each of these hexoses can be converted into any other by a series of reactions that change the position and bonding of certain hydrogen and oxygen atoms.

In addition to the hexoses and pentoses in our diet, we eat a great deal of double-hexose carbohy-

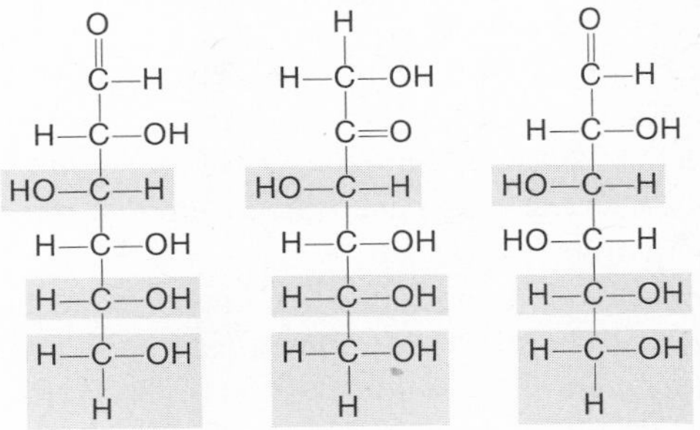

Figure 2-1. Three common hexoses.

drates, which are *disaccharides* that usually contain one glucose combined with another glucose molecule, or with galactose or fructose. The most common disaccharide is *sucrose*, or "table sugar," which contains one molecule of glucose and one of fructose. *Lactose*, the carbohydrate of milk, is a combination of glucose and galactose. *Maltose*, which is found in a variety of plant foods, contains two glucose units.

Because of their chemical bonding, disaccharides such as sucrose contain 12 carbon atoms and 11 water units. When disaccharides are broken down into hexose units during digestion (Chapter 4), a molecule of water enters the reaction process. This process is called *hydrolysis* (*hydro-*, or "water"; *-lysis*, or "breaking down").

All monosaccharides and disaccharides are considered by nutritionists to be simple sugars. These carbohydrates are found in many foods that are not generally associated with the commonly used term *sugar*. Sucrose, along with fructose and glucose, is a component of many fruits and vegetables. On the other hand, cereals, meats, and beans contain very little or none of this type of carbohydrate.

Complex Carbohydrates. About one-sixth of the energy in the average American diet is provided by simple carbohydrates. An approximately equal amount of dietary energy comes from complex carbohydrates called *polysaccharides* (*poly-*, or

15

"many"; *saccharide,* or "sugar"). Most complex carbohydrates consist of many glucose units chemically bonded to each other. One water molecule is required to hydrolyze each glucose unit of the large carbohydrate molecule.

Complex carbohydrates are classified according to several characteristics, including the length and arrangement of their glucose units. The *starch* carbohydrates consist primarily of long chains containing several hundred or even a thousand glucose units. Starch is stored in the seeds of plants, and so cereals and grains are a good dietary source of carbohydrate energy. Beans and other vegetables also provide starch.

Amylopectin and *amylose* represent the different types of glucose chains in starch molecules. Amylopectin is the insoluble component of starch, as present in flour, that causes gravy to thicken as it is heated. Amylose is the straight chain portion of starch and is soluble in water.

Dextrins are relatively small complex carbohydrates (approximately five glucose units) that are found in the leaves of starch-forming plants. During the processing of corn to make corn syrup, the starch of corn is partially hydrolyzed to produce dextrin. Only polysaccharides no larger than dextrin exhibit the sweet taste associated with sugars but not with starch.

While plants produce starch as their major type of complex carbohydrate for storage of energy, animals form *glycogen*—a different polysaccharide for energy storage. Glucose is the basic building unit in both starch and glycogen, but the glucose units in glycogen are arranged in complex patterns that contain many branches of short-chain glucose units attached to the main part of the molecule. Starch molecules contain fewer branches than does glycogen.

Some dietary sources of carbohydrates are shown in Table 2-1. The relative amounts of simple and complex carbohydrates in plants vary because at different stages of development and under differ-

ent environmental conditions, plants hydrolyze starch to simpler forms or synthesize polysaccharides from glucose. Therefore, the sweetness and texture of many fruits and vegetables vary with their age or degree of ripeness. The proportions of sugar and starch within the cells of some plants continue to change after the plants have been harvested, but these changes occur more slowly at cold temperatures. For this reason, the time and the conditions of storage during transportation, in the supermarket, and at home alter the carbohydrate composition of some foods.

Nondigestible Carbohydrates. Some of the polysaccharides formed of chains of glucose units cannot be digested by humans. This group of carbohydrates, commonly called *fiber* or *roughage,* includes *cellulose, hemicellulose, lignin,* and *pectin.*

Cellulose is the most abundant carbohydrate in nature. Flax and cotton are more than 97 percent cellulose; wood, more than 40 percent; and cereal straw, at least 30 percent. (Crude and dietary fiber in plant foods is discussed in Chapter 24.)

Cows and other ruminants can derive energy from the cellulose contained in straw and in ground-up corn cobs, but humans would starve on such a diet. Cellulose travels through the human gastrointestinal tract largely undigested, and is excreted in the feces. The stomach and intestines of a cow are no better able to digest cellulose than are these same organs in the human. The crucial difference between these two species is that the digestive system of a cow includes an additional organ, commonly called a "second stomach." This organ is analogous to a fermentation vat because its temperature and other internal conditions are ideal for the growth of bacteria that break down cellulose into glucose.

Why can a primitive form of life such as bacteria release energy from cellulose, while the more developed human life form cannot? The answer to this question involves the process by which the

TABLE 2-1. Sucrose, Other Simple Carbohydrates and Complex Carbohydrates in Various Foods

Food	Sucrose (grams per 100 grams of food)	Other Monosaccharides and Disaccharides (grams per 100 grams of food)	Complex Carbohydrate (grams per 100 grams of food)
Apple	3.1	8.3	0.6
Banana	8.9	8.4	1.9
Cantaloupe	4.4	2.3	—
Orange	4.6	5.0	—
Raisins	—	70.0	—
Prunes	2.0	47.0	0.7
Tomatoes	—	6.9	—
Cabbage	.3	3.4	—
Carrots	1.7	5.8	—
Peas	5.5	—	4.1
Potatoes	0.1	6.8	17.0
Sweet potatoes	4.1	2.4	16.5
Milk	—	4.9	—
Peanuts	4.5	4.7	6.5
Corn	—	—	62.0
Oats	—	—	56.4
Rice	0.4	2.0	73.8
Wheat flour	0.2	2.1	74.3
Corn syrup	—	47.5	34.7
Honey	1.9	74.2	1.5
Molasses	53.9	16.5	—

SOURCE: Adapted from M. G. Hardinge, J. G. Swarner, and H. Cook, "Carbohydrates in Foods," *Journal of The American Dietetic Association* 46 (1965): 198–201. Copyright The American Dietetic Association. Reprinted by permission.

glucose-to-glucose bonds in polysaccharides are broken during digestion. A simple example may help you to understand this phenomenon.

You can chew on a toothpick for an hour, but the cellulose in the wood will not change. However, if you put a small amount of cornstarch in your mouth and hold it there for a while, you will detect a sweet taste. Although the necessary ingredients, water and polysaccharide, are present in both cases, one polysaccharide is hydrolyzed but the other is not.

Starch is hydrolyzed in the mouth to sweet-tasting dextrin by an enzyme called *amylase*, which is found in saliva. Because of its unique configuration, amylase can slip into the characteristic bonds between two glucose units of starch and facilitate the insertion of a hydrogen and a hydroxyl unit, thus

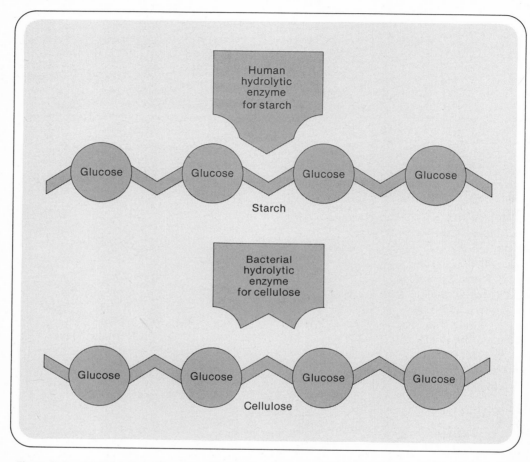

Figure 2–2. How enzyme configurations fit the characteristic glucose bonds in starch and in cellulose.

lysing the starch into smaller, carbohydrate units. Amylase does not, however, "fit" the bonds characteristic of cellulose. Although starch and cellulose are both chains of glucose units, their hexoses are linked together at different angles (Figure 2-2). Amylase can therefore aid in the digestion of starch but not of cellulose, which is hydrolyzed by a specific enzyme that is produced only by certain bacteria. Because of its uniquely bonded glucose units and because humans lack the cellulose-digesting enzyme, the energy trapped in cellulose cannot be tapped directly as human food.

What Is a Fat?

Consumers are bombarded with vocabulary related to fats. New products are marketed on the merits implied in "low-fat content" or in "contains

Saturated fatty acid

Unsaturated fatty acid

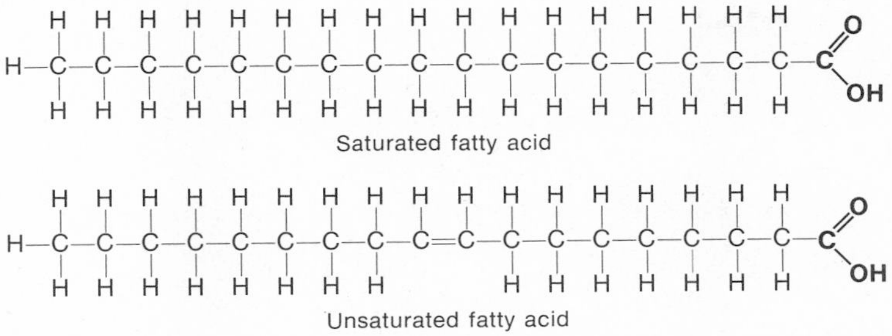

Figure 2–3. Structural representation of a saturated fatty acid and an unsaturated fatty acid.

no animal fat." The terms *saturated fatty acids* and *polyunsaturated fatty acids* are used often in newspapers, magazines, and food advertisements. We hear that fat and cholesterol have something to do with heart attacks, but most of us are confused about which foods contain either or both of these constituents. Many brands of margarine list ingredients such as partially hydrogenated soy and cottonseed oils, vegetable mono- and diglycerides (and lecithin), sodium benzoate (as a preservative), artificial flavoring and coloring, carotene, and vitamins A and D. These ingredients are listed on the label supposedly to inform the consumer, but what do they mean?

Fats are a class of nutrients within the group of plant and animal substances called *lipids*. The physical properties that distinguish most lipids from other compounds are their oiliness and their inability to dissolve (insolubility) in water. The lipid group includes *fats, fatty acids, phospholipids, waxes,* and a broad group of specialized substances called *nonphosphorylated lipids.*

Most dietary lipids are fats or fatty acids. Phospholipids are a minor component of meat, and waxes are rare in foods. Although nonphosphorylated lipids account for little of the total diet, this group includes important *sterols,* such as *cholesterol* and vitamin D. Many of the male and female sex hormones (*estrogen, progesterone, androgens*) are nonphosphorylated lipids.

Fatty Acids. These building blocks of fats are analogous to the hexose building blocks of polysaccharides. Fatty acids, however, are usually three to four times larger than simple sugars.

Although fatty acids, like hexoses, are composed of carbon, hydrogen, and oxygen, they contain much less oxygen than do hexoses. Each fatty acid molecule contains only two atoms of oxygen, regardless of the number of its carbon and hydrogen atoms. In Figure 2-3, you can see how these two oxygen atoms are linked to the terminal, or end, carbon atom to form the acid unit of all fatty acids.

Most of the fatty acids in our diet contain 16 or 18 carbon atoms, but there may be as few as four, or as many as 24 or more. Milk fat and coconut oil contain short-chain fatty acids. Goat cheese, with its sharp, pungent aroma, contains four to six carbon atoms in its fatty acid chains. Rancidity of some fats is due to the breakdown of long-chain fatty acids into acetic acid (two carbon atoms) and butyric acid (four carbon atoms), which produce the vinegary and acrid flavors of spoiled fats.

The word *saturated* is often used to refer to something like a cloth that is drenched with water or some other fluid. A fatty acid molecule, however, contains no units of water; its only two oxygen atoms are in the acid part of the molecule. What, then, does saturated or unsaturated mean in referring to fatty acids?

The answer to this question lies in a comparison

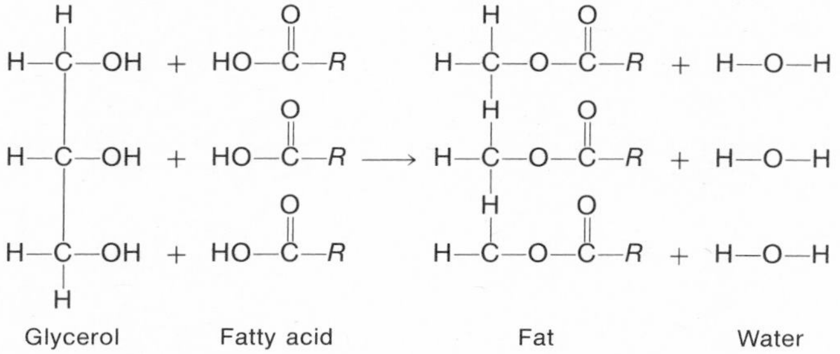

NOTE: *R* stands for a part of a molecule. *R* groups vary in size, composition, and configuration. The *R* groups of the fatty acids shown in this figure may be the same or different.

Figure 2–4. Formation of a fat.

of the two fatty acid structures represented in Figure 2-3. In the saturated fatty acid, every carbon atom except the terminal carbon atom is linked to four atoms—either to other carbon atoms or to hydrogen atoms. There is no place in the chain of the saturated fatty acid molecule where more atoms can be added. In the unsaturated fatty acid represented in Figure 2-3, two of the carbon atoms are linked to fewer than four other atoms and are held to each other by a *double bond*. These two carbon atoms are said to be *dehydrogenated* because they are holding fewer hydrogen atoms than they would hold in a saturated state. The double bond represents the unsaturated part of the fatty acid. In *polyunsaturated* fatty acids, hydrogen atoms are missing from several pairs of adjacent carbon atoms, each pair of which is joined by a double bond. The polyunsaturated fatty acids that occur most often in foods have two, three, or four such linkages.

Removing six hydrogen atoms from an 18-carbon fatty acid causes some rather remarkable changes. When saturated, an 18-carbon fatty acid is a solid at room temperature; when triunsaturated, it is a *viscous*, or thick, liquid at room temperature. All saturated fatty acids melt at higher temperatures than do their corresponding unsaturated counterparts (those containing the same number of carbon atoms). The melting point of a fatty acid is also affected by the length of the molecule. Shorter ones change from a solid to a liquid at a lower temperature than do longer ones. Thus, both the length and the degree of hydrogenation or saturation determine whether a fatty acid can be poured or must be scooped.

The unsaturated bonds of fatty acids react with oxygen and are easily ruptured, resulting in two or more shorter segments. The compounds thus formed often taste rancid. Many foods that contain unsaturated fatty acids would become rancid quickly if their double bonds were not protected by additives that reduce this oxidation tendency. Adding hydrogen to, or *hydrogenating*, some of the unsaturated bonds also reduces the occurrence of rancidity.

Fats.   When one, two, or three fatty acids are combined with *glycerol*, the resulting compound is classed as a *fat*. Fats are called either *monoglycerides*, *diglycerides*, or *triglycerides*, depending on whether one, two, or three fatty acids are bonded to the glycerol molecule. The characteristic glyceride structure distinguishes fats from other lipids.

Glycerol belongs to the class of organic compounds called *alcohols*, which are characterized by one or more hydroxyl (OH) groups. Figure 2-4 shows how fatty acids combine with the hydroxyl groups of glycerol to form fat. The chemical connection point is called the *glyceride linkage* and involves the OH part of the acid group in the fatty acid and the OH group in glycerol. When a fat is formed, one molecule of water (HOH) is released for each fatty acid that joins to glycerol by sharing an oxygen atom.

When fats are eaten, they are digested to form fatty acids and glycerol by the process of hydrolysis, similar to the hydrolytic digestion of complex carbohydrates to glucose. Most of the fats we eat are composed of combinations of fatty acids of varying lengths and different degrees of saturation. Vegetable oil contains more polyunsaturated fatty acids than saturated fatty acids; animal products contain proportionately more saturated fatty acids. Neither vegetable nor animal dietary fat, however, is completely saturated or completely unsaturated.

The proportion of polyunsaturated to saturated fatty acids in a fat can be expressed as a *P/S ratio.*

For example, a food that contains three times as much polyunsaturated as saturated fatty acids will have a P/S ratio of 3/1, which means that of the total four parts, one part (25 percent) is saturated fatty acids.

The approximate P/S ratios for several vegetable and animal fats are given in Figure 2-5. Most of the polyunsaturated fatty acids in the American diet come from the oil of corn, safflower, cottonseed, peanut, and soybean. These foods have a high P/S ratio, generally in the range of 2/1 to 4/1. Among the animal products listed, the relative amount of saturated fatty acids is greater in beef than in chicken and fish. Recent research indicates that altering the diet of farm animals can change the P/S ratio of the fat in meat.

Phospholipids. This class of lipids is similar in structure to a diglyceride except that a terminal

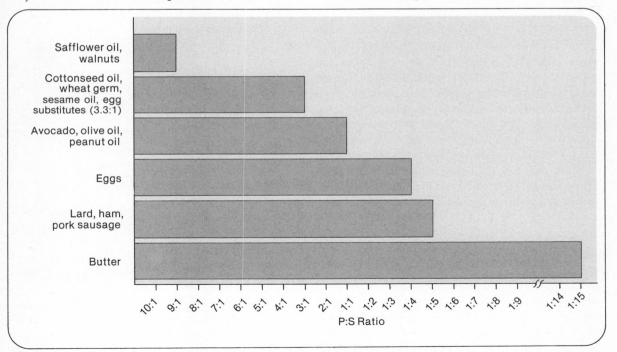

Figure 2–5. P/S ratios of some foods.

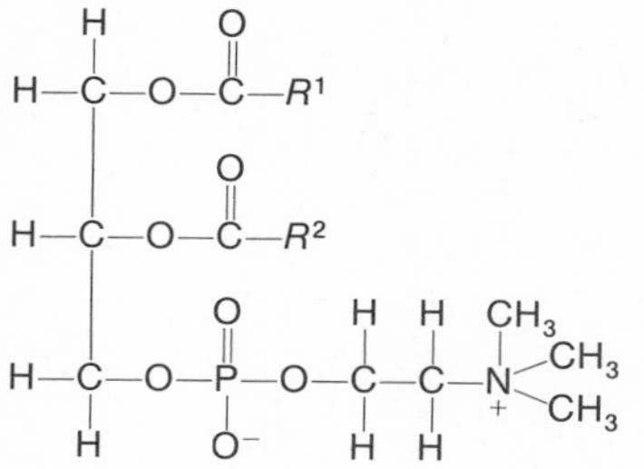

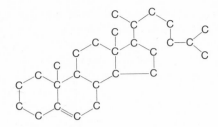

Figure 2–6. Lecithin, a phospholipid.

Figure 2–7. Carbon skeleton of sterols. Cholesterol, bile acids and salts, vitamin D, and steroid hormones are built around this basic carbon skeleton.

carbon atom is linked to a *phosphate group* (phosphorus and oxygen), which can react or combine with other chemical groups.

The body contains only small amounts of *phospholipids*, which have important functions. They are part of the membranes around cells and around small specialized compartments within cells. *Lecithin* (Figure 2-6) is an example of a phospholipid.

Sterols. The basic configuration of *sterols* is different from the straight-chain fatty acids or the prong-shaped fats and phospholipids. The carbon atoms of sterols are arranged in hexagons, which touch each other in such a way that they share some of the same carbon atoms (Figure 2-7). Despite their basic structural similarity, the sterols—such as *steroid* hormones, cholesterol, bile salts, and vitamin D—have different biological properties because of differences in the position and arrangement of their side chains, hydroxyl groups, or double-bonded oxygen atoms.

Dietary Sources. The foods that contain the highest percentages of lipid substances are the oils used in cooking and for making salad dressing (Figure 2-8). Butter and margarine are primarily lipids, but they contain a small percentage of water. The other major sources of lipids in the American diet are meat, poultry, fish, and dairy products. Beef and pork contain more lipids than do fish and poultry.

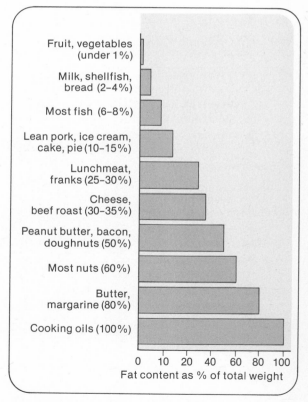

Figure 2–8. Some typical foods and the percentage of fat they contain.

The first two carbons of all amino acids are surrounded by a similar arrangement of oxygen, hydrogen, and amino groups.

Although only about 1 gram of the approximately 100 grams of fat we eat daily is cholesterol, the cholesterol content of various foods is an important consideration in diet planning for many people. The amount of cholesterol in various foods, and the relationship of cholesterol, total fat, and fatty acids to cardiovascular disease are discussed in Chapter 25.

What Is a Protein?

Proteins, like complex carbohydrates and lipids, are constituted of smaller units. These units are the *amino acids;* they are called the building blocks of proteins.

Structure of Proteins. About 20 different amino acids are commonly found in the proteins of food and of the body. Their structures vary widely in size and shape, but common to all amino acid structures is the group shown in Figure 2-9. Note that the end carbon atom and its surrounding hydrogen and oxygen atoms constitute an acid group, as in the fatty acids; next to the acid group is a carbon atom bonded to an amino group consisting of one nitrogen atom and two hydrogen atoms (NH_2). The uniqueness of each amino acid results from the composition and configuration of the various molecular segments attached to the group shown as *R* in the figure. *R* is not an abbreviation for any specific element; it is used to denote the "remainder" of the amino acid molecule.

Almost all types of amino acids are used to synthesize the various long chains that make up proteins. In one step of protein synthesis, a bond is

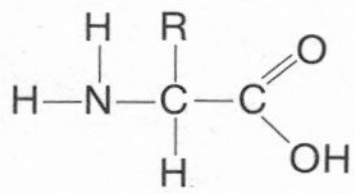

Figure 2–9. Structural group characteristic of amino acids.

formed between the amino group of one amino acid molecule with the acid group of another identical or different amino acid. As happens in synthesis reactions of other nutrients, water is released when the bond, or linkage, is formed. This linkage is called an *amide bond* (Figure 2-10). Two bonded amino acids form a *dipeptide;* three together form a *tripeptide;* chains of several amino acids are called *polypeptides.*

Proteins are large molecules that may contain several hundred amino acids. Because there are about 20 common amino acids from which proteins can be made and because each of them can react with itself or with any other amino acid, the sequences and configuration of their combinations are almost limitless. Each of these different combinations constitutes a unique protein. Some unique proteins are listed in Table 2-2. The various names of these proteins are given primarily to emphasize that all proteins are not alike. There are differences in structure and function, for example, among the proteins of blood, of fingernails, of wheat, and of egg.

Protein Quality. Although the sequence and configuration of the amino acids in proteins influence protein properties such as biological function, solubility, digestibility, and texture, these factors are not the crucial determinants of the nutritional value

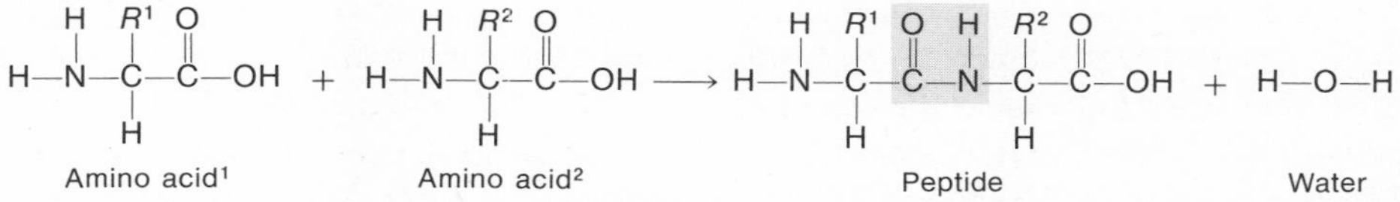

Figure 2–10. Formation of a dipeptide.

TABLE 2-2. Various Proteins Found in Foods and the Body

Protein	Body or Food Source
Albumins	Blood, milk, egg white
Casein	Milk
Collagen	Gelatin, bones, cartilage, connective tissue
Elastin	Arteries, ligaments, tendons
Gliadin	Wheat, rye
Globulins	Blood, muscle, potato, lentils
Histones	Glandular tissue
Keratin	Hair, fingernails
Protamines	Salmon, mackerel, herring
Zein	Corn

of protein. The efficiency or degree to which dietary proteins can be used for building the cellular components of the human body is determined principally by the type and relative amounts of the amino acids in the particular protein molecule.

Some dietary proteins are made up largely of amino acids whose R portions can be interconverted within the body. Therefore, if a particular amino acid is in short supply, it can be formed internally by the transfer of amino groups (-NH$_2$) from an amino acid in excess supply to a nonamino organic acid that contains the required R group. Certain amino acids can also be synthesized within the body by adding or removing parts of the R group of another amino acid.

If this internal synthesis were possible for all amino acids, the nutritive value of proteins would not be influenced by which amino acids they contain. However, there are eight amino acids needed for making body proteins that cannot be made internally because the human body lacks the required enzymes. These eight *essential amino acids* (Figure 2-11) must therefore be supplied by the food we eat. The amino acids that can be synthesized internally

are called *nonessential.* (Some nutritionists prefer the term *dispensable* amino acids.) Children require a ninth dietary amino acid—*histidine;* this amino acid can be synthesized in the body, but not in sufficient quantities to meet the needs of rapidly growing children. Researchers are still studying whether adults also need dietary histidine.

The nutritive value of dietary protein is determined by the amounts of the eight essential amino acids the food contains. However, the body does not need exactly the same amount of each essential amino acid. By feeding human subjects diets that contain known amounts of purified amino acids along with all other essential nutrients, researchers have determined the proportion of amino acids the body needs. The ideal proportion of amino acids is quite similar to the amino acid composition shown in Figure 2-12 for meat and egg protein and for *casein,* a milk protein. Soybeans also contain a good balance of amino acids, but their total protein content is lower than that of meat.

The protein of cereals, most beans, and vegetables contains all the essential amino acids, but the relative amounts of amino acids in these plant foods is less "ideal" than the amino acid composition of animal protein. Plant protein is therefore of lower nutritive value than an equivalent amount of animal protein.

The capacity of the body to build the proteins it needs from dietary proteins depends upon the simultaneous availability, in proper amounts, of all essential amino acids. If one amino acid is in short supply during production of a protein requiring that amino acid, then the amount of protein that can be produced will be limited. For example, wheat contains all eight essential amino acids but only about 31 percent of the amount of *lysine* needed for maximal utilization of the other essential amino acids to build protein (Figure 2-12). When wheat is digested, its essential amino acids are used up by the cells of the body in an amount proportional to the ideal amino acid ratio. When all of the available lysine has been incorporated into body protein with the

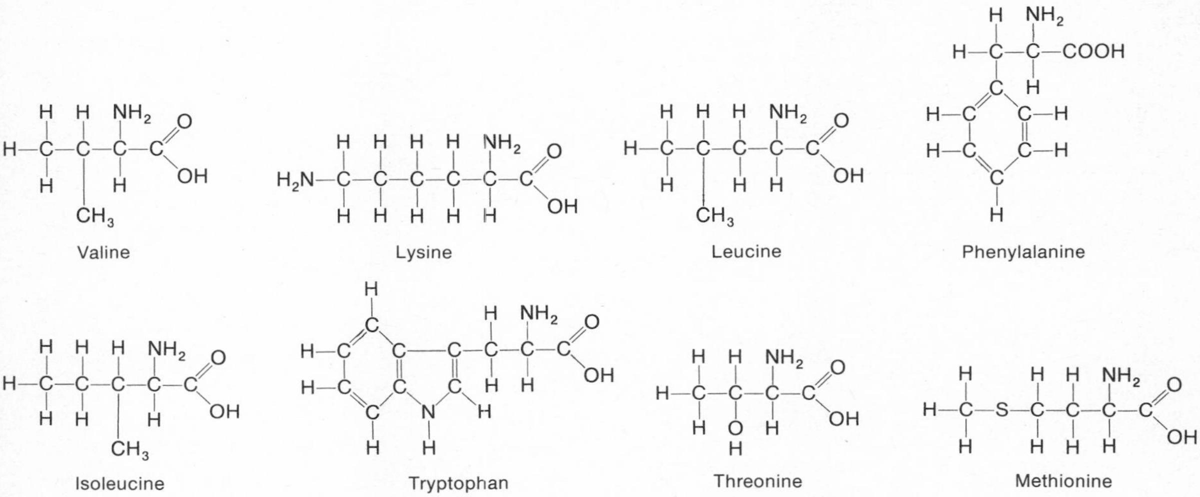

Figure 2–11. The essential amino acids.

other essential amino acids from the digested wheat, no more of that particular protein can be formed.

An inventory of only seven of the eight essential amino acids is useless for protein synthesis. It would be like trying to build a car with a carburetor, battery, transmission, gas tank, radiator, wiring, and ignition system, but without pistons—or like trying to read a novel in which every eighth page was missing. However, if you could get the missing auto part from another car, or those missing eighth pages from another copy of the same book, the product would be functional. In terms of amino acids, the body can, and does, do this with complementary foods.

An essential amino acid in short supply from one food can be provided by a *complementary* food that contains an ample supply of the required amino acid. Black-eyed peas have a high lysine content, and when they are consumed along with wheat, the nutritive value of the combined proteins increases. Protein production from two complementary foods eaten at the same meal is better than it is when the same two foods are eaten at different meals during the same day. As you can see from Figure 2-12,

eating pork-and-beans with a sandwich, black-eyed peas with corn bread, beef with corn or wheat, and eggs with beans and peas are other examples of how to put the complementary-amino-acid concept into practice.

The nutritive value of proteins is measured by an index called the *protein efficiency ratio,* or *PER.* This value is determined by feeding a specific amount of a protein source to young rats for four weeks and then dividing the weight gained by the rat during that time by the amount of protein eaten. The PER of eggs is almost 4; for fish it is about 3.5, and for milk about 3 (Table 2-3). Beef and soybeans have a PER around 2.3, other beans and nuts are in the range of 1.4 to 1.8, and bread is only about 1. It is important to note, however, that these PER values were determined by including only one protein source in the total diet, which contained all other nutrients.

The primary consideration in selecting dietary sources of protein is usually the absolute amount of protein provided by a given quantity of a food. The percentage of protein in several different foods is shown in Figure 2-13. Meat, fish, poultry, cheese,

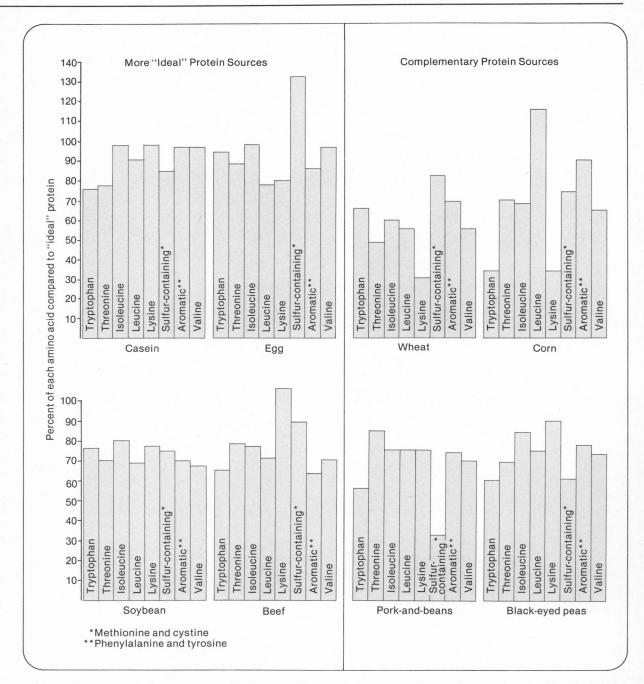

Figure 2–12. Amino acid content of foods of animal and vegetable origin compared to amino acid content of ideal protein.

TABLE 2-3. Protein Efficiency Ratios of Several Foods

Food	Protein Efficiency Ratio
Egg	3.9
Fish	3.6
Milk	3.1
Soybeans	2.3
Beef	2.3
Rice	2.2
Peanuts	1.7
Various beans	1.4–1.9
Corn	1.2
Breads	0.9–1.1

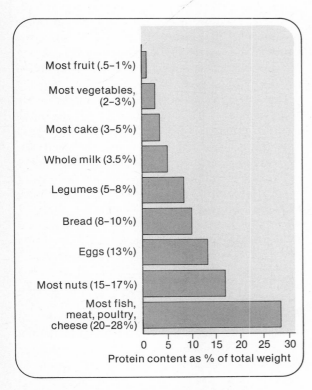

Figure 2–13. Dietary sources of protein.

nuts, and eggs provide the greatest percentage of protein; the smaller amounts of protein supplied by foods such as cereals and beans can help to meet daily needs.

On the average, Americans eat almost twice as much protein as their bodies need, and therefore few people in the United States need be concerned about combining protein from plant foods in order to optimize the body's utilization of this nutrient. However, if one omits animal protein, then planning meals around plant foods that contain complementary amino acids can help one make optimal use of these proteins while permitting flexibility in choosing foods.

What Is an Alcohol?

Alcohol is a chemical class of substances that is characterized by the presence of a hydroxyl (-OH) unit joined to a carbon atom. Alcohol molecules vary in size and shape. The alcohol in beer, whiskey, and wine is *ethanol,* or "grain alcohol." The ethanol molecule contains only two carbon atoms, which are linked to several hydrogen atoms and one hydroxyl group. *Methanol,* or "wood alcohol," contains only one carbon atom; it is harmful because it is changed in the body to the toxic substance *formaldehyde.* The relatively minor difference in the chemical structures of ethanol and methanol belies the major difference in their physiological properties—ethanol is a common source of energy and a mild toxin, whereas (in equal amounts) methanol is a potent poison.

Beer is about 4 to 7 percent alcohol; and wine, between 12 and 20 percent. Dividing the *proof* of "hard liquor" by 2 gives the approximate percentage of alcohol it contains. Many over-the-counter drugs such as cough syrups and "tonics" contain some alcohol.

Macronutrient Composition of Foods

To many people, the words *fat, carbohydrate,* and *protein* conjure up mental images of certain foods.

The word *fat* is associated with butter, cooking oils, and salad dressing. *Carbohydrate* connotes bread, pastries, potatoes, and perhaps candy. *Protein* is equated with meat, and possibly milk and eggs. But in what category do you put beans, avocados, or peanut butter? The classification becomes even more difficult when one considers stew, pancakes, and pizza. Each of these difficult-to-categorize foods contains some carbohydrate, fat, and protein. A similar varied composition applies to salad dressing, bread, meat, milk, and eggs. Although fat, protein, or carbohydrate may predominate in a certain food, most foods contain at least a small amount of all three macronutrients. In order to select a diet that supplies the proper proportion of carbohydrate, protein, and fat, it is helpful to know how these nutrients are distributed in foods.

Single-Nutrient Foods   Of the thousands of foods on the market, few contain only one macronutrient, although some are composed primarily of one macronutrient. Candy, soft drinks, honey, sugar, molasses, cornstarch, and some fruits consist almost exclusively of carbohydrate; but few foods contain only fat or only protein. More often, foods are composed primarily of a single macronutrient; they derive 70 percent or more of their energy from a single nutrient (Figure 2-14).

Macronutrient Partners.   Another way to mentally organize foods in terms of nutrient composition is to pick out the dietary items that supply substantial amounts of two macronutrients, but very little of the third. These foods are shown along the sides of the triangle in Figure 2-14. Although most people realize that meat is a source of protein, they are often unaware that, in general, beef and pork contain as much fat as they do protein. Another misconception is that beans provide only carbohydrates; these foods also provide protein. Wheat and other grains are primarily carbohydrate, but they also contain protein. Many combination foods such as pizza, macaroni and cheese, or a hamburger with

bun provide approximately the same amounts of all three macronutrients. Whole milk contains almost equal amounts of protein, fat, and carbohydrate.

Dietary Perspectives.   Tables of food composition that list the percentage of fat, carbohydrate, and protein in a food help us to see the relative amount of each macronutrient in foods. Several other factors, however, must be kept in mind when evaluating the contribution that specific foods make toward meeting daily nutrient needs.

The amount of food eaten has major dietary significance. Although 100 grams of milk contain only 3.5 grams of protein, a glass of milk (240 grams) at breakfast and at lunch, plus a cup of hot chocolate for a study break in the evening, adds up to a little more protein than is contained in 3 ounces of steak. Similarly, 2 teaspoons of sugar (10 grams) in coffee may seem hardly worth considering in the diet, but a person who drinks five cups of sugared coffee a day gets as much carbohydrate from drinking coffee as from eating a piece of pie.

The water content of a food also provides a clue to the amount of its energy-containing macronutrients. For example, hard candy contains very little water—it is almost solid carbohydrate. Peanut butter, margarine, nuts, and seeds are almost devoid of water and therefore are concentrated sources of protein, fat, and/or carbohydrate. Fruits and most vegetables, however, contain so much water that 1 cup of these foods supplies only about 2 tablespoons of the three principal macronutrients. Differences in water content explain why a cup of cooked beans provides much less protein and carbohydrate than a cup of dried beans.

Dairy products provide an example of why one should consider both the water content and the amount of food eaten. Butter is a high-fat food; milk is a low-fat food containing only about 3.5 percent fat. However, the amount of fat in 2 teaspoons of butter is about equal to the amount of fat in one glass of milk.

The contribution made by a food to meeting nutrient needs depends upon its macronutrient composition, the amount of food eaten, its water content, and its micronutrient composition.

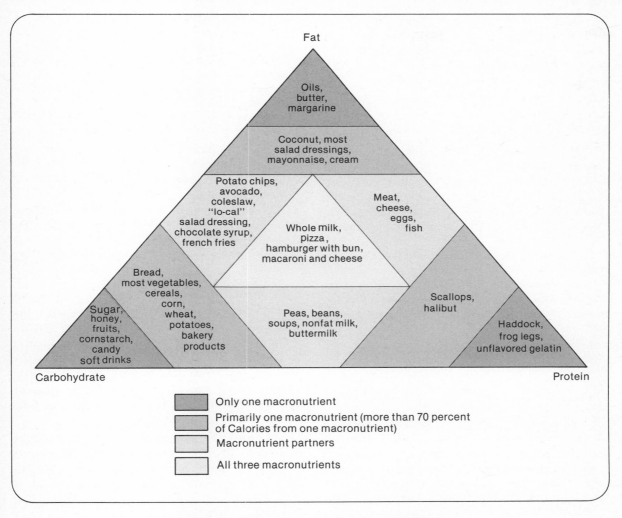

Figure 2–14. Mixed macronutrient composition of foods.

THE MICRONUTRIENTS

Micronutrient content should be kept in mind when considering dietary sources of carbohydrate, protein, and fat. To make comparisons among foods, we need to know what the vitamins and minerals are, and how they are distributed among foods.

Most people know that their bodies need vita-mins—for example, vitamin A has something to do with healthy eyes, and insufficient vitamin C can cause bleeding gums. Fewer people, however, are conscious of their need for minerals, although they may have learned from their dentist or from advertisements for milk to associate calcium with strong teeth and bones. Many people correlate iron and "good blood." However, nutrition knowledge regarding which foods provide these and other micronutrients is rather scanty among consumers in general, who would find it difficult to name good micronutrient sources other than wheat germ, milk, liver, and vitamin–mineral pills or tonics.

What Is a Vitamin?

The term *vitamin* refers to a number of unrelated organic substances that occur in many foods in small amounts and that are necessary for the normal metabolic functioning of the body but cannot be synthesized by the human body. This description delineates several important characteristics of vitamins:

1. "Organic substances" means that vitamins are made primarily of carbon, hydrogen, and oxygen. In terms of chemical composition, therefore, vitamins are similar to fats, carbohydrates, and proteins. (*Minerals,* such as calcium and iron, are *inorganic elements* rather than organic substances.)

2. Although vitamins do indeed "occur in many foods," synthetic vitamins function in the body in the same way that naturally occurring vitamins do. Synthetic vitamins include those available as capsule or tablet supplements, as well as those added to fortified or enriched foods.

3. "In small amounts" distinguishes vitamins from macronutrients, which are other organic substances that occur in food. The total weight of all the vitamins needed in one day is less than 100 milligrams (mg)—less than one-six-thousandth of the average total daily intake of fat, protein, and carbohydrate. Furthermore, our daily need for vitamins is less than one-twentieth of the recommended total daily intake of minerals.

4. "Necessary for the normal metabolic functioning of the body" distinguishes vitamins from the many organic compounds in food that are not vital for life but that provide flavor and color. Minerals and macronutrients are necessary for the normal metabolic functioning of the body, but the specific functions of micronutrients and macronutrients are quite different, as we shall see in the next chapter.

5. Because vitamins cannot be synthesized by the human body, they must be provided from some outside source—either food or as supplements. This crucial difference distinguishes vitamins from many other metabolically active organic compounds that occur in small amounts in foods. Cholesterol, for example, has important functions in the body and is present in many foods, but we do not require it in our diets because it can be synthesized internally.

Although each of the five properties of vitamins also describes other substances that we eat, only vitamins meet all these criteria.

Unlike macronutrients, vitamins cannot be grouped according to chemical structure. Vitamins vary in size and shape from the simple six-carbon vitamin C molecule to the complex vitamin B_{12} molecule. Vitamins can be classified, however, according to their solubility in water or in fat.

Fat-Soluble Vitamins. Although we might expect the fat-soluble vitamins (Figure 2-15) to occur in the greatest concentrations in high-fat foods, this assumption does not always hold true, as can be seen in Table 2-4. Some high-fat foods contain one of the fat-soluble vitamins but little of the others, and some low-fat foods contain the fat-soluble vitamins A and E. Furthermore, low-fat foods may be fortified with fat-soluble vitamins.

Vitamin A is provided in relatively large amounts by animal products such as egg yolk, organ meat (liver, kidney, and so forth), and fish oil. Dietary sources of vitamin A include prepared foods such as custard and liverwurst.

Vitamin A needs can also be met by eating fruits and vegetables that contain vitamin A *precursors*—pigments that can be converted to vitamin A by the body. The most common of these pigments, *carotene,* is yellow, but this color is sometimes masked by other pigments in the same food. The yellow color of apricots, peaches, mangoes, sweet potatoes, and carrots indicates that these foods are good sources of carotene. Deep-orange squashes contain more carotene than do lighter varieties. Yellow cornmeal provides some carotene, but white corn-

Fat-soluble vitamins (A, D, E, and K) are not necessarily concentrated in high-fat foods.

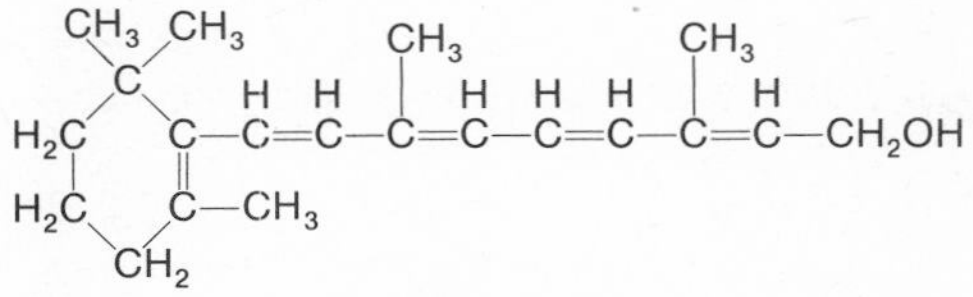

Vitamin A

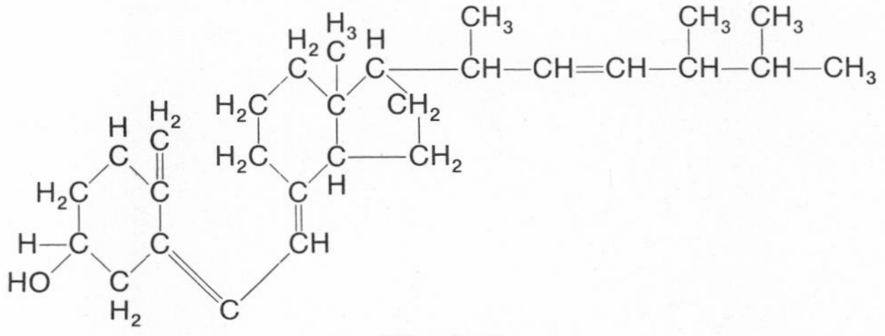

Vitamin D

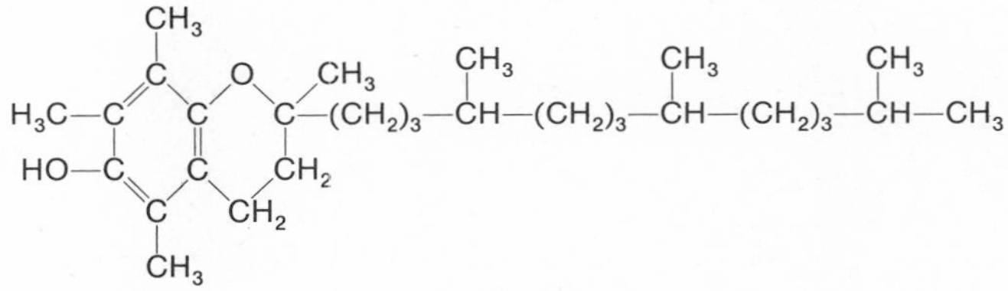

Vitamin E

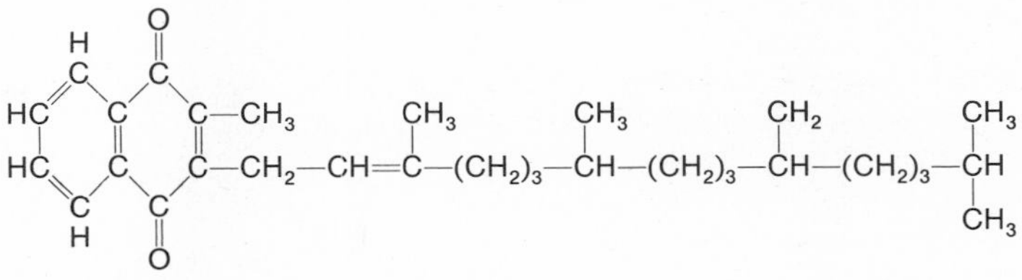

Vitamin K

Figure 2–15. Fat-soluble vitamins.

meal supplies very little. Other excellent sources of vitamin A precursors are dark-green foods such as spinach, kale, and broccoli, and the green tops of turnips and beets (which are discarded by many people). Vitamin A precursors are contained in the red foods tomatoes, watermelons, and strawberries, but not in beets or red (purple) cabbage.

Milk and other dairy products are usually good sources of vitamin A regardless of their fat content. Federal regulations require that if these foods are transported across state borders, their vitamin A and D content must meet minimum government standards. Some dairy products that are produced and sold in the same state, however, may not be fortified with vitamins A and D. (Dairy products are often labeled "Grade A"; this label indicates a quality standard and does not mean that the product is fortified with vitamin A.)

Although it is important to know which foods are good sources of certain nutrients, it is equally im-

TABLE 2-4. Dietary Sources of Vitamins

Vitamins	Sources		
	Good	Moderate	Poor
Fat-Soluble Vitamins			
Vitamin A or precursors of vitamin A	Egg yolk, dairy products, organ meat, fish oils, most yellow and orange fruits and vegetables, dark-green (especially leafy) vegetables	Other fruits and vegetables	Egg white, muscle of meat and fish, cereals, beans, citrus fruit, nonfortified imitation dairy products
Vitamin D	Egg yolk, butterfat, fortified dairy products, fish oils, organ meat		Egg white, vegetable oils, nonfortified dairy products, fruits, vegetables, cereals, beans, muscle of meat and fish, nonfortified imitation dairy products
Vitamin E	Vegetable oils, wheat germ, peanuts, almonds, eggs, organ meat	Some fruits and vegetables	Animal fat, muscle meat, cereals, dairy products
Vitamin K	Dark-green and yellow vegetables	Intestinal synthesis by bacteria	Meat, cereals, dairy products

portant to know which foods are not good sources of a particular nutrient. For example, the muscle portion of meat and fish, cereals, citrus fruits, and most beans are not good sources of vitamin A. Imitation dairy products made with vegetable oils contain vitamin A only if it has been added during processing.

Vitamin D, commonly called the "sunshine" vitamin, is provided by relatively few foods. It is found primarily in egg yolk, butterfat, organ meat, and the oil of fish such as tuna and salmon. But if we had to rely solely upon these foods to meet our need for vitamin D, rickets (the disease caused by a defi-

ciency of this nutrient) would be rampant throughout the world. The reason for the relative rarity of this disease is that a sterol in our skin can be converted by sunlight into vitamin D.

Adults need less vitamin D than children because they are no longer growing. Therefore adults who are occasionally in the sunshine get enough of this vitamin by internal synthesis from the skin sterol. However, children, teen-agers, pregnant women, nursing mothers, and people who spend most of their time indoors cannot meet their need for vitamin D unless they eat foods that supply this nutrient. A quart of milk to which vitamin D has

TABLE 2-4. Dietary Sources of Vitamins (*continued*)

Vitamins	Sources		
	Good	Moderate	Poor
Water-Soluble Vitamins			
Moderate amounts in wide variety of foods			
Thiamin	Organ meat, pork, nuts	Enriched cereal products, whole-grain cereal products, dairy products, beans, peas, lentils, fruits, nonleafy vegetables, green leafy vegetables, muscle meat other than pork	Fats and oils
Riboflavin	Dairy products, organ meat	Similar to thiamin	Fats and oils
Niacin	Organ meat, poultry, fish, pork, beef, lamb	Similar to thiamin	Fats and oils
Pyridoxine	Meat, poultry, fish, egg yolk, bananas, tomato juice	Similar to thiamin but excluding enriched cereal products	Fats and oils, enriched as well as nonenriched refined cereals, fruits
Folacin	Green leafy vegetables and asparagus	Fruits, dairy products, nonleafy vegetables, beans, cereals	Fats and oils, meat
Widespread			
Pantothenic acid and biotin	Yeast, organ meat, eggs, wheat germ, peas, beans	Almost all other foods	Fats and oils
Relatively large amounts but in few foods			
Vitamin C	Citrus fruit, tomatoes, potatoes, peppers, broccoli	Other vegetables and fruits	Cereals, beans, meats, dairy products
Vitamin B_{12}	Liver, muscle meat, fish, eggs	Dairy products	Foods of plant origin

been added at the level required by federal regulations, can supply the recommended daily amount of this nutrient. Vitamin D is added to many other dairy products and to a few fortified nondairy foods.

Vitamin E is provided primarily by vegetable fats in margarine, salad dressings, and cooking oils. The few other concentrated sources of vitamin E include wheat germ, peanuts, and almonds. Eggs and liver can also help to satisfy our need for this nutrient. Although fruits and vegetables contain relatively little vitamin E, several portions of this type of food supply about 10 percent of our average daily dietary intake.

Vitamin K is not generally supplied by foods high in fat. Dark-green and yellow vegetables are the best dietary sources of this nutrient.

Vitamin K is similar to vitamin D in that both of these vitamins can be made within the body. Bacteria in the intestinal tract synthesize some vitamin K, which is then absorbed into the blood. The amount of vitamin K from bacterial synthesis is a relatively small part of our total daily needs, whereas the amount of vitamin D formed by the action of sunlight on skin sterol represents a comparatively large part of our dietary requirement.

Water-Soluble Vitamins. Although the water-soluble vitamins (Figure 2-16) are sometimes presented in alphabetical and numerical order, these nutrients can be grouped more logically according to similarities in the types of foods that supply them, and according to whether they occur in concentrated amounts in a few foods or are distributed in small amounts in a wide variety of foods. This perspective on vitamin distribution patterns in food is helpful for planning a nutritionally complete diet and for evaluating whether a food is a good, moderate, or poor source of a certain vitamin.

Thiamin, riboflavin, and *niacin,* for example, are distributed among many different foods in moderate amounts and in varying proportions. Many cereals and flour used in baked goods have been "enriched" by the addition of this nutrient group, and are therefore good sources of these three B vitamins. Whole-grain cereal products contain approximately as much thiamin and niacin as do enriched milled products, but only about half as much riboflavin. Meat, poultry, fish, and beans also supply all three of these vitamins, but more of them are contained in organ meat than in muscle meat. One serving of most fruit or nonleafy vegetables usually provides less than 10 percent of the daily need for these three vitamins, but the contribution of such foods to the total diet may be significant. Dairy products are a much better source of riboflavin than of thiamin or niacin, and pork is a better source of thiamin than of riboflavin or niacin.

Niacin can be made in the body from the amino acid *tryptophan.* Sixty milligrams of tryptophan are needed to make 1 milligram of niacin, but when the diet contains several hundred milligrams of tryptophan in several grams of dietary protein, a relatively large proportion of the niacin needed in the total diet can be supplied from synthesis by the body.

Pyridoxine is found in relatively small amounts in a wide variety of foods. One serving of only a few foods provides more than 10 percent of the pyridoxine needed daily by an adult. Meat, poultry, fish, egg yolks, bananas, and tomato juice provide this vitamin in larger amounts, but most of our total daily intake is simply the summation of small amounts of pyridoxine supplied by a variety of vegetables, cereals, beans, peas, and dairy products. Fruits contribute only a small proportion of the pyridoxine in the diet. Enriched cereal products do not contain added pyridoxine, and are therefore inferior to whole-grain cereals as a source of this vitamin.

Folacin is provided by a broad variety of foods, but there are comparatively few concentrated sources of this nutrient. (*Folic acid* is one of several forms of folacin present in food and in the body.) Liver, asparagus, and green leafy vegetables are among its better sources; moderate amounts of folacin are found in nonleafy vegetables and in beans, peas, orange juice, and whole-grain cereals. Potatoes, dairy products, fruits, and orange-flavored breakfast drinks contain little, if any, folic acid.

Pantothenic acid and *biotin* are found in almost all types of foods, but their better sources are brewer's yeast, organ meat, eggs, wheat germ, nuts, and peas. Because these two water-soluble vitamins are so widely distributed among foods, our diets are not likely to be deficient in pantothenic acid or

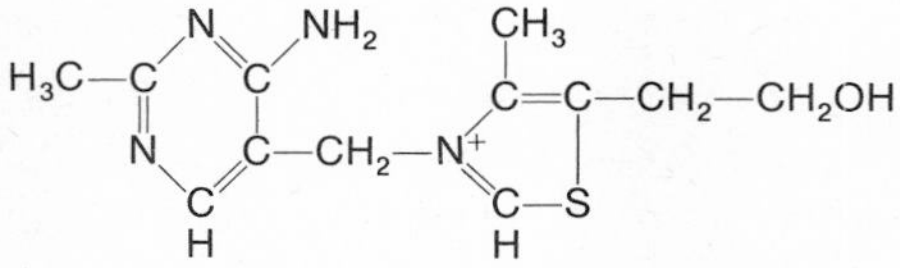

Thiamin (vitamin B_1)

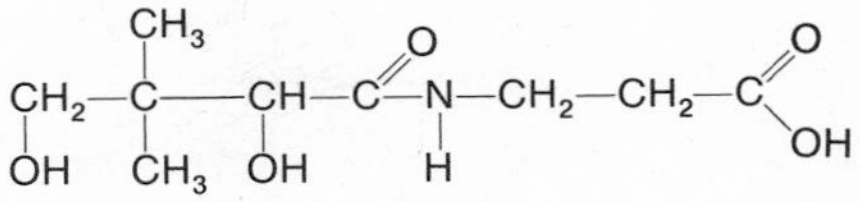

Pantothenic acid

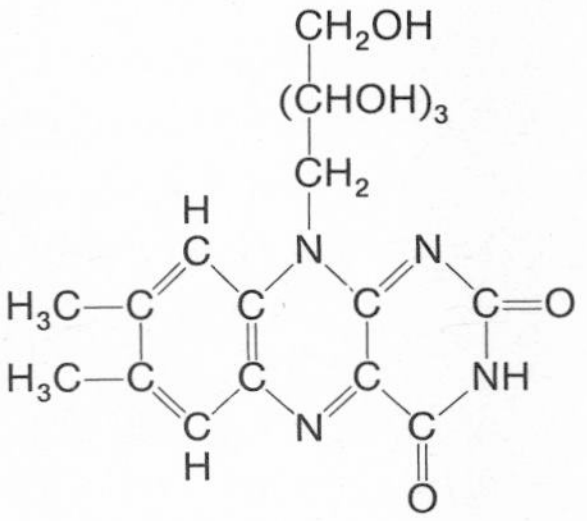

Riboflavin (vitamin B_2)

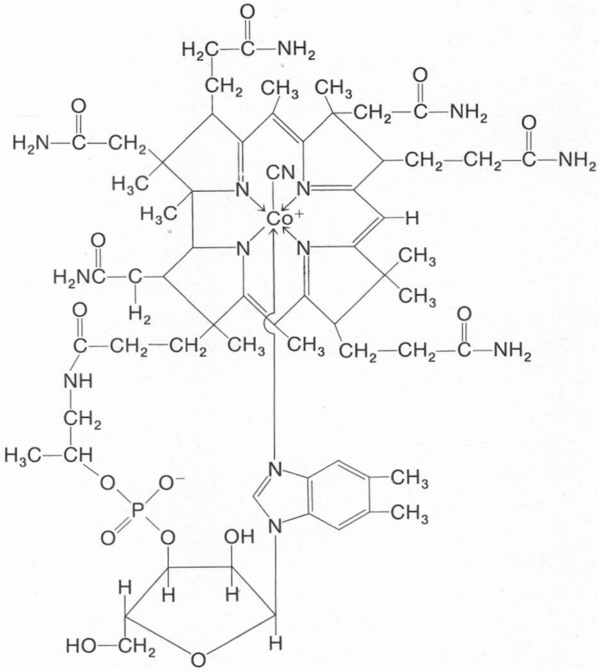

Vitamin B_{12}

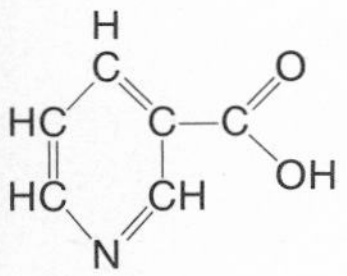

Niacin

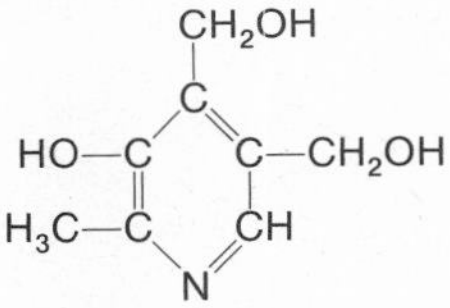

Pyridoxine (vitamin B_6)

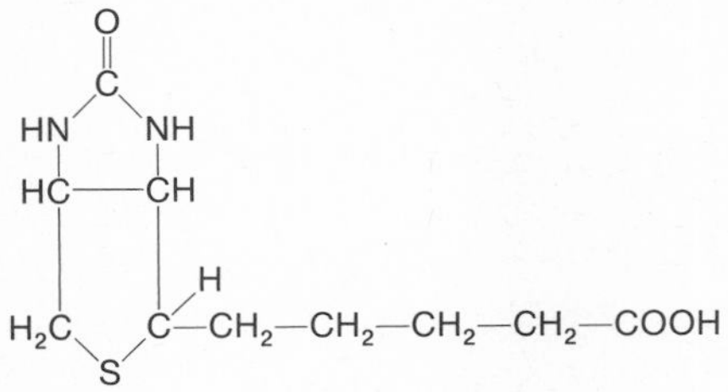

Biotin

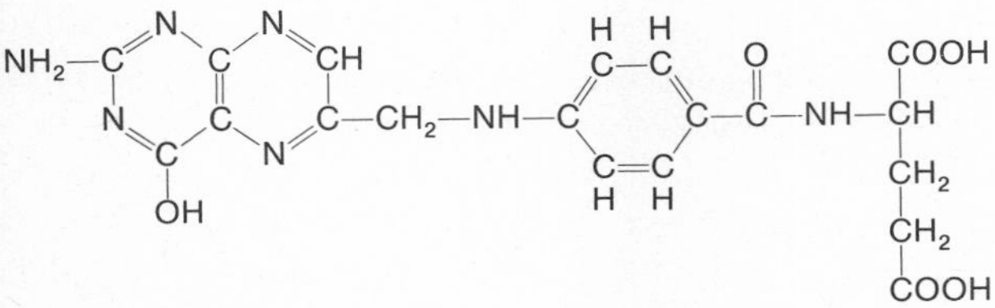

Folic acid (a form of folacin)

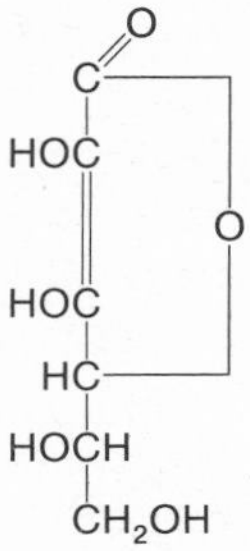

Vitamin C

Figure 2-16. Water-soluble vitamins.

TABLE 2-5. Dietary Sources of Certain Minerals

Minerals	Sources		
	Good	Moderate	Poor
Widely distributed in food and generally consumed in excess of minimum need			
Sodium	Table salt and foods to which it is added; seasoning salts; foods preserved with sodium salts; baking soda, baking powder, MSG, cheese, some leafy vegetables	Salt substitutes	Fruits, beans, vegetables other than leafy greens
Potassium	Salt substitutes, bananas, oranges, cranberries, dried fruits	Vegetables (Some potassium dissolves into cooking water and is lost.)	Cereal products
Chloride	Often present in foods as sodium chloride and other chloride salts		
Needed in relatively large amounts (400–1200 mg)			
Calcium	Dairy products, fish bones, broccoli, dark-green leafy vegetables low in oxalate	Whole-grain cereals, other vegetables	Refined cereals, beans, peas, lentils
Phosphorus	Dairy products, fish bones, meat, some soft drinks	Whole-grain cereals, peas, beans, lentils	Refined cereals
Magnesium	Meat, peas, beans, lentils, dark-green leafy vegetables	Whole-grain cereals, dairy products	Refined cereals

NOTE: The following elements are consumed as part of macronutrients or vitamins: carbon, oxygen, hydrogen, nitrogen, sulfur, cobalt. The biological necessity for the following minerals has been demonstrated in experimental animals but not in humans: nickel, tin, vanadium, silicon.

TABLE 2-5. Dietary Sources of Certain Minerals (*continued*)

Minerals	Sources		
	Good	Moderate	Poor
Added to the water or food supply			
Fluoride	Fluoridated water, tea, other beverages		Nonfluoridated water
Iodine	Iodized salt	Seafood, foods to which iodine is added during processing	Freshwater fish
Needed in small amounts			
Iron	Organ meat, leafy vegetables low in oxalate phytate, egg yolk, beans, nuts	Muscle meat, dried fruits, other vegetables, whole-grain cereals, enriched cereals, seafood	Fresh fruits, fats and oils, milk and dairy products
Zinc	Organ meat, oysters, egg yolk, beans, nuts	Muscle meat, dried fruits, whole-grain cereals, vegetables	Fresh fruits, fats and oils, enriched refined cereals

biotin unless our total food intake is severely restricted.

The distribution pattern of two other vitamins in foods is quite different from that of the vitamins discussed above. Relatively few foods contain *vitamins C and B_{12}*, but these foods are often very concentrated sources of these vitamins. For example, one glass of citrus fruit juice provides enough vitamin C for the entire day. Tomatoes, potatoes, peppers, broccoli, and a few other fruits and vegetables are also good sources of this vitamin. One serving of these foods contains enough vitamin C to meet at least half of the daily needs of an adult. However, a diet that contains only milk, dairy products, eggs, cereals, beans, and meat is almost completely lacking in vitamin C.

Vitamin B_{12} also has a limited distribution in nature and is found only in foods of animal origin. It is added to a few plant foods during processing.

Vegetarians must give careful consideration to sources of vitamin B_{12} (Chapter 12).

What Is a Mineral?

Unlike vitamins, minerals are *inorganic* elements. Dietary minerals that are necessary to support life are listed in Table 2-5. These mineral groupings can provide some guidelines for determining which minerals deserve special attention in diet planning and which foods supply them.

Elements Combined with Macronutrients or Vitamins. There are six minerals that exist as parts of nutrient molecules.

Carbon, hydrogen, and *oxygen* are the elements from which macronutrients—carbohydrates, lipids, proteins—and vitamins are made.

Nitrogen is not generally considered to be an

essential nutrient, but it is an essential part of amino acids and therefore of protein. It must be supplied in the diet to support growth and to replace nitrogen used up by the body and lost in urine, feces, and cells of the skin, nails, and hair.

Sulfur is present in thiamin, pantothenic acid, and biotin, and in the amino acids *cysteine, cystine,* and *methionine.*

Cobalt has a central place in the structure of *cyanocobalamine,* or vitamin B_{12} (Figure 2-16). It is also found in small amounts in foods that contain little or no vitamin B_{12}.

Widely Distributed Minerals. Three minerals—sodium, potassium, and chloride—are so readily available that there is little likelihood of a deficiency occurring. They are consumed in relatively large amounts. The average American diet contains 2.5 to 7.5 grams of sodium and 2.0 to 6.0 grams of potassium; chloride intake is probably in about the same range. A minimum dietary requirement has not been established for any of these three elements, but animal experiments indicate that the daily need of humans is probably less than 1 gram.

Sodium is readily available in our diets as table salt (sodium chloride), which is about one-third sodium and two-thirds chloride by weight. One teaspoonful of salt weighs about 5 grams and therefore contains about 1.6 grams of sodium and 3.4 grams of chloride. You can estimate how much sodium is added to food in the kitchen or at the table by putting one, two, or more shakes of salt into your hand and measuring or visually comparing that amount with a teaspoonful.

Sodium also enters our diet in less obvious ways. It is a part of baking soda and baking powder, and is therefore contained in most pastries, crackers, and breads, and in some cereals. MSG, or *monosodium glutamate,* is used to enhance the flavor of many foods, especially Chinese and Japanese dishes. Other forms of sodium added to food are listed as ingredients on some product labels.

A glass of milk contains about 125 milligrams of sodium, but when the water is removed from milk to make cheese, the sodium becomes more concentrated. Sodium is also found in meat, poultry, fish, eggs, and olives. Sodium nitrite is added to many "cured" foods, such as ham. Many leafy green vegetables are high in sodium, but there is relatively little of it in other vegetables, fruits, or beans.

Commercially available substitutes for sodium chloride are usually mixtures of potassium chloride and sodium chloride. These products, however, should not be confused with onion salt, celery salt, and similar seasonings, which are high in sodium.

Low-sodium diets prescribed by physicians for certain patients may contain 500 milligrams or less of sodium. Although it is not necessary for healthy people to restrict their sodium intake this drastically, moderating sodium intake is considered by many health professionals to be one step toward reducing the risk of *cardiovascular* disease (Chapter 25).

Potassium, like sodium, is found in meat, poultry, and fish; unlike sodium, potassium is provided in relatively large amounts by fruits and vegetables such as bananas, oranges, cranberries, and dried fruits. Baked goods and dairy products, however, are low in potassium.

Since some potassium is lost from food during cooking while sodium is usually added, the ratio of sodium to potassium may increase greatly from market to mouth. This distortion of the sodium–potassium balance of many foods complicates dietplanning for persons on low-sodium diets.

Chloride is supplied in the diet mainly as sodium chloride (table salt) added either at the table, in the kitchen, or during processing. There is no indication that chloride intake is either deficient or excessive in American diets. The safety of several chloridecontaining preservatives in food is presently under investigation.

Minerals Required in Relatively Large Amounts. The three minerals calcium, phosphorus, and magnesium are needed in relatively large

Some minerals are needed in relatively large amounts (calcium, phosphorus, magnesium); two minerals are commonly added to water (fluoride) or food (iodine).

amounts (400 to 1200 mg per day) and are often found in the same foods in varying amounts. A quart of milk, for example, provides enough calcium and phosphorus to meet the daily needs of most adults, but it supplies only about one-third of the needed magnesium. Meat, however, is rich in phosphorus and magnesium but provides relatively little calcium. Beans, peas, and other legumes are among the better sources of magnesium, but they provide only moderate amounts of phosphorus and relatively little calcium.

The distribution of calcium, phosphorus, and magnesium in food is partly explained by the functions these minerals had when the food was "alive." Meat is a good source of phosphorus and magnesium, the minerals required in high concentration by metabolically active muscle cells. The soft bones of cooked salmon have a mineral composition similar to our own skeleton. Green leafy vegetables are high in magnesium because this mineral is contained in chlorophyll, the green pigment of plants that is responsible for photosynthesis. Vegetable peelings and outer layers of grains are good sources of calcium because this mineral is part of plant cell walls.

Whole grain cereals contain some magnesium, calcium, and phosphorus, but much of the phosphorus of grain is in a form called *phytate*. Large amounts of phytate in the diet combine with some of the calcium to form a calcium–phosphorus complex that cannot permeate the intestinal wall and thus be absorbed into the bloodstream. Much phytate, as well as the magnesium of whole grain, is lost during milling.

Spinach, chard, rhubarb, and beet greens contain a carbon–oxygen complex called *oxalate*, which ties up some of the calcium as does the phytate in cereal. Broccoli and dark-green, leafy vegetables such as turnip greens and kale are low in oxalate, and are therefore good sources of absorbable calcium.

The diet should contain approximately equal amounts of calcium and phosphorus; an excess of one of these two nutrients impairs the utilization of the other by the body. For example, one bottle of a phosphoric-acid-containing soft drink may contain as much as 50 percent of the daily need for phosphorus. Excessive use of this type of beverage can have a detrimental effect on the availability of calcium to body cells.

Added to Food or Water. Two minerals—fluoride and iodine—are often added to food or water. *Fluoride* is frequently added to municipal water supplies in amounts that vary among communities. Mineral concentration in fluids is often expressed as *parts per million* (ppm). This measurement corresponds to *milligrams per kilogram* and *micrograms per gram*. If the fluoride content of the water supply is 1 ppm, 1 milligram of fluoride is present in 1 kilogram (approximately 1 quart) of water.

Tea and other beverages made with water are good sources of fluoride. The amount of fluoride in a total daily diet, exclusive of drinking water, ranges from 0.3 mg to 3.0 mg depending upon the amount of fluoride in the soil where the foods are grown.

Excessive intakes of fluoride can be harmful. An intake of 20 to 80 mg each day for several years causes toxic (poisonous) effects. Mottling or dark streaking of the teeth has occurred in children who grew up in communities where the fluoride concentration of the drinking water is between 2 and 8 ppm.

Iodine concentrations in plant foods are strongly influenced by the iodine content of the soil and water where the plants are grown. Iodine concentration in vegetables, for example, may vary fivefold depending upon where they are grown. Seafood is one of the best sources of iodine; freshwater fish contain much less of this mineral.

The daily need for iodine is only about 0.1 gram. The best way to assure that iodine needs are met is to use iodized salt, one-fifth teaspoon of which supplies the total daily adult dietary need. The amount of available iodine in the diet is also increased by the addition of iodine salts in some food-processing methods.

Some minerals are needed in very small, known amounts (iron, zinc); some are needed in very small, unknown amounts (copper, selenium, manganese, chromium, molybdenum); the need for some minerals is yet to be determined (nickel, tin, vanadium, silicon, and arsenic).

Trace Minerals Needed in Known Amounts. At the present time dietary recommendations (see Chapter 8) have been established by nutritionists for only two trace minerals—iron and zinc—which are needed by the body in amounts smaller than 2 percent of our need for calcium and phosphorus. Meat, egg yolk, beans, and nuts are among the better sources of these minerals; milk and dairy products contain very little of either of them. Liver and other organ meats are better sources of iron than are muscle meats, but zinc is about equally distributed in organ and in muscle meats. Oysters are one of the best sources of zinc.

Broccoli and dark-green, leafy vegetables are good sources of iron, but their zinc content is not especially high. Among cereal products, oats and whole wheat are better sources of both iron and zinc than are rye and corn. The iron content of enriched, refined cereals is restored to the level found in whole-grain cereals, but zinc lost during processing is not replaced in these products. Fresh fruits are not generally noted for their iron content, but dried fruits are a much more concentrated source of iron.

The iron content of the American diet has decreased during the last hundred years. This decrease is due partly to changes in food selection patterns, losses during milling of cereal products, and the smaller quantity of food eaten by a more sedentary population. Another factor is that cast iron pots and pans are rarely used today; some of the iron in these utensils dissolves into foods during their preparation. Another reason for lower intakes of iron today is simply that the food we eat is cleaner than it used to be. Dirt contains iron and other minerals as well as bacteria, some of which cause disease. As the safety of our food supply has increased, the iron content has decreased.

Trace Minerals Needed in Small but Unknown Amounts. Our daily requirement for five trace minerals—manganese, copper, selenium, chromium, and molybdenum—has not been established. Our average daily intakes are about 5 mg for manganese, 2 mg for copper, and less than 0.5 mg for each of the other three elements. Table 2-6 lists foods that contain high, moderate, and low concentrations of these minerals.

Minerals of Unknown Value in Human Nutrition. Although they are required for biological functions in experimental animals, the need for *nickel, tin, vanadium, silicon,* and *arsenic* in human nutrition is still undetermined.

One of the major research needs in the science of nutrition is for experiments that will determine the amounts of these minerals that are needed to support health. A second research need is for more complete information about the trace mineral content of various foods. Although there is little evidence that deficiencies of these trace elements exist among Americans, such a possibility cannot be dismissed until we have the knowledge necessary for comparing nutrient needs to nutrient intake, and until methods are developed to detect physiological abnormalities caused in humans by a deficiency of each trace element.

TABLE 2-6. Relative Concentrations of Trace Minerals Needed in Small but Undetermined Amounts

Trace Mineral	Relative Concentrations in General Food Categories		
	High	Moderate	Low
Chromium	Nuts, grains and cereals, condiments and spices		Seafood, meat, dairy products, oils and fats, fruits and vegetables
Manganese	Similar to chromium	Green leafy vegetables	Same as for chromium except for green leafy vegetables
Copper	Nuts, meat, oils and fats, condiments and spices	Seafood, dairy products, legumes, grains and cereals	Fruits, most vegetables
Selenium	Meat	Seafood, nuts	Grains and cereals, condiments and spices, fruits and vegetables, dairy products
Molybdenum	Legumes, nuts, fruits	Meat, condiments and spices	Seafood, dairy products, fruits and vegetables, oils and fats

NOTE: This classification system ranks general categories of food according to the limited values available for trace element content.

STUDY QUESTIONS

1. Approximately how much protein, lipid, carbohydrate, vitamins, and minerals are eaten by an average adult each day?

2. What are three simple carbohydrates and three complex carbohydrates that contain glucose?

3. What is the difference between a lipid and a fat?

4. In what way are all amino acids similar in chemical composition?

5. What determines the nutritional value of a dietary source of protein?

6. Describe the macronutrient composition of five foods you ate yesterday.

7. What factors other than macronutrient composition determine the contribution made by a food to meeting nutrient needs?

8. Name five characteristics of vitamins. Name one other component of food that has each of these five characteristics.

9. In what low-fat foods do fat-soluble vitamins (A, D, E, and K) occur?

10. What are the primary sources of vitamin C and vitamin B_{12} in your diet?

11. Of the minerals listed in Table 2-5, which might be deficient in your diet?

SUGGESTED READING

1. C. F. Adams, *Nutritive Value of American Foods in Common Units.* Agriculture Handbook No. 456. Washington, D.C.: U.S. Department of Agriculture, Agricultural Research Service, 1975.

2. B. K. Watt and A. L. Merrill, *Composition of Foods: Raw, Processed, Prepared.* Agriculture Handbook No. 8. Washington, D.C.: U.S. Department of Agriculture, Agricultural Research Service, 1963, reprinted 1975.

3. *Nutritive Value of Foods.* Revised USDA Home & Garden Bulletin. No 72. Washington, D.C.: U.S. Department of Agriculture, Agricultural Research Service, 1970.

4. M. L. Orr and B. K. Watt, *Amino Acid Content of Foods.* Home Economics Research Report No. 4. Washington, D.C.: U.S. Department of Agriculture, Agricultural Research Service, 1957.

5. M. L. Orr, *Pantothenic Acid, Vitamin B_6 and Vitamin B_{12} in Foods.* Home Economics Research Report No. 36. Washington, D.C.: U.S. Department of Agriculture, Agricultural Research Service, 1969.

6. B. P. Perloff and R. R. Butrum, "Folacin in selected foods," *Journal of the American Dietetic Association* 70(1977):161–71.

7. E. W. Murphy, B. W. Willis, and B. K. Watt, "Provisional tables on the zinc content of foods," *Journal of the American Dietetic Association* 66(1975):345–55.

8. J. T. Pennington and D. H. Calloway, "Copper content of foods: Factors affecting reported values," *Journal of the American Dietetic Association* 63(1973):143.

9. P. S. Kidd, F. L. Trowbridge, J. B. Goldsby, and M. Z. Nichaman, "Sources of dietary iodine," *Journal of the American Dietetic Association* 65(1974):420.

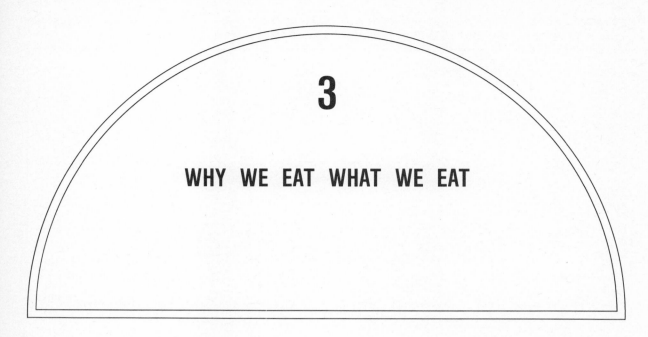

3

WHY WE EAT WHAT WE EAT

Having considered in a general way why food is necessary for life, what the nutrients are, and which foods supply these nutrients, we shall now proceed to develop some basic concepts about the energy needs of the body and about the energy value of different foods, and to discuss in greater detail the specific functions of each group of nutrients.

ENERGY INTAKE

A *calorie* is the basic unit for measuring the energy value of macronutrients and the energy used by our bodies. One calorie is the amount of energy that will raise the temperature of one gram of water one degree centigrade. Since one calorie is a small amount of energy compared to what our bodies need each day, it is more practical in nutrition discussions to use a unit that stands for one thousand times as much energy as a calorie represents. This larger unit is called a *kilocalorie* (kcal) and is often signified by the word *Calorie* (spelled with a capital "C"). However, many nutrition articles in the popular press use *calorie* to mean *Calorie* (Cal) or kilocalorie. American scientists are gradually shifting to a more universal system that represents food

energy in units called *kilojoules* (kJ). One Calorie equals 4.18 kilojoules.

Energy Value of Macronutrients

Energy values of macronutrients are determined in an apparatus called a *calorimeter* (Figure 3-1). A weighed sample of a macronutrient (or a food) is placed inside the chamber; after the door is closed securely, the contents are ignited and burned. The energy released from the macronutrient heats the water surrounding the chamber, just as the heat from a stove burner makes water boil in a pan. The exact amount of energy released from the burned sample can be calculated from the weight in grams of water heated, and from the increase in the water's temperature.

Energy values determined by a calorimeter are slightly higher than the amount of energy released from food taken into the body. In the calorimeter, food is burned completely; but in our bodies, a small fraction of the food we eat is not digestible and is therefore excreted without releasing its energy. Energy values must therefore be adjusted to reflect the fact that approximately 5 percent of the carbohy-

One gram of fat provides slightly more than twice as much energy as does a gram of carbohydrate or protein; the energy value of alcohol is intermediate between the energy value of fat and carbohydrate or protein.

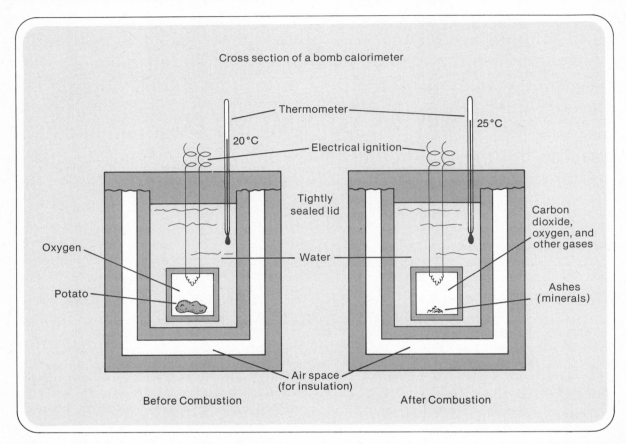

Figure 3–1. Use of a bomb calorimeter to determine the number of Calories contained in a potato. If the combustion of a potato causes a 5° Centigrade increase in the temperature of 20 litres (20 kilograms or 20,000 grams) of water, we know that the potato contained 100 Calories of energy.

drate, 8 percent of the protein, and 2 percent of the fat, in our diet are not normally digested. Corrected macronutrient energy values are as follows: One gram of carbohydrate or of protein provides 4 Cal (17 kJ); and one gram of fat, 9 Cal (38 kJ). One gram of alcohol provides 7 Cal (29 kJ).

Energy Value of Food

It is difficult to keep track of how much energy we consume each day because there is no easy,

practical method for us to know exactly how much energy is provided by all the foods we eat. There are thousands of foods, each with a different energy value.

Caloric values cannot be estimated simply by multiplying the weight of a food in grams by a constant factor because some food components have no energy value. In order to make caloric estimations, the weight of water, nondigestible macronutrients, and minerals must first be subtracted from the weight of the food portion. (Factors for converting cups and other household measures to grams are given in Appendix A3-1). If the only energy-providing macronutrients in a food are protein and/or carbohydrate, the dry weight in grams (weight of the food minus weight of the water) can be multiplied by 4 to approximate the energy value in calories, as in the following example:

$$
\begin{array}{rl}
100 \text{ grams} & \text{Weight of one small orange} \\
-86.8 \text{ grams} & \begin{cases} \text{Weight of water} = 86.3 \text{ grams} \\ \text{Weight of fiber} = 0.5 \text{ grams} \\ \quad \text{(negligible amount of fat,} \\ \quad \text{protein, and minerals)} \end{cases} \\
\hline
13.2 \text{ grams of carbohydrate} \\
\times\ 4 \text{ Calories per gram of carbohydrate} \\
\hline
52.8 \text{ Calories in one small orange}
\end{array}
$$

Similar estimates of energy value can be made for vegetables, cereals, or other foods that are primarily carbohydrate and/or protein. For foods that are primarily fat, such as butter or salad oil, the multiplication factor is 9. This method is cumbersome, however, for foods of mixed macronutrient composition, such as milk, meat, or pizza.

Other sources of food-energy values are tables such as those in Appendix Table A3-2, and pocket-sized calorie-counters or booklets. Although the latter references are convenient to carry, they rarely include total nutrient composition, which is vitally important in making food choices. Food labels sometimes state not only the energy value but also the nutrient content of one serving of that food. It is useful to memorize the approximate energy value of the foods you eat most often so that you can make a rough tally of the Calories supplied by the major items in your diet.

Energy values for some alcoholic beverages are given in Appendix Table A3-3. The proof of "hard" liquor is approximately equal to the number of Calories in one ounce of the liquor, and so 2 ounces of 80-proof vodka, for example, contain approximately 160 Cal (670 kJ) of energy. The sugar and mixes in some alcoholic drinks increase their caloric value.

ENERGY EXPENDITURE

Energy needs vary from one person to another. Even within a single individual, certain circumstances increase or decrease the body's need for energy. Knowing the amount of energy needed from the diet each day enables one to adjust food intake so that the body's energy reserves become neither excessive nor exhausted.

Total bodily energy needs are calculated from three factors: (1) basal metabolism, (2) the specific dynamic activity of the diet, and (3) physical activity or exercise. Several variables determine the contribution each factor makes to an individual's total energy requirement (Figure 3-2).

Basal Metabolism

Basic body functions continue to operate even when a person is in a state of complete rest. The lungs expand and contract, the heart beats, and chemical reactions occur within the body when you are asleep as well as when you are awake. These and other energy-requiring processes that occur involuntarily constitute the *basal metabolism*. In an adult, liver function accounts for about one-third of basal metabolism; brain function, one-fifth; and heart function, one-tenth.

The rate at which involuntary energy utilization or basal metabolism occurs is called the *basal metabolic rate (BMR)*. Basal metabolic rates are measured by a special laboratory procedure where the subject breathes through a mask attached by a hose to a machine that measures the amount of oxygen in air being inhaled and exhaled; the difference is retained oxygen. The rate of oxygen utilization for metabolic reactions is the basis for determining the BMR for a resting person. The rate of basal metabolism during the test period is used to calculate total daily basal metabolism just as distance traveled can

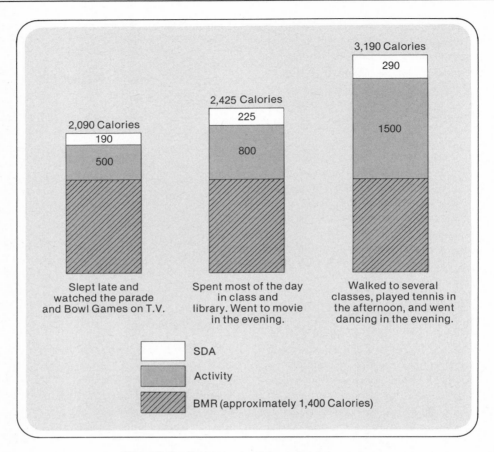

Figure 3–2. Components of energy requirements.

be calculated from the speed of a car for a given number of hours.

Accurate measurement of basal metabolic rate requires that several conditions be met. The person must not eat for 12 to 18 hours before the test. The subject must be comfortably relaxed, at rest, in quiet surroundings, and under no nervous stress. The temperature of the room must be carefully controlled, and the height and weight of the subject must be measured at the time of the test. Each of these conditions is necessary because several factors (discussed next) affect basal metabolism.

Body Size and Composition. The rate at which basal metabolism occurs depends upon cellular activity. Since the number of body cells is proportional to body weight, larger people generally have a higher BMR than do smaller people.

Body composition influences BMR because more energy-requiring reactions occur in muscle cells than in fat cells, even when a person is at rest. Since men normally have fewer fat depots and more muscle tissue than do women, a man usually has a higher BMR than does a woman with the same body weight. Differences in body composition also ac-

BMR varies among individuals depending upon body size and composition, body surface area, air temperature, age, hormones, and various health states.

count for variations in the BMRs of people of the same sex and body weight. For example, athletes and heavy laborers whose bodies contain little fat but many muscle cells have a higher BMR than do sedentary people of equal body weight.

Body Surface Area. Since some body heat is released through the skin, the amount of energy required to maintain normal internal temperature is proportional to body surface area. People of the same weight and body composition whose skin surface areas are different, have different BMRs. For example, a short, broad-shouldered football player is spherical, whereas a tall, lanky basketball player is oblong. The basketball player has a greater surface area and loses more body heat than does the equally muscular football player, who weighs the same as the basketball player but is shorter and broader. The basketball player therefore has a higher BMR.

Air Temperature. Since energy is used to maintain internal body temperature within a fairly narrow range, extremes of environmental temperature can alter the BMR. In cold weather, more body heat is lost than in warm weather; the lost body heat must be replaced by the release of metabolic energy. Most of the time, however, people are in buildings where the temperature is not extreme, or they wear clothing appropriate to the weather. Therefore, extreme climatic variations in temperature usually cause only minor differences in BMR.

Growth and Metabolism. Children have lower BMRs than do adults because of their smaller body size, but their rate of metabolism per pound of body weight is greater because more chemical reactions take place in growing tissues than in adult tissues. The BMR of a child fluctuates in response to growth spurts and growth plateaus.

BMR begins to decrease gradually during the third decade of life, and may be 20 percent lower for a seventy-year-old than it was when that person was twenty. It is not known whether the BMR

decreases with age because of reduced cellular activity, fewer metabolizing cells, or both.

Hormones. To a certain degree, factors associated with the hormones may contribute to the difference in BMR.

Thyroxine, a hormone made in the thyroid gland from the amino acid *thyronine* and from iodine, facilitates the metabolic utilization of energy. Variations in amounts of this hormone secreted by the thyroid gland affect the BMR. In the past, the BMR was frequently used to diagnose an overactive or underactive thyroid gland. Another classic technique for evaluating thyroid-gland activity involves determining the protein-bound iodine (a measure of thyroxine and related hormones) in the blood. Today, however, sophisticated radioisotopic techniques provide a more accurate assessment of thyroid function.

When a person is frightened or under other stress, the BMR is increased by the release of the hormones *cortisol* and *epinephrine* from the adrenal glands, which are located just above the kidneys. These hormones are therefore referred to as the "fright-and-flight" mediators for energy release.

Abnormal Conditions. An increase in body temperature from 37°C to 38°C is accompanied by a 10 percent increase in BMR. Energy needs are greater, therefore, when you have an illness accompanied by a fever. Abnormal metabolic rates are also associated with malnutrition.

Average BMR Values. The laboratory procedure for measuring BMR is tedious and costly, and it is rarely used today except for nutrition research. Since body size is the most significant variable influencing the BMR of healthy adults, the most practical way of estimating a BMR is from tables based on weight and height. The BMR for women usually ranges from about 1,300 Cal (5,460 kJ) to 1,500 Cal (6,300 kJ); for men, from about 1,500 Cal (6,300 kJ) to 1,800 Cal (7,560 kJ). (See Appendix Table A3-4.)

Specific Dynamic Activity

Just as a match or lighter is usually required to start a fire, a certain amount of energy must be invested before the energy in macronutrients can be released. Digestion of food, absorption of nutrients, and the metabolic reactions that release energy from macronutrients are processes that require some energy input. The energy required for the conversion of food into metabolic energy is called the *specific dynamic activity* (*SDA*). It might be thought of as the "postage and handling charge" that must be included in the "order" for food energy.

SDA usually amounts to about 10 percent of the energy needed for basal metabolism. It is less for carbohydrate and fat than it is for protein, which requires more processing within the body in order to be broken down. Although SDA varies slightly depending upon the macronutrient composition of the diet, it usually ranges from 200 Cal (840 kJ) to 300 Cal (1260 kJ) per day.

Physical Activity or Exercise

The component of the total energy requirement that varies most among individuals is the energy used for exercise or physical activity.

Body Size. This factor influences the amount of energy expended during exercise. For example, two people who tie in a swimming race use different amounts of energy during the contest if one weighs 120 pounds and the other weighs 140 pounds. The smaller racer propels less body weight through the water and therefore uses less energy than does the larger swimmer.

Exercise Rate. Energy expenditure is also affected by the rate at which exercise is performed. The swimmer who finishes last may weigh the same as the winner, but because the loser swam more slowly, he or she used less energy during the race than did the winner.

Climate. Extreme weather temperatures can alter the amount of energy used during various activities. A skier uses slightly more energy on very cold days than on mild days to perform identical maneuvers.

At the opposite temperature extremes, more energy is required to perform a particular exercise in 100° weather than in 70° weather. On a hot day, extra energy is required to dissipate body heat. This is accomplished by circulating blood to the skin at faster rates and by producing sweat, which during evaporation helps cool the body.

Activity Patterns. The total amount of energy used daily depends on a person's activities. Table 3-1 lists some specific activities and the energy expended on each depending upon a person's body weight. Because the energy values apply only to the activity and do not include energy needed at the same time for BMR and SDA, this table is useful primarily for comparing energy expenditures on very active days with those on less active days. For example, we can compare the extra energy (above BMR and SDA) used during one hour by a person weighing 60 kilograms (132 lb.) who is engaged in any of the following activities:

lying still, awake	0.1 Cal × 60 kg =	6 Cal
typing rapidly	1.0 Cal × 60 kg =	60 Cal
bicycling (moderate speed)	2.5 Cal × 60 kg =	150 Cal
swimming (2 mph)	7.9 Cal × 60 kg =	475 Cal

Adjusting total energy expenditure to avoid gaining or losing weight is discussed in greater detail in Chapter 9.

FUNCTIONS OF MACRONUTRIENTS

Protein, carbohydrate, and fat have other important functions in the body besides supplying energy.

Protein Functions

The roles of protein in helping children to grow

Energy utilization during activity depends upon body size, the rate of exercise, climate, and the strenuousness of the activity.

TABLE 3-1. Energy Cost of Activities (Exclusive of Basal Metabolism and Influence of Food)

Activity	Cal/kg/hr	Activity	Cal/kg/hr
Light indoor activities		Transportation	
Crocheting, knitting	0.4–0.7	Bicycling (moderate speed)	2.5
Dressing and undressing	0.7	Driving car	0.4
Eating	0.4	Horseback riding (walk)	1.4
Lying still, awake	0.1	Horseback riding (gallop)	6.7
Reading aloud	0.4	Running	7.0
Playing piano	0.8–2.0	Walking (3 mph)	2.0
Playing violin	0.6	Walking (4 mph)	3.5
Sewing, by hand or machine	0.4	Walking (5.3 mph)	9.3
Singing loudly	0.8		
Sitting quietly	0.4	Recreation (moderate to	
Standing relaxed	0.5	heavy exercise)	
Writing	0.4	Boxing	11.4
		Dancing (waltz)	3.0
Work tasks		Playing table tennis	4.4
Carpentry (heavy)	2.3	Rowing in race	16.0
Dishwashing	1.0	Skating	3.5
Laundry, light	1.3	Swimming (2 mph)	7.9
Painting furniture	1.5		
Paring potatoes	0.6		
Sawing wood	5.7		
Sweeping, vacuuming	1.4–2.7		
Typewriting rapidly	1.0		
Washing floors	1.2		

SOURCE: Adapted from C. M. Taylor and G. McLeod, *Rose's Laboratory Handbook for Dietetics*, 5th ed. (New York: The Macmillan Company, 1949). Copyright 1949 by Macmillan Publishing Co., Inc., renewed 1977 by Clara Mae Taylor. Used by permission.

and in building muscles represent only two of the many important functions of this macronutrient. Muscle is, indeed, primarily made of protein, but so are kidneys, liver, and many other vital organs. About 15 percent of our entire body weight is protein. Protein is important not only because our bodies contain so much of it, but also because our bodies contain so many different proteins, each of which has special functions.

Functional Classification. Although there are thousands of body proteins—no one knows how many—most of them can be grouped according to similarities in function. *Enzymes* are an example of the amazing capacity of the human body to manufacture innumerable specialized protein structures; each of the hundreds of enzymes is precisely shaped to slip into a special position between body chemicals during metabolic reactions, and each contains a slightly different arrangement of amino acids. Perhaps even more amazing is that the body's defense system can synthesize specific *antibodies* (which are protein) to combat each of the myriad types of bacteria, viruses, molds, pollens, toxins, and other foreign substances that can enter the body and upset its normal functioning.

Carriers are specialized proteins whose function is to combine with minerals, vitamins, and other chemicals so that these substances can be carried across cellular membranes and be transported in the body fluids from one area to another. For example, much of the lipid that circulates in the blood is bound to protein carriers as *lipoprotein* molecules.

Other important proteins with unique functions include *hemoglobin,* which binds oxygen in the red blood cells for oxygen transport throughout the body; *fibrinogen* and *prothrombin,* two of several blood proteins that function together in blood clotting; *opsin,* a protein in the eye that combines with vitamin A and enables us to see in dim light; and *insulin,* a hormone produced by the pancreas that is necessary in order for glucose to pass from the blood into some body cells. Muscle tissue is made of different proteins—including *myoglobin,* to which oxygen is bound, and *actin* and *myosin,* which are involved in muscle contraction.

Buffering of Body Fluids. Every body fluid, except urine and bile, contains proteins. The *R* portions of the amino acids in proteins contain both acid and alkaline groups. These groups can react with and neutralize other acidic or alkaline body chemicals that are produced during cellular reactions. This ability of proteins to help maintain the acid–base balance of the body within its ideal range is called *buffering capacity.* (The importance of maintaining a normal acid–base balance in the body fluids is discussed in Chapter 7.)

Intracellular Concentrations and Pressure. Proteins help to maintain the proper environment for cellular reactions. The fluid within a cell is separated from the fluid surrounding it by a *cell membrane* (Figure 3-3). This membrane has tiny pores through which water and small molecules can easily pass. Inside the cell are certain cellular proteins, while other proteins exist in the fluid outside the cell. The cell membrane is said to be *selectively permeable*—water, minerals, and other small particles can pass through the membrane but large molecules such as proteins cannot.

If a person is severely deprived of water or perspires excessively, water and minerals may be lost from the body so rapidly that the body cells cannot function properly and may eventually dry up and die. However, cells and body functions are protected to a considerable extent by the ability of proteins to attract and hold water molecules within the cells. The protein–water affinity is important in maintaining a proper concentration of minerals and other small dissolved particles in and outside the cells. By moderating the flow of water across the cell membrane, proteins help the cells maintain the size, shape, and internal pressure required for proper cellular functioning. This characteristic is called the *osmotic effect* of proteins.

Carbohydrate Functions

Carbohydrates do not have as many specialized functions as do proteins, but their importance should not be underestimated. Simple carbohydrates are structural components of larger, complex molecules such as the *cerebrosides* in the nervous system and the *mucopolysaccharides* of the skeletal system. Glucose is the primary fuel of the brain. If glucose is in short supply in the cerebral circulation, drowsiness results; if severe glucose depletion occurs in the brain, coma and death follow.

Role in Fat Utilization. The release of energy from fat depends upon certain chemicals that are created during the breakdown of carbohydrate. This metabolic relationship between fat and carbohydrate is sometimes of great significance. If, for example, a person does not eat for a day or more, body stores of fat are used as a source of energy because very little carbohydrate is stored in the body. Therefore, the special chemicals produced during carbohydrate metabolism and required for complete

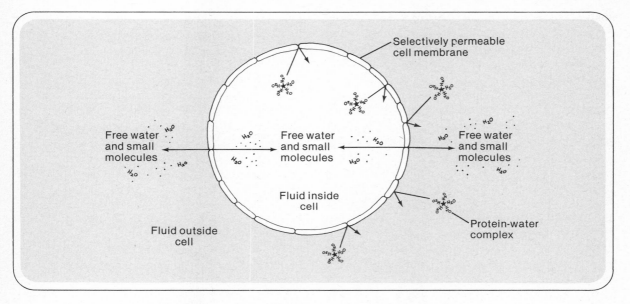

Figure 3–3. Protein reduces flux of water into and out of cells.

metabolism of the stored fat are unavailable. This situation causes the accumulation in body fluids of small acid molecules that are formed from the incomplete breakdown of fat; some of these substances are called keto-acids. If the concentration of these small acid molecules becomes too great to be neutralized by the body's buffering capacity, the acid–base balance of body fluids may be dangerously disturbed and a condition called *ketosis* may result.

Protein Sparing. When food intake is severely restricted, the predominant function of all available macronutrients, including protein, is to supply enough energy to sustain life. The need for energy takes priority over other unique but less vital functions of proteins. It is important, therefore, that the diet supply enough carbohydrate and fat to "spare" protein for functions other than providing energy.

Intestinal Motility. Although nondigestible carbohydrates are not a source of energy for humans,

their presence in the gastrointestinal tract affects the movement of its contents. This type of carbohydrate soaks up water (similarly to a sponge) as it passes through the digestive tract, thus making the feces larger and softer, and enabling them to move more rapidly and easily through the intestinal tract. For this reason, a diet including beans, fruits, vegetables, whole-grain cereal, and other foods that contain nondigestible carbohydrates is recommended for persons bothered by constipation.

Lipid Functions

A primary function of lipids is to provide energy and, like carbohydrates, to "spare" protein; but there are many other reasons for maintaining both adequate intakes and sufficient body reserves of this macronutrient.

Fat Depots. Stored body fat is more than an energy reserve. The bodies of men who are not obese are approximately 15 percent fat; female bodies contain approximately 20 percent fat. This fat helps to insulate the body, thus preventing loss of body heat. Fat depots also act as protective cushions to prevent damage to vital organs such as the liver and kidneys.

Satiety Value. Fat normally stays in the stomach longer than carbohydrate and protein. It therefore helps to diminish the sensation of hunger.

Essential Fatty Acids. Most lipids can be made in the body, and cannot therefore be considered essential dietary nutrients. However, one of the unsaturated fatty acids, *linoleic acid,* cannot be made by the body; it is therefore called an *essential fatty acid (EFA).* Deficiency of this fatty acid limits growth and causes a skin condition generally called *dermatitis.*

An adult needs approximately 5 grams of linoleic acid per day; this amount can be provided by some of the foods shown in Table 3-2. Part of the dietary requirement for linoleic acid can be met by foods containing *linolenic acid,* a related unsaturated fatty acid. Linolenic acid supports growth but does not protect against dermatitis. Another unsaturated fatty acid, *arachidonic acid,* cures the skin abnormality but does not support growth. Vegetable fats supply some linolenic acid; some animal tissues contain arachidonic acid.

Linoleic, linolenic, and arachidonic acids can be converted into *prostaglandins,* a group of hormone-like substances. Recent research suggests that prostaglandins may affect important biological functions including heart contractions, normal blood flow, and the amount of cholesterol in the blood. Linoleic acid may therefore prove to be of importance in preventing heart disease.

Specialized Lipids. Other lipids mentioned in Chapter 2 have important functions but do not have to be provided by the diet because they can be synthesized internally. The nervous system, including the brain, contains phospholipids and complexes

TABLE 3-2. Linoleic Acid Content in Average Servings of Certain Foods

Food	Linoleic Acid (grams)
Black walnuts, ½ cup	14.0
Oil, 1 T.	
Safflower	10.0
Corn	7.0
Soybean	7.0
Cottonseed	7.0
Sesame	6.0
Peanut	4.5
Olive	1.0
French salad dressing, 1 T.	5.0
Avocado, whole	4.0
Bacon, 4 strips	6.0
Pork loin, lean and fat, 3 oz.	2.8
Beef roast, average cut, 3 oz.	2.7
Ham, 3 oz.	2.0
Lamb leg, lean and fat, 3 oz.	0.6
Wheat germ, 1 T.	0.5
Polyunsaturate-rich margarine, 1 T.	0.9 to 3.0
Butter, 1 T.	0.5

of lipids with proteins (lipoproteins) or with simple carbohydrates (gangliosides and cerebrosides). Other lipid-containing molecules are part of cell membranes. Many hormones, including *estrogens, androgens,* and *cortisone,* are steroids. The bile acids, which help digest fat, are also lipids.

Vitamin Carrier. Fat is important as the medium in which fat-soluble vitamins A, D, E, and K are dissolved. Omission from the diet of foods that contain fat may make it difficult to meet the body's need for vitamin E, which is supplied primarily by vegetable oil. However, an adequate supply of vitamins A and K is not necessarily threatened by low-fat diets because these fat-soluble vitamins can be supplied by carefully selected fruits and vegetables.

Low-fat dairy products are usually fortified with vitamins A and D.

Alcohol Functions

Alcohol holds a unique place in the diet. Like protein, fat, and carbohydrate, it can be used for energy. Unlike these macronutrients, however, it is not required for any body function.

Alcohol is formed as an intermediate product during the conversion of certain small molecules into other molecules. A minute amount of alcohol is therefore found even in the bodies of people who have never consumed alcoholic beverages.

An explanation of the toxic effects of alcohol, especially on the liver and the nervous system, would go too far for this text into the medical sciences of physiology and pathology. However, the dual attributes of alcohol—that is, as an energy source and as a toxin—should be kept in mind in diet planning.

FUNCTIONS OF MICRONUTRIENTS

In one way or another, vitamins and minerals are involved in almost every macronutrient function. Several vitamins and minerals are necessary for specific steps in the series of reactions whereby energy is released from carbohydrates, fats, proteins, and alcohol. Many vitamins are involved in the synthesis of proteins and other specialized molecules required for growth and for maintaining normal body functions. The interdependence of these functions—how nutrients operate as a team within the body—will become more apparent in Chapters 4 through 7, which explain how the body uses food.

Functions of Water-Soluble Vitamins

Although there are important exceptions, most functions of water-soluble vitamins fall into two categories: (1) energy shuttles, and (2) metabolic cofactors.

Energy Shuttles. The release of energy from macronutrients involves dozens of reactions, each causing subtle changes in the arrangement of carbon, hydrogen, and oxygen atoms. During these reactions, a hydrogen atom is removed from a macronutrient molecule and linked to a specialized molecule, which simultaneously accepts a portion of the energy within the macronutrient. Some of these specialized molecules acting as hydrogen–energy shuttles contain the vitamins riboflavin or niacin (Table 3-3). Without these vitamins, energy would remain locked within the macronutrient molecules; with them, however, food energy can be harnessed, shuttled around the body, and ultimately used for muscle contraction, synthetic reactions, or the numerous other energy-requiring processes that sustain life.

Cofactors. Water-soluble vitamins participate with minerals, enzymes, and energy shuttles in the *catabolic* (tearing down) and *anabolic* (building up) phases of metabolism. A substance that activates an enzyme is called a *cofactor.* Many B vitamins either alone or as parts of larger molecules, are important cofactors. (Occasionally a vitamin combines with an enzyme during a metabolic reaction; under these circumstances, the vitamin acts as a co-enzyme.)

In some reactions, a vitamin combines with one of the reacting substances or by-products of a reaction. For example, when carbon dioxide is removed from certain molecules during the metabolism of glucose, it is first linked to thiamin. Pantothenic acid and biotin are also necessary for carbon dioxide transfer. Pyridoxine has a similar role in the transfer of amino groups to and from amino acids.

Specific Metabolic Functions. Each water-soluble vitamin has specific metabolic functions (Table 3-3). Thiamin, pantothenic acid, and biotin are primarily involved in energy release and in removal of carbon dioxide during the metabolism of carbohydrates and fats. Pyridoxine participates in many reactions involving amino acids. Folacin and

TABLE 3-3. Functions of Vitamins

Participant	Process or Reaction
Water-Soluble Vitamins	
Riboflavin	Energy transfer involving flavin mononucleotide (FMN) or flavin adenine dinucleotide (FAD)
Niacin	Energy transfer involving niacinamide adenine dinucleotide (NAD) or niacinamide adenine dinucleotide phosphate (NADP)
Thiamin	Energy release and removal of carbon dioxide from breakdown products of carbohydrates and fats
	Formation of DNA (genetic material within cells) and RNA (necessary for synthesis of body proteins)
Pyridoxine	Transfer of amino groups to and from amino acids; synthesis of nonessential amino acids and removal of amino groups from amino acids used for energy
	Synthesis of niacin from tryptophan
	Transfer of sulfur groups
	Removal of carbon-oxygen groups
	Conversion of amino acids into specialized molecules such as neurohormones
	Synthesis of hemoglobin
	Conversion of stored carbohydrate (glycogen) to glucose for energy release
Folic acid	Transfer of one-carbon groups during breakdown of larger molecules and synthesis of specialized substances such as DNA and hemoglobin
Vitamin B$_{12}$	Synthesis of active forms of folic acid
	Some reactions involving folic acid, and similar one-carbon-unit transfers not requiring folic acid
Pantothenic acid	Transfer of acetyl groups (as component of coenzyme A)
	Removal from macronutrient of breakdown products that have only two carbon atoms plus oxygen and hydrogen atoms
	Synthesis of hemoglobin
	Synthesis of cholesterol and other sterols
Biotin	Release of energy and removal of carbon dioxide from carbohydrates and fats
	Synthesis of fatty acids
	Removal of amino groups from some amino acids
Vitamin C	Formation of an amino acid in collagen, the intracellular protein that binds cells together
	Synthesis of active form of folic acid
	Absorption of iron and calcium
Fat-Soluble Vitamins	
Vitamin A	Maintenance of cells lining canals into body
	Resistance to bacterial infection
	Normal structure and secretions of skin and eye
	Growth and reproduction
	Taste sensitivity
Vitamin D	Control of amount of calcium and phosphorus in body fluids and amount deposited in hard tissues
Vitamin E	Antioxidant protection of vitamin A, vitamin C, unsaturated fatty acids, and other sensitive substances
Vitamin K	Formation of specialized proteins necessary for blood-clot formation

vitamin B_{12} sometimes participate together in the same reaction or separately at different steps in a reaction series. Vitamin C is used to synthesize an amino acid called *hydroxyproline,* a constituent of the protein *collagen.* Deficiency of this vitamin ultimately affects the quality of bone, teeth, blood vessels, and other collagen-containing tissues.

Functions of Fat-Soluble Vitamins

Unlike the water-soluble vitamins, the fat-soluble vitamins are not energy shuttles or metabolic cofactors. Although their influence is not so broad in terms of overall metabolism, their specific roles are equally important.

Vitamin A. This vitamin is necessary for maintaining the cells that line the cavities, tubes, and openings inside the body, such as the gastrointestinal tract, the genitourinary tract, and the respiratory tract. This contributes to our resistance to bacterial infection. Vitamin A also helps to maintain the cells of the skin, which becomes dry if the diet is deficient in vitamin A. Furthermore, vitamin A is vital to growth and reproduction, and for normal functioning of the taste buds.

That our eyes need vitamin A is well known. When we walk into a dark theater, vitamin A enables us to adjust our vision to dim light. In this process, a form of vitamin A called *retinaldehyde* combines with the protein *opsin* in the *retina* (internal lining of the eye) to form *rhodopsin* (Figure 3-4). When light strikes rhodopsin, the complex degenerates into opsin and retinaldehyde, and a stimulus is sent along the *optic nerve* to the brain. Since some retinaldehyde is lost during this process, an adequate supply of vitamin A is needed to replenish the rhodopsin in the eye.

Vitamin D. The ability of the body to maintain proper amounts of calcium and phosphorus in blood and other tissues, such as bone and developing teeth, depends upon vitamin D. This vitamin, with calcium and phosphorus, acts together with parathy-

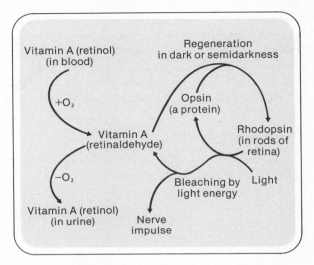

Figure 3–4. Vitamin A and the visual process.

roid and thyroid hormones to influence growth in children, and to control the continuous breakdown and formation of bone tissue. The active forms of vitamin D contain one or two hydroxyl groups and are synthesized primarily in the liver and kidneys.

Vitamin E. The chemical structure of vitamin E enables it to combine easily with oxygen. Many substances, including vitamins A and C and unsaturated fatty acids, also react with oxygen; but in their oxidized form, they cannot function properly. Because vitamin E protects these substances from oxidation by "soaking up" oxygen from the environment, it is called an *anti-oxidant.*

Vitamin E also plays a part in the formation and maintenance of normal red blood cells.

Vitamin K. This vitamin was named by a Danish scientist who discovered that it is necessary for blood coagulation (*koagulation* in Danish) and is therefore essential to the prevention of potentially lethal hemorrhages. Many years passed before scientists understood the role of this vitamin in coagulation. Vitamin K is not actually present in coagulated blood, but it is necessary for the synthesis in the liver of a protein called *prothrombin*. This protein is subsequently changed into the protein *thrombin*. The formation of thrombin sets off a dominolike series of reactions involving the protein *fibrinogen* and calcium; the end result is the formation of a fibrin clot.

Functions of Minerals

Minerals cannot be clearly categorized according to their functions. One mineral often has several functions, such as in body structures (teeth and bones or cell membranes), as a metabolic cofactor (often acting with vitamins), in maintaining the optimal cellular environment, or in controlling the performance of nerves and muscles.

Minerals do not generally act as energy shuttles or combine with metabolic by-products, but the efficiency and speed of metabolic reactions depends upon the concentration of certain minerals in the body tissues where the specific reactions occur (see Appendix Table A3–5). In some cases, one mineral such as manganese may substitute for another such as magnesium. However, high levels of certain minerals may block the effectiveness of other minerals. Mineral imbalances (high or low intake of any one mineral combined with normal intakes of all other minerals) can have serious metabolic consequences; therefore it is dangerous to take high dosages or supplements of any one mineral.

An excess or an insufficiency of a necessary mineral can slow down or even stop a metabolic reaction. In normally functioning cells, there is a finely tuned mechanism for bringing in additional minerals or pumping out those in excess. However, if the diet is not supplying the minerals in the amounts required, the reactions proceed sluggishly or, in severe imbalances, simply cease.

Calcium and Phosphorus. These minerals are the most abundant ones in the body. A 150-pound body contains about 2.2 pounds of calcium and 1.5 pounds of phosphorus. Approximately 99 percent of the calcium in the body is in bones and teeth. The remaining 1 percent (10 grams, or about two-thirds tablespoon) is essential for many vital functions such as blood clot formation, muscle contraction, and transmission of nerve impulses. Absorption of vitamin B_{12} is dependent upon the presence of calcium. This mineral is a metabolic cofactor for many reactions, including the release of energy from macronutrients, and the conversion of prothrombin to thrombin. Calcium in cell membranes helps to control the concentration of many substances on either side of the cell membrane.

Phosphorus is more widely distributed throughout the body than is calcium. Between 10 and 15 percent of the phosphorus in the body is found in body fluids and soft tissues, whereas only 1 percent of the body's calcium is found in these tissues. The wider distribution of phosphorus correlates with the multitude of metabolic reactions in which it participates, usually in one of several oxygen–phosphorus complexes called *phosphates*. The active forms of several vitamins (including thiamin and pyridoxine) are complexes containing phosphates. The nucleic acids DNA and RNA, which are required for cell division (reproduction) and protein synthesis contain phosphate. Many lipids become soluble in water by combining with phosphorus to form phospholipids. In order to participate in certain metabolic reactions, glucose and other simple sugars must be combined with phosphate. Many substances can be absorbed in the intestine or across membranes only in the phosphorylated forms. Phosphorus, oxygen, and hydrogen atoms can bond together in different ratios, and these complexes vary in acidity. Changes in their concentration help maintain the acid–alkali balance in the body.

Two of the most important phosphates are adenosine diphosphate (ADP) and adenosine triphosphate (ATP). These molecules serve as high-energy storage batteries and power a great many important metabolic reactions in the body.

Magnesium. Like calcium and phosphorus, magnesium is found primarily in bones and teeth, but in much smaller quantities. The adult body contains about one ounce of this element, approximately half of which is present in hard tissues.

Magnesium is needed for some metabolic functions that also require calcium and phosphorus. Like calcium, magnesium has roles in nerve transmission, in muscle contraction and relaxation, and in blood coagulation. It is also required for the interconversion of ATP and ADP during many processes of energy release, transfer, or storage. Many of the reactions necessary for protein synthesis will not operate without sufficient magnesium.

Sodium, Potassium, and Chlorine. These three minerals have several functions, in common, including the maintenance of the proper acid–base balance and pressure within cells.

Potassium is present in greater concentrations within cells, while sodium is found mainly in the surrounding fluid. The movement of these two elements across the cell membrane occurs during nerve transmission. The automatic, rhythmic contraction of the heart muscle is extremely sensitive to changes in the potassium content of its cells. Potassium is involved in muscle relaxation (calcium participates primarily in muscle contraction), and in the release of insulin from the pancreas. Sodium affects the transport of glucose and other substances across cell membranes. The ratio of sodium to potassium is important to many reactions, including protein synthesis.

Chlorine is part of hydrochloric acid in the stomach. In this form, it aids digestion and helps to inactivate disease-causing microorganisms that enter the stomach.

Sulfur. This mineral is important because it is contained in several essential nutrients, including some vitamins. Sulfur-containing amino acids are found in relatively high concentrations in hair, skin, and nail protein. Some important enzymes and hormones contain sulfur groups, as do some complex carbohydrates.

Iron. Many biologically important molecules, including several enzymes, contain iron. Hemoglobin of blood and myoglobin of muscle both contain iron at the center of a uniquely fashioned complex molecular part called *porphyrin*. The iron within the porphyrin of both hemoglobin and myoglobin is the only point within the structure of these extremely large proteins to which oxygen can be attached. Without the iron in these molecules, oxygen could not be circulated through the body or made available to muscle cells.

Trace Elements. Only recently have researchers begun to identify the functions of trace elements. For years these studies were impossible because laboratory instruments were not sensitive enough to measure these minerals in the low concentrations at which they are found in the body and in foods. Today, the topic of trace elements is one of the most active areas of nutrition research, although little is currently known about their functional relationships.

- *Cobalt* is part of the vitamin B_{12} molecule, but there are no other known roles for this mineral.
- *Selenium*, like vitamin E, is an anti-oxidant. It can substitute for sulfur in certain sulfur-containing amino acids. It is a part of several enzymes.
- *Iodine* is part of thyroxin and other thyroid hormones, which affect the rate of metabolism.
- *Fluoride* strengthens the calcium- and phosphorus-containing protein matrix of bones and teeth.
- *Molybdenum* and *zinc* are components of certain enzymes; zinc also has a role in wound healing and in sexual maturation.
- *Manganese* is a component of an enzyme and has a role in bone development.
- *Chromium* is necessary for the action of the hormone insulin.

57

STUDY QUESTIONS

1. How do the energy values of fat, carbohydrate, protein, and alcohol compare?

2. How can you find out the energy content of foods?

3. How can total energy needs be determined?

4. What factors influence basal metabolic rate?

5. Define *specific dynamic activity*.

6. What factors affect energy utilization during activity?

7. Name five body proteins and their functions.

8. What functions do carbohydrates serve in the body?

9. What are the functions of lipids in the body?

10. What do water-soluble vitamins do in the body?

11. How do the general functions of fat-soluble vitamins differ from the general functions of water-soluble vitamins?

12. What are some of the functions of minerals in the body?

SUGGESTED READING

1. F. H. Mattson, "Fat," Chapter 4 in *Present Knowledge in Nutrition*. 4th ed. New York and Washington, D.C.: The Nutrition Foundation, 1976.

2. W. E. Connor and J. L. Connor, "Sucrose and carbohydrates," Chapter 5 in *Present Knowledge in Nutrition*. 4th ed. New York and Washington, D.C.: The Nutrition Foundation, 1976.

3. M. C. Crim and H. N. Munro, "Protein," Chapter 6 in *Present Knowledge in Nutrition*. 4th ed. New York and Washington, D.C.: The Nutrition Foundation, 1976.

4. M. W. Blackburn and D. H. Calloway, "Basal metabolic rate and work energy expenditure of mature, pregnant women," *Journal of the American Dietetic Association* 69(1976):24–28.

5. L. M. Maffia, H. E. Clark, and E. T. Mertz, "Protein quality of two varieties of high-lysine maize fed alone and with black beans on mild-to-normal and depleted weanling rats," *Journal of the Dietetic Association* 29(1976):817–24.

6. F. Konishi, *Exercise Equivalents of Foods: A Practical Guide for the Overweight*. Carbondale, Ill.: Southern Illinois University Press, 1975.

7. R. B. Bradfield, "Assessment of typical daily energy expenditure," *American Journal of Clinical Nutrition* 24 (September and December, 1971).

8. *Amino Acid Content of Food and Biological Data on Proteins*. FAO Nutritional Studies No. 24. Rome: Food and Agriculture Organization, 1970.

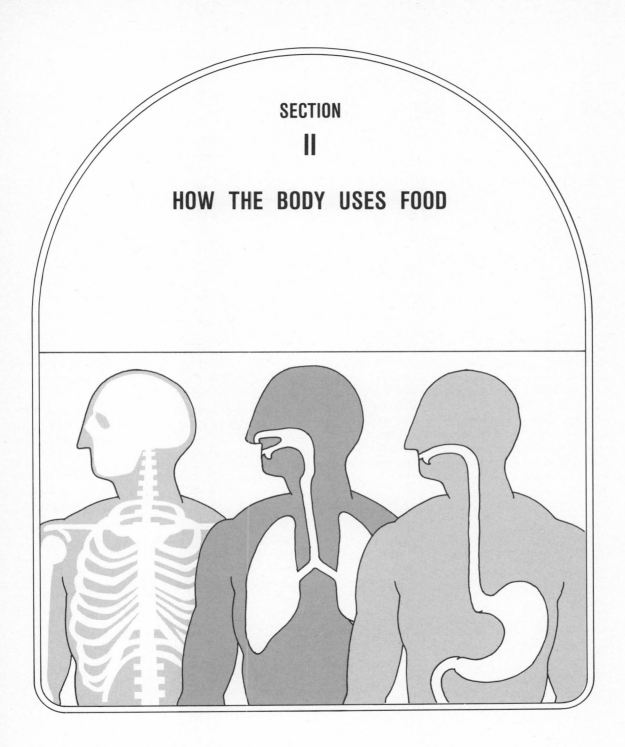

SECTION

II

HOW THE BODY USES FOOD

HOW THE BODY USES FOOD

Food cannot benefit our bodies unless several conditions are met. Food must first be digested, and the nutrients within it absorbed from the gastrointestinal tract. The energy of food is not accessible to the body until it is released by a series of reactions within body cells. Furthermore, every nutrient works cooperatively with water and other nutrients to accomplish many functions in the body. Section II contains information regarding what happens inside our bodies to the food we eat.

CHAPTER 4 FROM MOUTH TO CELL explains how food is digested and nutrients are absorbed, and how the gastrointestinal tract helps to protect the body.

CHAPTER 5 ENERGY RELEASE AND BIOLOGICAL SYNTHESES discusses the process by which energy is released from macronutrients, and explains other functions of macronutrients within the body.

CHAPTER 6 INTEGRATED NUTRIENT FUNCTIONS IN BODY SYSTEMS describes how the nutrients work together to support the functions of several systems within the body.

CHAPTER 7 MAINTAINING BODY FLUIDS explains the function of water and how it is distributed within the body, how the body maintains the proper water content, and the importance of controlling the proper alkalinity of body fluids.

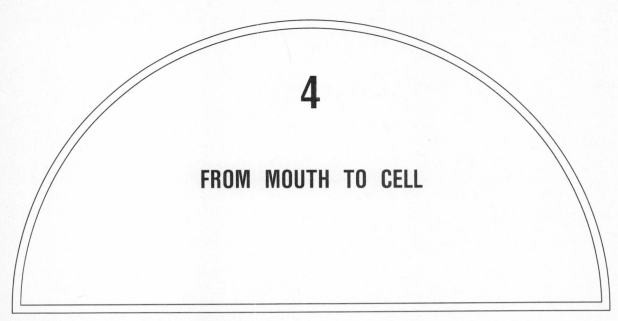

4

FROM MOUTH TO CELL

The potential benefits of dietary nutrients and their contribution to the maintenance of body functions hinges upon their successful passage from the mouth to the cells that use them. This journey involves more than the swallowing of food, the flow of digested food slowly through the gastrointestinal tract, and the gradual soaking up of nutrients by body cells. The digestion of food and the subsequent absorption of its nutrients involve a variety of active processes and reactions, which occur in organized progression within a carefully controlled environment. Food must be changed in a step-by-step fashion along the pathway to the cells, until its macronutrient parts become small enough and soluble enough to pass through the intestinal wall.

THE GASTROINTESTINAL TRACT

Food is changed into absorbable nutrients within the *gastrointestinal tract*, which comprises several organs linked by *sphincters*, or valves, that control the flow of food and water. The gastrointestinal tract can be visualized as a tube winding through the body from mouth to anus. (Figure 4-1). It is rather like a long tunnel that contains various ducts opening into it to bring in fresh air, remove exhaust

fumes, and drain away water that seeps in. The gastrointestinal tract has a duct that brings in metabolic waste products from the liver by way of the gallbladder and another duct that brings in digestive fluids and enzymes from the pancreas. At this point, however, the GI tract–tunnel analogy ends. While the tile walls of a tunnel have supportive and aesthetic functions, the cells that line the gastrointestinal tract have many active functions. The vital roles of these cells include absorption of digested food as well as excretion and secretion of other substances—all for the purpose of bringing needed nutrients, including water, into the interior of the body while selectively excluding harmful or unnecessary substances.

The gastrointestinal tract has four general, simultaneous functions:

1. *Digestion,* or the transformation of food into absorbable nutrients
2. *Absorption,* or the selective transfer of substances across the membrane of intestinal cells
3. *Protection,* or the exclusion of harmful substances from the interior of the body
4. *Excretion,* or the removal of nondigestible food components and waste products formed during metabolism and the normal destruction of dead cells

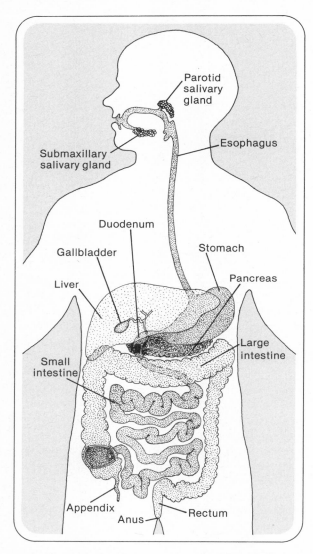

Figure 4–1. The gastrointestinal tract. (Adapted with permission of Macmillan Publishing Co., Inc. from *Man and the Natural World* by C. J. Goin and Olive B. Goin. Copyright © 1970 by Coleman J. Goin and Olive B. Goin.)

DIGESTION

The ultimate purpose of digestion is to break down the structure of food and to change the macronutri-ents it contains to their simplest units without releasing their stored energy. Starch, protein, and fat molecules are too large to pass through cell membranes. Most of the glucose-to-glucose bonds within complex carbohydrates are broken during digestion, leaving glucose molecules dissolved in the watery contents of the gastrointestinal tract. Digested proteins are hydrolyzed to form small peptide chains, which break down into a mixture of amino acids. Some fats are broken down into glycerol and fatty acids before absorption occurs, but monoglycerides and to a lesser extent diglycerides can be absorbed intact.

The complex forms of all three macronutrients usually enter the body together. A hamburger, for example, provides protein and fat; the hamburger bun is predominantly starch. Such food mixtures generally move as *chyme*, a semiliquid slush, through the gastrointestinal tract. There are no separate channels for fat, protein, and carbohydrate. Each type of macronutrient is broken down at a slightly different rate at different sites along the gastrointestinal tract and by different enzymes.

Digestive Processes

Digestion of food is accomplished by the cumulative effects of several different processes. The simplest of these processes is the mechanical breakdown of food in the mouth by chewing. *Lubrication* or *solubilization* occurs when the chewed food (*bolus*) is mixed with saliva and other fluids that flow from various ducts and cells into the gastrointestinal tract. The contractions of muscles in the walls of the gastrointestinal tract mix the bolus with water, mucus, and digestive juices, and propel it through the intestines. These mechanical processes do not break the chemical bonds in macronutrient molecules, but they increase the exposure of the macronutrient molecular surfaces to the specific bond-breaking substances in the digestive juices.

Other factors are involved in digestion. For example, hormones control the production and secretion of digestive substances (Appendix Table A4-1). Bile salts and bile acids that are made in the liver and stored in the gallbladder are released in a controlled manner into the gastrointestinal tract, where they help emulsify dietary lipids.

Bonds within protein, triglyceride, and complex carbohydrate molecules are broken (hydrolyzed) by chemical and enzymatic digestive processes. Chemical digestion results from the action of acid in the stomach or of *alkaline*, or *basic*, substances in the intestine. Some macronutrient bonds are sensitive to acids; others, to bases.

There are many different enzymes that aid in digestion. Each enzyme is named for the nutrient it helps to split plus the suffix *-ase*. For example, a *lipase* hydrolyzes, or breaks bonds in, lipids; a *protease*, proteins; a *disaccharidase*, disaccharides.

The shift from acid to alkaline conditions along the gastrointestinal tract maximizes the efficiency of the specific enzymes that are secreted at various points. Gastric (stomach) enzymes do not function in the alkaline environment of the intestine; intestinal enzymes do not function in the acidic environment of the stomach. For example, *amylase*, the starch-cleaving enzyme in saliva, is active in the mouth. When it is swallowed with the food mixture, however, amylase is chemically digested, along with dietary protein, by the acid in the stomach. Other enzymes that break down carbohydrates are secreted in the intestines. These enzymes, some of which act specifically on smaller carbohydrates, operate with optimal efficiency under alkaline conditions.

Functions of the Digestive Organs

The digestive processes operate uniquely at various places and within the organs of the gastrointestinal tract. Referring to Figure 4-2, we can trace the stepwise digestion and ultimate absorption of the nutrients contained in food.

Mouth. Digestion begins in the mouth, which is more than just the doorway to the gastrointestinal tract. The teeth are important for chewing; and the tongue, for mixing food. Saliva (which contains water, some salts, a mucus lubricant, and the enzyme amylase) is secreted by the salivary glands.

Esophagus. This sophisticated organ is more than a simple conduit from the mouth to the stomach. Its walls contain muscles that squeeze and move the bolus of food along as it is swallowed. At each end of the esophagus is a delicately controlled "trapdoor," or valvelike structure, that opens and closes with precise timing, ensuring that food is not misdirected into the lungs but goes down into the stomach and stays there. The contraction and relaxation of the valve between the esophagus and the stomach is governed by pressure changes and nervous stimuli. If this valve were to leak, the acidic contents of the stomach would flow back into the esophagus, and ulcerate or scar the sensitive cells lining the esophagus. If acidic fluid were to back up from the stomach and into the lungs, pneumonia or even death might result.

Stomach. Sensors in the stomach are activated by the presence of certain types of food—especially proteins, caffeine, spices, and alcohol. These sensors cause the release into the bloodstream of various hormones. The most extensively researched of these hormones is *gastrin*, which recirculates to the stomach and stimulates specialized secretory cells to produce *gastric acid*. The acidity of foods such as grapefruit, vinegar, or tomatoes is mild compared to the strength of gastric acid; the acid contained in some cola beverages, however, approaches gastric acid in strength.

The stomach cells also secrete *gastric lipase* and a protein-digesting enzyme called *pepsin*. (Infants secrete an enzyme called *rennin*, which digests milk protein.) The contents of the stomach are lubricated by a watery, slippery solution called *mucin*, a protein–carbohydrate complex, which is secreted by the mucous glands of the stomach. *Intrinsic factor*,

Each organ from mouth to large intestine and the organs linked by ducts to the gastrointestinal tract have specific roles in the digestive process.

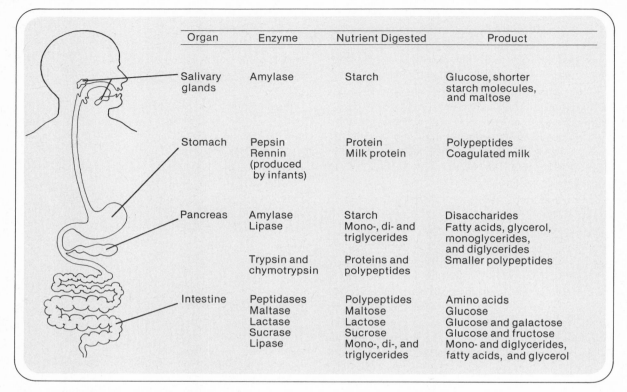

Organ	Enzyme	Nutrient Digested	Product
Salivary glands	Amylase	Starch	Glucose, shorter starch molecules, and maltose
Stomach	Pepsin	Protein	Polypeptides
	Rennin (produced by infants)	Milk protein	Coagulated milk
Pancreas	Amylase	Starch	Disaccharides
	Lipase	Mono-, di- and triglycerides	Fatty acids, glycerol, monoglycerides, and diglycerides
	Trypsin and chymotrypsin	Proteins and polypeptides	Smaller polypeptides
Intestine	Peptidases	Polypeptides	Amino acids
	Maltase	Maltose	Glucose
	Lactase	Lactose	Glucose and galactose
	Sucrase	Sucrose	Glucose and fructose
	Lipase	Mono-, di-, and triglycerides	Mono- and diglycerides, fatty acids, and glycerol

Figure 4–2. Digestive enzymes, glands that produce digestive enzymes, the nutrient each digests, and the products. (Adapted with permission of Macmillan Publishing Co., Inc. from *Man and the Natural World* by C. J. Goin and Olive B. Goin. Copyright ©1970 by Coleman J. Goin and Olive B. Goin.)

which is necessary to the absorption of vitamin B_{12}, is also released by stomach cells.

At the lower end of the stomach is an important valve, or sphincter, that controls the flow of partially digested food, water, and acid into the *duodenum*, which is the first portion of the small intestine.

Pancreas and Gallbladder. Although these organs have separate functions, the ducts from them make a Y-shaped connection leading into the duodenum, where their secretions are simultaneously mixed with the chyme.°

° The connection between these ducts is important to people with gallstones. If a stone is above the junction of the Y, the flow of gallbladder secretions is impeded; a stone located below the

The pancreas is a soft, elongated organ shaped like a hand with the fingers together. It lies deep in the abdomen behind the stomach, tapering off to the left. As pancreatic juice, which is alkaline, mixes with the chyme, it neutralizes the acid from the stomach, so that the intestinal enzymes can function. The pancreas secretes peptidases, amylases, and lipases—thus aiding in the digestion of all three macronutrients.

The gallbladder resembles a small, thin-walled pouch. It is located in the upper right side of the abdomen, tucked under the liver. It stores and con-

junction stops the passage of digestive secretions from both organs. In some people, the ducts from these organs lead directly into the duodenum and are not connected to each other.

centrates the bile that the liver produces. Bile is an alkaline fluid containing bile salts, bile acids, and metabolic waste products. At any given time, the gallbladder holds only about one-fourth cup of bile; but during one day, almost a quart of bile flows through this organ.

The release of bile from the gallbladder into the duodenum is controlled by the hormone *cholecystokinin.* When fatty foods as well as acid and amino acids reach the duodenum, they trigger the release of cholecystokinin into the bloodstream; the hormone travels to the gallbladder, which then contracts and releases bile.

Bile salts and bile acids do not hydrolyze fats, but they do have an important role in the utilization of these macronutrients by the body. Digestion of fat and related substances is complicated by the fact that lipids do not dissolve in water, and lipases do not dissolve in fat. In order for the lipases to digest a lipid such as butter, the lipid must be dispersed in a watery fluid. Bile salts and bile acids perform this function (*emulsification*) in much the same way that soap makes it possible to wash grease or oil out of clothes. Like bile salts and bile acids, soap has long molecules, one end of which is soluble in water and the other end of which is soluble in fat or oil. The oil-soluble end of soap is attracted to the grease from clothes while the water-soluble end stays in the wash water. The fat-soluble end of a bile salt is attracted to a lipid globule, while the water-soluble part stays in the watery fluid of the intestine. In both cases, tiny oil particles become surrounded by, or dispersed in, water (Figure 4-3). The water-soluble lipid complex is called a *micelle.*

Small Intestine. Cells of the small intestine produce numerous digestive enzymes. By the time food reaches this region of the gastrointestinal tract, some of the larger nutrient complexes have been broken down into molecular components of intermediate or small size. Some intestinal enzymes are specific for hydrolyzing disaccharides; others act on small protein units such as polypeptides or on vari-

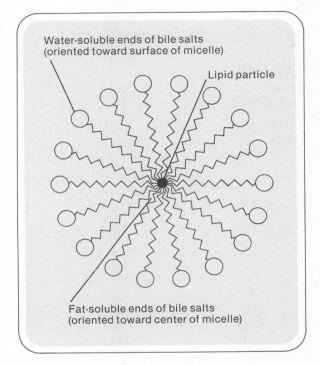

Water-soluble ends of bile salts
(oriented toward surface of micelle)

Lipid particle

Fat-soluble ends of bile salts
(oriented toward center of micelle)

Figure 4-3. Formation of a micelle—solubilization of a lipid in a water solution.

ous lipids such as monoglycerides and diglycerides. Most of the macronutrients are digested and reduced in size and complexity in the small intestine so that they can be absorbed into the bloodstream.

Large Intestine. Secretions of the large intestine, or colon, contain *mucus* but no digestive enzymes. Most of the macronutrients have been absorbed before the contents of the gastrointestinal tract reach this organ. Some of the nondigestible food residue is utilized as an energy source by *microorganisms* that normally reside in the large intestine.

ABSORPTION

Digestion and absorption are often discussed together because these two functions are closely interrelated. Absorption of most nutrients is impossible without digestion, but digestion is purposeless unless it is followed by absorption.

Intestinal Anatomy

Although water and some drugs—for example, alcohol and aspirin—can be absorbed into the bloodstream from the stomach, other nutrients are absorbed only in the intestine. Absorptive processes cannot be appreciated without some knowledge about the anatomy of the small intestine.

Macroanatomy. "Small intestine" seems to be a misnomer, considering that this tube in its relaxed state is about 30 feet long—or about the same length as a garden hose. How can so much intestine fit inside a human being? The small intestine, like the heart or the biceps in your arm, is a very muscular organ; in its normal state of contraction, it is only about 10 feet long. Furthermore, only a small portion of the intestine is full of food at a given time.

There are two separate sets of muscles within the walls of the intestine: one set contracts and relaxes lengthwise like a rubber band; the other set alternately contracts and relaxes around the circumference of the intestinal tube, thus decreasing the tube's diameter and then allowing it to distend. The intestinal muscles squeeze the mixture of digesting food in a highly coordinated manner, relaxing in front of and contracting behind the advancing bolus of digesting food. This rhythmic, muscular action propels food through the intestine, a process called *peristalsis.*

Microanatomy. The inner surface or lining of the small intestine is called the *intestinal mucosa.* To the unaided eye, the mucosa appears somewhat rough, but under a magnifying glass, thousands of fingerlike projections called *villi* can be seen in the mucosa (Figure 4-4). Each of these projections is

about one millimetre long and contains *microvilli* (little villi), which can be seen under a more powerful microscope. One side, or *pole*, of a cell containing microvilli faces the interior, or *lumen,* of the intestine and is therefore in contact with the digested macronutrients. The other pole of the cell faces inward toward the center of the villus, where a membrane separates the cell from a series of vessels. One set of vessels comprises the *capillaries* of the blood circulatory system; the other is a network of vessels of the lymphatic system, which are called *lacteals.*

Tiny slips of muscle allow the villi and microvilli to move back and forth. Running your finger across the top of a thick pile carpet might convey an idea of how these villi move around the swirling contents of the intestine. These specialized structures of the mucosal cells increase the total absorptive area of the intestine about 600-fold. If all of the intestinal microvilli were pressed flat, they would cover an area half the size of a basketball court.

Absorptive Processes

The smaller nutrient molecules released during digestion permeate the intestinal mucosa by several different mechanisms. The factors that determine how each molecule is absorbed include its size, its solubility in water, whether or not energy is required for its absorption, and its concentration in the intestine relative to its concentration in the bloodstream. The following five key words identify the absorptive processes: pores, porters, pumps, pinocytosis, and particularization.

Pores. It has been postulated that there are tiny pores 0.0000005 millimetres (mm) in diameter through which water and very small substances can pass. Movement through these pores is possible for some substances if their concentration in the intestine is greater than it is in the blood. This process of *downhill diffusion* (or *passive absorption*) occurs

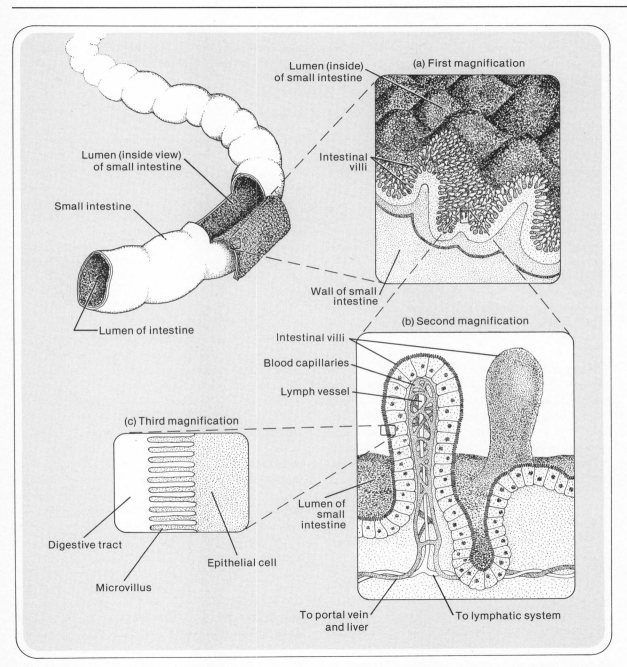

Lumen (inside)
of small intestine

(a) First magnification

Lumen (inside view)
of small intestine

Small intestine

Intestinal
villi

Lumen of intestine

Wall of small
intestine

(b) Second magnification

Intestinal villi

Blood capillaries

Lymph vessel

(c) Third magnification

Lumen of
small
intestine

Digestive tract

Epithelial cell

Microvillus

To portal vein
and liver

To lymphatic system

Figure 4–4. Three stages of increasing magnification of the small intestine showing the lining (a), villi (b), and microvilli (c).

when a substance moves from a region where its concentration is high to a region where its concentration is low. Energy is not required for passive absorption through pores.

Porters. Many end-products of digestion, such as monosaccharides and amino acids, are too large to pass through the tiny pores. Some of these substances can be transported through the cell if they are first attached to specialized carrier molecules that might be thought of as *porters*. Some vitamins and minerals are also absorbed in this way.

Pumps. Absorption by *pumps* is energy dependent. This process allows nutrients to travel against a *concentration gradient*—from a region of low concentration to a region of high concentration. Pumps are known to exist for the movement of sodium and glucose, and they have been postulated for other nutrients. Some nutrients of similar structure, such as the simple sugars, may even compete for the same pump.

Pinocytosis. In this process, a segment of the cellular membrane gradually wraps itself around a tiny droplet of intestinal contents, ultimately forming a *vacuole* (or small cavity) containing the nutrient. The walled-off particle is then transported across the cell. While inside the vacuole, the nutrient may or may not undergo further digestion before being released at the opposite pole of the villus into the blood or lymph vessels.

Particularization. This process, which is unique to lipids, involves the dispersion of fatty acids and monoglycerides in water. The molecular products of lipid digestion are surrounded by the soaplike bile salts and phospholipids to form the water-soluble complexes or micelles. When these tiny droplets come into contact with the intestinal lining, the fatty acids and monoglycerides are released from the micelles and pass into the villi. The bile acids are then freed to move further down the small intestine,

where most of them are absorbed into the blood, recirculated to the liver and gallbladder, and later dumped back into the first part of the intestine to perform the same digestive and absorptive functions again.

Reactions in Mucosal Cells

Some of the digestive enzymes synthesized by the intestinal mucosa are located at the border of the mucosal cells. They hydrolyze small nutrient complexes such as disaccharides when the nutrient comes into contact with the cell membrane and enters the cell.

Other enzymes inside the mucosal cells reverse the fat-digestion reaction and resynthesize triglycerides, which are then solubilized by lipoproteins to form *chylomicrons.*

Transport Systems

Absorbed nutrients are conveyed by the blood and lymph systems to other cells of the body. The tiny vessels of both systems begin inside the villi, from which different digested nutrient molecules enter one or the other of these transport systems.

Short-chain fatty acids (those containing only 6, 8 or 10 carbons), along with most other nutrients, enter the blood capillaries of the villi. The nutrient-rich blood leaves the villi and flows through the capillaries, which converge to form veins. As these veins receive blood from greater segments of the intestine, they converge and become larger until finally they become visible as fingerlike projections on the outer surface of the intestine (Figure 4-5). These veins converge to form the *portal vein,* which carries the nutrients from the small intestine to the liver.

The portal vein terminates in the liver as many tiny capillaries. As nutrient-rich blood flows through these liver capillaries, some of the nutrients are further processed or converted into other substances by the actively metabolizing liver cells, and released

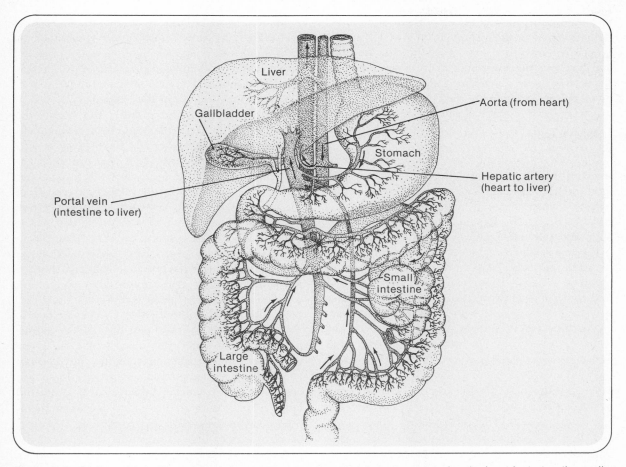

Figure 4–5. Major veins and arteries of the circulatory system that help transport absorbed nutrients to other cells.

into the blood for use by the body. Some nutrients carried to the liver by the portal vein leave the liver unchanged or only partially processed. These nutrient substances are circulated to the capillaries of all tissues and organs—including skin, kidneys, muscles, lungs, heart, gastrointestinal tract, and even bones and teeth.

The chylomicrons that are formed in the microvilli travel a more circuitous route before reaching the blood circulatory system. These lipid-rich particles pass into the lymphatic capillaries, which travel upward from the intestines, unite to form larger vessels, and then form a single vessel, or duct, which leaves the abdominal cavity and passes through the diaphragm and into the chest cavity. The fatty contents of this duct enter the blood circulatory system just above the heart, near the point where the jugular vein joins one of the major veins behind the collar bone. These fluids subsequently circulate with the blood throughout the rest of the body.

The lymphatic system is not a closed, or circulatory, system. It collects lipid substances from the intestinal cells and funnels them into the blood without carrying them through the liver. The chylomicrons make their first cycle through the body and are very quickly removed from the blood by *lipoprotein lipase,* an enzyme found in tissue such as heart muscle and *adipose* (fat) tissue.

Fluid Transfer

The water absorbed from the gastrointestinal tract not only consists of the water contained in food and beverages but also includes the water from digestive juices. The daily volume of these fluids is between 8 and 10 litres (about 2 to 2.5 gallons)—approximately one-fourth of all body water.

Feces normally contain less than one cup (240 ml) of water per day. Most gastrointestinal water is absorbed primarily from the colon or large intestine into the blood. However, large amounts of water may be lost by people who have severe diarrhea. Under these circumstances, some of the fluid lost comes from a reverse flow of both water and small molecules from the blood into the intestine; thus, the total volume of blood in the body is reduced. In order to compensate for this loss of water from the blood, water moves out of the cells and into the circulatory system. The cells become dehydrated, and their contents more concentrated. The consequences of this intracellular imbalance can be fatal if not corrected.

PROTECTION MECHANISMS

The gastrointestinal tract protects the body in three ways: the first way is related to digestion; the second, to absorption; and the third, to the immune system and its specialized collections of cells that produce antibodies. (The latter aspect of intestinal function is not directly related to digestion and will be covered in Chapter 21.)

If most dietary proteins, fats, or complex carbohydrates were infused directly into the bloodstream, they would cause serious allergic or other often fatal reactions.° Such allergic reactions occur because the body's protective mechanisms (*immunologic machinery*) can recognize differences between the arrangement of building blocks in most dietary macronutrients and those in the macronutrient molecules normally found in the body.

The digestive process protects the body from "foreign" proteins, complex carbohydrates, and fats. When these large molecules have been broken down to simple building blocks, they are no longer harmful. Normally the body does not have either the enzymes or the blueprint (DNA) to reconstruct foreign substances that are biologically dangerous. Furthermore, stomach acid is so strong that many, but by no means all, bacteria and other living organisms are destroyed and subsequently digested.

The membrane of the intestinal cells constitutes a mechanical barrier that protects the body from invasion by harmful organisms. For example, if certain bacteria that constantly thrive and reproduce in the large intestine were to pass through the intestinal lining and enter the bloodstream, an overwhelming, life-threatening infection (*septicemia*) could result. Under normal circumstances, such a condition does not occur because bacteria are too large to pass through the intact intestinal membrane. Under two abnormal conditions, however, bacteria may be able to penetrate the walls of the gastrointestinal tract: (1) the bacteria may produce toxins that damage intestinal cells, causing a microscopic abscess through which penetration can occur; and (2) the gastrointestinal tract may be weakened and easily torn as a result of colitis or various tumors, thus allowing bacteria, undigested macronutrients, or toxins to pass through.

Some liver enzymes provide a protection mechanism by participating in *detoxification* reactions.

° The fluid used in hospitals for most *intravenous* (IV) feeding is not only sterile but also free of proteins, fats, and complex carbohydrates. Short-term IV feeding solutions usually contain glucose for energy, minerals in amounts similar to those found in human blood, and vitamins. Special preparations of amino acids and fatty acids are occasionally added to IV solutions.

Many harmful substances that are not destroyed during digestion and that slip through the intestinal membrane are changed in the liver into a nontoxic form. Alcohol is an example of a potentially harmful substance that is not digested by the intestinal tract but is ultimately detoxified by the liver.

DIGESTION AND ABSORPTION OF MICRONUTRIENTS

In general, the basic structure of vitamins and minerals is not altered during their passage from mouth to cell. In many cases, the micronutrients we eat are in a form that is biologically active. There are, however, some important exceptions to this generalization. Furthermore, certain factors can enhance or impair the absorption of micronutrients.

Table 4-1 summarizes information about both the digestion and absorption of vitamins and minerals. Not all nutrients are absorbed in the same part of the small intestine. For example, most of the water-soluble vitamins are absorbed in the initial part of it; vitamin B_{12}, however, enters the bloodstream near the terminal segment of the small intestine.

Nutritionists have much to learn about the dietary and physiological conditions that affect the efficiency of nutrient absorption. Research is hampered by the fact that results of experiments in one species, such as rats, sometimes differ from those observed in another species, such as chickens. Studies of humans can be done, but they are often difficult and expensive. One of the most accurate ways to measure absorption of very small amounts of a nutrient is to feed its radioactive form to the experimental animal; however, many radioactive substances cannot be used in human studies. As safer and more sensitive techniques are refined by nutritionists and gastroenterologists, many of the gaps in Table 4-1 will be filled.

Information about nutrient absorption is important not only for people with intestinal and *endocrine* (hormonal) diseases but also in diet planning for people who have had part of the gastrointestinal tract surgically removed because of ulcers, cancer, or other diseases. Such information will also help those concerned with food production and processing, and those concerned with improving the nutrient content of foods and the nutrient intake of active people.

Water-Soluble Vitamins

Most of the information in Table 4-1 is self-explanatory, but a few of the listings merit further explanation.

Vitamin C. The absorption of vitamin C (ascorbic acid) into the intestinal mucosal cells apparently occurs by means of a pump that is affected by the presence of sodium. The popularization of self-medication with large doses of vitamin C has increased the importance of learning how this nutrient is absorbed. Whether some absorption-related mechanism exists to protect the body against harm from high doses of vitamin C and whether large concentrations of this vitamin affect the digestion and absorption of other nutrients, need to be determined.

Thiamin, Riboflavin, and Niacin. These vitamins are absorbed in the upper part of the small intestine. Thiamin must be combined with phosphate groups in order to be absorbed; on the other hand, phosphate groups must be removed from riboflavin before it can be absorbed.

Folacin. This vitamin is found in food in several forms, all of which contain the basic structure called *folic acid.* Biologically active folacin includes folic acid and several forms with slightly different chemical structures. In food, folic acid is generally combined with one to seven *glutamic acid* groups (similar to the amino acid *glutamine*). All except one (or possibly two) of these groups must be removed by a specific digestive enzyme prior to absorption of the

TABLE 4-1. Absorption of Vitamins and Minerals

Micronutrient	Region Where Absorption Occurs	Prior Digestive Process	Process	Factors That Increase Absorption	Factors That Decrease Absorption
Ascorbic acid	Terminal part of small intestine		Sodium-dependent pump (varies among species)		
Thiamin	Initial part of small intestine (rapid but incomplete absorption)	Phosphate must be added.	Pores and pumps		Malnutrition in alcoholism
Riboflavin	Initial part of small intestine	Phosphate must be removed.	Pores (?) (Phosphorus is added back within intestinal cells.)	Age	
Pyridoxine	Mainly in initial part of small intestine but some in middle part		Pores (?)		Might be interrelated with amino acid absorption
Folacin	Initial part of small intestine beyond area where most pyridoxine is absorbed	All except one (or possibly two) glutamic acid group must be removed.	Pores (?) Porters (?)		Lack of glutamate-cleaving conjugase
Vitamin B$_{12}$	Terminal part of intestine	If bound to protein, vitamin must be released before absorption. Must be bound to intrinsic factor (produced by stomach cells)	Porter in intestinal cells (?) Pinocytosis (?) Calcium has role in absorptive process.		Fish tapeworm sequesters this vitamin for its own growth. Lack of intrinsic factor Pancreas has undermined role in absorption.

Nutrient		Site of absorption	Mechanism	Substances needed	Factors that decrease absorption
Vitamin A and vitamin A precursors	Acid groups must be removed.	Initial and middle part of small intestine	In some species, vitamin A precursors are split within intestinal cell. Fatty acid group is added back within intestinal cell.	Bile salts	Low intake of dietary fat; Disorders that impair fat absorption; Vitamin E deficiency and protein deficiency
Vitamin D		Middle part of small intestine	Pumps (?) or porters (?)	Bile salts	Disorders that impair fat absorption
Vitamin E				Pancreatic juice and bile	
Vitamin K				Pancreatic juice and bile; Vitamin K that is synthesized by intestinal bacteria is absorbable.	Disorders that impair fat absorption; Antibiotics that kill intestinal bacteria reduce amount of vitamin K formed.
Calcium		More in initial and middle than in terminal part of small intestine	Energy required; Calcium-binding protein porter; Sodium and hexoses may have role.	Amount absorbed adjusts to body needs (deficiency, pregnancy, growth spurts). Lactose. Vitamin D. Acidic conditions	Oxalate; Phytate (but body adjusts to this); Laxatives; Imbalance between calcium and phosphorus; Abnormalities related to thyroid and parathyroid hormones
Iron	Stomach acid changes chemical state.		Bound to protein porter (ferritin) in intestinal cell	Amount absorbed adjusts to body needs.	Phytate; Oxalate; Fiber (?)

NOTE: Question marks indicate processes that have been hypothesized.

TABLE 4-1. Absorption of Vitamins and Minerals (continued)

Micronutrient	Region Where Absorption Occurs	Prior Digestive Process	Process	Factors That Increase Absorption	Factors That Decrease Absorption
Iron (continued)			Energy required	Ascorbic acid	Iron from meat is better absorbed than iron from plant sources.
Magnesium					Phytate Oxalate
Copper	Stomach and initial part of small intestine		Bound to a protein porter		High concentrations of zinc, cadmium, molybdenum, and silver compete for this protein porter.
Zinc			Bound to a protein porter		Cadmium and calcium compete for this protein porter. Phytate
Manganese			Bound to a protein porter		Iron may compete for this protein porter. Excess calcium and phosphorus
Chromium			Appears to pass through pores but depends upon chemical state		
Iodine					Goitrogenic substances in some foods

vitamin. When this enzyme is in short supply or is not fully active, as in people who have gastrointestinal disease, folic acid absorption is impaired.

Vitamin B$_{12}$. This vitamin cannot be absorbed unless it is first combined with intrinsic factor, which is secreted by the stomach cells. Before the role of intrinsic factor was discovered, many people died of *pernicious anemia,* a condition in which stomach cells fail to secrete intrinsic factor. Today, people with pernicious anemia can live a normal life as long as they receive vitamin B$_{12}$ injections, thus bypassing the need for the absorption factor.

Absorption of vitamin B$_{12}$ is also reduced in cases of fish tapeworm infestations, found more commonly in Japan, Scandinavia, Canada, and Alaska than in other parts of the world. Fish tapeworm sometimes occurs among Jewish women who taste gefilte fish as they prepare it prior to cooking. This tapeworm has an enormous affinity for vitamin B$_{12}$, and it uses the vitamin for its own growth before the vitamin can be absorbed into the blood of its "host."

Fat-Soluble Vitamins

The absorption of fat-soluble vitamins is reduced by conditions that impair the absorption of fat, such as lack of bile salts, disease of the pancreas, or stones blocking the duct from the gallbladder and/or pancreas. Such conditions often lead to a deficiency of vitamins A, D, E, and K.

Minerals

Calcium absorption is enhanced by the presence of lactose, or milk sugar, and by the acidic conditions that exist where the stomach joins the duodenum. Calcium absorption is impaired in conditions involving vitamin D deficiency; certain hormonal imbalances; excess amounts of dietary oxalates, phytates, and laxatives; and an imbalance in the dietary intake of calcium and phosphorus.

Iron exists in food in several different chemical states. The acid conditions in the stomach change dietary iron to the chemical form that is most efficiently absorbed. Iron absorption is enhanced by vitamin C but impaired by high intakes of oxalates and phytates. Large amounts of fiber may also reduce the absorption of iron as well as zinc, but it is not yet known whether the amount of fiber normally in the diet is sufficient to impair mineral absorption. The iron in meat products is better absorbed than is the iron in vegetable products.

To a certain extent, the amount of iron absorbed depends on a person's needs and reserves. For example, approximately 10 percent of dietary iron is absorbed in people who have adequate stores of this mineral, whereas people who have low body stores or an increased specific need for this mineral absorb iron more efficiently. The absorption of certain minerals increases during pregnancy when nutrient needs are greater.

With the exception of calcium and iron, the absorption of minerals has not been studied in as great detail as has the absorption of vitamins. We do know, however, that the absorption of iodine is impaired by certain substances called *goitrogens,* which occur naturally in a limited number of foods (see Chapter 27).

Many minerals are bound to protein porters or carriers, which facilitate their absorption but usually require energy. Two or more minerals often compete for a place to attach themselves to the same carrier—for example, strontium competes with calcium. This competition is of vital significance if a body has been exposed to the long-lived radioisotope *strontium-90.* This isotope can substitute for calcium during absorption and actually replace it in bone tissue, where it remains for years giving off dangerous radiation.

STUDY QUESTIONS

1. What must happen before the nutrients in foods can be absorbed into the body?

2. What four general functions does the gastrointestinal tract simultaneously serve?

3. What happens to proteins, fats, and complex carbohydrates during digestion?

4. What specific roles do the organs in the gastrointestinal tract and the organs linked to it play in the digestive process?

5. Describe how the macroanatomy and the microanatomy of the small intestine are specialized to optimize the absorptive process.

6. What are the five processes involved in nutrient absorption?

7. What is the difference between the two systems that carry nutrients from the intestinal mucosal cells to other body cells?

8. Why can malabsorption of fluids be life-threatening?

9. How does the gastrointestinal tract protect the interior of the body?

10. What differences are known to exist in the absorption of various vitamins and minerals?

SUGGESTED READING

1. F. J. Ingelfinger, "The esophagus, not an uninteresting tube but a fascinating organ," *Nutrition Today* 8(1973):4–13.

2. F. J. Ingelfinger, "Gastrointestinal absorption," *Nutrition Today* 2(1967):2–10.

3. F. J. Ingelfinger, "Gastric function," *Nutrition Today* 6(1971):2–11.

4. E. Bjòrn-Rasmussen et al, "Measurement of iron absorption from composite meals," *American Journal of Clinical Nutrition* 29(1976):772–78.

5. S. Babu and S. G. Srikantia, "Availability of folates from some foods," *American Journal of Clinical Nutrition* 29(1976):376–79.

6. "Calcium transport in the ileum," *Nutrition Reviews* 33(1975):84–85.

7. "Intestinal malabsorption of iron," *Nutrition Reviews* 34(1976):270–71.

8. "Gastric emptying, pancreatic and biliary secretion during digestion," *Nutrition Reviews* 33(1975):169–70.

9. "Effects of oral and parenteral feeding on pancreatic enzyme content," *Nutrition Reviews* 33(1975):187–88.

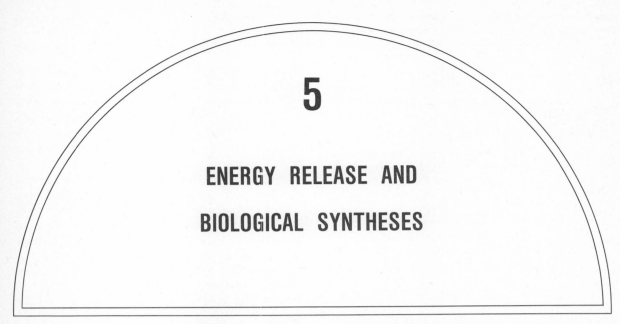

5

ENERGY RELEASE AND

BIOLOGICAL SYNTHESES

The energy stored in macronutrients can be released only after amino acids, simple carbohydrates, fatty acids, and glycerol reach those cells of the body that have the enzymes and other conditions necessary for *catabolism,* or metabolic breakdown of nutrients. Energy is released through a series of reactions in which oxygen is consumed and carbon dioxide is given off by the cells. This process is called *chemical* or *cellular respiration.*

During the energy-releasing process inside cells, other products, besides carbon dioxide, are formed; these products may be used for the synthesis of more complex and unique constituents of body cells—a process called *anabolism.* The mechanism of energy release in the body and the process of anabolism for the construction and repair of body tissues from nutrients are the subjects of this chapter.

ENERGY RELEASE
AND CELLULAR REACTIONS

In the energy-releasing process, oxygen and the small units formed by the digestion of macronutrients enter the cell, where low-energy molecules are waiting to be recharged. The products of this process are carbon dioxide, water, and high-energy mol-

ecules. The overall cellular energy-releasing process can therefore be summarized as follows:

macronutrients, oxygen, and low-energy molecules

↓

carbon dioxide, water, and high-energy molecules

The carbon dioxide released from the cells is carried by the blood to the lungs, where it is exhaled. The water formed during catabolism enters the body's pool of fluids and is excreted. Approximately 1 cup of "new" water is added daily to the fluid pool from the processing of an average diet.

The carbon dioxide and water formed during the energy-releasing process retain no utilizable energy. All the energy from the cellular reactions is transferred to low-energy molecules within the cells. The high-energy molecules thus formed power many functions, including growth, repair, and maintenance of the body.

The energy-releasing process streamlines the availability of energy within the body by channeling energy from many macronutrient molecules—about two dozen amino acids, several different hexoses, alcohol, glycerol, and fatty acids of all sizes and degrees of saturation—into the same high-energy molecules that are utilized in all cells of the body.

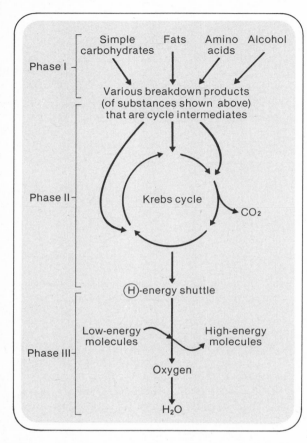

Figure 5–1. The three phases of the energy-releasing process.

Figure 5-1 summarizes the three phases of the energy-releasing process that will be explained in greater detail later in this chapter. In Phase I, the various macronutrient molecules are converted into one of several units that can be used in Phase II. Most of the simple macronutrients are broken down in Phase I to a two-carbon unit that combines with a molecule called coenzyme A (CoA) and enters Phase II in this form. Some macronutrient breakdown products formed in Phase I enter Phase II by other routes.

Phase II is actually a cycle of reactions, the pur-

pose of which is to rearrange incoming molecular units to form other compounds and simultaneously to release carbon dioxide and an energized hydrogen particle. The carbon dioxide is exhaled; the hydrogen particle is bound to an "energy shuttle"—a molecule containing either riboflavin or niacin (Chapter 3).

In Phase III, the hydrogen-containing energy shuttle transfers its energy to low-energy molecules; the hydrogen particle is released and combines with oxygen to form water. The energy shuttle returns to the Phase II cycle, where it can harness another hydrogen particle and repeat the process. The high-energy molecules formed in Phase III are used for energy-requiring reactions.

With this general view in mind, let's examine the details of what happens in each phase of the energy-releasing process.

Phase I: Macronutrient Rearrangement and Breakdown

In Phase I, all macronutrients are broken down and their structures rearranged to form various molecules that can enter the Phase II reaction cycle at certain points. Simple carbohydrates, alcohol, fatty acids, and glycerol are all broken down into the same two-carbon unit that is combined with a CoA molecule to form a complex called acetyl CoA. Portions of some amino acids are converted into acetyl CoA; others follow different pathways and are converted into molecules that enter at alternate points of the Phase II reaction cycle.

Carbohydrates. Figure 5-2 shows how several simple carbohydrates all flow into a central pathway leading to the formation of acetyl CoA. (Many intermediate steps have been omitted from this figure.)

Glucose is converted to glucose-6-phosphate, or glucose-6-P, by the addition of a phosphate to the terminal (sixth) carbon in its structure. Galactose and glycogen, the storage form of glucose, are con-

There are three phases in the energy-releasing process, each yielding distinct products: (I) the atoms of the absorbed macronutrient molecules are rearranged to form one of several intermediate molecules; (II) the intermediate molecules are transformed into carbon dioxide and hydrogen energy complexes; (III) low-energy molecules are converted into high-energy molecules; and hydrogen particles combine with oxygen to form water.

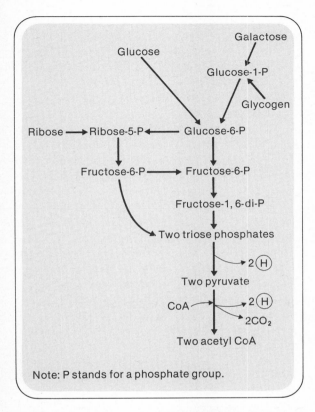

Note: P stands for a phosphate group.

Figure 5–2. Phase I for carbohydrates (conversion of some carbohydrates into acetyl CoA). Many intermediate steps are not shown in this diagram.

verted to glucose-1-P and then to glucose-6-P. Fructose can be converted to fructose-6-P, an intermediate product in the central carbohydrate pathway. Pentoses (five-carbon sugars such as ribose) enter the central pathway by a complex series of reactions leading to the formation of a phosphate–three-carbon sugar or triose-P. Triose-P is an intermediate product in the pathway used by all of the hexoses. Triose-P is converted in several steps to a three-carbon acid called *pyruvate* or pyruvic acid. In the final step, pyruvate combines with CoA; this results in the formation of acetyl CoA, and at the

same time carbon dioxide is released and two hydrogen particles are transferred to energy shuttles.

The rearrangements of the molecules and the formation of phosphate complexes in the central pathway require energy input for several steps, but energy is released at other steps. The total net yield of energy varies slightly, depending upon whether glucose, fructose, galactose, glycogen, or pentose enters the central pathway, and whether these carbohydrates are combined initially with phosphate. These differences are insignificant, however, because the total amount of energy released from carbohydrates in Phase I is less than 5 percent of the energy ultimately released during the entire catabolic sequence.

Fatty Acids. Like carbohydrates, fatty acids enter the Phase II cycle as acetyl CoA. During Phase I, fatty acids are broken down by a repeated sequence of reactions; each sequence shortens the fatty-acid chain by a two-carbon unit, which is released in combination with CoA as a molecule of acetyl CoA (Figure 5-3). In order to break down an 18-carbon saturated fatty acid, for example, the sequence must be repeated eight times; the eighth or last sequence produces two acetyl CoA molecules, and so nine molecules of acetyl CoA are formed from the whole process.

Figure 5-3 shows another important by-product of this reaction sequence: each sequence yields four hydrogens attached to energy shuttles, and so eight sequences yield 32 hydrogen-energy shuttle complexes. This greater release of energy during Phase I catabolism of fatty acids (compared to energy release during Phase I catabolism of protein or carbohydrate) explains the greater amount of calories provided by 1 gram of fat compared to 1 gram of protein or carbohydrate. Approximately half of the total energy of fatty acids is released as hydrogen energy complexes during Phase I. (Unsaturated fatty acids are broken down by a slightly different sequence, but the overall energy yield does not vary greatly.)

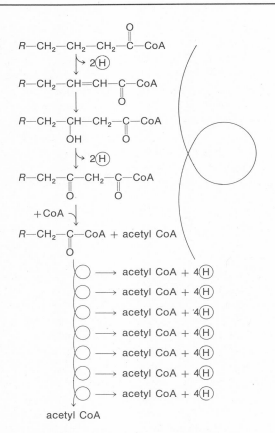

Figure 5–3. Phase I for fatty acids (conversion of an 18-carbon fatty acid into acetyl CoA).

Amino Acids. Each of these building blocks of protein follows a slightly different Phase I pathway, depending upon the structure of its *R* portion. Ultimately, however, all amino acids are converted into one of the intermediate products of the Phase II cycle (Figure 5-4). The entry point for a particular amino acid depends upon its length and structure. Each amino acid and the intermediate formed from it often contain the same number of carbon atoms and have similar configurations. For example, several three-carbon amino acids are converted into the three-carbon acid, pyruvate, and then into acetyl CoA.

The pathways along which amino acids are converted into cycle intermediates may involve only a few structural rearrangements, or may be quite complicated. Some of the reactions require energy input; others release energy.

Before entering the Phase II cycle, the amino acids must give up their amino groups ($-NH_2$). This process occurs by either *transamination* or *deamination*. Transamination involves the transfer of an amino group from an amino acid to an organic acid in return for an oxygen atom from the organic acid (Figure 5-5a). For example, the three-carbon amino acid *alanine* is converted into pyruvate (an acid with oxygen on its second carbon) by giving its amino group to the five-carbon organic acid *ketoglutarate*, which then becomes the five-carbon amino acid *glutamate*. When this transfer has been accomplished, the stage is set for releasing the energy that entered the body as alanine, perhaps in the protein of a hamburger. Pyruvate enters Phase II of the energy-releasing process. The glutamate, carrying the amino group from alanine, enters a complex pathway in the liver that leads to the formation of *urea*. Urea is an amino-containing compound that is released by the liver into the blood, and is then filtered by the kidney and excreted into the urine.

In deamination reactions, which also take place in the liver cells, certain amino groups are removed from amino acids and converted to ammonia (NH_3) or to a charged form of ammonia called an ammonium ion (NH_4^+), which is excreted in the urine. The vitamin pyridoxine participates in both transamination and deamination reactions. The niacin-containing cofactors, NAD and NADP, have a role in deamination.

Alcohol. There are two Phase I pathways for the rearrangement of alcohol, both of which end in acetyl CoA. Alcohol contains only two carbon atoms, and its conversion to acetyl CoA is therefore rather simple. During this process, two hydrogen atoms are removed and form hydrogen energy complexes, which (like those formed in fatty acid break-

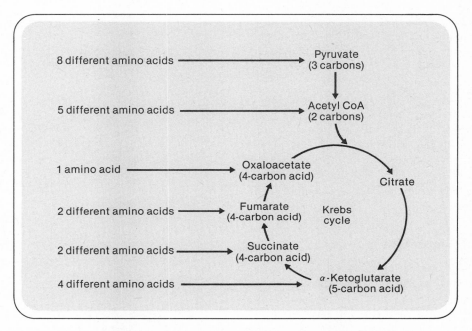

Figure 5–4. Phase I for amino acids (conversion of amino acids into Phase II cycle intermediates).

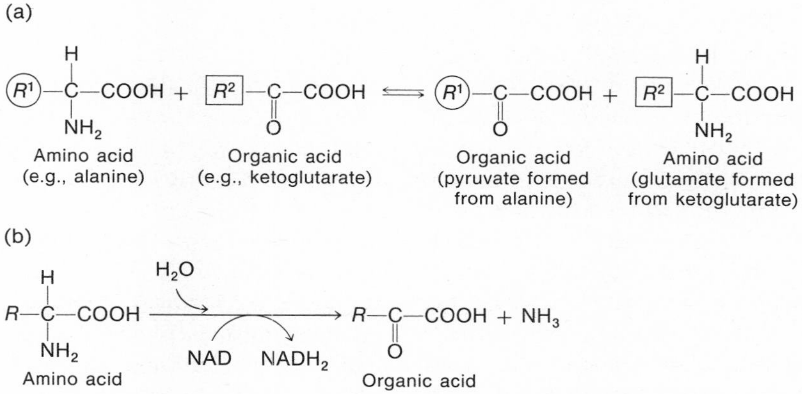

(a)

R^1—C(H)—COOH + R^2—C—COOH ⇌ R^1—C—COOH + R^2—C(H)—COOH

| Amino acid (e.g., alanine) | Organic acid (e.g., ketoglutarate) | Organic acid (pyruvate formed from alanine) | Amino acid (glutamate formed from ketoglutarate) |

(b)

R—C(H)(NH$_2$)—COOH $\xrightarrow[\text{NAD} \quad \text{NADH}_2]{\text{H}_2\text{O}}$ R—C(O)—COOH + NH$_3$

Amino acid   Organic acid

Figure 5–5. Transamination (a) and deamination (b).

down) bypass the Phase II cycle and proceed directly to Phase III. The acetyl CoA from alcohol metabolism enters the Phase II cycle along with acetyl CoA from the Phase I metabolism of carbohydrates, fats, and many amino acids.

Alcohol metabolism occurs in the liver, not in muscle cells, and so its energy is not directly available for muscle contractions. Because exercising cannot speed up the utilization of alcohol, people who are drunk cannot lower their blood alcohol level by "walking it off." The liver metabolizes alcohol at a rate of about two-thirds ounce of 90-proof alcohol per hour.

Phase II: The Krebs Cycle

This cycle is named for Sir Hans Krebs, whose laboratory studies proved the existence of this series of energy-releasing reactions. It is also called the citric acid cycle because it contains citrate (a synonym for citric acid) as an important intermediate.

Like Phase I, this phase of the energy-releasing process consists of a series of reactions; however, Phase II reactions occur in a repeating cycle rather than in a straight line. Figure 5-6 shows what happens to one molecule of acetyl CoA as it moves through the Krebs cycle; in reality, there are myriads of molecules continuously being catabolized through thousands of cycles occurring simultaneously in millions of cells. Consider that one gram of glucose (about one-fifth teaspoonful) contains approximately, 2,000,000,000,000,000,000,000 molecules, which become twice as many acetyl CoA molecules, which in turn enter the Krebs cycle.

At various intermediate stages in the Krebs cycle, certain molecules enter and others exit. As long as there is a supply of intermediate products from Phase I, the cycle is self-perpetuating. During one complete cycle, acetyl CoA enters the reaction sequence, and one CoA and two molecules of carbon dioxide and eight hydrogen-energy shuttles are released. The CoA can return to be used in Phase I; the carbon dioxide travels from the cell where it was

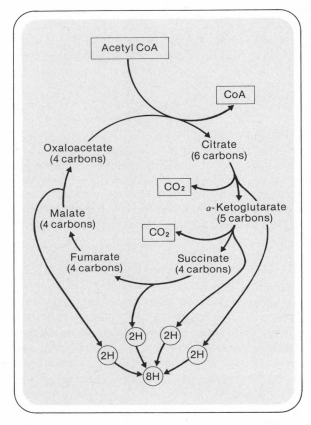

Figure 5–6. Phase II of the energy-releasing process: the Krebs cycle. Details of this cycle are shown in Appendix Figure A5-1.

produced to the blood (where it combines with hemoglobin) and is ultimately released in the lungs and exhaled; the hydrogen-energy shuttles flow into the final Phase III series of reactions.

Closer examination of Figure 5-6 shows how this breakdown of acetyl CoA occurs. This diagram indicates the number of carbons in each of the intermediate products of the cycle. The two carbons of acetyl merge with a compound that contains four carbons, thus forming a six-carbon complex. As this molecule progresses through the sequence of reactions, it is shortened by one, then another, carbon, so

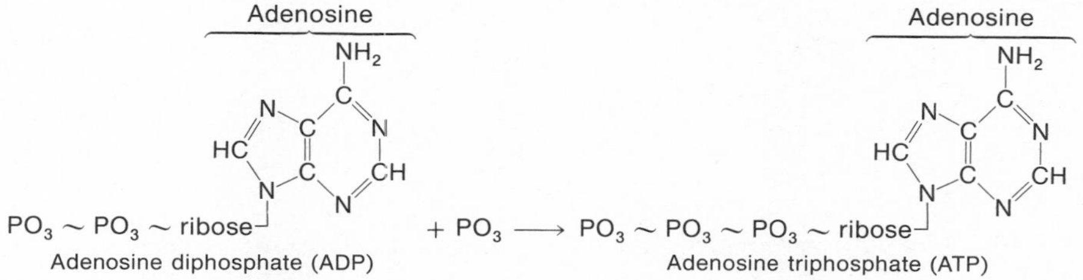

Adenosine

NH_2

$PO_3 \sim PO_3 \sim$ ribose

Adenosine diphosphate (ADP)

$+ PO_3 \longrightarrow$

Adenosine

NH_2

$PO_3 \sim PO_3 \sim PO_3 \sim$ ribose

Adenosine triphosphate (ATP)

Figure 5–7. Structures of ATP and ADP (adenosine triphosphate and adenosine diphosphate).

that it is ultimately changed into a specific four-carbon product, which can combine with another acetyl CoA entering the cycle.

As shown in Figure 5-6, neither carbon dioxide nor hydrogen is released at the steps that have no side arrows. Actually, several structural shifts not shown in the diagram do occur in the basic molecule during the steps of this cycle: water goes in and comes out; hydrogens and oxygen move from one carbon to another. More detailed reactions are shown in Appendix Figure A5-1, but if you are simply trying to get an idea how food energy is converted to biologically utilizable energy, Figure 5-6 will suffice.

Phase III: Formation of High-Energy Molecules

During Phase II of the energy-releasing sequence of reactions, almost all of the energy that originated in food is transferred to hydrogen energy shuttles. During Phase III, hydrogen particles are passed from one carrier to another in a chain of reactions until they combine with oxygen to form water. These transfers do not occur randomly but in a well-ordered procession. As a hydrogen particle moves along this procession, the energy that is needed to bind it to each subsequent carrier decreases. Simultaneously, a portion of the hydrogen energy is gradually released.

Some of the energy escapes as heat, which maintains normal body temperature but cannot power cellular reactions or other processes. Other energy is used along the Phase III pathway to convert a low-energy molecule (*adenosine diphosphate*, or ADP) into a high-energy molecule (*adenosine triphosphate*, or ATP) by the addition of a phosphate group (Figure 5-7).°

Not all of the body's energy is derived from the Phase III reactions. A small amount of ATP is formed directly by the release of energy during Phase I and Phase II. Also, some of the hydrogen energy complexes formed during these phases can be used directly to power certain biological processes that are designed to accept energy from these complexes. Many reactions, however, can accept energy only when it is provided by ATP.

ROLE OF MICRONUTRIENTS

Earlier chapters pointed out that most body functions require macronutrients and micronutrients working together. The three phases of energy re-

° The transfer of energy from hydrogen particles to the high-energy bonds of ATP takes place through a process called *oxidative phosphorylation*. The transfer of hydrogen from a high-energy state to a lower one involves the electron transport system. The hydrogen-energy shuttles that contain the vitamins niacin and riboflavin, together with several minerals and enzymes, have important roles in this system.

The energy of ADP is low only in relation to the energy of ATP. Adenosine monophosphate (AMP), the lowest-energy adenosine phosphate compound, accepts a phosphate group to form ADP in a manner similar to the formation of ATP from ADP. Conversions of AMP to ADP occur in the body but with much less frequency than those of ADP to ATP.

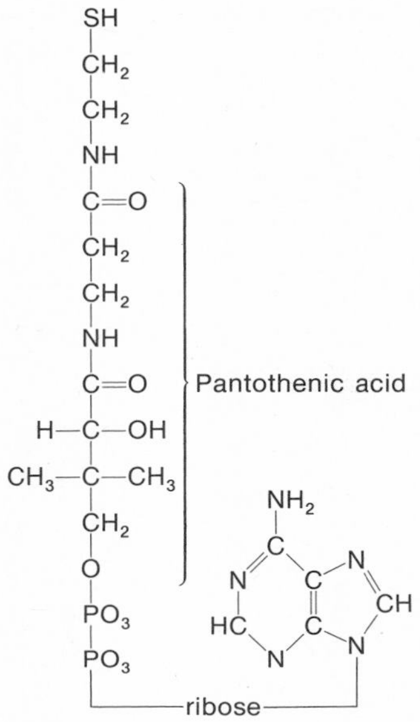

SH
|
CH$_2$
|
CH$_2$
|
NH
|
C=O
|
CH$_2$ ⎤
| |
CH$_2$ |
| |
NH | Pantothenic acid
| |
C=O |
| |
H—C—OH |
| |
CH$_3$—C—CH$_3$
|
CH$_2$
|
O
|
PO$_3$
|
PO$_3$
|
—ribose—

NH$_2$
|
C
N   N
C
HC   CH
C
N   N

Figure 5–8. Structure of Coenzyme A.

lease provide an excellent example of the collaborative roles vitamins and minerals play. Understanding these interrelationships is basic to an appreciation of why a diet that supplies adequate macronutrients but lacks micronutrients may fail to provide the energy the body needs.

Vitamins

Several vitamins are required for amino acid breakdown. Folic acid and vitamin B$_{12}$ are necessary for the addition or removal of one-carbon units during the transformation of amino acids into compounds that subsequently participate in the Phase II cycle. Pyridoxine is necessary for transamination and deamination reactions and for the removal of carbon dioxide units from amino acids. This vitamin is so important in amino acid metabolism that dietary recommendations for it are based on the body's protein requirements.

Thiamin compounds are cofactors in reactions where carbon dioxide is removed from a molecule, such as when pyruvate is converted to acetyl CoA in the central pathway of glucose metabolism. Thiamin is also used in one of the pathways that converts alcohol to acetyl CoA.

Biotin participates in carbon dioxide transfers; it is particularly important in reactions that remove carbon groups from long-chain fatty acids during fat metabolism. CoA, which is needed for the synthesis of acetyl CoA and for the breakdown of fatty acids, is made of pantothenic acid, phosphorus, sulfur, and other small subunits (Figure 5-8).

The importance of riboflavin and niacin in molecules that form energy shuttles with hydrogen particles was discussed in Chapter 3. The molecule that contains riboflavin is called flavin adenine dinucleotide, or FAD; the one containing niacin is called nicotinamide adenine dinucleotide, or NAD (Figure 5-9). These hydrogen carriers all contain phosphate groups. NADP is NAD with a third phosphate group.

Minerals

Minerals, like vitamins, participate in many steps of the energy-releasing process. Many of the intermediate products formed during the carbohydrate breakdown of Phase I are complexed with phosphorus. This mineral is also part of both ADP and ATP molecules, and the hydrogen energy complexes.

Concentrations of magnesium, manganese, potassium, iron, and cobalt must be maintained within critical limits in order for certain reactions in all three phases to proceed. Iron and copper are especially important in Phase III reactions. Iron is part of one of the enzymes in this reaction series.

Zinc and chromium are necessary for the passage of glucose from the blood into many body cells. The energy of glucose cannot be released until this passage is accomplished. Zinc is needed for the first step in the conversion of alcohol to acetyl CoA.

(a) Nicotinamide adenine dinucleotide (NAD)   (b) Flavin adenine dinucleotide (FAD)

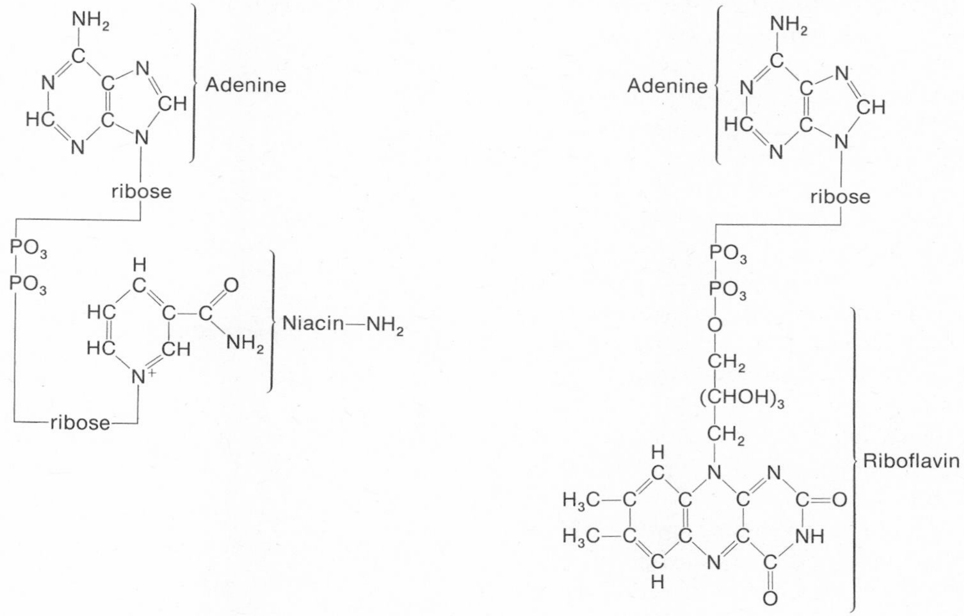

Figure 5–9. Structure of the hydrogen energy complexes containing niacin (a) and riboflavin (b).

ROLE OF OXYGEN

Oxygen in the air we breathe is not considered a nutrient, but it is essential to the energy-releasing reactions of the Phase III chain and to other metabolic reactions.

A small portion of the oxygen we breathe crosses the membranes of the tiny air sacs in the lungs and enters the blood vessels that lie adjacent to the air sacs. The oxygen then enters the red blood cells and combines with hemoglobin. As oxygen is carried in the red blood cells throughout the body and through the tissues, it is taken into the tissue cells, where it can participate in various reactions.

Insufficient oxygen can halt the final step in the energy-releasing process—the combining of oxygen with the hydrogens that are passed from carrier to carrier in Phase III. If the carriers are filled up but unable to transfer hydrogens to oxygen, high-energy molecules cannot be formed in Phase III. Oxygen deprivation can also cause an imbalance in the concentration of the many Phase II intermediate products, because their flow into the final step in the process is blocked when oxygen is lacking. When oxygen is deficient in the final phases of energy release, the buildup of hydrogen particles eventually quenches or smothers all other reactions in the cells of the body.

There are many examples of cellular oxygen starvation. A scuba diver whose tank is almost empty is very aware of the importance of oxygen. Drowning or strangulation can result in death because of oxygen deprivation. Carbon monoxide poisoning causes oxygen starvation but through a different mechanism. The carbon monoxide gas links to hemoglobin in the red blood cells up to two hundred times more tenaciously than does oxygen. Inhaled carbon monoxide fills the sites in the hemoglobin molecule that usually bind oxygen, thus crowding oxygen out of the blood.

Less severe oxygen deprivation occurs when people travel from a low to a high altitude, where the air contains less oxygen. Travel in airplanes and other spacecraft would be difficult if the cabins were not pressurized to ensure an adequate supply and tension of oxygen.

In an anemic person, the supply of red blood cells and hemoglobin is inadequate to transport oxygen to tissue cells. Even if there is enough oxygen to allow energy-releasing reactions to occur, the formation of high-energy ATP molecules cannot keep pace with the energy needs of the muscles. For this reason, anemic people tire easily and cannot perform or sustain strenuous activities.

A tourniquet, such as would be applied to reduce the spread of poison after a snakebite or to stop excessive bleeding, can prevent adequate supplies of oxygen and nutrients from reaching tissue cells. If the blood supply is cut off for too long, gangrene can result. In a similar manner, damage from a stroke is caused by a marked reduction or cessation of the flow of oxygen to the brain.

ALTERNATE SOURCES OF ENERGY

The energy-releasing process we have just described provides energy from digested food to the cells of the body. The food intake of people who maintain a constant body weight supplies the amount of energy their bodies need and use, and such people do not have to call upon their *fat depots* (reserves of energy) nor do they add to them.

Most of the energy of the food we eat is released rather than stored, but the release need not occur instantaneously. There are slightly different pathways that macronutrient molecules can follow between the time of their absorption and the release of their energy.

Daily Variations

The amount of energy that can be stored in the body as high-energy molecules is exceedingly small. These molecules are used up rapidly and must constantly be resupplied by Phase III of the energy-releasing process.[*] However, it is not necessary to nibble food or sip beverages continuously throughout the day in order to maintain a constant flow of high-energy molecules, because not all of the macronutrients we eat at one meal or snack are metabolized immediately after they enter the body cells.

Several body processes spread out the release of food energy over several hours between meals, and the concentration of absorbed nutrients circulating in the blood can fluctuate within certain limits. For example, the amount of glucose in the blood shortly after a high-carbohydrate breakfast may be almost twice what it was when the person awoke. During the next couple of hours, much of the glucose from breakfast is gradually siphoned out of the blood and into the cells, and the concentration of glucose in the blood returns to a lower level. Some of the glucose inside the cells is channeled into the energy-releasing process; but some glucose molecules are linked together to produce *glycogen,* a complex carbohydrate that is then stored in the liver and muscles. Between meals and during the night, the body converts glycogen back into glucose, which is then metabolized to release energy. However, the maximum amount of energy that can be stored in the body as glycogen is barely enough to meet all the needs of a sedentary adult for one day. If food is not eaten, these glycogen stores are quickly depleted, and energy needs must then be met by other means.

[*] The energy of ATP can be used for the formation of another high-energy molecule called creatine–phosphate. This substance is a temporary storage form of energy, and it is an important energy source during exercise.

When formation of high-energy molecules cannot keep pace with the energy demands of actively contracting muscles, hydrogen energy complexes formed by the conversion of pyruvate to lactic acid can be used directly for certain energy needs.

When Energy Intake Is Inadequate

Most of our energy reserves are stored in the fatty acids of fat molecules. When stored glycogen is used up, low blood glucose causes the release of hormones, which in turn stimulate the release of fatty acids from the cells where they are stored. These fatty acids are broken down in the same way as dietary fatty acids that have not been stored.

If the energy deficit continues and fat stores are depleted, the only remaining source of energy is the protein within body cells. This protein is not supposed to be an energy store—it is part of tissues that have important functions. When the body must resort to using cellular protein in order to meet the body's energy requirements, the consequences are serious and, if prolonged, can be fatal.

The various forms of body energy might be compared to financial resources. High-energy molecules are financially liquid like the pocket change we carry. Glucose circulating in the blood might be compared to a dollar bill, which can be broken when we run low on change. Glycogen is analogous to a checking account—fairly frequently we make deposits and write checks, which increase and decrease this ready reserve of money. Fat stores are comparable to a savings account, which is built up more slowly and generally not used except under special circumstances. If we have unusual expenses and no savings, we can take out a loan—this is comparable to the breakdown of body protein. A certain amount of financial overextension can be tolerated, but as we get deeper and deeper in debt, we are threatened by bankruptcy. At this point, the energy–money analogy ends, because when the body declares "energy bankruptcy," death occurs.

When Oxygen Intake Is Inadequate

Although oxygen is not itself a source of energy, it must be present in the cells for the formation of high-energy molecules, which are usually generated at a rate fast enough to maintain normal body functions. However, when a person exercises strenuously for prolonged periods, the circulatory system cannot satisfy the oxygen needs in the cells, and the production of high-energy molecules falls behind the needs of the vigorously contracting muscles. Under these circumstances, a reserve system or auxiliary pathway for energy production comes into play (Figure 5-10).

The central pathway for metabolism of simple carbohydrates operates up to the pyruvate-formation reaction, regardless of the oxygen supply. Beyond this point, however, if Phase III is oxygen-starved and therefore proceeding slowly, the Phase II reaction cycle becomes backlogged with intermediate products. Under these conditions, pyruvate can be converted into another acid called lactic acid (*lactate*). This reaction releases energy and a hydrogen particle, complexed with a niacin-containing energy shuttle. This hydrogen energy complex can be used in several energy-requiring reactions without the need to transfer its energy to a low-energy (ADP) molecule.

The net energy yield from this reserve mechanism is only about 5 percent of the energy released when pyruvate proceeds through Phase II and Phase III. However, because oxygen is not required for the pyruvate-to-lactate conversion, this auxiliary pathway furnishes some energy to help meet immediate muscle demands. Furthermore, because less acetyl CoA is being formed and fed into the Krebs cycle, cycle intermediate products do not accumulate.

The pyruvate–lactate interconversion can occur in many cells that have high-energy demands; but lactate cannot be converted back to pyruvate in muscle cells, because they lack the necessary enzyme. Therefore, lactate accumulates in muscle cells during prolonged exercise and contributes to muscle fatigue. When high energy demands lessen and as lactate is gradually released into the blood, muscle fatigue decreases. The released lactate circulates to the liver cells, which do have the enzyme

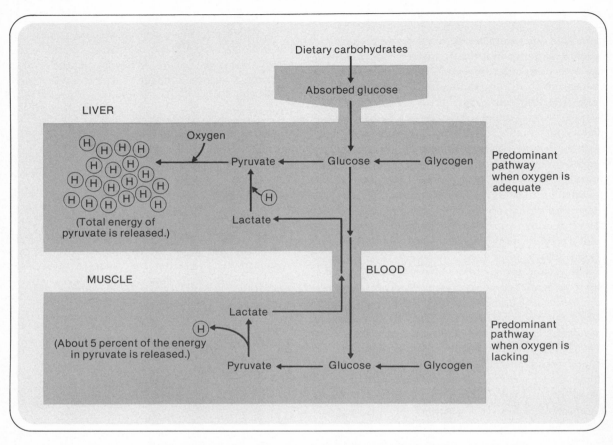

Figure 5–10. Alternate pathways of energy release (when oxygen is adequate or lacking).

necessary to convert lactate back into pyruvate. When the oxygen supply again becomes adequate, pyruvate energy can be released by the Phase II and III processes.

In reality, both energy-releasing processes operate continuously, but at varying rates. For example, although lactate builds up in vigorously exercising muscles, it continuously leaks out of the muscle cells and circulates to the liver. Because of the oxygen deficit, the pyruvate regeneration process in the liver is sluggish, but it does continue to operate. Once the exercise ends, the rates of these reactions reverse. The muscle reactions diminish, and the liver reactions increase.

This phenomenon is only one of many examples of how the body is engineered to cope with changing physiological demands and environmental conditions. Meeting these challenges requires an adequate supply and reserve of both micronutrients and macronutrients.

Understanding the body's need for both protein and energy can help you select the diet that is most economical but that also meets nutritional needs and avoids overweight.

PROTEIN–ENERGY INTERRELATIONSHIPS

The interrelationship between the body's need for energy and its need for protein is based on nutrition concepts that have broad practical applications. The person who masters these concepts can make better decisions about planning a diet to ensure that physiological needs are met, to make the most of the food budget, and to avoid becoming overweight.

Fundamental Concepts

The interrelationship between protein and energy can be summarized as follows:

1. The body needs an absolute amount of energy; this requirement can be met by any macronutrients—carbohydrate, fat, protein—alone or in combination, or even from alcohol.
2. The body requires a minimum amount of protein, which is needed for the many functions described in Chapter 2.
3. All of the functions of protein are dependent both upon having adequate dietary protein building blocks and upon meeting energy needs. Both of these conditions must be met in order to construct muscles, hormones, and enzymes; to replace worn out cells; to maintain cellular pressure; and so forth.

The protein requirement is not exactly the same for each individual, but for most adults, it is approximately 50 grams per day. This amount of protein supplies about 200 Cal (840 kJ), or from 7 to 10 percent of total energy needs.

Although energy requirements increase with activity, protein needs are fundamentally related to body size and growth—not to exercise. A bus driver needs the same amount of dietary protein as does a construction worker, if their bodies are the same size and have similar composition. An active teen-ager who spends leisure time dancing and participating in sports needs more energy, but the same amount of protein, as does a classmate of the same body size who spends leisure time watching television, reading, or doing sedentary crafts. The protein needs of teen-agers vary only slightly from those of adults. (More quantitative recommendations regarding energy and nutrient intakes are discussed in Chapter 8.)

Analysis of Dietary Patterns

The fate of dietary protein—whether it is "spared" and used specifically for unique protein functions or whether it is metabolized for energy along with other macronutrients—depends simultaneously upon two factors: (1) protein intake compared to protein need, and (2) energy intake compared to energy need.

Figure 5-11 shows how the body uses dietary protein, depending upon the quantity of protein eaten and nutrient composition of the entire diet. Situation A is an example of the most economically planned diet pattern. It satisfies both energy and protein needs of the body. Protein intake is sufficient to accomplish the unique function of this nutrient; carbohydrate, fat, and alcohol supply the remaining requirement for energy.

In Situation B, protein intake is greater than needed, and the excess protein is used to meet energy needs. Although this situation is acceptable nutritionally, it does not represent an economical distribution of the food dollar because most foods that are high in protein are also high in price. The excess protein is broken down to amino acids, which enter Phase II of the energy-releasing process in the same manner as do fats and carbohydrates from foods that are usually cheaper than protein sources. If a person prefers to eat a high-protein diet and can afford to do so, there are normally no ill effects. However, one should not think that protein in amounts above what the body needs, has any beneficial effect other than providing energy.

In situation C, protein intake equals protein requirements, but the dietary protein cannot be used to meet the body's specific needs for this nutrient.

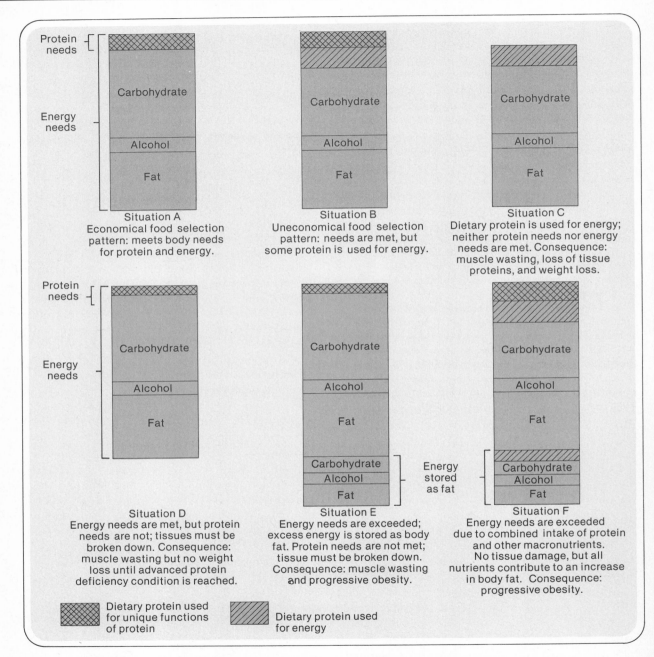

Protein needs
Energy needs

Carbohydrate
Alcohol
Fat

Situation A
Economical food selection pattern: meets body needs for protein and energy.

Carbohydrate
Alcohol
Fat

Situation B
Uneconomical food selection pattern: needs are met, but some protein is used for energy.

Carbohydrate
Alcohol
Fat

Situation C
Dietary protein is used for energy; neither protein needs nor energy needs are met. Consequence: muscle wasting, loss of tissue proteins, and weight loss.

Protein needs
Energy needs

Carbohydrate
Alcohol
Fat

Situation D
Energy needs are met, but protein needs are not; tissues must be broken down. Consequence: muscle wasting but no weight loss until advanced protein deficiency condition is reached.

Carbohydrate
Alcohol
Fat
Carbohydrate
Alcohol
Fat

Energy stored as fat

Situation E
Energy needs are exceeded; excess energy is stored as body fat. Protein needs are not met; tissue must be broken down. Consequence: muscle wasting and progressive obesity.

Carbohydrate
Alcohol
Fat
Carbohydrate
Alcohol
Fat

Energy stored as fat

Situation F
Energy needs are exceeded due to combined intake of protein and other macronutrients. No tissue damage, but all nutrients contribute to an increase in body fat. Consequence: progressive obesity.

Dietary protein used for unique functions of protein

Dietary protein used for energy

Figure 5–11. Six situations showing the interrelationship between protein needs and energy needs.

The body's need for energy takes priority over the body's need for protein; and when energy intake from fats and carbohydrates is inadequate, protein will be used primarily for energy—not for body building. This concept is important for a person on a low budget to know; otherwise that person might invest most of the grocery money in high-protein foods and not have money left to buy cheaper, high-energy foods. Such a food selection pattern fails to meet either the protein needs or the energy needs of the body.

Certain variations of this situation can modify the fate of dietary protein. Within certain limits, stored body fat can be used to compensate for inadequate energy intake and thus permit protein to be used for its unique functions. However, if the energy intake drops too low (such as on very strict weight reduction diets), special protein functions cannot occur. For example, there will not be enough amino acids available to make new proteins for replacing body cells, which normally die and are rebuilt from dietary proteins. The crash dieter, therefore, may lose protein tissue such as muscle, rather than losing only body fat.

Situations D and E represent what happens when protein intake is lower than the amount needed by the body. In situation D, energy needs are met by carbohydrates, fats, and alcohol, but there is not enough dietary protein to maintain body functions. Under these circumstances, the only way the body can get enough amino acids to build or replace critical body proteins is by tearing down body protein that is less critical, such as the protein in muscles. Situation E is comparable to the diet patterns of people who are overweight and whose diets contain excessive amounts of fats, carbohydrates, and alcohol, but insufficient proteins. The excess supply of energy is stored as fat, while muscles are whittled away to meet protein needs.

Either situation D or situation E can result from a diet that contains primarily cereal products, alcoholic beverages, butter or margarine, fruits, vegetables, sugar, and soft drinks, but that lacks protein sources such as beans, meat, nuts, and dairy products. Whether weight is maintained or gained depends upon the amount eaten; but in either case, muscle tissue wastes away.

Situation F also leads to overweight, but it usually occurs in affluent people who erroneously think that protein is "not fattening." Their intake of excess protein, combined with other macronutrients in the diet, results in excessive energy intake. Stored fat is synthesized from acetyl CoA, which can come from amino acids of protein as well as from glucose, fatty acids, or alcohol—none is more "fattening" than the other.

OTHER USES OF MACRONUTRIENTS

Although all the macronutrients can be used as a source of energy, all of them also produce breakdown products that can be used for building the variety of substances of which our bodies are made.

Macronutrient Combinations

Amino acids, simple carbohydrates, glycerol, and fatty acids can be joined to each other in various combinations. For example, when fatty acids are released from cells into the blood, they are solubilized by combining with the protein *albumin*. Lipoproteins are lipid–protein combinations that are present in the blood, and in the milk of humans and cows. Lipoproteins are also structural components of cell membranes.

Glucose and several of the other hexoses combine with lipids to form *gangliosides* and *cerebrosides*, components of the brain. Hexose–amino group complexes include *sialic acid* and *hyaluronic acid*, which are important for nerve cells and for cement-like substances.

Carbohydrate–protein combinations are important constituents of bones, cartilage, and tendons. They are also the substances that determine whether your blood is type A, B, AB, or O.

Intermediate Products

The intermediate products in the energy-releasing process can be used for biological syntheses as well as energy release.

Acetyl CoA. Bile acids, steroid hormones, and sterol compounds such as cholesterol can be synthesized from acetyl CoA. It can also be used in the producton of fatty acids, which combine with glycerol to form stored fat. Such is the fate of those extra Calories or kilojoules that find their way onto our plates!

Pyruvate. The many biosynthetic reactions that use pyruvate generally (but not exactly) retrace the Phase I breakdown pathways. Within each sequence, there exists at least one step that is regulated by one of several metabolic control factors; this control point determines whether the reactions occur in the direction of breakdown or synthesis.

Gluconeogenesis (glucose-new-birth) is basically the reverse process of the glucose central pathway. It differs at several critical points from glucose breakdown; but under the proper conditions, it is possible to synthesize glucose from pyruvate. Therefore, pyruvate that is made from certain amino acids that were consumed as hamburger or peanut butter, for example, can become part of internally synthesized glucose—identical to glucose from fruits and vegetables.

Cycle Intermediates. Although essential amino acids cannot be made in the body, nonessential ones can be made from cycle intermediates by transamination. The amino acids thus formed may be used for protein synthesis or for other synthetic reactions.

Protein Synthesis

Proteins are made of hundreds and sometimes thousands of amino acids. The sequence and configuration of the amino acids in these huge molecules is determined by the nucleic acids *deoxyribonucleic acid* (DNA) and *ribonucleic acid* (RNA). These nucleic acids are both made of similar subunits called *nucleotides;* the nucleotide subunits of DNA contain less oxygen than do RNA subunits. There are only a few other structural differences between the two substances, but they have vastly different roles in the body.

DNA is the basic mammalian genetic substance and is present in every cell of your body. It is a replica of the DNA that was present in the fertilized ovum from which you originated. As that cell divided into 2, then 4, then 8 cells, replicas of the original strands of DNA were created and incorporated into each newly formed cell. Although an adult human body contains trillions of strands of DNA, the sequence and composition of the nucleotides in each of those molecules is unique to each person. Portions of these long chains are similar to portions of the DNA in other people, but no other person has exactly the same DNA that is in your body.

The body uses DNA as a pattern from which to make numerous strands of RNA, just as a seamstress can use a dress pattern in various ways. A dress pattern often contains pieces to make either long or short sleeves, and various necklines; it might also include pieces for making slacks, a skirt, and a jacket. In a similar way, different segments of the DNA molecules are used as patterns for making various proteins—hormones, hemoglobin, enzymes, and so forth. In fact, within a single strand of DNA are the patterns for making the entire "wardrobe" of biological proteins needed by your body.

There are three steps in the synthesis of a particular protein needed by the body:

1. The portion of DNA that controls the synthesis of that protein is used as a pattern to make a corresponding strand of RNA called messenger RNA.

2. The nucleotides of that strand of RNA attract smaller units of RNA (transfer RNA) to which specific amino acids are linked (Figure 5-12). These smaller units

DNA is used as a pattern for making RNA; the sequence of nucleotides in RNA determines the sequence of amino acids linked together to form each unique protein molecule.

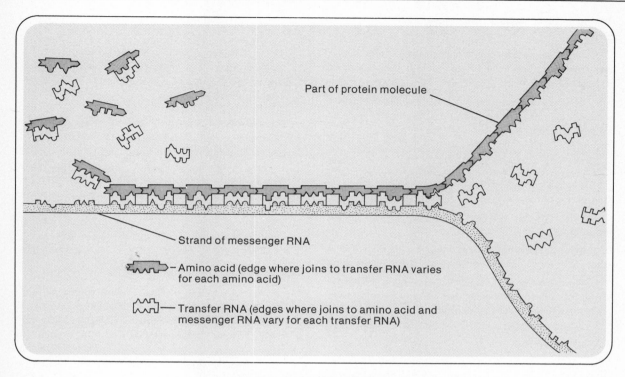

Figure 5–12. Protein synthesis.

of RNA contain only three nucleotides; each amino acid complexes with a specific transfer RNA unit. The sequence of amino acids in the newly formed protein is built up in conformity with the pattern designated by the sequence of nucleotides in messenger RNA, which conforms to the sequence in the DNA.

3. The amino acids are joined together as a straight or a branching chain, thus forming the needed protein. Once the specific protein molecule is formed, it drops off the RNA assembly line and another copy is run off. This process is repeated simultaneously in millions of like cells until the desired production schedule has been met; then the process slows or temporarily ceases.

STUDY QUESTIONS

1. What happens to simple carbohydrates, fatty acids, amino acids, and alcohol in Phase I of the energy-releasing process?

2. What are the products that enter and leave Phase II of the energy-releasing process? What happens to each of the products of this cycle of reactions?

3. How and why does oxygen deprivation affect the body?

4. Explain how vitamins and minerals are involved in each phase of the energy-releasing process.

5. How is energy provided to the body between meals and at night?

6. What does the body use as energy sources when food is not eaten for 12 hours? For three days? For one month?

7. How does the body acquire energy when the formation of high-energy molecules cannot keep pace with the energy demands of actively contracting muscles?

8. Which of the situations in Figure 5-11 best describes your diet yesterday?

9. How are simple macronutrients and the intermediate products of the energy-releasing process used for the synthesis of biological substances?

10. Why are DNA and RNA necessary for protein synthesis?

SUGGESTED READING

1. D. M. Hegsted, "Energy needs and energy utilization," Chapter 1 in *Present Knowledge in Nutrition*. 4th ed. New York and Washington, D.C.: The Nutrition Foundation, 1976.

2. R. H. Barnes, "Energy," Chapter 2 in *Present Knowledge in Nutrition*. 4th ed. New York and Washington, D.C.: The Nutrition Foundation, 1976.

3. D. M. Hegsted, "Protein needs and possible modifications of the American diet," *Journal of the American Dietetic Association* 68(1976):317–20.

4. H. P. Broquist, "Amino acid metabolism," *Nutrition Reviews* 34(1976):289–93.

5. "Protein sparing produced by proteins and amino acids," *Nutrition Reviews* 34(1976):174–76.

6. A. Theologides, "Anorexia producing intermediary metabolites," *American Journal of Clinical Nutrition* 29(1976):552–58.

7. K. S. Jaya Rao and L. Khan, "Basal energy metabolism in PCM and vitamin A deficiency," *American Journal of Clinical Nutrition* 27(1974):892–96.

8. D. E. Fulton, "Basal metabolism rate of women: An appraisal," *Journal of the American Dietetic Association* 61(1972):576.

6

INTEGRATED NUTRIENT
FUNCTIONS IN BODY SYSTEMS

A person can understand the benefits of selecting a nutritionally balanced diet without having mastered the intricate biochemical and physiological mechanisms that underlie each nutrient-dependent reaction in the body. To apply sound dietary practices, however, one must know more than simply the general effects of nutrients on the whole body. In this chapter we shall briefly examine which nutrients are needed for the optimal performance of each system of the body, such as the circulatory system, the skeletal system, the gastrointestinal system, and several others.° This discussion does not exhaust the known relationships between nutrients and their effects on body systems, but it does offer examples of the better known interactions.

Several dietary factors are needed together within each system of the body for optimum performance. This is why it is important to select a diet that contains sufficient amounts of all essential nutrients. The interdependency of the nutrient functions precludes a single nutrient from assuring the healthful harmony of a body system—just as one violinist cannot perform a symphony, and a lone quarterback cannot assure victory without the cooperation of other team members. It is the cooperation of the players, each fulfilling a special role in concert with the others, that ultimately determines a person's nutritional and health status or the quality of a symphonic performance or the outcome of a game.

CIRCULATORY SYSTEM

The circulatory and nervous systems are the major communication networks in the human body. The blood circulatory system comprises the heart and a network of blood vessels—arteries, veins, and capillaries—which wind their way throughout the body like a series of underground tunnels (Figure 6-1). The lymphatic system is a specialized portion of the overall circulatory system, and it generally parallels the blood vessels. The circulatory system exists primarily for the transport of materials to and from the cells of the body; blood serves as the major transport medium, or carrier of these materials. Lymph is the fluid that drains from tissues and ultimately joins the blood. The circulatory system bathes every tissue cell with blood *plasma* (the fluid portion of whole blood that remains after the blood cells have been

° Micronutrient deficiency diseases are discussed in Chapter 27.

95

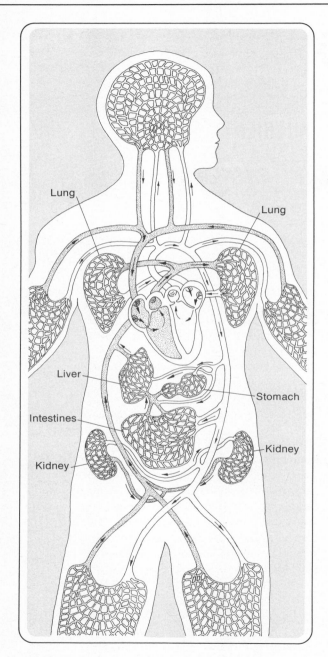

Figure 6–1. The human circulatory system. Arrows indicate the direction of blood flow through the blood vessels.

removed). Plasma contains vitamins, minerals, small and large macronutrient molecules, hormones, hydrogen energy complexes, high-energy molecules, and many hundreds of other substances. Blood carries away from the cells metabolic waste products and also important substances such as hormones that are synthesized in one tissue but needed in another.

The concentration of the many substances transported by the circulatory system varies somewhat, depending upon the time interval between meals, the nutrient composition of the diet, the rates of internal metabolic processes, and the conditions within the cells and the body as a whole. However, sophisticated mechanisms that are controlled primarily by hormones maintain the concentration of these substances in the blood within a fairly narrow range.

Table 6-1 shows the interrelationship of various nutrients with functions of the circulatory system, which we will now discuss.

Red Blood Cell Formation

Of all the substances transported by the blood, oxygen is the substance upon which the body is most dependent. The blood contains minute amounts of dissolved oxygen, but most of the oxygen is complexed with the iron portion of *hemoglobin,* a protein in red blood cells. The transport of oxygen throughout the body is impaired by certain dietary deficiencies or by unusual requirement for or loss of iron or other nutrients.

Hemoglobin is a large protein that is synthesized inside red blood cells during the later stages of their formation. The *heme* part of hemoglobin is a complex structure containing at its core an atom of iron, to which oxygen is bound. The incorporation of iron into heme depends upon the presence of copper and molybdenum. Pyridoxine, folic acid, and pantothenic acid are cofactors in the reactions by which heme is synthesized. The *globin* part of hemoglobin is made of protein; its formation is dependent upon

Vitamin C, vitamin K, calcium, and magnesium are needed to maintain the integrity of the vessels of the circulatory system; many other nutrients are necessary for delivering hemoglobin-bound oxygen to the cells in proper amounts.

TABLE 6-1. Macronutrients and Micronutrients Associated with the Circulatory System

Activity, Role, or Function Involving Blood	Substances Derived from Macronutrients	Micronutrient	
		Vitamin	Mineral
Red Blood Cell Formation			
Form structure of hemoglobin	Globin		Iron
Synthesize hemoglobin		Pyridoxine, folic acid pantothenic acid	
Mobilize iron stores			Molybdenum
Increase utilization of iron			Copper
Produce DNA and RNA for red blood cell division and maturation		Folic acid, vitamin B_{12}, vitamin C	Magnesium, manganese
Stabilize cell membrane; prevent chemical or toxin damage		Vitamin E	
Maintaining blood supply to tissues			
Maintain elasticity and strength of capillaries	Collagen	Vitamin C	
Maintain blood clotting process	Prothrombin, thrombin	Vitamin K	Calcium

an adequate supply of amino acids and of all the nutrients needed for protein synthesis.

Red blood cells live only about 120 days and must be continuously resupplied by repeated divisions of specialized cells in the bone marrow. Although red blood cells of most mammals lose their nuclei when the cells are released into the circulatory system, the parent cells contain nuclei. Within these nuclei are the nucleic acids DNA and RNA, which are necessary for cell division (whereby new red blood cells are created), and for red blood cell maturation. Folic acid and vitamin B_{12} play important roles in the synthesis of DNA and RNA; magnesium, manganese, and vitamin C are also necessary for red blood cell production; and vitamin E protects the lipids within the membranes of red blood cells from oxidation and therefore helps to maintain the stability of the cell membrane.

Maintaining Blood Supply to the Tissues

Two vitamins and one mineral are particularly important in maintaining the integrity of the circulatory system. Both the strength and elasticity of the capillaries are dependent upon an adequate supply of vitamin C. This vitamin is necessary for the synthesis of *collagen*, a protein contained in capillary walls and in other supporting tissues. Collagen functions much like the steel girders that make up the framework of buildings.

When a blood vessel is torn or cut, the capacity of blood to clot is impaired if there is an inadequate supply of vitamin K or calcium (Figure 6-2). These nutrients, therefore, help to prevent leakage of blood—either internally or externally—from the circulatory system. The proteins prothrombin and thrombin also are needed for blood clotting.

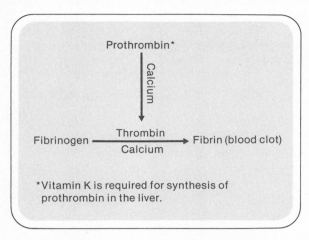

Prothrombin*

Calcium

Fibrinogen ⟶ Thrombin ⟶ Fibrin (blood clot)

Calcium

*Vitamin K is required for synthesis of prothrombin in the liver.

Figure 6–2. Role of calcium in blood clotting.

Anemias caused by nutritional disorders are discussed in Chapter 22.

NEUROMUSCULAR SYSTEM

The nervous and muscular systems operate together intimately. Both systems run on electric currents. The nervous system conducts and interprets stimuli from inside and outside the body; the most readily observable response to these stimuli involves a muscular action. Many similarities exist in the effects of vitamins and minerals upon the functions of these two systems. For these reasons, the nervous and muscular systems are frequently considered together as one *neuromuscular* system.

Table 6-2 shows the way various nutrients interact with the neuromuscular system, which we will now discuss.

Nerve Impulse Transmission

Stimuli to the nervous system cause *electrochemical impulses* to be transmitted along the membranes of nerve cells. These membranes can be compared to the capacitor of a battery. Negatively charged elements are lined up against the inside of the cell;

and positively charged elements, along the outside. The lipid material in the cell membrane acts as the dielectric (nonconductor), similar to the role of mica in an electrical capacitor. When an impulse is transmitted along a nerve, high-energy molecules release energy, which enables sodium and potassium ions (charged particles) to change places across the membrane—sodium moves into the cell, and potassium moves out. After the impulse is transmitted, the original distribution of electrochemical charges is reestablished.

Impulses are transmitted from one nerve to another, or from a nerve to a muscle, across a junction called a *synapse* (Figure 6-3). The influx of calcium ions across the membrane of a nerve cell stimulates the release of an excitatory substance, which increases the permeability of the membrane to sodium.

Several specialized substances known as neurohormones (Table 6-2) are synthesized from amino acids by a series of reactions that require pyridoxine. These substances control the speed of nerve transmission and the ability of a nerve to continue to respond to rapid and repeated stimuli. One of these, gamma-amino butyric acid, is of primary importance in the normal functioning of the brain.

Muscle Contraction and Relaxation

Skeletal muscles are composed of numerous muscle fibers, each of which contains hundreds of *myofibrils,* which are made up of hundreds of protein filaments called *actin* and *myosin.* The myofibrils are suspended in a matrix of tissue fluid much like plasma. This fluid contains calcium, sodium, potassium, magnesium, phosphate, enzymes, and other substances. When a muscle contracts, actin and myosin filaments combine to form *actomyosin,* a protein of more compact configuration than either of its constituent proteins. These filaments slide together in a manner somewhat analogous to slipping together the fingers of both hands.

The coming together and breaking apart of actin

TABLE 6-2. Macronutrients and Micronutrients Associated with the Neuromuscular System

Activity, Role, or Function Involving Muscles and Nervous System	Substances Derived from Macronutrients	Micronutrient	
		Vitamin	Mineral
Structural Components			
Form structure of myoglobin	Globin		Iron
Form structure of myelin sheath	Lipids		Copper
Form structure of cerebrosides and gangliosides	Lipid–carbohydrate complexes		
Nerve impulse transmission			
Maintain electrical potential on each side of the cell membrane			Sodium, potassium, chloride
Control rate of transfer of sodium and potassium through cell membranes			Calcium
Synthesize neurohormones (epinephrine, norepinephrine, and gamma-amino butyric acid)	Amino acids	Pyridoxine	
Muscle contraction and relaxation			
Contract muscles	Actin, myosin		Calcium
Relax muscles	Actin, myosin		Magnesium
Sensory functions			
Maintain taste and smell acuity		Vitamin A	Zinc, other trace elements
Synthesize rhodopsin for vision, help rods and cones adapt to light changes, and maintain tear duct cells		Vitamin A	

and myosin are controlled by calcium and magnesium in the fluid of muscle tissue. Magnesium normally keeps the myofibrils in a relaxed state by inhibiting any reaction between actin and myosin. When a stimulus or contractile signal passes through a muscle fiber, calcium is released into the muscle cell fluid. Stimulated by the presence of calcium ions, myosin causes high-energy molecules (ATP) to release energy, which enables actin to combine with myosin. A continuous circulation of "fresh" tissue fluid around all cells washes away free calcium so that the actin and myosin remain interlaced only

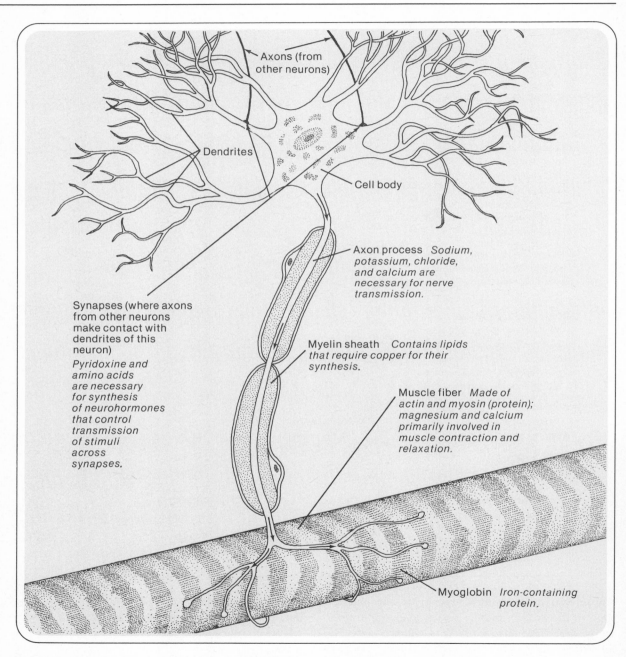

Figure 6–3. Role of nutrients in neuromuscular system. (Adapted with permission of Macmillan Publishing Co., Inc. from *Man and the Natural World* by C. J. Goin and Olive B. Goin. Copyright © 1970 by Coleman J. Goin and Olive B. Goin.)

momentarily after each stimulus. This fluid circulation also brings in magnesium, which maintains muscles in a relaxed state between stimuli.

Structural Roles of Nutrients

Nutrients have structural functions in the neuromuscular system. Some nerve cells are surrounded by a *myelin sheath,* a membrane that contains lipids; copper is required for the synthesis of the myelin sheath (Figure 6-3). Muscles contain the protein *myoglobin,* which, like hemoglobin, is constructed around the mineral iron. Lipids and carbohydrates combine to form gangliosides and cerebrosides, which are components of the nervous system.

Effects of Deficiencies

Many nutrient deficiencies adversely affect the nervous and muscular systems. In some cases, the metabolic bases for these effects are understood; in others, the specific dysfunction is not known.

Abnormal brain waves can be shown on an electroencephalogram (EEG) and convulsions may result from a severe deficiency of pyridoxine. Thiamin deficiency may cause tingling and numbness in the fingers and toes, a jerking of the eye muscles when looking to either side, and an absence of nervous reflexes. A deficiency of niacin, folic acid, vitamin B_{12}, or vitamin A also causes abnormalities in the nervous system.

Abnormal concentrations of sodium and potassium in body fluids can cause muscle cramping, and fluctuations in magnesium, calcium, and phosphorus levels can lead to muscle spasms or to decreased muscle tone and paralysis. The crucial and interrelated roles of these minerals is illustrated by *tetany,* a syndrome manifested by severe, constant muscle spasms of the face and jaw, spine, hands, or other muscle groups, or by muscle twitching or irritability. In severe cases, respiratory failure and death result. The underlying cause may be low blood calcium, low magnesium, low potassium, or excessive alkalinity of the blood due to loss of chloride from vomiting, to loss of carbon dioxide from *hyperventilation* (rapid, shallow breathing), or to excessive intake of antacids.

Although pantothenic acid deficiency has never been reported in people eating normal diets, persons who were fed specially prepared experimental diets lacking this vitamin exhibited personality and nervous system abnormalities under experimental conditions. In laboratory experiments with monkeys, a type of muscular dystrophy (unlike human muscular dystrophy) resulted from vitamin E deficiency.

Sensory Functions

Sensory functions are mediated by the nervous system, but certain nutrients have unique sensory functions. Taste and smell acuity are impaired by a deficiency of vitamin A, zinc, and possibly some trace minerals.

Several nutrients have a role in the visual process. Inadequate intakes of riboflavin may be related to a type of cataract formation, but there is no evidence that large dosages of this vitamin affect cataracts caused by more common diseases or disorders. The nutrient most commonly associated with vision is vitamin A. The role of this vitamin in enabling the eye to see in dim light was discussed in Chapter 3. Vitamin A is needed for maintenance of the *epithelial cells* that line the tear ducts. A deficiency of this nutrient leads to the cessation of tear production; the eyes become dry and cannot readily rid themselves of bacteria and debris. Minor eye irritations become easily infected, leading to ulcers of the cornea and blindness due to scar tissue. In a severe deficiency, the lens of the eye may actually become detached from the iris.

INTEGUMENTARY SYSTEM

The integumentary system comprises the skin and all its outgrowths and ingrowths. Tissues lining the

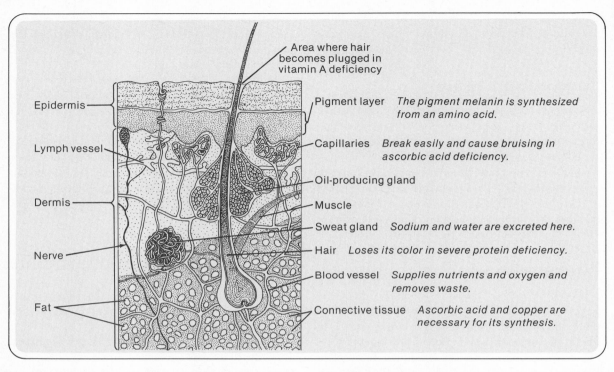

Figure 6–4. Role of nutrients in integumentary system. (Adapted with permission of Macmillan Publishing Co., Inc. from *Man and the Natural World* by C. J. Goin and Olive B. Goin. Copyright © 1970 by Coleman J. Goin and Olive B. Goin.)

outer edges of internal passages at the nose, ears, lips, anus, and the openings of the urinary and reproductive tracts are part of this system.

Many nutrients affect the integumentary system, as shown in Figure 6-4 and Table 6-3. The skin is a complex, metabolically active tissue—not simply a covering or container for vital organs. The skin is the site of vitamin D formation from the sterol *7-dehydrocholesterol.* Specialized glands within the skin produce and excrete certain lipids, which lubricate the skin and keep it from becoming dry and flaky.

The integumentary system controls body temperature by regulating the loss of heat from the body. If you exercise strenuously on a hot day, the blood capillaries near the skin's surface enlarge in diameter, a greater than normal volume of blood flows

through these capillaries, and more body heat escapes. (On a cold day, these capillaries contract, thereby permitting less blood flow to the skin, and so less heat can be lost. As water evaporates from the skin, there is a cooling effect on the body since heat is lost as water is vaporized. Water and sodium chloride are excreted through the skin as perspiration.)

Structure of Skin

Skin consists of two different structures: (1) the outer layer, or *epidermis,* and (2) the deeper layer or *dermis.*

The epidermis is composed primarily of a protein called *keratin,* which consists of a large proportion of sulfur-containing amino acids. (A harder type of

Maintenance of normal skin cells requires vitamin C, copper, vitamin A, and several other nutrients.

TABLE 6-3. Macronutrients and Micronutrients Associated with the Integumentary System

Activity, Role, or Function Involving Skin	Substances Derived from Macronutrients	Micronutrient	
		Vitamin	Mineral
Structural components			
Synthesize collagen	Amino acids	Vitamin C	
Synthesize elastin	Amino acids		Copper
Inhibit excess keratin formation		Vitamin A	
Form keratin for nails and hair	Amino acids, especially those containing sulfur		
Synthesize melanin	Tyrosine	Pyridoxine	Copper
Lubricate skin	Lipids		
Heal wounds		Vitamin C	Zinc
Cool body temperature by evaporation	Water		

keratin is found in fingernails and toenails.) Since there are no blood vessels nourishing this layer of skin, its cells continuously die. During a lifetime, 40 to 50 pounds of these epidermal cells are shed, and replaced by cells that originated in the dermis, or the deeper layer of skin.

The dermis contains a nonliving *ground substance* composed of hexose chains to which nitrogen and sulfur groups are attached. This substance functions much like mortar in holding together the structural elements of tissues. Intertwined through the ground substance are the protein fibers *collagen* and *elastin*. The former are tough and inelastic, whereas the latter can be stretched but will snap back into their original shape, much as a rubber band would. Vitamin C and copper are required for the synthesis of collagen and elastin, respectively.

The redness of skin is determined by red blood cells flowing through the vessels of the dermis. The darkness of skin, however, is determined primarily by the concentration of the pigment *melanin* in the pigment layer at the junction of the dermis and the epidermis. Melanin is synthesized from the amino acid tyrosine by a series of reactions requiring pyridoxine and copper.

Effects of Deficiencies

Deficiencies of riboflavin, niacin, pyridoxine, and essential fatty acids cause slightly different types of dermatitis, or inflammation of the skin. Lack of vitamin A causes keratin to accumulate near the base of the follicles from which hairs grow; the skin there becomes bumpy, dry, and scaly. Lack of vitamin C first causes small bruises where capillaries are broken; as the deficiency worsens, bruising becomes more extensive. Both vitamin C and zinc are necessary to the normal wound-healing processes.

Severe protein deficiency is characterized by depigmentation of the hair and skin due to reduced production of melanin. *Albinism,* the condition manifested by absent pigment in hair or skin, is a genetic disorder caused by an inborn lack of one of the enzymes necessary to convert tyrosine to mela-

Bones and cartilage are made of proteins, calcium, phosphorus, fluoride, magnesium, manganese, and other minerals; vitamins D and A are important for the normal formation of bone.

TABLE 6-4. Micronutrients Associated with the Skeletal System

Activity, Role, or Function Involving Bone and Cartilage	Micronutrient	
	Vitamin	Mineral
Synthesize collagen	Vitamin C	
Synthesize elastin		Copper
Comprise bones and teeth		Calcium, phosphorus, fluoride, magnesium, manganese, and other minerals
Harden hydroxyapatite		
Maintain bone-forming cells		Fluoride
Prevent rickets and softening	Vitamin A	Copper
and thinning of bones	Vitamin D	Calcium, phosphorus, fluoride

nin—not by a deficiency of the amino acid or micronutrients necessary for melanin synthesis.

SKELETAL SYSTEM

The skeletal system is characterized by two kinds of tissue: bone and cartilage (Table 6-4). In both types of tissue, living cells exist in small spaces that are scattered through a nonliving matrix of collagen, elastin, and calcium salts. Synthesis of collagen is impaired when vitamin C is lacking; synthesis of elastin is impaired when copper is lacking.

Cartilage is flexible and acts as a cushion between bones, as in the knees, elbow, or spinal column. Cartilage supports the nose and ears. In developing embryos and infants—and in children up through the age of physical maturity—cartilage is the precursor of bone and is the main component of parts of the skeleton.

Bone is hard because crystals of calcium and phosphate are embedded between its rows of well-ordered collagen fibers. The presence of fluoride within these fibers adds to the hardness of bone. Magnesium, manganese, and small amounts of other minerals are also part of bone structure. Bone is constantly being broken down and restructured. In this process, optimal performance of the bone-forming cells depends upon the availability of vita-

min A and copper as well as of the minerals found in bone.

A deficiency of vitamin D results in rickets, a condition characterized by bowed legs and knobby, bead-like deposits on the breastbone. Excess fluoride can cause the spine to become stiff and inflexible, but a deficiency of fluoride, calcium, phosphorus, or vitamin D can cause the bones to become thin or soft or both. Hormones also affect bone structure. Prolonged periods of inactivity cause minerals to be lost from bones. High protein intakes increase the body's need for calcium.

GASTROINTESTINAL SYSTEM

In order for the gastrointestinal system to digest food and perform its other functions, the cells lining this tract must have an adequate supply of nutrients (Table 6-5).

Maintenance of Cells and Functions

Because mucosal cells have a short lifespan and must be rapidly replaced, there must be an adequate and steady source of folic acid and vitamin B_{12}—nutrients needed for cell division and maturation. A deficiency of either nutrient results in blunting of the villi, a condition that drastically reduces the

The gastrointestinal tract is particularly sensitive to lack of iron, folic acid, and vitamin B_{12}; digestion and absorption are also impaired by a deficiency of other nutrients.

TABLE 6-5. Micronutrients Associated with the Gastrointestinal System

Activity, Role or Function Involving GI Tract	Micronutrient	
	Vitamin	Mineral
Prevent blunting of intestinal villi	Folic acid, vitamin B_{12}	
Maintain mucosal epithelium	Vitamin A	
Maintain muscle tone of GI tract	Thiamin	
Maintain gums, tongue, and mucosal membrane	Vitamin C, niacin, riboflavin, folic acid, vitamin B_{12}	
Maintain gastric acidity		Chloride (in hydrochloric acid)
Part of a protein-digesting enzyme		Zinc
Activate a lipid-digesting enzyme		Calcium
Regulate pump mechanism for absorption of glucose		Sodium

absorptive surface of the intestinal tract. In people who do not consume or are unable to absorb enough of these vitamins, a steady deterioration of nutritional status results from the decreased absorption of all other nutrients.

The gastrointestinal tract and the ducts that channel secretions into it are lined with epithelial cells. These cells are somewhat different from the epithelial cells of the integumentary system, but both the integumentary and the gastrointestinal systems require an adequate supply of vitamin A.

Maintenance of the muscular tone of the intestinal walls for the propulsion of nutrients and fluids through the tract are dependent upon an adequate supply of thiamin. Lack of appetite occurs in many nutritional disorders but is especially characteristic of thiamin deficiency.

Nutrients Needed for Digestion and Absorption

Several components of digestive fluids are nutrients. Chloride is a part of the hydrochloric acid in the gastric juice of the stomach. Zinc is part of the protein-digesting enzyme *carboxypeptidase*. Calcium activates lipase, which is secreted by the pancreas. Vitamin B_{12} cannot be absorbed in the intestine unless it is combined with intrinsic factor (described in Chapter 4), which is secreted by stomach cells. Glucose is absorbed by a pump that is influenced by the presence of sodium ions.

Signs of Nutrient Deficiencies

Abnormalities of the mouth are the clue to many nutritional deficiencies. Scurvy, a disease caused by vitamin C deficiency, is characterized by bleeding of the gums, especially around the base of the teeth. A scarlet-red inflammation of the tongue is characteristic of acute *pellagra*, a multinutrient deficiency disease that is primarily associated with lack of niacin. This inflammation is also seen in *sprue*, a condition associated with folic acid deficiency and vitamin B_{12} deficiency. Soreness and ulceration of the mouth may accompany these deficiencies. A darker, beef-red tongue is caused by less severe niacin deficiency or by a lack of other B vitamins. A purplish or magenta tongue is often a symptom of riboflavin deficiency, which can also cause sores and inflammation at the corners of the mouth (*cheilosis*).

Diarrhea and inflammation of the intestinal tract occur when the diet is severely deficient in folic acid, niacin, protein, or energy.

ENDOCRINE SYSTEM

The endocrine system is composed of several glands, each of which produces one or more hormones (Figure 6-5). These hormones are transmitted in the blood from the organs that produce them to their target organs—those that respond to a particular hormone. Several glands produce hormones that signal other endocrine organs to retain or release their own hormones. The endocrine system carefully fine-tunes numerous metabolic, muscular, excretory, and other processes by turning on, or turning off, the production and release of specific hormones.

Hormone Synthesis and Action

The functioning of the endocrine system is dependent upon many dietary essentials (Table 6-6). Vitamin A and pantothenic acid are required for the synthesis of the hormone *corticosterone*, which is produced by the adrenal glands. Essential fatty acids are necessary for the synthesis of a group of hormonelike substances called *prostaglandins. Thyroxine* is synthesized in the thyroid gland from two molecules of the amino acid tyrosine, which are combined with iodine. Chromium is part of a recently identified substance called *glucose tolerance factor* (GTF). This factor is required to activate insulin (produced by the pancreas). One manifestation of chromium deficiency is abnormal glucose metabolism. The release of insulin is stimulated by glucose, potassium, fatty acids, and the amino acids leucine and arginine.

Vitamin D is converted in the kidneys and liver to two substances called hydroxycholecalciferol (HCC) and dihydroxycholecalciferol (DHCC). Research within the last decade has shown that HCC and DHCC function more like hormones than like vitamins. These substances, along with the thyroid and parathyroid hormones, maintain proper amounts of calcium and phosphorus in blood and other tissues such as bone and teeth. This is accomplished by regulating the amounts of these minerals absorbed and excreted and by causing minerals to be either added to or withdrawn from bone (Figure 6-6).

Interrelationships between nutrients and endocrine function in reproduction are less well understood. A deficiency of zinc causes delayed sexual maturation and stunting of growth (a type of dwarfism). In severely deficient experimental animals, lack of zinc, vitamin A, riboflavin, and several other micronutrients causes spontaneous abortions or birth defects. Vitamin A is necessary for formation of sperm cells and maintenance of a normal menstrual cycle.

Hormonal Influences upon Metabolism

Hormones affect digestion and absorption (Chapter 4) and the metabolism of many nutrients. Insulin and growth hormone have *anabolic* effects—that is, they direct the cells to store energy and conserve tissue protein. Glucagon and hormones from the adrenal glands (cortical hormones) have a *catabolic* role—they cause energy release and the breakdown of carbohydrate, fat, and protein. Thyroxine controls the general pace of metabolic reactions. Aldosterone stimulates the kidneys to excrete potassium and to retain sodium, chloride, and water within the body. Cholecystokinin, a hormone released by the duodenum, stimulates the release of bile from the gallbladder, thus enhancing the absorption of some lipids.

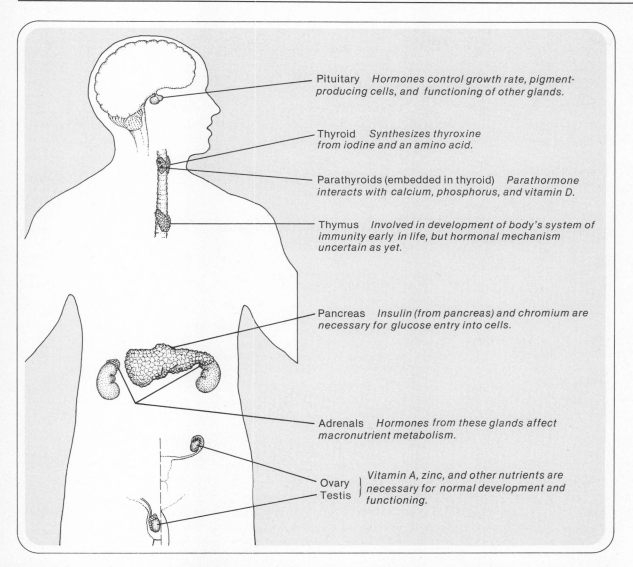

Figure 6–5. Role of nutrients in endocrine system. (Adapted with permission of Macmillan Publishing Co., Inc. from *Man and the Natural World* by C. J. Goin and Olive B. Goin. Copyright © 1970 by Coleman J. Goin and Olive B. Goin.)

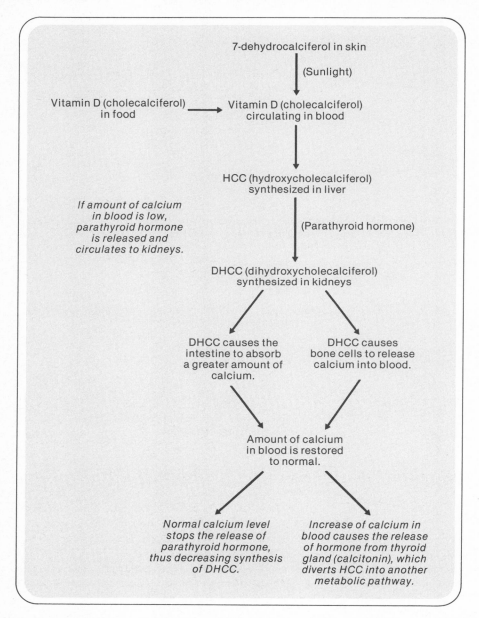

Figure 6–6. How vitamin D, its active forms, and hormones maintain normal calcium levels in the blood. (Adapted from *Introductory Nutrition,* 3d ed., by Helen Andrews Guthrie. The C. V. Mosby Co., St. Louis, 1975. Also used by permission of the author.)

TABLE 6-6. Macronutrients and Micronutrients Associated with the Endocrine System

Activity, Role, or Function Involving Hormones	Substances Derived from Macronutrients	Micronutrient	
		Vitamin	Mineral
Hormone synthesis and action			
Synthesize corticosterone		Vitamin A, pantothenic acid	
Synthesize norepinephrine	Tyrosine	Pyridoxine	
Synthesize prostaglandin	Essential fatty acids		
Synthesize thyroxine	Tyrosine	Pyridoxine	Iodine
Synthesize glucose tolerance factor			Chromium
Stimulate insulin release	Leucine, arginine, fatty acids, glucose		Potassium
Interact with parathyroid and thyroid hormones		Vitamin D (HCC and DHCC)	Calcium, phosphorus
Reproduction			
Aid in sexual maturation			Zinc, other trace elements
Prevent birth defects		Vitamin A, riboflavin	Zinc
Maintain normal menstrual cycle and spermatogenesis		Vitamin A	

NOTE: Metabolism of carbohydrates, fats, and proteins is regulated by epinephrine, insulin, glucagon, cortisol, and growth hormone. The body's salt and water balance is regulated by aldosterone from the adrenal gland and by antidiuretic hormone from the brain and the pituitary gland.

OTHER INTERDEPENDENT ROLES

Macronutrients and micronutrients complement each other in many ways that are not unique to any one system of the body.

Metabolic Reactions

Optimal conditions for many metabolic reactions depend upon several nutrients being available at the same moment and in the same place. Vitamins are necessary for the transfer of numerous chemical groups to and from the intermediate products of metabolic pathways. For optimal activity, these reactions often require the presence of a mineral, either as part of the enzyme or in a critical concentration in the cellular fluid. Since enzymes are proteins, their synthesis depends upon the availability of all the nutrients involved in protein synthesis.

Structural Interrelationships

There are several important structural interrelationships among micronutrients: *sulfur* as a component of thiamin and biotin; *cobalt* as a component of vitamin B$_{12}$; and *phosphorus* as a part of the active forms of pyridoxine and thiamin, of the hydrogen

TABLE 6-7. Interdependent Roles of Micronutrients

Activity	Related Micronutrient
Transfer one-carbon units among various forms of folic acid	Vitamin B_{12}
Convert folic acid to active folinic acid	Vitamin C, niacin
Convert tryptophan to niacin	Pyridoxine, thiamin
Substitute for vitamin E in some metabolic reactions	Selenium
Protect vitamin A, carotenes, vitamin C, and unsaturated fatty acids from oxidation	Vitamin E
Maximize absorption and utilization of iron	Ascorbic acid, hydrochloric acid, copper

energy complexes that contain riboflavin and niacin, of high-energy ATP, and of the nucleic acids DNA and RNA.

Optimal Activity or Utilization

In many cases, one micronutrient is necessary for the activity or optimal utilization of another. For example, there are several metabolically active forms of folic acid, each of which is a cofactor for different reactions. The basic molecule may be modified by the addition of a nitrogen-containing subunit or several slightly different subunits containing one carbon atom. Vitamin B_{12}, vitamin C, and niacin are required for some of these intercon-versions. Several other examples of this type of interdependence have been mentioned in earlier chapters. They are summarized in Table 6-7.

OTHER SYSTEMS

The above discussion does not cite all of the body systems in which nutrients function. Other examples are included in Section V ("Diet and Health"). The interdependence of nutrient function is particularly evident in the discussion of how the body resists infection and invasion by foreign substances (Chapter 21) and how diet helps maintain oral health (Chapter 28).

STUDY QUESTIONS

1. Why does taking a vitamin–mineral capsule not replace the need for selecting a nutritionally balanced diet?

2. What micronutrients are needed to keep the circulatory system intact?

3. What micronutrients are important in nerve transmission and in muscle contraction and relaxation?

4. What micronutrients are necessary for sight, taste, and smell?

5. What micronutrients are needed to maintain normal, healthy skin cells?

6. What macronutrients and micronutrients compose bones and cartilage or are essential for their formation?

7. Lack of folic acid and vitamin B_{12} has what effect on the gastrointestinal tract?

8. How are nutrients and hormones related?

9. Give four examples of how one micronutrient affects the functioning of another micronutrient.

SUGGESTED READING

1. J. G. Bieri and R. P. Evarts, "Tocopherols and fatty acids in American diets: The recommended allowance for vitamin E," *Journal of the American Dietetic Association* 63(1973):147.

2. D. M. Hegsted and L. M. Ausman, "Sole foods and some not so scientific experiments," *Nutrition Today* 8(1973):22–27.

3. P. V. Johnston, "Nutrition and neural development," *Food and Nutrition News* 45(Feb.-March 1974).

4. R. J. Wurtman and J. D. Fernstrom, "Effect of diet on brain neurotransmitters," *Nutrition Reviews* 32(1974):193–200.

5. "Skeletal fluorosis and dietary calcium, vitamin C, and protein," *Nutrition Reviews* 32(1974):13–15.

6. "Relation of zinc to calcium in bone," *Nutrition Reviews* 34(1976):294–95.

7. E. L. R. Stokstad, "Vitamin B_{12} and folic acid," Chapter 20 in *Present Knowledge in Nutrition.* 4th ed. New York and Washington, D.C.: The Nutrition Foundation, 1976.

8. O. A. Levander, "Selenium and chromium in human nutrition: A review," *Journal of the American Dietetic Association* 66(1975):338–44.

9. S. Margen et al, "Studies in calcium metabolism: I. The calciuretic effect of dietary protein," *American Journal of Clinical Nutrition* 27(1974):584.

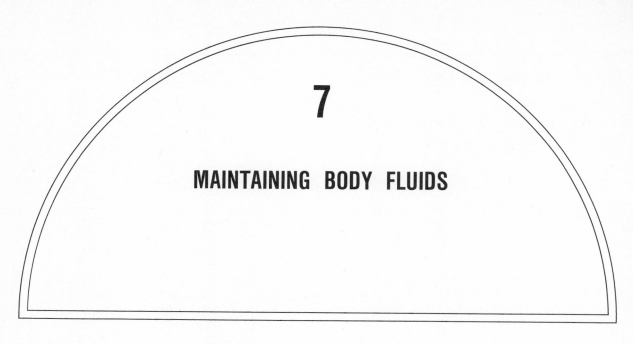

7

MAINTAINING BODY FLUIDS

Surprising as it may seem, about 60 percent of the adult human body is water. Deprivation of this nutrient upsets the life-supporting processes within the body more quickly than does a deficiency of any vitamin or mineral. For example, hikers lost in the wilderness may have adequate food sources, but unless they can find drinkable water, they will live only a few days.

This chapter discusses why it is vitally important to maintain the proper amount of fluid in the body and the correct composition of body fluids.

CHARACTERISTICS OF BODY FLUIDS

Water is the basis for all body fluids—blood, lymph, digestive juices, urine, and spinal fluid. It is also present in every living cell, including those in bones and growing teeth. Water does not, however, exist in the body in a pure state; pure water administered intravenously to the body is fatal.

The water in the body always contains dissolved substances, much as a soft drink contains invisible sugar particles. Other ingredients of body fluids may be held in solution as minute particles; for example, lipids may be solubilized by a protein coating. The macronutrients within a cell, as well as all other components of cells, are either surrounded by or dissolved in water.

Water Content of the Body

The amount of water in an average man's body is enough to fill a 10-gallon fish tank. The body of a woman who is the same weight contains slightly less water; breast tissue and other more substantial fat deposits are mainly lipid, and contain a smaller proportion of water than does muscle tissue. The body of an obese person contains more lipid and less water than does the body of a muscular person of the same weight.

Butter floats on water because butterfat (a lipid) is less dense than water. For the same reason, fat people can float in a swimming pool more easily than thin people can. A body that is 40 to 45 percent fat rises to the water's surface, whereas a lean body sinks because it does not have enough low-density fat to support the weight of high-density tissues such as bone. One of the laboratory tests for measuring body fatness is based on the principle that fat bodies are more buoyant than lean bodies.

Lack of water impairs body functions more quickly than does lack of a micronutrient or energy-containing macronutrient. Water content of the body is inversely proportional to fat content.

Distribution of Water in the Body

The major compartments into which body water is distributed are the *intracellular* spaces and the *extracellular* spaces (Figure 7-1). The intracellular space comprises the fluids contained within the trillions of cells of the body. The extracellular space consists partly of the fluids within the blood and lymph vessels, the juices of the gastrointestinal tract, the fluid within the eye, and the cerebrospinal fluid. These extracellular fluids are contained within definite boundaries in the body. The major portion of fluid in the extracellular space is, however, more difficult to locate; this fluid fills the spaces between cells in tissues such as muscles, skin, liver, and kidneys. Remember that no two cells of the body actually touch each other; they are separated and surrounded by a thin film of tissue fluid. This tissue fluid is in a dynamic state of circulation, exchanging nutrients and wastes with the blood and lymph.

Blood accounts for about 5 to 6 quarts of the fluid

in an adult's body. The water within the red and the white blood cells is part of the intracellular fluid; the plasma surrounding these cells is extracellular fluid.

Nutrient Ions in Body Water

Many of the substances within body fluids are present as ions, or charged particles, which are formed when a molecule dissolves in water. For example, table salt is made of molecules in which sodium and chloride are tightly held together. When we sprinkle salt in water, it disappears, but we know it is there because we can taste it. What happens in the water is that the sodium and chloride in salt move apart, thus destroying the solid salt that we can see. The dissolved chloride forms negatively charged ions called *anions* and the sodium forms positively charged ions called *cations*. These oppositely charged particles are attracted to each other, just as a cation will move to a negatively charged *electrode* (electrical pole) and an anion to a positively charged electrode.

The cations in a particular body fluid must balance out the anions in that fluid. (It is physically impossible for a fluid to contain only anions or only cations.) Certain nutrients are crucial to maintaining the cation–anion balance.

The major positively charged ions in body fluids are sodium, potassium, calcium, and magnesium. The major negatively charged ions are chloride and the complexes of carbon, phosphorus, and sulfur with oxygen (carbonates, phosphates, and sulfates). These complexes sometimes contain hydrogen. Proteins can exist as either positive or negative ions, depending on the charge of their constituent amino acids and on the acidity of the body fluid.

The components of the various body fluids are specially tailored to facilitate the metabolic reactions and physiological functions characteristic of each fluid. For example, gastric juice has a different composition from the fluid secreted by the pancreas, and spinal fluid differs from plasma.

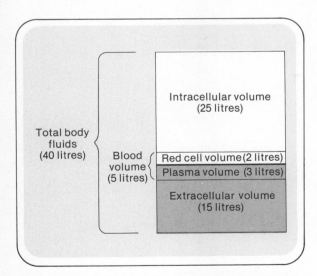

Figure 7–1. Distribution of body fluids. Extracellular fluids are found in tears, spinal fluid, the gastrointestinal tract, eyes, lymph tissues, and between cells. Intracellular fluids (the greater portion of body fluids) are located only within cells.

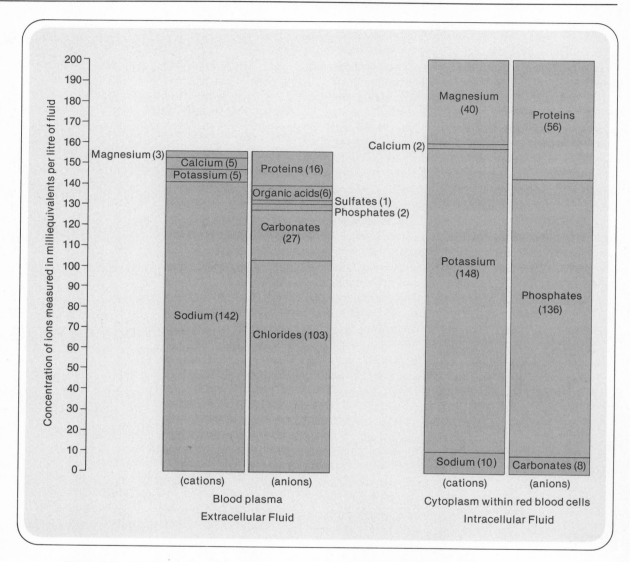

Figure 7–2. Distribution of anions and cations in examples of intracellular and extracellular fluids.

Figure 7-2 graphs the principal differences in ion composition between blood plasma (an extracellular fluid) and the cytoplasm inside red blood cells (an intracellular fluid). These graphs show that although the negative ions equal the positive ions in both fluids, the concentrations of specific anions and ca-

tions are markedly different. Sodium and chloride ions predominate in plasma, whereas red blood cells contain much more potassium, phosphates, and protein.

The pattern of ion distribution shown in Figure 7-2 is maintained by intricate control mechanisms that operate within the body to prevent random ionic shifts that would impair the efficiency of metabolic reactions in each compartment. The relative concentrations in body fluids of many ions—sodium, potassium, manganese, magnesium, and calcium ions in particular—influence the rates of anabolic and catabolic reactions and the availability of energy from high-energy ATP molecules.

Ionic control mechanisms allow small but crucial quanities of ions to move across cellular membranes to maintain a balance of positive and negative charges within each cell. As we saw in Chapter 6, the concentration and movement of certain ions is critical for many physiological functions, such as nerve transmission and muscular contraction.

Functions of Body Water

Body fluid is not a stagnant pool enclosed by cell membranes, but a constantly circulating medium that transports many substances and serves other "transfer" functions.

Metabolism. Perhaps the most important but least obvious function of body water is as the medium in which metabolic reactions occur. For example, when amino acids link together to form protein, and when energy is released from macronutrients, these substances as well as the enzymes, minerals, and cofactors necessary for their reactions are dissolved in water.

In addition to being a reaction medium, water is a participant in many reactions. The reactions of the energy-releasing process and the synthesis of carbohydrates, lipids, and proteins involve the addition or the removal of water molecules.

Digestion. Water has several roles in digestion. It participates in the hydrolytic cleavage of complex carbohydrates into hexoses, of proteins into amino acids, and of fats into fatty acids and glycerol. Water is a major component of the fluids that carry the various digestive enzymes into the gastrointesti-

nal tract; these fluids also adjust the acidity or alkalinity of the intestinal contents. Water also moves in and out of the gastrointestinal tract to facilitate the passage of chyme and the mixing of nutrients with enzymes.

Transport. Water is the medium in which vitamins, minerals, macronutrients, and other substances are carried by the circulatory system throughout the body. It is therefore the principal vehicle of the physiological transportation and communication network.

Retention of excessive amounts of water in the body can place a burden on the circulatory system. For this reason, many people who have heart disease are given *diuretics* ("water pills"), which increase urine output and thereby reduce body water and the circulatory burden.

Lubrication. Saliva, tears, and mucus (all of which are largely water) are the lubricants of the body. Joints between bones are cushioned by a layer of *synovial* fluid, which is largely water.

Temperature Control. Water participates in the regulation of body temperature. When water evaporates from the skin surface, and when it is exhaled as water vapor from the lungs, the body is cooled.

Excretion. When water leaves the body as urine, it carries with it many substances that are no longer needed by the body, as well as substances that are toxic in high concentrations. Accumulation within the body of the components of urine can have disastrous effects upon acid–base balance and ion balance.

WATER BALANCE

Several litres of water enter and leave the body every day (Figure 7-3). Small imbalances between intake and output alter body weight; but if they are only temporary, they have little consequence. For

The amount of water consumed in foods and beverages plus the water formed during metabolism normally equals the amount of water lost through the lungs and the skin and as part of urine and feces; water imbalances cause either edema or dehydration.

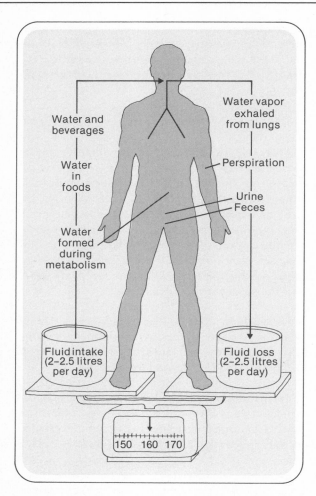

Figure 7–3. Normal water balance in the body. (Adapted from *Nutrition and Physical Fitness,* 9th ed., by L. J. Bogert, G. M. Briggs, and D. H. Calloway. © 1973, Saunders Publishing Company. Used by permission.)

example, many women retain water (which affects their body weight) for several days immediately prior to menstruation, but they experience only minor, if any, ill effects from this increase in body fluid.

Prolonged imbalances of a minor degree or severe imbalances that occur quickly can be dangerous. If

excessive amounts of water are lost and not replaced, the cells become dehydrated. If the amount of water consumed exceeds the amount of water lost, the excess water is retained within and between cells, thereby causing parts of the body (usually those in the lower or dependent portions of the body) to swell. This condition is called *edema.*

Intake

The amount of water entering the body as part of foods and beverages varies according to individual diet preferences, but averages about 2.5 quarts (2,400 ml) each day. Foods such as meat, potatoes, and vegetables contribute approximately 1 quart of the daily fluid intake. Water intake from beverages depends upon personal habits such as stopping at water fountains, drinking with meals, sipping while studying or watching television, and so forth. In addition to the water intake from foods and beverages, approximately 1 cup (240 ml) of water is formed within the body from an average adult daily diet during the energy-releasing process (Chapter 5).

Output

Approximately 1 quart (960 ml) of water leaves the body daily through the lungs, skin, and gastrointestinal tract, without our being aware of it. Some water is excreted in feces, but most of the water the body loses is in the form of urine.

Lungs. A surprisingly large amount of water— approximately 200 to 500 millilitres (ml) per day— is contained in the air that is exhaled from the lungs. Only on a cold day, or when one breathes on a cold window pane or a mirror, does this lost water become visible.

Skin. Water is lost from the skin as perspiration, or sweat, in varying amounts that depend upon certain conditions. Evaporation of sweat is most effective when the surrounding air is cooler than the skin temperature, when humidity is low, and when air velocity is high—such as when you sit in front of a fan or ride a motorcycle. Sweating increases during exercise, especially in a hot, humid environment. Sweat may evaporate in a dry climate without accumulating sufficiently to be noticed, or it may soak the clothing and drip off the brow. Only sweat lost through evaporation (rather than dripping) lowers the body temperature. When one gram of body water lost as sweat evaporates, 0.59 Calorie of heat is removed from the body. When a person is resting in a comfortable environment, about 25 percent of the total amount of heat lost from the body is due to the evaporation of sweat and the water exhaled from the lungs.

Feces. Water is normally lost in the feces at the rate of about 100 to 200 millilitres per day. However, severe diarrhea can cause a shift of water from intracellular to extracellular compartments and then into the gastrointestinal tract. The resulting cellular dehydration and increased cellular ion concentration can seriously alter the body's internal balance. When these conditions become extreme, as in *cholera* and similar intestinal (*enteric*) infections, death may result.

Urine. The volume of water excreted as urine approximately parallels the water intake from beverages. The water lost from the lungs, skin, and gastrointestinal tract is about equal to the water consumed in solid food together with the water formed from macronutrients during the energy-releasing process. A minimum of approximately 600 millilitres of urine must be formed in order for the body to have enough fluid to dissolve toxic waste products and rid itself of them.

Contrary to popular opinion, the smaller the volume of urine excreted per day, the greater the work load on the kidneys (under normal conditions). Therefore, it is recommended that a normal individual consume sufficient fluids to assure a urine output of at least twice, and preferably three times, the minimum volume required to dissolve all wastes, salts, toxins, and so forth. For an average-sized person, this volume amounts to between 1,200 and 1,800 millilitres of urine every 24 hours.

Composition of Urine

Urine is usually about 96 percent water, but its concentration varies greatly in response to fluid intake, loss of water by other routes, and body waste production. Of the total amount of substances dissolved in urine, about half is *urea* (Table 7-1), a nitrogen-containing product formed from amino acid breakdown. A high-protein diet, which causes the production of more urea than do other diets, requires greater urinary volume to carry this breakdown substance out of the body. One hazard of a high-protein weight-reduction diet is the buildup of urea and other protein wastes in the body; this hazard becomes more threatening if the dieter fails to drink an increased amount of water.

Other nitrogen-containing waste products in urine are *ammonia* and *creatinine*. The urinary component *uric acid* is formed from the breakdown of the DNA and RNA of cells that die.° Urine also contains several grams of sodium, potassium, chloride, sulfur, and phosphorus, and smaller quantities of calcium, magnesium, and other minerals. Normally urine contains little or no protein or glucose.

The amount of vitamins in urine depends upon body stores and the quantity of vitamins consumed. The body can store only small amounts of water-soluble vitamins and most minerals. Therefore, people who eat an adequate diet but who prescribe for themselves supplements of water-soluble vitamins and minerals, are simply channelling these micro-

° Abnormalities in the breakdown of RNA and DNA nucleotides result in the condition called gout. Excessive turnover (replacement) of cells, as in psoriasis or malignancies, results in excessive production of uric acid and in the possibility of kidney or bladder stones.

Within the kidneys, the components of blood that are not needed or are potentially harmful are separated from the components of blood that should be retained by the body.

TABLE 7-1. Normal Constituents of Urine

Substance	Amount Excreted Daily (grams)
Nitrogen-containing substances	
Urea	20.0–35.0
Creatinine	1.0–1.5
Ammonia	0.4–1.0
Uric acid	0.5–0.8
Minerals	
Chloride	10.0–15.0
Sodium	2.0–5.0
Sulfur	2.0–5.0
Phosphorus	2.0–2.5
Potassium	1.5–2.5
Calcium	0.1–0.3
Water-soluble vitamins	Variable; depends upon amount consumed and person's nutritional status
Macronutrients	Normally none, but small amounts of glucose may be excreted after a meal very high in carbohydrate
Total Solids	55.0–70.0

nutrients from the mouth to the blood, to the kidneys, and into the urine. Their bodies get no benefits from these excessive vitamin intakes, and the money spent on these supplements buys nothing but vitamin- and mineral-rich urine.

Kidney Function

Urine excretion is far more complex than a simple dumping of extra water and waste products not needed by the body. Strange as it may seem, excretion can be compared to the work involved in panning for gold. In both cases, there is first a mixture containing some compounds that one wants to keep, and some that must be discarded. Gold is mixed in creek water with pebbles and mud; glucose, protein, amino acids, and other vital chemicals are mixed in the blood with waste products and potentially toxic materials. The separation of the wanted from the unwanted components of blood occurs in the approximately one million filtering units, called *nephrons*, of each kidney (Figure 7-4).

The first separation step is filtration, where larger molecules are segregated from smaller ones. Liquid is filtered through the pores of the tuft of blood vessels in each kidney nephron and into a cup surrounding the tuft. The blood cells and larger molecules, such as most proteins, remain within the blood of the tuft because they are too big to pass through the pores of the blood vessels. Water and small molecules, both good and bad, cross over into the urinary collection tubules to form *urinary filtrate*.

The second separation step represents a "fine-tuning" of the filtrate. The urinary filtrate flows through a series of microscopic urinary tubules that are closely intertwined with blood capillaries. It thus collects further wastes, and at the same time

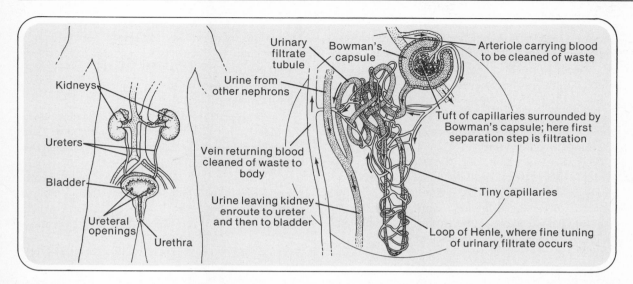

Figure 7–4. The human excretory system and an enlarged diagram of a kidney nephron. (Adapted with permission of Macmillan Publishing Co., Inc. from *Man and the Natural World* by C. J. Goin and Olive B. Goin. Copyright © 1970 by Coleman J. Goin and Olive B. Goin.)

useful materials are reabsorbed by the tubule cells out of the filtrate and returned to the blood. As the urinary filtrate flows down and then back up through the loop of the urinary tubule, important substances are almost fully recovered and greater amounts of wastes are added. This is the process called countercurrent exchange, whereby wastes are moving into the filtrate from one direction and other substances are being recovered in the opposite direction of flow. By the time the filtrate leaves the loop, it has the characteristics of urine. Ultimately, the filtrates from the two million nephrons flow together into the bladder and are excreted through the urethra (Figure 7-4).

This give-and-take between the blood and the urinary filtrate is one of the most important processes for protecting the ion and acid–base balances within body fluids. The entire volume of blood in the body circulates through the kidneys and is cleaned up about 16 times every day. More than a quart (about 960 ml) of blood flows through the kidneys every minute, and about 10 percent of the fluid of blood goes into the initial urinary filtrate. The total daily filtrate volume in the first separation step weighs more than twice as much as the body. Fortunately, about 99 percent of this filtrate is absorbed back into the blood by the tubule cells of the kidneys.

Effects of Alcohol

The volume of urine excreted is determined partly by how much of the water in the urinary filtrate is reabsorbed by the tubule cells and returned to the blood. The rate of body water retrieval by the kidney tubule cells is accelerated by a hormone called ADH (antidiuretic hormone), which is synthesized in the hypothalamus and stored in the pituitary gland at the base of the brain. Alcohol blocks this hormone and thus decreases the amount of filtrate water that is brought back into the blood by the tubule cells. Therefore, the rate of urine excretion is increased by alcohol.

The thirst that a person may experience on the

morning after a drinking bout is the physiological sign that the body needs more fluid to compensate for excess urine lost the night before. Since the alcohol in beer is accompanied by more water than is the alcohol in hard liquor, thirst is less after a beer party than after drinking low-volume cocktails, although the quantity of alcohol consumed may be the same in both cases.

The effect of alcohol on the excretion of body water explains why drinking alcoholic beverages could make worse the fate of a person who has limited access to drinking water. For example, whiskey has no place in the rations of people who might be stranded in a lifeboat.

Effects of Sodium

Salty foods such as ham, pretzels, and potato chips affect urination much as do alcoholic beverages but for different reasons. The body rids itself of excess sodium by filtering it into the urine. This movement of sodium, however, must be accompanied by water molecules, thus increasing the volume of urine excreted. At the same time, the initially high sodium content of the blood stimulates the thirst center of the brain. More fluids are consumed, thus providing the water necessary for urinary excretion of sodium.

Water Deprivation

The most serious complications of water deprivation are cellular dehydration and accumulation of toxic waste products. Rapid water loss may accompany certain conditions such as diarrhea and vomiting.

A baby is especially vulnerable to dehydration. The body of an infant contains a higher percentage of water (about 75 percent) than does an adult's. However, since the total body water content of an infant is relatively small, babies cannot tolerate as great a water loss as can adults. Furthermore, the ratio of an infant's body surface to body weight is greater than this ratio is for an adult. Therefore, water loss due to fever and excessive perspiration from the skin can be much more dangerous for a baby than for an adult.

Water deprivation is potentially hazardous for the elderly, because the percentage of body water normally decreases as people grow older. Diarrhea caused by food poisoning might be fatal to an older person, whereas a young adult who ate the same contaminated food might survive. (Other factors, such as heart disease or diabetes in an older person, also affect survival rates in the face of dehydration.)

ACID–BASE BALANCE IN BODY FLUIDS

The concentration of many substances in body fluids can vary within certain limits without creating a hazard for normal performance of body functions. For most constituents of blood, there is an upper and a lower limit to what is considered a safe concentration level. Some substances, such as blood glucose, may vary 200 percent; others, such as blood calcium, have a narrower range—about 20 percent—of safe variability.

The balance between the acidic and the alkaline (basic) components of body fluids cannot vary beyond a very narrow range, and must be carefully controlled at all times. If the acid–base balance fluctuates outside safe limits, the consequences to the body are serious.

The acidity or alkalinity of any solution is related to the hydrogen ion concentration, which is measured on a logarithmic scale of pH units ranging from 0 (most acid) to 14 (most alkaline). The midpoint of 7.0 represents neutrality—neither acidic nor alkaline. Blood is normally within the narrow range of 7.35 to 7.45—slightly alkaline (Figure 7-5). Outside the range of 7.0 to 7.6, life is threatened. A blood pH of less than 6.8 or greater than 7.8 is almost always fatal.

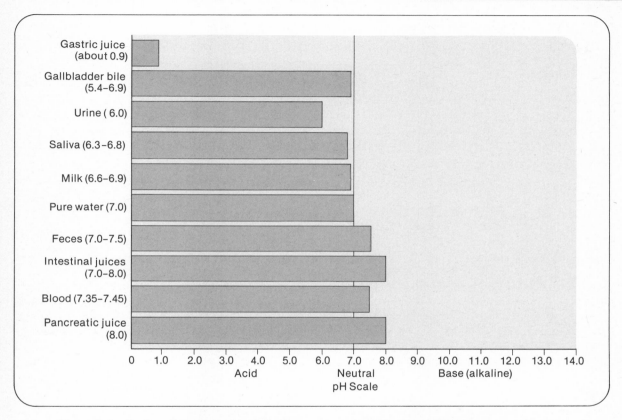

Figure 7–5. On the pH scale most body fluids are concentrated in the middle range, near neutrality.

Consequences of Imbalance

The ill effects of an abnormal blood pH are not caused by macronutrient destruction—the damage is not analogous to what occurs under the more extreme conditions of acidity and alkalinity during digestion. Rather, a high or low pH of blood or tissue fluids impairs body functions because the enzymes that facilitate metabolic reactions can operate optimally only in solutions of a specific alkalinity. As the pH of body fluids deviates from normal, enzyme-catalyzed reactions take place more slowly—synthesis of specialized molecules de-

creases, production of high-energy ATP molecules is impaired, intermediate metabolic products accumulate—and ultimately the entire metabolic machinery of the body breaks down.

Balancing Mechanisms

The alkalinity of body fluids is determined by the relative concentrations, or balance, of positively charged hydrogen ions (H^+) and several types of negatively charged ions, including bicarbonate (HCO_3^-). When hydrogen ions predominate, the

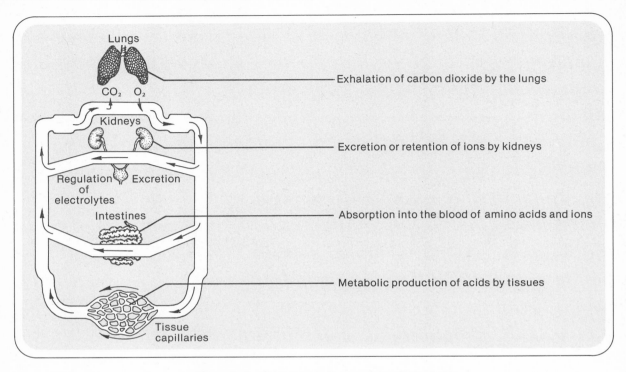

Figure 7-6. Mechanisms for the control of body pH.

fluid is acidic; when bicarbonate and similar ions predominate, the fluid is alkaline. The balance between these ions is affected by several mechanisms:

1. Excretion or retention of ions by the kidneys
2. Metabolic production of acids by tissues
3. Concentration of proteins in the blood
4. Exhalation or retention of carbon dioxide by the lungs

These mechanisms are illustrated in Figure 7-6.

Excretion or Retention of Ions. One way of maintaining the balance between hydrogen ($+$) and bicarbonate ($-$) ions is for the kidneys to excrete selectively whichever ion occurs in excess and to retain the other ion. Although the excretion of posi-

tively charged ions (cations) must be accompanied by equal numbers of opposite ion charges (anions), the kidneys are able to select from a large variety of each type so as to maintain ionic balance while correcting acid–base imbalances. This is because different types of ions have different degrees of acidity or alkalinity and different numbers of charges.

Metabolism. Many nutrients and intermediate metabolic products are acids. Fatty acids, pyruvate (pyruvic acid), and lactate (lactic acid) all contribute hydrogen ions to body fluids and thus increase the acidity of these fluids. The acid–base balance is therefore affected by the production, breakdown, or accumulation of these acids that are intermediate products of macronutrient metabolism.

The pH of body fluids is affected by excretion through the kidneys, release of carbon dioxide through the lungs, metabolism, concentration of proteins and other ions in body fluids, diet, and drugs.

Proteins. The many amino acids that are found in the body are categorized as acidic, alkaline, or neutral, depending upon whether their R groups donate or accept hydrogen ions when they dissolve in water. The ability of the R groups of their amino acids to donate or receive hydrogen ions enables proteins to play a major role in helping to buffer or maintain the body's acid-base balance.

Exchange of Carbon Dioxide. Carbon dioxide from the air we breathe and carbon dioxide produced during Phase II of the energy-releasing process can combine with the water of blood or of tissue fluids to form *carbonic acid.* This acid is very weak, but it can dissociate to form positively charged hydrogen ($+$) and negatively charged bicarbonate ($-$) ions. This chain of events is reversible—it can proceed either toward the formation of hydrogen and bicarbonate ions, or toward the formation of carbon dioxide and water.

$$H_2O + CO_2 \rightleftharpoons H_2CO_3 \rightleftharpoons H^+ + HCO_3^-$$

At any given moment, the reaction will proceed in the direction that produces end-products that are then needed in the body fluid. (These reactions depend on the presence of a zinc-containing enzyme called *carbonic anhydrase.*)

When you breathe hard and rapidly from strenuous exercise such as running up a long flight of stairs, carbon dioxide leaves your body rapidly in the air you exhale. The preceding reaction is therefore moving from right to left. The quickest way for the body to get rid of excess hydrogen ions (those produced by the energy-releasing process accelerated during exercise) is to combine them with bicarbonate, if it is available, forming carbonic acid, which can be converted to water and carbon dioxide. Carbon dioxide is easily released from blood in the lungs, and exhaled.

When you hold your breath while swimming under water, carbon dioxide that is produced in muscles builds up in the blood—it cannot be exhaled from the lungs while you hold your breath.

The high levels of carbon dioxide cause the reaction to proceed from left to right—toward the formation of hydrogen ions—and the acidity of the blood increases. Increased acidity and increased carbon dioxide dissolved in blood tend to impair metabolic reactions, especially energy release, and so fatigue sets in quickly. A good swimmer therefore learns to coordinate his or her breathing so as to prevent carbon dioxide buildup.

Breathing into a paper bag or holding your breath to try to stop hiccups is another way to increase carbon dioxide in the blood. This maneuver shifts the reaction in the acid direction. The consequent change in blood pH stops the muscle spasms of hiccups by altering the calcium balance at the irritable site in the muscle of the diaphragm.*

Dietary Influences. Certain foods increase or decrease the alkalinity of blood. Acid-forming foods include meat, poultry, fish, eggs, cheese, legumes, cereals, cranberries, plums, prunes, almonds, chestnuts, and coconuts. Alkali-forming foods include most fruits, vegetables, milk, peanuts, and walnuts. Normally the body can compensate easily for any slight shift caused by eating these foods, but they might occasionally affect a person who is ill with a condition accompanied by disturbance of the acid–base balance mechanisms.

Collaborative Action. Normally the lungs and the kidneys work together quickly to neutralize or excrete excess acidic or alkaline ions. The body has an enormous capacity to absorb excesses of either type of ion without the body pH being changed significantly, whether the excess results from dietary sources, breath-holding, exercise, drugs or toxins, disease, or any other factor. The capacity of pro-

*Emphysema and other lung diseases cause the blood to become more acidic than normal. This shift in pH is due either to a decreased number of functioning air sacs through which carbon dioxide can diffuse from the blood and out through the lungs, or to the inability of the lungs to exchange their "stale" carbon dioxide-laden air freely with atmospheric or fresh air.

teins and of ions such as bicarbonate to maintain acid–base balance, and the capacity of the lungs and kidneys to regenerate these ions, represent a complex and integrated series of processes only touched on in this chapter. The interested student is referred to textbooks in physiology for a fuller discussion of this topic.

STUDY QUESTIONS

1. Why is lack of water life-threatening?

2. Why is the water content of a woman's body less than that of a man who weighs the same?

3. Why are babies and elderly people particularly sensitive to water deprivation?

4. How does the ion composition of intracellular fluid differ from that of extracellular fluid?

5. In what metabolic and physiological processes does water play a role?

6. Under what conditions does edema or dehydration occur?

7. Why does urine composition change when protein intake increases?

8. How is urine formed from the components of blood?

9. How do alcohol and sodium cause increased urine output?

10. What processes control the pH of body fluids?

SUGGESTED READING

1. J. R. Robinson, "Water, the indispensable nutrient," *Nutrition Today* 5(1970):16.

2. J. Mayer, "Water: You can't live without it," *Family Health* 6(1974):27.

3. G. R. Meneely and H. D. Battarbee, "Sodium and potassium," Chapter 26 in *Present Knowledge in Nutrition*. 4th ed. New York and Washington, D.C.: The Nutrition Foundation, 1976.

4. "Water and electrolytes in malnutrition," *Nutrition Reviews* 33(1975):74–75.

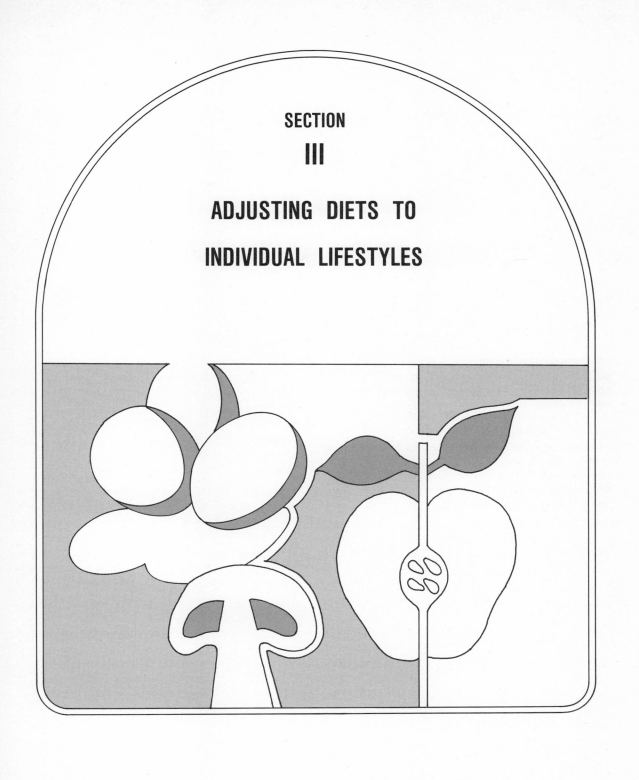

SECTION

III

ADJUSTING DIETS TO

INDIVIDUAL LIFESTYLES

ADJUSTING DIETS TO

INDIVIDUAL LIFESTYLES

The concepts presented in the preceding chapters laid the groundwork for making food choices that meet physiologically defined needs. Mastering this information is comparable to memorizing multiplication tables, but nutrition, like math, yields the greatest benefits when it is actually used in our daily lives.

In this section we begin to put nutrition knowledge into practice. We discuss the conditions and situations that affect the food choices of an individual—regardless of age or sex. (Adjustment of the diet during the lifespan is the subject of Section IV of this book.)

CHAPTER 8 FOOD SELECTION GUIDES considers the amounts of nutrients and energy recommended for different groups of people and how these recommended intakes can be met by choosing the appropriate variety and amounts of food.

CHAPTER 9 ADJUSTING DIET TO BODY WEIGHT AND ACTIVITY discusses how to adjust your diet to the amount of exercise you get and to your body weight.

CHAPTER 10 SNACKING AND EATING OUT shows how to select the diet you need if your way of life means that some foods are eaten as snacks or mini-meals and if you frequently eat away from home.

CHAPTER 11 STRETCHING THE FOOD BUDGET shows how to select an economical diet—low in price but nutritionally appropriate.

CHAPTER 12 DIET AND PERSONAL PRIORITIES suggests how to use nutritional criteria when selecting from among the foods you prefer because of your own value system.

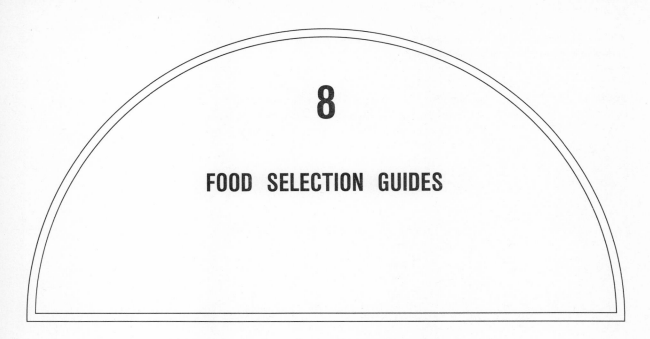

8

FOOD SELECTION GUIDES

The preceding chapters that described the metabolic and physiological functions of nutrients may motivate you to seek a diet that supplies the proper amounts of energy and essential nutrients. To obtain this type of diet, you must know how much of these nutrients you need and how to get the appropriate amounts and types of these nutrients from the foods that fit your way of life. In this chapter we discuss several ways to plan your food selections to meet your nutrient needs.

RECOMMENDED DIETARY ALLOWANCES

"How much of each nutrient do I need?" The best available guide for approaching an answer to this question is the Recommended Dietary Allowances, commonly referred to as the RDA (Table 8-1). This standard contains about 400 numbers—the amounts of energy, protein, 10 vitamins, and six minerals recommended daily for 15 groups of people, males and females of all ages. Because the RDA is the basis of several simpler and more convenient food selection guides, it is important to understand both the derivation and the appropriate application of the RDA.

Derivation of the RDA

The 125-page paperback book entitled *Recommended Dietary Allowances* (the eighth edition of which was published in 1974) tells how the RDA table should be used. It explains the scientific basis for the allowances for each nutrient. The RDA table is often misused because people fail to remember what is stated in the first chapter of this book:

> The Recommended Dietary Allowances are the levels of intake of essential nutrients considered, in the judgment of the Food and Nutrition Board on the basis of available scientific knowledge, to meet the known nutrition needs of practically all healthy persons.

These words were not chosen casually, and several of the phrases merit discussion.

"**. . . Levels of Intake of Essential Nutrients. . .**" RDA values refer to the amounts of nutrients actually eaten. No consideration is made for nutrients destroyed by improper storage and cooking or for nutrients in food that is served but not eaten. Furthermore, no allowance is made for the

The Recommended Dietary Allowances (RDA) are established by a committee of nutrition scientists and are revised periodically on the basis of the latest research.

TABLE 8-1. Recommended Daily Dietary Allowances[a]
Designed for the maintenance of good nutrition
of practically all healthy people in the United States

	Age (years)	Weight (kg)	Weight (lbs)	Height (cm)	Height (in)	Energy (kcal)[b]	Protein (g)	Vitamin A Activity (RE)[c]	Vitamin A Activity (IU)	Vita-min D (IU)	Vita-min E Activity[e] (IU)
Infants	0.0–0.5	6	14	60	24	kg × 117	kg × 2.2	420[d]	1,400	400	4
	0.5–1.0	9	20	71	28	kg × 108	kg × 2.0	400	2,000	400	5
Children	1–3	13	28	86	34	1,300	23	400	2,000	400	7
	4–6	20	44	110	44	1,800	30	500	2,500	400	9
	7–10	30	66	135	54	2,400	36	700	3,300	400	10
Males	11–14	44	97	158	63	2,800	44	1,000	5,000	400	12
	15–18	61	134	172	69	3,000	54	1,000	5,000	400	15
	19–22	67	147	172	69	3,000	54	1,000	5,000	400	15
	23–50	70	154	172	69	2,700	56	1,000	5,000		15
	51+	70	154	172	69	2,400	56	1,000	5,000		15
Females	11–14	44	97	155	62	2,400	44	800	4,000	400	12
	15–18	54	119	162	65	2,100	48	800	4,000	400	12
	19–22	58	128	162	65	2,100	46	800	4,000	400	12
	23–50	58	128	162	65	2,000	46	800	4,000		12
	51+	58	128	162	65	1,800	46	800	4,000		12
Pregnant						+300	+30	1,000	5,000	400	15
Lactating						+500	+20	1,200	6,000	400	15

[a] The allowances are intended to provide for individual variations among most normal persons as they live in the United States under usual environmental stresses. Diets should be based on a variety of common foods in order to provide other nutrients for which human requirements have been less well defined.

[b] Kilojoules (kJ) = 4.2 × kcal.

[c] Retinol equivalents.

[d] Assumed to be all as retinol in milk during the first six months of life. All subsequent intakes are assumed to be half as retinol and half as β-carotene when calculated from international units. As retinol equivalents, three fourths are as retinol and one fourth as β-carotene.

[e] Total vitamin E activity, estimated to be 80 percent as α-tocopherol and 20 percent other tocopherols.

fact that intake of certain nutrients varies more from day to day than does intake of certain other nutrients. Protein intake, for example, is relatively constant for each person, but intake of vitamin A may be double the RDA on a day when an average serving of liver, carrots, sweet potatoes, or spinach is eaten and low on a day when such foods are not eaten.

". . . In the Judgment of the Food and Nutrition Board. . ." Each edition of the RDA is prepared by an expert committee of the Food and Nutrition Board (FNB) of the National Academy of Sciences (NAS). New editions are published every five or six years. The numbers in the RDA table are decided upon after extensive review of the latest nutrition research and lengthy discussion by the scientists on

	Water-Soluble Vitamins							Minerals					
Ascorbic Acid (mg)	Folacin[f] (µg)	Niacin[g] (mg)	Riboflavin (mg)	Thiamin (mg)	Vitamin B$_6$ (mg)	Vitamin B$_{12}$ (µg)	Calcium (mg)	Phosphorus (mg)	Iodine (µg)	Iron (mg)	Magnesium (mg)	Zinc (mg)
35	50	5	0.4	0.3	0.3	0.3	360	240	35	10	60	3
35	50	8	0.6	0.5	0.4	0.3	540	400	45	15	70	5
40	100	9	0.8	0.7	0.6	1.0	800	800	60	15	150	10
40	200	12	1.1	0.9	0.9	1.5	800	800	80	10	200	10
40	300	16	1.2	1.2	1.2	2.0	800	800	110	10	250	10
45	400	18	1.5	1.4	1.6	3.0	1,200	1,200	130	18	350	15
45	400	20	1.8	1.5	2.0	3.0	1,200	1,200	150	18	400	15
45	400	20	1.8	1.5	2.0	3.0	800	800	140	10	350	15
45	400	18	1.6	1.4	2.0	3.0	800	800	130	10	350	15
45	400	16	1.5	1.2	2.0	3.0	800	800	110	10	350	15
45	400	16	1.3	1.2	1.6	3.0	1,200	1,200	115	18	300	15
45	400	14	1.4	1.1	2.0	3.0	1,200	1,200	115	18	300	15
45	400	14	1.4	1.1	2.0	3.0	800	800	100	18	300	15
45	400	13	1.2	1.0	2.0	3.0	800	800	100	18	300	15
45	400	12	1.1	1.0	2.0	3.0	800	800	80	10	300	15
60	800	+2	+0.3	+0.3	2.5	4.0	1,200	1,200	125	18+[h]	450	20
80	600	+4	+0.5	+0.3	2.5	4.0	1,200	1,200	150	18	450	25

[f] The folacin allowances refer to dietary sources as determined by *Lactobacillus casei* assay. Pure forms of folacin may be effective in doses less than one fourth of the recommended dietary allowance.

[g] Although allowances are expressed as niacin, it is recognized that on the average 1 mg of niacin is derived from each 60 mg of dietary tryptophan.

[h] This increased requirement cannot be met by ordinary diets; therefore, the use of supplemental iron is recommended.

SOURCE: Food and Nutrition Board, National Academy of Sciences-National Research Council, *Recommended Dietary Allowances,* 8th ed. (Washington, D.C.: National Academy of Sciences, 1974).

this committee of the various human and animal experiments.

"... On the Basis of Available Scientific Knowledge. . ." The number of nutrients that are considered essential keeps changing as more is learned about nutritional needs. The first edition of the RDA included only energy, protein, two minerals, and six vitamins; since 1943, many of the recommended allowances for these nutrients have changed on the basis of new research. Changes in America to a more sedentary lifestyle necessitated a reduction in the RDA for energy from 4,500 Calories for an active adult male in the early 1940s to only 2,700 Calories for an average adult male in 1974. (Since the need for thiamin parallels energy intake, the RDA for this vitamin decreased proportionately.)

In 1968, four vitamins and three minerals were

added to the RDA table. In 1974, an RDA for zinc was established and the values for several other nutrients were revised slightly. The current edition of the RDA discusses other nutrients that are known to be essential (such as copper, selenium, manganese, chromium, and molybdenum) but for which insufficient information exists to develop recommendations.

Allowances are determined primarily on the basis of the nutrient needs of healthy people. However, because research on human subjects is expensive and is limited by ethical considerations, allowances are also extrapolated from the results of animal experiments. As we noted in Chapter 2, for example, animal experiments indicate that nickel, tin, vanadium, and silicon are essential nutrients for some animals and therefore may also be necessary in human diets. Periodic changes in the RDA reflect the fact that knowledge regarding nutritional needs is constantly expanding.

". . . Practically All Healthy Persons. . ." The RDA values have been selected to meet, or even exceed, the nutrient needs of most individuals. The RDA takes into account not only the experimentally determined average requirement for a nutrient but also a statistically determined increase that allows for individual variation in nutrient needs.

The distinction between an *average requirement* and a *recommended intake* is an important concept. The average requirement is considered to be equal to, or greater than, the amount of a nutrient required by approximately half of the subjects studied in an experiment.* Statistical analysis of the results of the same experiment shows the percentage of the population that requires the nutrient in larger or smaller amounts, and how much more or less. The RDA are recommended intakes—they are higher than an average requirement. A very small percentage of the

population may require even more nutrients than the amounts stated in the RDA; most people actually require less than the RDA.

Let us look at the RDA for protein to clarify the distinction between an average requirement and an RDA (Figure 8-1). Human experimentation determined that the average daily protein requirement for a male adult is 43 grams of mixed animal and vegetable protein. In other words, it can be statistically predicted that if a thousand men each eat exactly 43 grams of protein daily, half of them have an adequate protein intake and half of them do not. Statistical evaluation of the data from the same experiments showed that increasing the average requirement by 30 percent (43 grams × 130% = 56 grams) would give a protein intake sufficient to meet the protein need of 97.5 percent of the adult male population. The RDA for protein for adult males was therefore set at 56 grams.

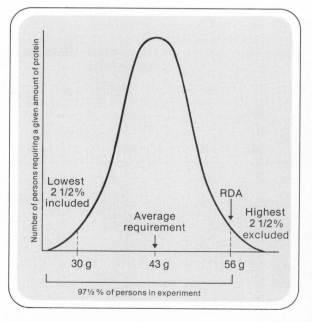

Figure 8–1. Protein requirements of a large population.

*This actually is the median value, not the mean value or arithmetic average.

The U.S. RDA was established by the Food and Drug Administration as a standard to be used for providing information on food labels about the nutritive value of a serving of food.

The U.S. RDA values are, in most instances, the highest values for any group of people shown on the RDA table.

The procedure for establishing the RDAs for energy is different from that for protein and micronutrients. The energy allowance is the lowest value thought to be consonant with good health. It is not an average requirement that has been increased to meet the needs of most of the population.

Use of the RDA

The RDA does not provide a definite answer about whether or not nutrient needs of an individual are met by a certain dietary intake. For example, if you eat 45 grams of protein daily, the only way to know whether your protein intake is greater or less than your protein requirement is to measure in a laboratory the nitrogen-containing protein waste products lost in your urine and feces. Such laboratory tests are rarely necessary. You should, however, keep in mind that, as the Food and Nutrition Board states, "the farther habitual intake of a particular nutrient falls below the RDA standard, and the longer the low intake continues, the greater is the risk of deficiency."

Although the RDA are not appropriate for determining the adequacy of individual daily diets, they can provide information regarding diets for groups of people. They can be used in various ways:

- Planning goals for projects such as the school lunch program
- Developing new food products
- Establishing standards for public assistance programs
- Studying trends in dietary intake
- Comparing the diets of different populations
- Designing human experiments to gain information about nutrient needs

U.S. RDA

The U.S. Recommended Daily Allowance (U.S. RDA) is the legal standard established by the Food and Drug Administration (FDA). It is used on the nutrition information panel on many food labels; its purpose is to inform shoppers about the nutritive value of foods. This is the most practical and accessible guide for comparing the nutrient content of a food to approximate nutrient needs of an adult. Although this guide is much less complex than the RDA, it can be misleading unless its derivation and proper use are understood.

Derivation of the U.S. RDA

The U.S. RDA (Table 8-2) is based on the RDA standard. The values are derived from the 1968 RDA, rather than from the 1974 RDA, because the 1974 edition of the RDA was published by the National Academy of Sciences during the development of the U.S. RDA standard by the FDA.

The 15 sets of values according to age group and sex in the RDA table were modified to give a single set of values in the U.S. RDA table. This single set of values applies to the entire U.S. population four years of age and over. The U.S. RDA is based on the highest RDA value for each nutrient given in any RDA category according to age and sex. Each value, therefore, is either equal to or greater than the RDA. An exception to this rule is that the U.S. RDA for calcium and phosphorus is an average of the RDAs for teen-agers (1,200 mg) and adults (800 mg). Another difference is that there are U.S. RDA values for three nutrients (copper, biotin, and pantothenic acid) not listed in the RDA. These U.S. RDA values are generally based on the average intakes of these nutrients by healthy people, as discussed in the RDA book. The percentages of the U.S. RDA that equal the 1974 RDA for each age/sex group are shown in Appendix Table A8-1.

Almost all foods on the market are labeled according to the adult U.S. RDA. Three other sets of U.S. RDA values (Appendix Table A8-2) are used for labeling products consumed primarily by infants, children aged one to four, and pregnant or lactating women.

TABLE 8-2. U.S. Recommended Daily Allowance (U.S. RDA)
(for use in nutrition labeling of foods)

Nutrient	Adults and Children over 4 years
Protein	65 g[a]
Vitamin A	5,000 IU
Vitamin C	60 mg
Thiamin	1.5 mg
Riboflavin	1.7 mg
Niacin	20 mg
Calcium	1.0 g
Iron	18 mg
Vitamin D	400 IU
Vitamin E	30 IU
Vitamin B$_6$	2.0 mg
Folacin	0.4 mg
Vitamin B$_{12}$	6 mcg
Phosphorus	1.0 g
Iodine	150 mcg
Magnesium	400 mg
Zinc	15 mg
Copper	2 mg
Biotin	0.3 mg
Pantothenic acid	10 mg

[a] If protein efficiency ratio of protein is equal to or better than that of casein, U.S. RDA is 45 g.

NOTE: Nutrients shown in italic type are required on all labels; inclusion of other nutrients is allowed but not required.

Use of the U.S. RDA

Although the U.S. RDA table states the recommended amount of each nutrient in grams, milligrams, micrograms, or international units, the consumer need not learn all these values. Food labels simply state nutrient content as a *percentage* of the U.S. RDA value. The reader must, however, keep in mind that the percentages of the U.S. RDA values given on packages are based on a *specific amount of food* noted on the label as the serving size (Figure 8-2). If you eat more or less than that amount, the percentage U.S. RDA of nutrients you consume is proportionately greater or smaller than the values stated on the label.

The U.S. RDA provide valuable information. They can help you do the following:

- Become familiar with dietary sources of specific nutrients
- Get an idea of the energy value of a food

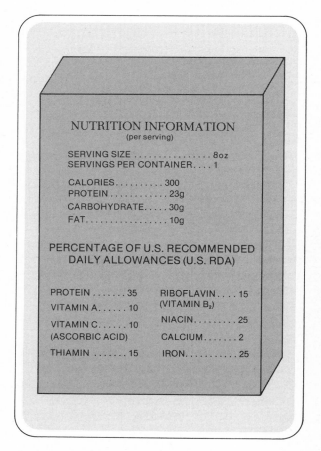

Figure 8–2. A sample label showing the nutrient content of a food.

relative to its protein, vitamin, and mineral content

- Compare the amount of a nutrient in different types of food or brands of the same product
- Plan meals that are nutritionally appropriate

For example, if you are considering two different foods, either of which might complete your dinner plans, U.S. RDA values on labels can help you select an iron-rich vegetable (such as lima beans) or one that is a better source of vitamin A (such as carrots), depending upon how much of these two nutrients have already been provided by the other foods chosen during that day.

The U.S. RDA is not practical, however, for totaling your daily nutrient intake to the last decimal point. There are several reasons for this:

1. Many food labels do not include nutrition information. Current FDA regulations apply only to foods if a nutrient is added to the product or if a claim is made by the manufacturer about the nutritional value of the product.

2. Most labels provide U.S. RDA information only for protein and seven micronutrients.

3. U.S. RDA values are not exact. They are rounded to the nearest 2 percent for values less than 10 percent; to the nearest 5 percent for values between 10 percent and 50 percent; and to the nearest 10 percent for values above 50 percent.

4. U.S. RDA values are higher than the corresponding (and more accurate) RDA values for many groups of people.

5. As with the RDA, one must still allow for nutrient losses in foods during storage and cooking, the variability in daily intake for some nutrients, and the need for trace minerals for which recommendations have yet to be developed.

The use of nutrition information on food labels is explained in greater detail in Chapter 29.

NUTRIENT DENSITY

Nutrient density refers to the ratio of nutrients to energy in a food. This way of evaluating foods was used as early as 1904 to express the "nutritive ratio" in rations for farm animals and it was applied to human diets in 1928. It is being used more widely in the 1970s as nutritionists seek precise ways of establishing criteria for comparing the nutritive values of foods.

The term *Index of Nutritive Quality* (*INQ*) was coined in 1973 as a way of expressing nutrient density.

$$\text{INQ} = \frac{\begin{array}{l}\text{Percent of the daily requirement for a specific}\\ \text{nutrient supplied by a quantity of food}\end{array}}{\begin{array}{l}\text{Percent of the total energy requirement sup-}\\ \text{plied by the same quantity of the same food}\end{array}}$$

If the INQ for a nutrient in a food is greater than 1.0, that food supplies relatively more of the nutrient (compared to the amount needed) than energy (compared to the amount needed). If the INQ is less than 1.0, the nutrient density of that food is below the nutrient density needed for the total day's diet.

Calculation of Nutrient Density

The percentages of U.S. RDA values for protein and several micronutrients given on food labels can be easily used in the numerator of the INQ formula. Since there is no U.S. RDA value for energy, you must consult the RDA table for the appropriate energy value for your sex and age.

Let's use the information given on the food label in Figure 8-2 to see how the system works for an adult woman and for an adult man. One serving of this food provides 300 Calories. From the RDA table we know that the energy value for adult women is 2,000 Calories; for men, 2,700 Calories.

$$\frac{300 \text{ Calories}}{2,000 \text{ Calories}} = 15\% \text{ of the energy needs of the average woman}$$

$$\frac{300 \text{ Calories}}{2,700 \text{ Calories}} = 11\% \text{ of the energy needs of the average man}$$

Therefore, the nutrients listed on the label at more than 15 percent of the U.S. RDA have an INQ greater than 1.0 for the adult woman, whereas those at a level greater than 11 percent have an INQ greater than 1.0 for the adult man.

Food Comparisons

Nutrient density calculations are helpful when comparing the merits of a food in the diet of people who have different energy needs, as we have seen for an adult woman versus an adult man. These calculations are also helpful for finding out which foods provide the most nutrients when consumed in calorically equal quantities. For example, Table 8-3 shows that broccoli has a higher vitamin C INQ than does asparagus, spinach, oranges, summer squash, carrots, or potatoes. However, spinach moves to the top of the list, as Table 8-3 shows, when these foods are ranked according to their vitamin A INQ. In other words, some foods are better sources of one nutrient, while other foods are better sources of another.

It is important to remember that INQ values do not tell you whether or not your nutrient needs are actually met by eating a certain food. That depends upon how much of the food you eat. For example, Table 8-3 shows that either a cup of summer squash or a baked potato provides about 36 percent of the U.S. RDA for vitamin C. However, squash that has a higher INQ provides fewer Calories per serving than does the potato.

Perhaps the most practical application of nutrient density is as an aid in the selection of food for people who choose to limit their energy intake. A person who is trying to lose weight needs to select foods of higher nutrient density. If a woman wishes to reduce her energy intake to only 1,000 Calories, she must select a diet that is twice as nutrient dense as she would need while eating 2,000 Calories each day. Her protein and micronutrient needs continue to be 100 percent of the RDA even though she may choose to cut her energy intake in half. Active

TABLE 8-3. Selected Foods Ranked According to Vitamin C INQ and Vitamin A INQ

	Vitamin C			Vitamin A	
Food	INQ*	Percent U.S. RDA per Serving	Food	INQ*	Percent U.S. RDA per Serving
Broccoli	134	270% per stalk (45 Cal)	Spinach, cooked	168	292% per cup (40 Cal)
Asparagus	49	63% per cup (30 Cal)	Carrot, raw	127	110% per medium carrot (20 Cal)
Spinach, cooked	48	83% per cup (40 Cal)	Broccoli	45	90% per stalk (45 Cal)
Orange	39	110% per orange (65 Cal)	Asparagus	20	26% per cup (30 Cal)
Summer squash	27	35% per cup (30 Cal)	Summer squash	13	16% per cup (30 Cal)
Potato, baked	9	37% per medium potato (105 Cal)	Orange	2	5% per orange (65 Cal)
Carrot, raw	8	7% per medium carrot (20 Cal)	Potato, baked	0	0% per medium potato (105 Cal)

*Based on an energy requirement of 2,300 Calories.

SOURCE: Adapted from R. G. Hansen, A. W. Sorenson, and A. J. Wittmer, "Index of Nutritional Quality Food Profiles" (Logan, Utah: Utah State University, 1975). © 1975, Utah State University. Used by permission.

people who use more energy (see Chapter 9) may select foods lower in nutrient density.

At this point in our discussion, we have two aids for selecting foods:

1. Percent U.S. RDA tells us how much of a nutrient (compared to approximately the amount we need) is provided by a specific amount—an average serving—of that food.

2. INQ tells us the most concentrated sources of nutrients. INQ values do not change, regardless of how much we eat.

THE BASIC FOUR FOOD GROUPS

The RDA, the U.S. RDA, and nutrient density values provide information related to nutrient needs and food selection, but none of these alone is a convenient guide for choosing a total daily diet without doing some arithmetic. Nutritionists have developed a daily food guide, based on the RDA, which (when combined with the other guides) can help you organize the thousands of available foods into a well-balanced diet. This guide sorts foods that are good sources of many of the same nutrients into one of four categories: fruits/vegetables, cereals, milk, and meat (Figure 8-3). Most people have already learned—perhaps in elementary school health class or through food advertising—about these categories. To make the system effective, however, several points must be understood concerning which foods and nutrients are in each group, the number of recommended servings from each group, and the serving sizes.

Sorting foods can be both simple and practical. The foods in the fruits/vegetables group are the ones you would expect from the group's name. The cereals group offers many options besides breakfast cereals. It includes the products made from enriched or whole-grain wheat, rice, and corn such as rolls, muffins, or biscuits. Pancakes, waffles, and pizza crust lend variety and flavor to this group. The milk group offers not only whole, low-fat, or

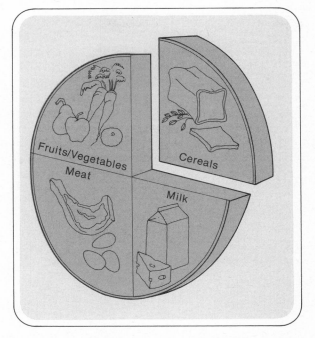

Figure 8–3. The basic four food groups—each is needed to make up a nutritionally adequate diet.

fat-free milk (whether fresh or dry), but also buttermilk, cheese, and yogurt. The meat group includes not only beef, pork, lamb, fish, and poultry but also eggs, peas, beans, and nuts.

Nutrient Profile of Each Group

The major nutrients provided in greatest concentration by each food group are:

- Fruits/vegetables—carbohydrate, vitamin C, vitamin A
- Cereals—carbohydrate, several B vitamins, iron, protein
- Milk—all three macronutrients, calcium, riboflavin, vitamin D
- Meat—protein, fat, iron, thiamin, riboflavin, niacin, vitamin B_{12}

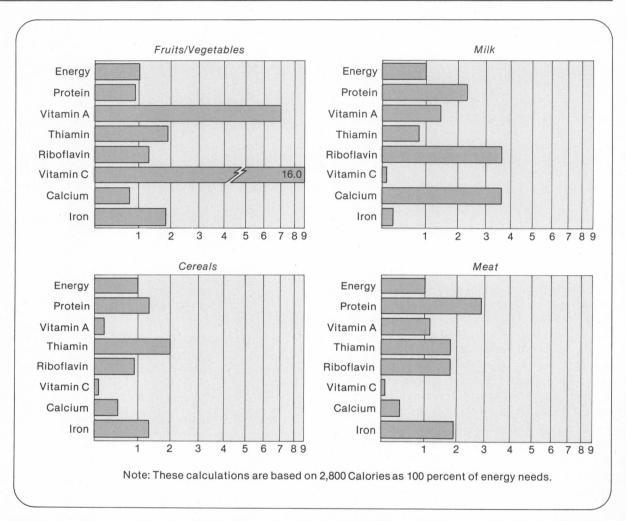

Figure 8–4. Average nutrient density of combinations of food in the basic four food groups. (Adapted from "Nutrient Density" by R. Gaurth Hansen, in *Nutrition Reviews* 31 (January 1973). © 1973, The Nutrition Foundation, Inc. Also used by permission of the author.)

Figure 8-4 shows the overall strengths and weaknesses of each group as indicated by the average INQ values of a combination of foods in each group. Although many nutrients are provided by more than one group of foods, omitting any one of the groups makes it difficult to get enough of certain nutrients.

Without fruits and vegetables, for example, it is almost impossible to get enough vitamin C. Avoiding cereal products makes it difficult to meet one's needs for iron, thiamin, niacin, and riboflavin. Peas, beans, and nuts are good sources of protein, iron, and many of the B vitamins found in meat; but since they do not contain vitamin B_{12} (obtainable only from foods of animal origin), they cannot substitute completely for meat products. Nondigestible carbohydrate is supplied by fruits, vegetables, cereals, and beans but not by meat or milk products.

Vitamin D comes almost exclusively from dairy products, but this food group is a poor source of iron and copper.

Number of Recommended Servings

For adults, the number of recommended servings is four (or more) of fruits/vegetables and cereals and two (or more) of milk and meat. This sequence can be coded as "4-4 and 2-2" for ease in remembering it.

Your four servings from the fruit/vegetable group should not be all fruits, which are generally not high in iron and calcium; many vegetables can contribute significant amounts of these minerals. Each day you should select from the fruit/vegetable group one good source of vitamin C such as citrus fruits, tomatoes, broccoli, Brussels sprouts, or spinach. At least every other day you should include from this group a food high in vitamin A. If you do not like spinach, sweet potatoes, summer squash, carrots, and the few other good vegetable sources of this nutrient, you may have a problem obtaining enough vitamin A in your diet and may need to look more carefully for sources of it.

Few people have trouble getting their quota of four cereal servings unless they avoid bread, thinking that it is fattening. A slice of bread supplies only about 70 Cal (294 kJ); it is the butter, margarine, mayonnaise, or jelly that increases the energy value of this type of food. In a similar way, breakfast cereals supply only about 120 Cal (500 kJ), but a tablespoon of sugar sprinkled on top adds another 45 Cal (190 kJ). Most of the Calories people associate with macaroni, noodles, or spaghetti come from the sauces added to them.

It is in the milk group that variations are made in the number of recommended servings depending on a person's age and physiological needs. The variations are as follows:

Children under 9	2 to 3 servings
Children 9 to 12	3 or more servings
Teen-agers	4 or more servings
Adults	2 servings
Pregnant women	3 or more servings
Nursing mothers	4 or more servings

For teen-agers, therefore, the basic four code is "4-4-4 and 2;" for children, it is "4-4-3 and 2."

Serving Size

The size of a serving for each food group can be approximated as shown in Table 8-4.

In the milk group, serving size equivalents of cheese and yogurt are based on the calcium content

TABLE 8-4. Approximate Serving Sizes for the Basic Four Food Groups

Food Group	Household Units	Metric Units
Fruits/vegetables	½ cup	120 grams
Cereals	1 ounce	30 grams
Milk	1 cup	240 millilitres
Meat	⅕ pound (approximately 3 ounces)	90 grams

TABLE 8-5. Meeting Nutritional Needs with Foods from the Milk Group

Portions of Milk-Substitute Foods	Calcium Equivalent of 1 Cup Milk	Fractional Equivalent
Cottage cheese, 1 cup	2 cups*	$\frac{1}{2}$
Cream cheese, 3 tablespoons	2 cups (32 T.)	$\frac{1}{10}$
Ice cream, $\frac{1}{2}$ cup	$1\frac{1}{2}$ cups	$\frac{2}{5}$
		Total 1 serving

*Calcium content of cottage cheese varies,; check the U.S. RDA value of the product you choose.

of each product. For example, the calcium provided by one cup of milk could be supplied by any one of the following: cheddar cheese, 1 inch × 1 inch × 2 inches; ice cream, $1\frac{1}{2}$ cups; or cream cheese, 2 cups. Fractions of servings added together can contribute to meeting nutritional needs for this group (Table 8-5).

Low-fat and fat-free milk contain all the vitamins, minerals, and protein of whole milk, but less fat and cholesterol; one glass of these beverages equals one serving from the milk group. Many dairy substitutes made from nonanimal products are low in fat and cholesterol, but you should compare the calcium, riboflavin, and protein content listed on the label of these products to see whether they can be counted as servings from the milk group. Similarly, before ordering a malt or shake at a fast-food establishment, you may want to ask the manager whether these drinks are made from milk there. Some fast-food restaurants sell malts and shakes that have a vegetable protein base and consequently have very little calcium, riboflavin, vitamin D, or other nutrients usually found in dairy products; other fast-food establishments include milk solids (which contain these nutrients) in their shakes.

In the meat group, the portion size of peas and beans must be larger than 3 ounces in order to be nutritionally equivalent to meat. One-half cup of dried beans equals one meat serving, but that equals about $1\frac{1}{2}$ cups of cooked beans. Two tablespoons of peanut butter, a more compact source of these nutrients, equals one serving. One-fourth cup of nuts or sunflower seeds provides about as much energy and protein as a serving of many types of meat.

Most fast-food restaurants serve 2 to 3 ounces of meat in regular hamburgers, the least expensive ones on the menu. An 8-ounce steak equals two servings of meat—all you really need from this group for an entire day if the rest of your diet follows the basic four guidelines.

Other Foods

Many frequently eaten foods are not included in any of the four food groups. These nutrient-dilute foods supply energy but few or no vitamins and minerals. However, they can improve the taste of foods in the four basic groups (Table 8-6). Butter, for example, helps make some vegetables more palatable; salads become more appealing with dressing; cream sauces are an important ingredient in many recipes. Other types of foods that dilute nutrients and add energy to the diet are harder to justify nutritionally, but they are important to some people for nonnutritional reasons. These include wine, cocktails, beer, soft drinks, hard candy, and cream and sugar with coffee or tea. The most common problem in many diets is overconsumption of nutrient-dilute foods. When people load their diet with these foods, either their total energy intake is excessive, or they fail to eat enough foods from the basic four groups to meet their nutrient needs.

TABLE 8-6. Energy Value of Nutrient-Dilute Foods

Nutrient-Dilute Food	Approximate Energy Value	
	(Cal)	(kJ)
Coffee with 1 t. sugar	20	84
Sugar on cereal, 2 t.	40	170
Soft drink, 12 oz.	150	630
Beer, 12 oz.	150	630
Whiskey, $1\frac{1}{2}$ oz. jigger	110	460
Mayonnaise, 1 T.	100	420
Blue cheese salad dressing, 1 T.	75	315
White sauce, $\frac{1}{4}$ cup	100	420
Tartar sauce, 1 T.	75	315
Fat for frying foods, 1 T.	100	420
Margarine or butter for vegetables, 1 T.	100	420

COMBINING FOOD SELECTION GUIDES

Each of the systems for selecting an adequate diet has certain advantages and limitations. Although none of the systems is perfect, the problems inherent in one guide can be minimized by using the others (Table 8-7). The following method, built around the basic four guide, is an example of how to use all four systems to plan a diet that meets your nutrient needs.

Build around the Basics

Although the basic four system is the easiest guide to diet planning, it does have some major problems:

1. Foods within each group have different INQ values for the nutrients primarily provided by that group.
2. Serving recommendations do not reflect the greater need for certain nutrients by some people (such as calcium for teen-agers and iron for women).
3. Some foods, such as pizza, overlap more than one group.
4. Specific guidelines for energy intake are not provided.

Let's see how we can deal with these problems.

Intragroup Nutrient Variations. We have already seen that the INQ for vitamins A and C of foods in the fruit/vegetable group vary, and that calcium INQ is different for milk and milk substitutes. Similar variations exist within the other two food groups. The U.S. RDA values of some food labels can help solve this problem. When comparing your food options within each group, you need not check every nutrient on the label; just concentrate on differences in the nutrients characteristic of a particular food group. For example, labels on canned or frozen fruits and vegetables can help you identify which foods are superior sources of vitamin A, which supply vitamin C, and whether or not calcium is provided.

Another example of how the U.S. RDA can help improve the basic four system is that you can easily identify which of two similar cereal products is enriched by comparing the percent U.S. RDA of iron, thiamin, niacin, and riboflavin on the labels of each. Within the milk group you can determine how much cheese is nutritionally comparable to a

Many of the problems inherent in the basic four system can be minimized by understanding the proper use and the limitations of the RDA, by using U.S. RDA values on food labels, and by learning which foods within each group have a nutrient density appropriate for you.

TABLE 8-7. Advantages and Limitations of Various Food Selection Guides

Food Selection Guide	Advantages	Limitations
RDA	Based on latest research Specific for age and sex Includes energy guide	Too complex to use in diet planning RDA not yet established for all essential nutrients (this limitation affects all guides)
U.S. RDA	Accessible on many food labels Much simpler than RDA	Not all foods labeled with U.S. RDA values Many nutrients not listed on labels No energy guide Not age and sex specific
Nutrient density	Helps adjust diet to individual needs for energy and nutrients needed in larger amounts by some people Shows which foods within each group are the best sources of certain nutrients	Does not tell whether total nutrient needs are met Initially requires pencil and paper to calculate values or accessible INQ tables
Basic four	Simple Based on RDA Takes into consideration several nutrients (such as folic acid and vitamins D and B_{12}) not on food labels	INQ variation within groups Little guidance for individuals with different nutrient needs Many foods overlap two or more groups No energy guide

glass of milk simply by looking at the calcium and riboflavin values if they are given on the label. Within the meat group U.S. RDA values are less accessible. At the time of this writing, labeling is rarely used for fresh or packaged meat. You must usually refer to food composition tables for the nutrient values of meat.

Individual Variations in Nutrient Needs The only way to handle this problem is to identify which nutrients are needed in higher amounts by men or women your age. Table 8-8 may be of some help; it is based on the RDA, but it gives the amount of nutrients recommended per 1,000 Calories (4,200 kJ), rather than in the total diet. If you scan each column vertically, comparing the value for your own group to values for other groups, you can determine which nutrients are needed in a higher density in your own diet. Planning appropriate diets for males and females throughout the lifespan is the topic of Section IV.

Overlap Foods in one group are often eaten in combination with foods from other groups—such as macaroni and cheese, sandwiches, pizza, cream soups, stews, chow mein, spaghetti and meatballs,

TABLE 8-8. Recommended Allowances per 1,000 Cal

Category	Protein (g)	Vitamin A (IU)	Vitamin D (IU)	Riboflavin (mg)	Thiamin (mg)	Calcium (mg)	Iron (mg)	Magnesium (mg
Infants								
0–5 months	18.6	2,000	570	0.57	0.43	510	14.0	86
5–10 months	18.5	2,060	412	0.62	0.52	560	15.0	72
Children								
1–3 yr.	17.8	1,540	308	0.62	0.54	615	12.0	115
4–6 yr.	16.7	1,390	222	0.61	0.50	445	5.5	110
7–10 yr.	15.0	1,370	167	0.50	0.50	333	4.2	104
Males								
11–14 yr.	15.7	1,790	143	0.54	0.50	427	6.4	125
15–18 yr.	17.9	1,666	133	0.60	0.50	400	6.0	133
19–22 yr.	19.2	1,666	133	0.60	0.50	267	3.4	117
23–50 yr.	20.7	1,850	147	0.59	0.52	296	3.7	130
51+ yr.	23.4	2,080	167	0.63	0.50	333	4.2	145
Females								
11–14 yr.	18.2	1,666	167	0.54	0.50	500	7.5	125
15–18 yr.	22.8	1,900	190	0.66	0.52	570	8.5	143
19–22 yr.	21.9	1,900	190	0.66	0.52	380	8.5	143
23–50 yr.	23.0	2,000	200	0.60	0.50	400	9.0	150
51+ yr.	25.6	2,220	222	0.61	0.55	445	5.5	157
pregnancy	31.7	2,080	167	0.63	0.54	500	7.5+	188
lactation	25.4	2,300	154	0.65	0.50	460	6.2	172

SOURCE: D. M. Hegsted, "Dietary Standards," *Journal of the American Dietetic Association* 66 (1975):13. Copyright The American Dietetic Association. Reprinted by permission.

and tacos. Nutrition labels may help when you buy these foods already prepared. When you prepare them yourself, however, the contribution these foods make to your 4-4 and 2-2 or (4-4-4 and 2 if you are a teen-ager) servings of the basic four probably will involve fractions based on your recipe, how much you eat, and some guesswork.

Energy Value. The approximate amount of energy you need can be ascertained from the RDA table, but this must be adjusted according to variables discussed in Chapter 3. Table 8-9 shows that the more nutrient dense foods selected from the basic four food groups—in the amounts designated—provide approximately 1,400 Calories (5,880 kJ). If you choose foods from each group that have the approximate energy value shown in Table 8-9, you can estimate how many "extra" Calories you might add to your diet and still not overeat. For example, a woman who needs 2,000 Calories of energy can consume approximately another 600 Calories of food in addition to the 4-4 and 2-2 basic four selections. A man who needs 2,700 Calories has an additional 1,300 Calories to use however he chooses if he takes care of his protein and micronutrient needs with 4-4 and 2-2 servings of nutrient dense foods.

TABLE 8-9. Approximate Energy Value of Nutrient-Dense Selections in Amounts Designated by the Basic Four System

Food Group	Number of Servings	Calories per Serving	Total Calories
Fruits/vegetables	4	50	200
Cereals	4	100	400
Milk	2	150	300
Meat	2	250	500
		Total	1,400

This energy may be acquired in several ways:

1. Larger portions or extra servings of the foods in the four food groups. For example, if you have an egg (70 Cal) for breakfast, two small hamburger patties (approximately 400 Cal) for lunch, a piece of chicken (approximately 200 Cal) for dinner, and one-fourth cup of peanuts (approximately 200 Cal) for a study break, then you have used about 870 Calories for five servings from the meat group. Since the basic four system calls for only two servings from this group, which provide about 500 Calories, the diet pattern just described uses up about 370 of your extra calories on foods from the meat group.

2. Selection of foods of lower nutrient density reduces the number of extra calories in your diet plan. For example, Table 8-9 allows 100 Calories per serving from the cereal group. The most nutrient-dense selection from this group is one slice of bread (approximately 70 Cal or 300 kJ); four servings of bread provide about 280 Cal (1,200 kJ). Suppose your selections from this group in one day are:

Toast	70 Cal
with ½ T. butter	50
and 1 T. jelly	60
Cereal	120
with 2 t. sugar	30
Sweet roll	250
Cake, 1 piece	300
Total	880 Cal

Then you are using approximately 480 Calories of your extra calories for nutrient dilute foods or food combinations from the cereal group.

Unless you are on a strict weight reduction diet, you have room in your diet for some extra large servings and nutrient-dilute foods. The important point is that you know how many Calories *you* can allot to them—it may be as low as 200 or 500 or as high as 1,500 (for very active people). After determining your own guidelines, be sure that consumption of these foods does not exceed the amount of energy you can use in this part of your diet. It is most important that nutrient-dilute foods not displace your 4-4 and 2-2 basic four servings.

Freedom and Responsibility. The system above is an example of the type of dietary freedom of choice possible if you know and use nutrition facts. Like all freedoms, however, it must be coupled with responsibility. This system works only if you select the appropriate amounts of foods from the basic four groups. Unless you are careful, your intake will exceed energy needs or you will fall short of meeting your needs for one or more nutrients.

Other Methods

If you are willing to take the time, you can daily tabulate everything you eat, add up the energy and nutrient content listed in food composition tables, and compare these values to your RDA.

Another approach is to carefully select enough sources of protein and vitamins and minerals. You may be able to eliminate some nutrients from your daily analysis if you habitually eat enough of the foods that supply those nutrients. For example, if you always have orange juice for breakfast, and meat and milk for both lunch and dinner, you can drop vitamin C, protein, and vitamin B_{12} from the list of nutrients you need to keep track of because you know that your needs for these three nutrients will be met by foods you habitually include in your diet. A limitation of this system is the lack of comprehensive food composition tables regarding the nutritive value of trace elements, folic acid, vitamin E, and several other nutrients.

Chapters 9 through 12 will provide many opportunities to practice ways of meeting nutrient needs depending upon individual circumstances. These examples and practice can help lead to whatever system or combination of systems works best for you.

STUDY QUESTIONS

1. How are Recommended Dietary Allowances (RDA) established?

2. If your dietary intake of riboflavin is only 90 percent of the RDA for your age-sex group, what does this tell you about the quality of your diet? What if it is 50 percent?

3. For what purpose was the U.S. RDA established?

4. How do the U.S. RDA values compare to the RDA values?

5. How can the nutrient density concept be used?

6. How did your diet yesterday compare with the number of servings recommended by the basic four system?

7. Describe the advantages and limitations of each food selection guide.

8. How can the problems inherent in the basic four system be minimized?

SUGGESTED READING

1. Food and Nutrition Board, *Recommended Dietary Allowances*. 8th ed. Washington, D.C.: National Academy of Sciences/National Research Council, 1974.
2. B. Peterkin, J. Nichols, and C. Cromwell, *Nutrition Labeling—Tools for its Use*. USDA Agriculture Information Bulletin No. 382. Washington, D.C.: U.S. Department of Agriculture, Agricultural Research Service, 1975.
3. A. A. Hertzler and L. W. Hoover, "Development of food labels and use with computers: Review of nutrient data bases," *Journal of the American Dietetic Association* 70(1977):20–30.
4. D. M. Hegsted, "Dietary standards," *Journal of the American Dietetic Association* 66(1975):13–21.
5. A. W. Sorenson, B. W. Wyse, A. J. Wittmer, and R. G. Hansen, "An index of nutritional quality for a

balanced diet," *Journal of the American Dietetic Association* 68(1976):236.

6. B. K. Watt, S. E. Gebhardt, E. W. Murphy, and R. R. Butrum, "Food composition tables for the 70's," *Journal of the American Dietetic Association* 64(1974):257.

7. E. F. Wheeler, "Who requires the requirement?" *Nutrition* (London) 29(1975):89–94.

8. D. H. Calloway, "Recommended dietary allowances for protein and energy," *Journal of the American Dietetic Association* 64(1974):157.

9. W. Mertz, "Recommended dietary allowances up to date—trace minerals," *Journal of the American Dietetic Association* 64(1974):163.

10. J. G. Bieri, "Fat-soluble vitamins in the eighth revision of the Recommended Dietary Allowances," *Journal of the American Dietetic Association* 64(1974):171.

11. M. M. Hill and L. E. Cleveland, "Food guides—their development and use," *Nutrition Program News,* U.S. Department of Agriculture (July-October, 1970).

9

ADJUSTING DIET
TO BODY WEIGHT AND ACTIVITY

Protein and micronutrient needs vary during our lifetimes and are different for men and women, but the RDAs for most nutrients do not change from day to day for the same individual. Your energy needs, on the other hand, might fluctuate considerably from one day to the next depending upon how much exercise you get. People who do not know how to adjust their diets to changes in energy needs are likely to be either overweight or underweight.

The information in this chapter can be used to help you (1) determine whether or not your weight is appropriate, (2) adjust your diet to changes in energy needs, and (3) lose weight (if you need to) while maintaining an adequate nutrient intake.

INDIVIDUAL VARIATION

An important part of applying nutrition knowledge is learning how to interpret for your own purposes the tables and charts that were developed for use with a general population. Such tables exist for both body weight and energy allowances.

Body Weight Reference Tables

A person's ideal weight is the one that is most conducive to health and long life. This weight cannot be found in body weight reference tables. Most such tables give average weights, which are not necessarily the same as ideal weights. For example, Table 9-1 is the table most often used as a standard of reference for weight by height and age, but it simply states the average weight of people (most of whom lived in urban centers on the Eastern Seaboard) who obtained life insurance policies at standard premium rates from about 1888 to 1905. The numbers do not take into account individual variables such as differences in body build; genetic, ethnic, or racial differences that influence body size, proportions, and rate of growth;° or differences in relative amounts of fat and muscle tissue.

___
° For instance, Black children have lower birth weights but later in life their average weights are equal to or greater than those of Caucasians.

Tables showing average body weights for heights can be used as guidelines, but they do not tell an individual his or her ideal weight.

Obesity means body fatness; it is most accurately measured by laboratory procedures or with skinfold calipers.

TABLE 9-1. Graded Average Weight in Pounds of Persons of Different Statures at Various Ages

Height, Inches	Age, Years							
	20	25	30	35	40	45	50	55
Men								
60	117	122	126	128	131	133	134	135
62	122	126	130	132	135	137	138	139
64	128	133	136	138	141	143	144	145
66	136	141	144	146	149	151	152	153
68	144	149	152	155	158	160	161	163
70	152	157	161	165	168	170	171	173
72	161	167	172	176	180	182	183	184
74	171	179	184	189	193	195	197	198
76	181	189	196	201	206	209	211	212
Women								
56	106	109	112	115	119	122	125	125
58	110	113	116	119	123	126	129	129
60	114	117	120	123	127	130	133	133
62	119	121	124	127	132	135	138	138
64	125	128	131	134	138	141	144	144
66	132	135	138	142	146	149	152	153
68	140	143	146	150	154	157	161	163
70	147	151	154	157	161	164	169	171
72	156	158	161	163	167	171	176	177

SOURCE: C. B. Davenport, *Body Build and Its Inheritance,* Publication 329 (Washington D.C.: Carnegie Institution of Washington, 1923). © 1923, Carnegie Institution of Washington. Used by permission.

Obesity and Overweight. The term *obesity* derives from the Latin verb meaning "to devour," and means overfat or excessive fatness. It is an index of *body composition* and not necessarily body weight for a specific height. Sedentary people can be excessively fat although their weight might coincide with the weight shown in reference tables for people of their height. In such cases, excessive fat tissue develops while muscle tissue wastes away from disuse.

Sometimes the term *overweight* is used for people whose weight is between 10 and 30 percent above the average shown in reference tables, while *obese* is reserved for persons more than 30 percent above the average. Another system classifies people as moderately obese if their weight is 25 to 50 percent above average, and grossly obese if 50 percent above the average. The percentage of Americans considered to be overweight in a recent government survey (see Chapter 13) is shown in Table 9-2.

Body fatness can be determined accurately by elaborate laboratory procedures that measure body density, water content, or the amount of a radioactive form of potassium (K^{40}) in the body. Equally useful information can be ascertained more easily

TABLE 9-2. Percentage of Obese People by Age, Sex, and Race, United States, 1971–72

Population	Age (years)	Percent Obese
Females		
Black	20–44	29.2
	45–74	32.4
White	20–44	18.9
	45–74	24.7
Males		
Black	20–44	10.6
	45–74	7.7
White	20–44	16.0
	45–74	13.4

SOURCE: *Preliminary Findings of the First Health and Nutrition Examination Survey, United States, 1971–72: Anthropometric and Clinical Findings,* U.S. Department of Health, Education and Welfare Pub. No. (HRA) 75-1229 (Washington, D.C.: Government Printing Office, 1975).

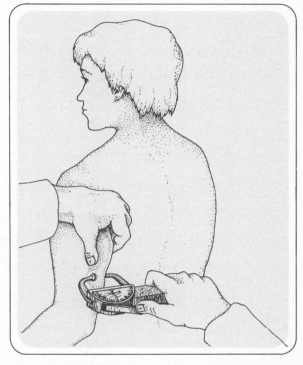

Figure 9–1. With a calipers, the thickness of a fold of skin plus subcutaneous tissue (but no muscle) is measured to the nearest millimetre. (Adapted from *Introductory Nutrition,* 3d ed., by Helen A. Guthrie.)

by comparing the length and circumference of arms or legs, and the dimensions of other parts of the body. A much more practical and sufficiently reliable measure can be made with calibrated pinchers called skin-fold calipers (Figure 9-1). A measure of the thickness of a fold of skin in several areas of the body provides a good index of body fatness.

The most convenient way to decide the appropriateness of your body weight might be called the "mirror test." It is hardly very scientific, but it can be more convincing than numbers from a chart. If you face yourself in front of a mirror without clothes selected to camouflage bulges and rolls, you probably do not need a weighing scale, reference tables or skin-fold calipers to tell you whether you are overweight. The advantage of the mirror test is that if you can be this honest with yourself about your weight, it will be easier to muster the self-discipline necessary to change the factors—dietary and nondietary—that caused the problem in the first place.

Underweight. Deviation from average weights in the direction of underweight is generally not as threatening to health or happiness as is overweight. Some range of weight below average values can indeed be compatible with health. The main danger in being moderately underweight is that the diets of such persons may be lacking in protein, vitamins, and minerals as well as energy. Underweight people who are very active and who select nutrient-dense diets may be eating enough of the right kinds of food to provide adequate nutrients even though their diets do not provide enough energy to main-

147

tain a normal body weight. Sedentary underweight people, however, probably are simply not eating enough food to provide either sufficient protein and micronutrients or sufficient energy.

Social Values. The values of a society play a large part in determining what is considered a desirable—though not always an ideal—body weight. Some cultures correlate fatness with prestige, respect, authority, and security, as well as beauty; others encourage people to strive for extreme leanness, perhaps influenced by fashions of dress. On a more philosophical basis, it is possible that in years to come leanness will be interpreted by society as an index of personal responsiveness to the world food problem and a willingness not to consume more of our limited food resources than each of us needs.

Within limits, you can select the body weight you prefer, for whatever reasons are personally meaningful. There is a point in both directions, however, when an increased probability of a detrimental effect upon health cannot be ignored.

Energy Needs

The values for energy needs in the RDA table (Table 8-1) provide a useful guide for estimating your energy needs. As we mentioned in Chapter 8, the energy allowance is the lowest value thought to be consonant with good health. It is not an average requirement that has been increased to meet the needs of most of the population. However, some people who follow these allowances gain weight while others lose weight. The Food and Nutrition Board states that many Americans are overweight and may require less energy than is recommended because they have sedentary living patterns.

Deviations from Average

From the above discussion of body weight and energy needs you can see that a body weight or an energy requirement that does not coincide precisely with standard tables is not necessarily cause for concern. These tables should be used as guides, not inflexible standards. Large deviations from them may indicate poor health, but small deviations should not be interpreted this way.

Fluctuations in body weight vary among individuals. For instance, a daily 500 Cal (2,100 kJ) deficit on the average will cause a person to lose 1 pound a week. If this does not work for you, it does not mean you should rush to a physician for fear there is something wrong with your metabolism; nor does it mean you should lose confidence in nutritional principles of energy balance. It simply means that you are not dead-center average—very few people are.

It is impossible to establish universal rules for what constitutes normal changes in body weight, yet each of us needs a semiquantitative handle for judging when to be concerned about weight deviations. If your weight changes rapidly, either up or down, an explanation should be sought. A gradual, but consistent, change in body weight should be taken as a warning, though not an alarm. You should also consider factors such as paleness, changes in hair, stomach pain or upsets, changes in character of stools, changes in emotional states, changes in menstrual pattern, and unusual localization of body fat. If these other warning signs occur, you should definitely seek medical help.

Pathological Causes of Weight Abnormalities

In most persons who are underweight or overweight, the cause is as difficult to identify as is the cause of smoking, though psychosocial factors probably underlie each condition. Apart from psychosocial disturbances, diabetes is the pathological condition most often associated with obesity. Still, obesity is more often the predecessor of diabetes than the converse.

There is a theory that obesity can result from glandular disturbances, such as an underactive thyroid gland (hypothyroidism), overactive adrenal glands (hypercortisonism or Cushing's syn-

Body weight changes when average daily energy intake does not equal average daily energy expenditure. Energy needs can be estimated using tables that show the amount of energy expended per hour (or minute) during various types of activities by a person of a certain body weight.

---

drome), or disturbance in growth hormone from the pituitary. Another more recently propagated explanation for obesity is that the appetite center in the hypothalamus of the brain or other brain centers have been damaged during birth or by infectious diseases. These conditions occasionally show up as causes of obesity, but even in persons whose obesity is traceable to such pathological conditions there are usually myriad other signs and symptoms of illness detectable by the physician.

It is impossible in this textbook to discuss fully the many potential causes of obesity and how to diagnose them. Suffice it to say that in the population at large, pathological conditions other than psychosocial disturbances are rarely identifiable as the cause of obesity. However, in each individual other causes should be sought through a careful medical examination by a competent physician at least once before any special diet therapies or practices are begun, and checkups should follow periodically until a desirable weight is attained.

ADJUSTING DIET TO ACTIVITY

A useful framework within which to begin practicing the application of nutrition knowledge is to examine situations that require modification of your diet because your activity pattern changes. Some circumstances that might increase your energy needs either now or later in life are:

- You start training for football, basketball, or track.
- You sell your car and start riding a bicycle.
- You move from a clerical job to a sales position.
- You retire from a desk job and begin working a garden and taking care of grandchildren.

On the other hand, your energy needs may decrease in any of the following situations:

- You have been active in school but take a desk job after graduation.
- You start playing bridge and stop giving tours of the art museum.

- You stop dating a dancer and start dating a movie fan.
- You stop waiting tables and start typing as a part-time job.

These specific situations may never occur in your life, but no doubt there will be other circumstances when you can put into practice the principles in the following discussion.

Estimating Changes in Energy Usage

A comparison of the way a college student lives during the summer versus during the school year can serve as an example of how to estimate changes in dietary energy needs.

Table 3-1 gives the rate of energy utilization attributable to specific activities—without including BMR and SDA (Chapter 3). This table is appropriate for identifying and calculating differences in energy needs due to changes in activity.

The procedure consists of several steps.

1. For two typical days—one in the summer and one during the school year—list your activities and their rate of energy expenditure (Table 9-3). Because not all of the activities in the two daily routines are listed in Table 3-1, we must guess at which activities are approximately equivalent to those for which energy expenditures are given. For example, energy expenditure while talking on the phone is probably about the same as that for reading aloud, whereas playing court tennis uses more energy than playing table tennis.

2. Omit activities that take about the same amount of time and energy on both days. In Table 9-3 we can therefore eliminate from our calculations time spent sleeping, dressing and undressing, and eating meals. Other cancellations can be made where the time and energy expended are the same even though the activities themselves are different. For example, we can cancel time spent changing clothes and snacking in the summer and browsing at the bookstore during the school day because both accounted for a half hour at 0.6 Cal/kg/h. Thanks to these cancellations, we need consider only 9 hours of activity (Table 9-4) instead of the entire 24 hours.

TABLE 9-3. Energy Expenditures (Exclusive of BMR and SDA) for Two Different Activity Schedules

	Summer				School		
Time	Activity	Total Time (hr)	Rate of Energy Expenditure (Cal/kg/hr)	Time	Activity	Total Time (hr)	Rate of Energy Expenditure (Cal/kg/hr)
7:00	Wake up			6:30	Wake up		
7:00	*Dress	1/2	0.7	6:30	*Dress	1/2	0.7
7:30	*Breakfast	3/4	0.4	7:00	*Breakfast	3/4	0.4
8:15	Bicycle to grocery	1/4	2.5	7:45	Walk to class	1/4	2.0
8:30	Stock shelves	1 3/4	1.4	8:00	Class	2	0.4
10:15	Coffee break	1/2	0.4	10:00	Walk to bookstore and to class;	1/2	2.0
					browsing at bookstore	1/2	0.6
10:45	Sweep	2	1.4	11:00	Class	1	0.4
12:45	*Lunch	1	0.4	12:00	Walk to apartment	1/4	2.0
1:45	*Cashier (standing)	1	1.0	12:15	*Lunch	1	0.4
2:45	*Break	1/4	0.4	1:15	Study	2 3/4	0.4
3:00	Stock shelves	1 1/2	1.4	4:00	Sit and talk at student center	1	0.4
4:30	Bicycle home	1/4	2.5	5:00	Eat dinner	1	0.4
4:45	*Change clothes; snack	1/2	0.6	6:00	*Watch TV and/or talk	1	0.4
5:15	Bicycle to courts	1/4	2.5	7:00	Study	1 1/4	0.4
5:30	Play tennis	1 1/2	5.5	8:15	*Drive to hamburger carry out	1/4	0.4
7:00	Bicycle home	1/4	2.5	8:30	*Eat	1	0.4
7:15	Help fix dinner	1/2	1.0	9:30	*Drive to apartment	1/4	0.4
7:45	*Eat dinner	1	0.4	9:45	*Type paper	1	1.0
8:45	*Wash dishes	1/4	1.0	10:45	*Undress	1/4	0.7
9:00	*Watch TV	1/2	0.4	11:00	Sleep	7 1/2	
9:30	*Talk on phone	1/4	0.4				
9:45	*Watch TV	1 1/2	0.4				
11:15	*Undress	1/4	0.7				
11:30	Sleep	7 1/2					

* Activities in one schedule that cancel out activities with similar energy values in the other schedule.

TABLE 9-4. Activities Contributing to Differences in Energy Needs for Two Different Activity Schedules

Summer			School		
Activity	Total Time (hr)	Rate of Energy Expenditure (Cal/kg/hr)	Activity	Total Time (hr)	Rate of Energy Expenditure (Cal/kg/hr)
Bicycle to grocery	¼	2.5	Walk to class	¼	2.0
Stock shelves	1¾	1.4	Attend class	2	0.4
Coffee break	½	0.4	Walk to bookstore and to class	½	2.0
Sweep	2	1.4	Attend class	1	0.4
Stock shelves	1½	1.4	Walk to apartment	¼	2.0
Bicycle home	¼	2.5	Study	2¾	0.4
Bicycle to courts	¼	2.5	Sit and talk at student center	1	0.4
Play tennis	1½	5.5	Study	1¼	0.4
Bicycle home	¼	2.5			
Help fix dinner	½	1.0			
Wash dishes	¼	1.0			
Total	9 hours		Total	9 hours	

A small imbalance between energy intake and energy expenditure can result in large changes in body weight if the imbalance continues for several months.

TABLE 9-5. Comparison of Total Energy Expenditures for Two Different Activity Schedules

Summer				School			
Activity	Total Time (hr)	Rate of Energy Expenditure (Cal/kg/hr)	Total Energy Expenditure (Cal/kg)	Activity	Total Time (hr)	Rate of Energy Expenditure (Cal/kg/hr)	Total Energy Expenditure (Cal/kg)
Coffee break	1/2	0.4	0.2	Attending class, studying, talking, eating	8	0.4	3.2
Fix dinner and wash dishes	3/4	1.0	0.75	Walking	1	2.0	2.0
Stocking shelves, sweeping	5¼	1.4	7.4			Total	5.2
Bicycling	1	2.5	2.5				
Playing tennis	1½	5.5	7.3				
		Total	18.15				

3. Tabulate the time during each day spent on activities that utilize energy at different rates. In the summer most of the entries remaining on Table 9-4 are at a rate of 1.0 Cal/kg/hr or more; on the school day most of the time is spent in activities that utilize only 0.4 Cal/kg/hr.

4. Calculate the difference in energy expenditure for the two routines. To do this, for each energy utilization category multiply the rate of energy expenditure times the hours spent; then add up all of these values (Table 9-5).

Energy expenditure was greater by approximately 13 Calories per kilogram of body weight during the summer. This may not sound like a large difference, but this equals 650 Calories for a person who weighs 50 kilograms (50 kg x 13.0 Cal/kg) or 910 Calories for a person who weighs 70 kilograms (70 kg x 13.0 Cal/kg). When these values are increased by 10 percent to compensate for SDA, the final values are between 715 and 1,001 extra Calories for people who weigh between 50 and 70 kilograms.

Dietary Adaptation

When you realize that changes in lifestyle affect energy needs, the logical response is to learn how to adjust food intake. The necessary diet modifications may seem small compared to total energy needs, but small imbalances can gradually add unwanted pounds.

Suppose, for instance, that a woman becomes accustomed to eating about 2,500 Cal (10,500 kJ) during the summer and maintains this food intake on campus when she is using only about 2,000 Cal (8,400 kJ) each day. The difference—500 Cal (2,100 kJ)—can lead to a weight gain of about a pound a week. No one notices this minor weekly increase, but by the time she changes to fall clothes, she knows that she is gaining weight. When she goes home for New Year's vacation, family and friends who have not watched this subtle accumulation of weight, are amazed to see the girl weighing 15 pounds more than when she left for college.

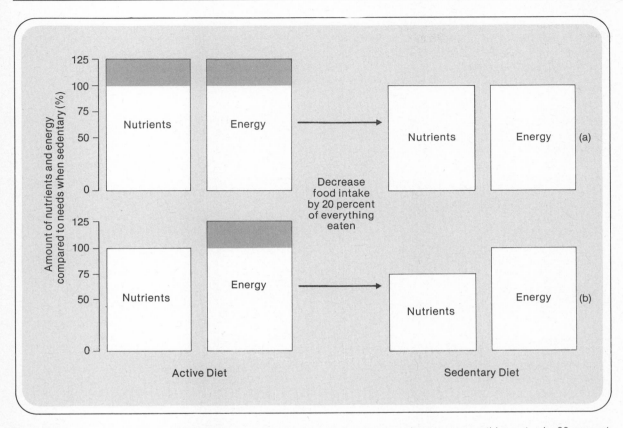

Figure 9–2. Effects upon nutrient adequacy of two different diets when a person decreases everything eaten by 20 percent.

This scenario need not happen to a person who knows and uses nutrition information. A crash diet could take off the pounds, but this method has several disadvantages:

1. It leaves you without a diet pattern to maintain your weight after the pounds are shed; you will undoubtedly slip back into the same cycle of gradual gain and crash diet.

2. Going on a strict weight reduction diet is an unpleasant experience. You feel hungry and often become unhappy, tired, and irritable.

3. Strict diets often require a change in lifestyle. People on such diets lack the energy to maintain routine activities, or their social life is restricted because they avoid the places and events where other people are eating.

Food intake can be reduced—before too many pounds go on—by any of several ways, alone or in combination. The main consideration in reducing energy intake is to ensure that your needs for protein and micronutrients are met by a diet that provides less energy.

Smaller Portions. If your current diet contains more protein and micronutrients than you need—for instance, 125 percent of your RDA for all nutrients, as shown in Figure 9-2a—you can reduce your

TABLE 9-6. Nutrient Density Variation

Food Group	Two INQs Characteristic of Group*		Combined INQs
Fruits/vegetables	Vitamin C	Vitamin A	
Spinach	48.0	167.0	215.0
Broccoli	134.0	45.0	179.0
Carrot	8.0	125.0	133.0
Strawberries	61.0	0.8	61.8
Tomato	40.0	19.0	59.0
Lettuce	23.0	32.0	55.0
Orange	39.0	2.0	41.0
Summer squash	27.0	13.0	40.0
Grapefruit	34.0	5.0	39.0
Sweet potatoes	6.0	26.0	32.0
Peach	7.0	17.0	24.0
Watermelon	10.0	10.0	20.0
Green beans	9.0	7.0	16.0
Potatoes, boiled	10.0	0	10.0
Corn, fresh	4.0	2.0	6.0
Potatoes, french fried	3.0	0	3.0
Apples	1.6	0.3	1.9
Applesauce	0.5	0.2	0.7
Cereals	Thiamin	Protein	
Bread, whole wheat	2.1	1.6	3.7
Oatmeal	2.2	1.4	3.6
Spaghetti	2.0	1.1	3.1
Rice, enriched	1.6	0.6	2.2
Corn flakes	1.6	0.5	2.1
Bread, rye	0.5	1.2	1.7
Corn muffin	0.8	0.8	1.6
Popcorn, plain	—	1.4	1.4
Brownie	0.7	0.4	1.1
Fig bar	—	0.7	0.7
Milk	Calcium	Riboflavin	
Milk, nonfat (skim)	7.6	6.6	14.2
Milk, lowfat (2%)	5.6	4.9	10.5
Yogurt made with skim milk	5.4	4.8	10.2
Milk, whole	4.1	3.5	7.6
Cheese, cheddar	4.2	1.5	5.7
Cheese, cottage	2.0	3.2	5.2
Ice cream	1.8	1.5	3.3
Sherbert	0.3	0.3	0.6

*Based on an energy requirement of 2,300 Calories.

SOURCE: From R. G. Hansen, A. W. Sorenson, and A. J. Wittmer, "Index of Nutritional Quality Food Profiles" (Logan, Utah: Utah State University, 1975). © 1975, Utah State University. Used by permission.

TABLE 9-6. Nutrient Density Variation (*continued*)

Food Group	Two INQs Characteristic of Group*		Combined INQs
Meat	Protein	Iron	
Liver, beef	4.9	4.9	9.8
Chicken, broiled without skin	6.2	1.6	7.8
Beef, lean hamburger	4.4	2.1	6.5
Tuna (drained)	5.0	1.2	6.2
Veal, roast	3.5	1.6	5.1
Beans, kidney	2.3	2.6	4.9
Egg	2.7	1.8	4.5
Lamb, roast	3.3	0.8	4.1
Pork, roast (lean/fat)	2.4	1.1	2.5
Beef, rib roast (lean/fat)	1.6	0.8	2.4
Frankfurter	1.5	0.6	2.1
Nuts, cashews	1.1	0.9	2.0
Peanut butter	1.5	0.4	1.9

energy intake by reducing everything you eat by about 20 percent. This is an easy way to reduce energy intake while not creating a problem with regard to protein, vitamins, and minerals. Under these circumstances, an across-the-board reduction in everything maintains the nutrient balance of your diet.

However, if your current diet barely meets your RDA for nutrients (Figure 9-2b), you must select a more nutrient-dense diet when you cut back your energy intake lest your nutrient intake fall below your RDA. Under these circumstances, most of the foods eaten in smaller portions must be those that primarily provide energy but small amounts of vitamins and minerals.

Increasing Nutrient Density. The nutrient density of your diet can be increased by making some substitutions within food groups and/or by cutting out some foods that primarily provide energy but little protein and few micronutrients.

Table 9-6 gives some examples of the range in nutrient density of foods within each food group.

Although each food group supplies several nutrients, the INQ's of only two primary nutrients per group are used as the basis for ranking foods in Table 9-6. A more extensive list of foods, along with their energy value per serving and the INQs of primary nutrients, is given in Appendix Table A9-1. Table 9-6 does not help you total your daily energy intake, but it can guide you toward the foods that supply the most nutrients per Calorie.

Fruits and vegetables are ranked in Table 9-6 according to the density of vitamin C and vitamin A; note, however, that few of these foods are concentrated sources of both. In the cereal group, thiamin INQ usually parallels the INQ of niacin, iron, and riboflavin, which are all added to enriched products; protein INQ is given as another indicator of the nutrient:energy ratio of these foods. In the milk group, calcium and riboflavin generally parallel each other in density. In the meat group, however, iron and protein are not always both high in the same foods.

The nutrient density of many foods depends upon the energy value of other foods consumed with

TABLE 9-7. Energy Value of Foods from Cereal Group and of Foods Commonly Added

Basic Food	Added Food	Energy Value of Basic Food (Cal)	(kJ)	Energy Value of Added Food (Cal)	(kJ)
Bread, 1 slice		70	300		
	Margarine, 1 T.			100	420
	Butter, 1 T.			100	420
	Mayonnaise, 1 T.			100	420
	Jelly			50	210
	Honey			60	250
Breakfast cereal, 1 oz.		120	500		
	Sugar, 1 T.			45	190
	Milk, ½ cup			75	320
	Raisins, ⅓ cup (1½ oz. pkg.)			120	500
Macaroni, 1 cup		190	800		
	Macaroni and cheese, 1 cup			430	1,800*
Noodles, 1 cup		200	840		
Spaghetti, 1 cup		190	800		
	Butter, 1 T.			100	420
	White sauce, ¼ cup			100	420
	Grated Parmesan cheese, 2 T.			50	210
	Chili sauce, ¼ cup			70	300
Pancakes, 3 four-inch		180	760		
	Butter, 1 T.			100	420
	Syrup, 1 T.			50	210
	¼ cup			200	840

*Value for combination of macaroni and cheese.

SOURCE: C. F. Adams, *Nutritive Value of American Foods in Common Units,* Agriculture Handbook No. 456 (Washington, D.C.: U.S. Department of Agriculture, Agricultural Research Service, 1975).

them—things added either in the kitchen or at the table. Many Calories can be saved by selecting items that taste good to you without having to add much butter, sugar, or nutrient-dilute sauces. Table 9-7 shows, for example, that the energy value of pan-

cakes is increased 150 Cal (630 kJ) by adding 1 tablespoon of maple syrup and 1 tablespoon of butter. Similarly, the energy value of boiled potatoes may be greater than for french fries, depending upon how much butter, sour cream, or bacon chips

Energy intake can be reduced by selecting smaller portions, choosing more nutrient-dense foods, omitting foods previously consumed in amounts greater than needed, and/or eating less frequently.

are added. The nutrient density of sweet potatoes is cut in half when butter and brown sugar are added.

Omitting Foods. Another way to reduce energy intake is to drop certain foods from your diet. Which foods should be omitted? The answer to this important question depends upon the total diet and how much your energy intake should be reduced.

The most likely candidates for omission are those that provide only energy, many of which are beverages, but this is not necessarily the only option. Suppose, for example, that an adult male who needs to reduce energy intake by 300 Calories is drinking each day three glasses of milk (150 Cal each) and two 12-ounce beers (150 Cal each). Cutting 300 Calories by omitting two glasses of milk makes it difficult to get enough calcium and riboflavin in the diet; cutting out both beers may be totally unacceptable to him. One solution, given that he will not abstain from beer, is to drop one serving of each beverage. The remaining two glasses of milk meet nutrient needs for an adult for this group of foods, and one beer may be an acceptable risk for a chance to take off excess weight as long as the remainder of the diet is wisely chosen. Making this type of decision takes some thought, but for some people it is worth the effort.

An easier way for this man to reduce energy intake may be to cut the necessary number of Calories from other foods besides beer that supply only energy. He can either reduce the amount he eats of several such foods or completely cut out a few, depending upon his food preferences and how quickly he wants to reduce.

Frequency of Eating. Another way to reduce energy intake is to stop eating so often. Frequency of eating depends mainly upon the pace for the day and the availability of food. The dormitory resident may not have access to a refrigerator—this alone might reduce total energy consumption. Regardless of housing facilities, however, there are always vending machines and foods that can easily be kept in the room. Practically speaking, decreasing the frequency of eating requires a conscious, voluntary change in food patterns. This type of dietary manipulation relies upon choices such as whether you go to the student center between classes; nibble while watching television; or eat on a study break.

WEIGHT REDUCTION

Many people reading this book are probably aware that they should reduce their weight and probably have tried many times to do so. The discussion to follow is not, however, written solely for these people. One area in which to apply nutrition knowledge is the prevention of obesity—a problem that may entangle even the slimmest young person at some point later in life. Knowing how to avoid becoming overweight is more important than learning how to correct the problem.

Causes of Overweight

The first step in correcting or preventing overweight is not to count Calories but to identify the reasons for energy imbalance.

Insidious Weight Gain. From age twenty on, many adults experience an annual weight gain because they fail to adjust their diet to decreased activity. Middle-age-spread is difficult to cope with simply because the weight gain can be very slight from year to year. The person gradually becomes accustomed to his or her appearance. Changing from a size 10 dress to a 12 to a 14 or from a trouser waist of 32 to a 34 to a 36 is not alarming if a few years intervene between each increment. The overweight is camouflaged psychologically by the euphemism that a different style of clothing is more "becoming" to the figure. Men who stop buying

Excessive energy intake (the cause of obesity) may be due to failure to reduce food intake when activity declines, unresolved psychosocial problems, preference for nutrient-dilute foods, too little time and thought given to food choices, or personal values.

tapered shirts or French-cut trousers for this reason are practicing denial just as are women who select dresses with vertical instead of horizontal stripes.

Psychosocial Factors. The psychological pathology that underlies many instances of obesity is discussed at length in many psychology textbooks. Here we will mention only a few examples.

Minor problems accumulating over time may set in motion a pattern of eating to obtain oral gratification. Once this pattern has started, breaking it is extremely difficult. The emotional repercussions of divorce, the loss of a job, or the death of a relative or friend may result in progressive obesity over a lifetime if the problem is not dealt with immediately.

More subtle psychological factors that lead to weight gain are influenced by changes in a person's self-image. For example, ten years after they are married, many people cannot fit into their wedding clothes. Home cooking and a more regular meal schedule may account for some of the weight gain, but many people gradually develop different standards for their own appearance as their roles in life change.

Overweight people sometimes develop crippling emotional problems that limit their social interaction, and ultimately lead to a more sedentary life—thus compounding the difficulty of losing weight. The overweight person may withdraw from group activities because of rejection (imagined or real) by others or embarrassment at not being able to perform as well as others in certain situations such as sports. People who do not have a weight problem might give some serious thought to how they treat overweight acquaintances. The subtleties—condemning or considerate—of social interactions between people of different body sizes may be the crucial factor in determining whether an overweight person participates in group activities that could be either psychologically intolerable or a pleasant opportunity to exercise off unwanted pounds.

Attitudes toward Food. A preference for high-energy types of food and a dislike for the more nutrient-dense foods compounds the weight reduction problem for many overweight people. If you anticipate having a less active lifestyle in the future, think now about learning to enjoy a wide variety of low-energy foods. Another way to avoid gaining weight is to learn to recognize when you are eating to satisfy hunger and when you are eating for other reasons. Failure to make this distinction leads many people down the road to obesity.

Some dieters use low-energy or noncaloric foods as token observations of a weight reduction diet. The best example of this behavior is the person who polishes off a martini, an 8-ounce steak, and a baked potato loaded with butter and sour cream, and then sanctimoniously sprinkles artificial sweetener into the after-dinner cup of coffee.

Schedule. It has been observed that fat people participating in sports move less and more slowly than do leaner players, but it is incorrect to classify all overweight people as lethargic. Many obese people are very busy, but with sedentary activities. Their days are spent behind the desk or the wheel of a car, or seated in an airplane. This busyness can partly explain their overweight because initially it takes some time and thought to plan a sound weight reduction diet. The busy person who cannot make time for such planning has more barriers to weight reduction than just the absence of an exercise routine.

Personal Values. Overweight sometimes results from a decision—conscious or subconscious—made by an individual. Many people who muster the self-discipline to stop smoking gain weight. Although both cigarettes and overweight are hazards to health, it is extremely difficult to cope with both at the same time. The new nonsmoker may be able to minimize weight gain by using nutrition knowledge. In some instances, however, the most realistic approach is to wait until the smoking problem is under control before starting a weight reduction program.

Consequences of Obesity

The overweight person hardly needs to be told about the consequences of obesity. This information, however, might help the person prone to overweight in later years to appreciate the merits of planning a diet today to avoid the problems tomorrow.

Quantity of Life. Excessive body fatness accompanies, and often complicates, several life-threatening disorders. Deaths from kidney disease, heart and circulatory diseases, diabetes, and hypertension are more common among obese people. Tuberculosis deaths, however, are less common among this population.

Overweight women often have more complications of pregnancy, especially if they are diabetics. Surgery is also more difficult if the doctor must probe through layers of fat to work, for example, on a gallbladder. Overweight puts an additional burden on the cardiovascular system. A bigger body has more tissue that must be supplied with blood—a function that can be accomplished only by the pumping of the heart. Each extra pound of body weight means that blood must be propelled through an additional mile of tiny capillaries and larger vessels.

Quality of Life. The obese person faces problems that, although not life threatening, make life less pleasant. To appreciate why fat people tire more easily, try carrying a 40-pound backpack for a day. The weight distribution is different, but a hiker who has had this experience understands why an overweight person might sit out the fast dances or prefer spectator sports to actually playing.

Obese people are more vulnerable to minor injuries. Their bodies are harder to coordinate, and they have to move heavier bodies to avoid accidents.

Overweight makes many people less tolerant of heat because the increase in body mass (metabolizing cells that generate heat) is greater than the increase in body surface (skin through which heat can be dissipated). The obese person is made even more uncomfortable by increased perspiration released along with the heat.

Social as well as physiological conditions make life difficult for overweight people. People of average weight give no thought to a turnstile in the sports arena; they nonchalantly select any sized chair in a restaurant or a friend's home; they quickly hop on and off buses. These and many other everyday experiences complicate life and decrease the potential pleasure of the daily routine for the overweight person.

NONDIETARY TREATMENT OF OBESITY

Unlike many other diseases, the cure for obesity is rarely permanent. It is much more likely to recur than other diseases because the predisposition to this condition involves a way of life. The best that can be hoped for is to control the condition through improved behavior, activity, and diet patterns that last a lifetime.

Behavior Modification

Dismally few people who try to lose weight are successful, and a high percentage of these few regain the lost pounds shortly after having reached their weight reduction goal. Many nutritionists feel that the most effective solution to the obesity problem requires broad changes in activity patterns and psychological factors—not simply modification of the diet.

Commercial weight reduction programs have for years used one-on-one counseling and group sessions to help overweight people understand their reasons for overeating. Peer encouragement and, to a certain degree, peer competition in the pounds-off race are effective motivation for some, though not all, people.

Several programs sponsored primarily by the Department of Health, Education and Welfare (DHEW) will probably in the near future broaden our expertise in diet-related behavior modification techniques. The MR. FIT (*Multiple Risk Factor Intervention Trial*) Program, the SCOR (Specialized Center for Research) Arteriosclerosis Program, and other projects are reporting higher success rates in weight reduction than many other efforts and fewer of their participants regain lost weight. The methods of these programs are still being investigated, but some early observations resulting from these programs may prove beneficial in efforts to help people lose weight through behavior therapy.

1. The factors that initially motivate a person to participate in a program differ to a certain degree from those that help a person continue in the program and avoid regaining weight.

2. Different motivation factors influence behavior depending upon whether people currently see themselves as sick, in a high-risk group, or disease-free.

3. Factors influencing the choice of appropriate behavioral therapy include degree of overweight, willingness of the entire family to participate in the program, and the interpersonal relationship between patient and therapist.

4. The success of a program seems to be influenced by the training and personality of the therapist, the intensity and continuity of the effort, the patient's nutrition knowledge and sustained awareness of certain problems, and pre-existing attitudes toward diet and health.

5. "Behavioral contracting" is effective with some people; others respond to environmental cues; the threat-to-health motivation technique may provoke harmful anxiety reactions in some people.

To both prevent and reduce obesity, behavior modification may in future years be expanded to the broader environment through programs such as more effective use of mass media, appropriate use of advertising, and education efforts to develop sound health beliefs and food behavior early in childhood.

Exercise

Some people find it easier to lose weight by increasing energy expenditure rather than reducing energy consumption. They would rather jog than juggle Calories. If your current diet is nutritionally adequate but provides too much energy, this is a sound way to lose weight. It may not be practical, however, unless your schedule allows a lot of time for exercising. Table 9-8 indicates how much vigorous exercise of various types it takes to use up the energy value of several foods.

There are many ways, however, within your normal routine to increase energy expenditure. Three flights of stairs can be climbed in as much time as you often spend waiting for an elevator. You may not want to jog to class or to work, but step up the pace whenever you walk. If it is too far to walk from home to school, at least get off the bus a couple of stops farther away or park your car a few blocks from your building.

A conscientious exercise program can improve the functioning of the circulatory system. There are many long-range benefits to be derived from making exercise part of your daily routine. Starting a vigorous program without the proper conditioning, however, can be dangerous, especially for older people who fail to discuss their exercise with their physician.

DIET MODIFICATION

Paperback books and magazines are filled with weight reduction diets. Some sound simple: eat only grapefruit, or cut out all starch, or eat only soups and beverages. Many of these diets are nutritionally inadequate and dangerous if continued for long. Furthermore, these diets do not help you learn how

Crash diets usually are simple, but they fail to provide sound guidelines for a lifetime of meeting nutrient needs and maintaining an appropriate body weight.

TABLE 9-8. Energy Cost of Various Activities Related to the Energy Value of Various Foods

Food	Energy		Walking (min.)	Cycling (min.)	Swimming (min.)	Jogging (min.)
	(Cal)	(kJ)				
Carrot, 1 large	42	184	8	6	5	4
Cheese, American, 1 ounce	112	407	22	17	13	11
Doughnut	125	525	24	19	15	13
Ice cream, ⅙ quart	186	681	36	28	22	19
Pork chops, 2 lean	260	1,092	49	39	31	26
Cheeseburger	462	1,940	89	69	55	46

SOURCE: *Exercise Equivalents of Foods—A Practical Guide for the Overweight,* by Frank Konishi. Copyright © 1973. Reprinted by permission of Southern Illinois University Press.

to plan a diet that meets your nutrient needs and your way of life, and that keeps the pounds off.

Crash Diets

As we learned in Chapter 3, energy needs must be met before protein can be used for body maintenance. For most people an intake of 1,200 Cal (5,000 kJ) is sufficient to spare body protein, while low enough to mobilize fat stores. At lower intake levels, most people begin to metabolize muscle protein to meet the body's need for this nutrient. If you choose to restrict your energy intake below 1,200 Calories, a doctor should plan and supervise your weight reduction program.

A more complex metabolic concept (discussed in Chapter 3) explains another danger of an extremely low energy intake. Stored fat that is mobilized to meet energy needs is first converted to acetyl CoA. If more acetyl CoA is produced than the Phase II (Krebs) cycle can metabolize for energy, the excess acetyl CoA is broken down into β-hydroxybutyric acid and acetoacetic acid. An accumulation of large amounts of these acids in the blood causes an acid–base imbalance in the body and ketosis.

The irony of crash dieting is its supposed success. The first few pounds come off quickly, but this loss is mostly water (not fat) sucked out of the normal body pool as the kidneys try to protect the body from the acids formed from excessive amounts of acetyl CoA. The formation of a small amount of these acids is not alarming; it is indeed an indication that fat is being mobilized, the objective of weight reduction. However, diets that drastically alter the acidity of body fluids and distribution of water within the body can be injurious to health.

Low-Carbohydrate and High-Protein Diets

Low-carbohydrate and high-protein diets are effectively the same. If you eliminate carbohydrate, you have only three other possible sources of energy: protein, fat, and alcohol. One problem of such diets (shown by an analysis of the Stillman diet in Table 9-9) is that most noncarbohydrate foods that provide protein almost always are high in fat, and often in cholesterol also.

High protein intake often causes a mild nausea that diminishes appetite. This nausea is associated with an increased concentration in the blood of

TABLE 9-9. Comparison of the Stillman Diet to the Average American Diet

	Average Daily American Diet	Stillman Diet
Calories	2,565	1,325
Total fat		
grams	115	73
% of total Calories	42	50
Protein		
grams	100	160
% of total Calories	16	48
Carbohydrate		
grams	261	7
% of total Calories	42	2
Cholesterol, grams	533	1,215

SOURCE: F. Rickman, et al., "Changes in Serum Cholesterol During the Stillman Diet," *Journal of the American Medical Association* 228 (1974):54. Copyright 1974, American Medical Association. Used by permission.

nitrogen-containing substances formed from amino acids when protein is used as a source of energy. The kidneys, therefore, must excrete more nitrogen-containing waste products. The kidneys of most people can handle this increased nitrogen load. However, some people have mild, undiagnosed kidney disease—their kidneys do not function optimally but perform adequately on a normal diet. Such people may have significant problems on a prolonged high protein diet. Muscle cramps, for example, are a signal that the body homeostasis has gone awry, but many other hazards of high-protein diets are not so easily detected without laboratory tests.

A Diet to Live With

An ideal diet is one that allows you to maintain not only a normal weight but also a normal daily routine. The foods in your diet should therefore (1) contain enough protein and micronutrients to meet your body's needs; (2) be readily accessible at home, at school, at work, and while socializing or traveling; and (3) supply enough energy that you are not constantly fatigued. To stay on the diet, you should not have to drastically alter your social life or your sleeping patterns.

If you are now overweight, check Table 9-10 for the energy deficits that will reduce body weight over various periods of time. How quickly you want to take off the pounds must be weighed against the degree to which you are willing to modify your energy intake. These decisions provide the basis for determining the total energy value of your weight reduction diet.

Start with foods that have the approximate energy value per serving outlined in the basic four guide (Chapter 8, Table 8-9). The 4-4 and 2-2 servings in the suggested amounts provide approximately 1,400 Cal (5,880 kJ). Subtracting 1,400 Calories from the total energy intake level you select tells you how many Calories can be allotted to additional foods in your weight reduction diet.

TABLE 9-10. Days Required to Lose 5 to 25 Pounds by Lowering Daily Calorie Intake

Reduction of Calories per Day (Cal)	Days to Lose 5 Pounds	Days to Lose 15 Pounds	Days to Lose 25 Pounds
100	150	450	750
300	50	150	250
700	22	66	110
1,000	15	45	75

SOURCE: *Exercise Equivalents of Foods—A Practical Guide for the Overweight* by Frank Konishi, Copyright © 1973. Reprinted by permission of Southern Illinois University Press.

TABLE 9-11. Similarities and Differences between Nutritionally
Adequate Weight Reduction and Maintenance Diets

Food Group	Reduction Diet	Transition Diet	Maintenance Diet
Fruits and vegetables	Tomato or vegetable juice Fresh fruit Vegetables seasoned mainly with herbs or vinegar	Orange or prune juice Apricot nectar Vegetables with a little butter Low-calorie salad dressing	Sweetened canned or frozen fruits Some sauces Regular salad dressing
Cereals	Breakfast cereal Toast Crackers or bread	Breakfast cereal with a little sugar Toast with a little butter	Toast with jelly or jam Some desserts
Milk	2 c. skim (use some for cereal)	2 c. whole and/or some cheese	Some cheeses or ice cream
Meat	Two 3-ounce portions lean meat, fish, or poultry, (or protein equivalent using beans, peas, or nuts)	Larger portions or extra servings	Some sauces Some fried foods Some bacon, sausage or cuts higher in fat
Other	Small amounts of butter and sugar	Occasional soft drink or alcoholic beverage	In amounts appropriate to energy needs

Once you reduce to the weight you desire, additional foods can be superimposed upon the basic reduction pattern of eating, or you can make more nutrient-dilute substitutions. If the scales start to swing upward, it is easy then to identify what food should go out of your diet or what portion sizes should be reduced until your weight gets back into line. For example, on your weight maintenance diet, one of your choices from the milk group might be a generous serving of ice cream. If your weight begins to climb, change back to the weight reduction diet by using nonfat or lowfat milk as one of your servings from the milk group.

People who manage to maintain a desired body weight never really stop dieting. They simply make a transition as needed between a weight reduction diet and a weight maintenance diet (Table 9-11). This system does not involve switching drastically from one way of eating to another. On the contrary, the core of both diets is the same.

Helpful Hints

Every smart dieter learns some practical tricks. Although none can substitute for a sound foundation diet, they can make weight control a little easier.

1. Smaller bites, chewing more, and sipping water help prolong a meal. You do not end up in front of an empty plate, watching everyone else eat.

2. Some vegetables are so low in energy per serving that they have very little effect upon the total daily intake. Spices, lemon, or vinegar improve the taste of many vegetables—explore these as an alternative to butter or margarine.

3. Nutrient-dense foods should be more easily accessible than other foods. Keep raw vegetables and skim milk in front of the cheesecake and left-over roast in the refrigerator. Be sure that the fruit bowl is in plain view and the cake box is closed.

4. Plan some of the basic four servings as snack items such as raw vegetables, cheese, or tomato juice.

5. Skipping meals is self-defeating for some dieters: they become so hungry that they snack on foods that do not fit the diet.

6. If you cannot stand the taste of coffee without sugar, try a complete switch to tea.

7. At parties drink something that can be mixed with water or sipped on the rocks. Stand next to the relish tray rather than the peanuts or hot meat hors d'oeuvres.

The final suggestion is simply to be prepared for the days when your willpower is weak. If you decide to splurge one day, enjoy it. Do not let guilt feelings destroy your motivation. Just pick up your diet on the next day, and keep shedding the pounds until you attain the weight you want to be.

STUDY QUESTIONS

1. Ten years from now, do you expect to have a higher or a lower energy requirement? Why?

2. What is the significance of having a body weight that does not conform to values shown on standard body weight reference tables?

3. Describe the ways of determining body fatness.

4. During last week, what was your greatest and your smallest daily energy expenditure?

5. If your daily energy intake is 100 Cal (420 kJ) greater than your energy expenditure, how much weight will you gain in one year?

6. Which of the four ways to reduce energy intake best fits your lifestyle?

7. What psychosocial factors contribute to excessive energy intake?

8. How does obesity affect the length and quality of life?

9. Why is behavior modification considered a promising approach for combating obesity?

10. How can you increase your energy expenditure without having to allot a certain amount of time each day for an exercise routine?

11. What are the dangers and disadvantages of crash diets?

SUGGESTED READING

1. S. F. Johnson, W. M. Swenson, and C. F. Gastineau, "Personality characteristics in obesity: Relation of MMPI profile and age of onset of obesity to success in weight reduction," *American Journal of Clinical Nutrition* 29(1976):629–32.

2. A. E. Thomas, D. A. McKay, and M. B. Cutlip, "A nomograph method for assessing body weight," *American Journal of Clinical Nutrition* 29(1976): 302–304.

3. S. Lewis et al, "Effects of physical activity on weight reduction in obese middle-aged women," *American Journal of Clinical Nutrition* 29(1976): 151–56.

4. E. M. Widdowson and M. J. Dauncey, "Obesity," Chapter 3 in *Present Knowledge in Nutrition*. 4th ed. New York and Washington, D.C.: The Nutrition Foundation, 1976.

5. T. B. Van Itallie and R. G. Campbell, "Multidisciplinary approach to the problem of obesity," *Journal of the American Dietetic Association* 61(1972):385.

6. B. K. Paulsen et al, "Behavior therapy for weight control: Long-term results of two programs with nutritionists as therapists," *American Journal of Clinical Nutrition* 29(1976):880–89.

7. S. M. Wishik and S. Van der Vynct, "The use of nutritional positive deviants to identify approaches

for modification of dietary practices," *American Journal of Public Health* 66(1976):38–42.

8. M. Weisenberg and E. Fray, "What's missing in the treatment of obesity by behavior modification?" *Journal of the American Dietetic Association* 65(1974):410.

9. Council on Foods and Nutrition, American Medical Association "A critique of low-carbohydrate ketogenic weight reduction regimens (A review of Dr. Atkin's Diet Revolution)," *Journal of the American Medical Association* 224(June 4, 1973).

10. *A Dozen Diets for Better or for Worse* (26 pages). California Dietetic Association, Los Angeles District, 1973.

11. D. A. Schanche, "Diet books that poison your mind . . . and harm your body," *Today's Health* 52(1974):56–61.

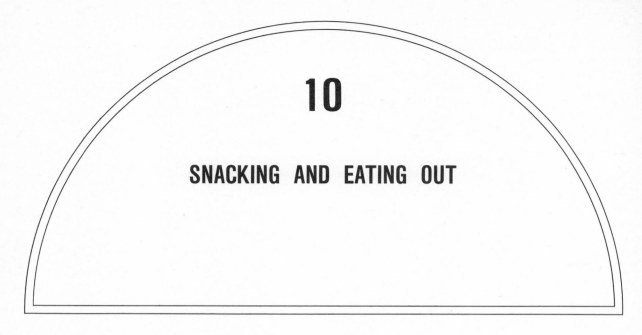

10

SNACKING AND EATING OUT

The nutrition information that many of us learned in elementary school and in our homes as children was based on a three-meals-a-day pattern of eating. For some of us, however, the pace of life today often makes it difficult to eat three meals a day, and many of the meals we do eat are prepared outside the home. Selecting an appropriate diet is not impossible under these conditions, but it does require giving more thought to food choices.

This chapter takes a look at how you can choose foods that balance the nutritional value of the total diet when you rely on snacks for a portion of your nutrient needs or often eat away from home.

PROBLEMS WITH SNACKING

The pace of life for many people influences their diet, which in turn is intimately related to health. Ignoring this relationship can lead to inappropriate diet modifications and impaired health. People who either by choice or of necessity eat few meals at the table are better prepared to make wise food choices and to protect their health if they realize the potential problems of snacking and take the necessary precautions to avoid these problems.

Stress

A lifestyle that bypasses regular sit-down meals is often also a lifestyle full of stress. Although stress cannot be precisely defined, it is related to certain behavior patterns, sociopsychological factors, and perhaps genetics or inheritance. Taken together, these traits are possible risk factors for the development of coronary heart disease (see Chapter 25).

Stress may also result in abnormal functioning of the gastrointestinal tract as evidenced by poor digestion, lack of appetite, or nausea. These problems may lead to nutrient deficiencies, which contribute to irritability, nervousness, and poor performance, which in turn accentuates stress. This cycle has not yet been fully proven scientifically, but it is a theory worth considering.

If you are a frequent snacker, ask yourself whether your pace of life so alters your nutrient intake that it leads to vitamin or mineral deficiencies and maybe even to weight loss or weight gain. Taking time for a meal and also for unwinding may have many benefits—some nutritional, others not related to nutrition—in terms of your overall health and your functional capacity.

The snacker (someone who eats few meals at the table at home) can still select an appropriate diet by applying knowledge of nutrition.

Energy Intake

Snacking may lead to overweight because:

1. Foods traditionally eaten as snacks tend to be nutrient-dilute or to provide only energy.
2. Many people snack simply out of habit, almost unconsciously; their food intake is not regulated by appetite.
3. It is more difficult to keep track of total energy intake when you eat frequently than if you eat only three or four times a day.

Being aware of these problems may help you keep your energy intake at the right level if you are a snacker.

Oral Health

The diet pattern chosen by a snacker may create another problem—dental caries and periodontal disease. Frequent eating of sticky foods without time for brushing afterwards increases the risk of developing oral diseases. Regular dental checkups are therefore crucial for people who eat frequently. Oral hygiene—both brushing and flossing—must not be neglected in spite of the pace of our lives. (Ways to help minimize oral diseases are discussed in Chapter 28.)

BROADENING YOUR CHOICES OF SNACK FOODS

Not as many foods can be eaten as snacks and minimeals as can be eaten at the table, but the variety of snack food options may be greater than you think. Expanding your snack choices may increase the chances of improving the quality of your diet.

The primary factor limiting which foods can be used as snacks is whether they remain safe to eat after being stored for several hours. In your enthusiasm for broadening the nutrient variety of your snacks, be careful not to compromise on the safety of foods. Foods made with eggs and mayonnaise such as potato salad can be an excellent snack for disease-causing bacteria, as well as for people. Likewise, fresh, cream-filled snacks or other protein foods contaminated by fingers or flies and allowed to sit as little as two hours at room temperature can be more hazardous than healthful (see Chapter 20).

Many foods that are safe as snacks are overlooked because they are too juicy or sticky; because they require kitchen utensils for preparation or eating; or because they lose their appealing appearance if left for long at room temperature. Almost all of these problems can be overcome if you give some thought to planning your snacks. Your choices expand quickly if you have a few basic utensils for the transporting, eating, and cleaning up of snack foods:

- Plastic containers—to protect fragile items such as grapes or tomatoes
- Plastic cup—for drinks of various kinds
- Fork, spoon (perhaps plastic)—for eating foods such as yogurt, cottage cheese, salads
- Peeler and/or paring knife—for raw vegetables such as carrots or even cucumbers
- Can opener—for items such as juices, fruits and vegetables that do not need to be heated
- Tissues or packaged damp towelettes—for cleaning up after eating a peach or orange

The utensils may be kept in your desk drawer or dormitory room or slipped into a backpack when you are bicycling. However, a word of caution again about food safety. Utensils that retain particles of food can quickly become a medium for bacterial growth. Common sense should outweigh the rush of any schedule—be sure to clean these tools both before and after using them.

Your snack food options also increase if you have a means of heating food or keeping it cold. If there is a small refrigerator at work or in the dormitory, stock it with cheese, fruit or vegetable juices, or raw vegetables that taste better cool and crisp. If you have a hot plate or even a coil for heating water for coffee, your snacks could include soups and a variety of beverages such as hot chocolate. An investment in a small thermos bottle or a can opener might improve considerably the quality of your diet

The snacker should realize that (1) a stressful lifestyle (often more common among people with little time to eat) can lead to impaired health, (2) it is more difficult for snackers to be aware of the total amount of energy they consume, and (3) their oral hygiene requires their special attention.

and ultimately reduce the cost of snacking and increase the likelihood of staying healthy.

BUILD AROUND THE BASICS

To make the most nutritionally of our snack choices, we need to consider our options within each food group. By keeping in mind the variations in nutrient density—as well as the energy value of food, the dental problem, and the safety of food—we can determine which foods are appropriate for each of us and the way we live.

Fruit and Vegetable Group

Fresh fruits (if washed) and dried fruits are ideal snacks, while canned fruits are also possible if you have a can opener and spoon. Vegetables, on the other hand, are the foods most often overlooked by snackers. Vegetable snacks need not be limited to potato chips, french fries, carrots, and celery. Most of the vegetables that go into a salad bowl can go into a plastic container and retain their taste appeal fairly well for a few hours—radishes, tomatoes, spinach, lettuce, cauliflower, cucumbers, peppers, shredded cabbage. Table 10-1 shows that vegetables provide less energy than do vegetable-containing soups; but both of these categories of vegetable snacks help meet your needs for micronutrients such as vitamin C, vitamin A, and folacin that may be lacking in a snacker's diet. Vegetable juices are perhaps the easiest way to ensure enough of this type of food in your snacks.

TABLE 10-1. Energy Value and Percent U.S. RDA for Vitamin C, Vitamin A, and Folacin for Snacks from Fruit and Vegetable Group

Food	Energy		Percent U.S. RDA		
	(Cal)	(kJ)	Vitamin C	Vitamin A	Folacin[a]
Apple juice, 1 cup	120	504	4	†	
Apricots					
Fresh, 3	55	231	17	58	†
Dried, ½ cup	180	756	16	165	†
Grapefruit juice, 1 cup					
Fresh	100	420	160	4	5
Canned*	100	420	140	†	‡
Frozen*	100	420	160	†	5
Grape juice, 1 cup	170	714	†	†	†
Grapes, 1 cup	65	273	5	2	2
Orange juice, 1 cup					
Fresh	110	462	210	10	15
Canned	120	504	170	10	‡
Frozen	120	504	200	10	15
Peaches					
Fresh, 1 medium	35	147	12	26	2
Dried, ½ cup	210	882	24	63	†

SOURCE: R. G. Hansen, A. W. Sorenson, and A. J. Wittmer, "Index of Nutritional Quality Food Profiles" (Logan, Utah: Utah State University, 1975). © 1975, Utah State University. Used by permission.

Options for snack foods should be based on consideration of a food's safety, texture, and the temperature at which the food tastes best; various utensils can be used to expand one's snack options.
Vegetables are the category of foods most commonly overlooked by snackers.

Table 10-1. Energy Value and Percent U.S. RDA (*continued*)

Food	Energy		Percent U.S. RDA		
	(Cal)	(kJ)	Vitamin C	Vitamin A	Folacin[a]
Pineapple juice, 1 cup					
Canned	140	588	40	2	‡
Frozen	130	546	50	†	‡
Potato chips, 10 medium	110	462	4	†	‡
Prune juice, 1 cup	200	840	8	30	‡
Prunes, 4	70	294	2	9	†
Raisins, 1½ oz. pkg.	120	504	1	0	†
Raw vegetables for salad					
Asparagus, canned, 1 cup	30	126	63	26	22
Bean sprouts, 1 cup	35	147	13	1	3
Beets, canned, 1 cup	85	357	12	0	35
Cabbage, shredded, 1 cup	20	84	70	2	15
Carrot, 1 medium	25	105	7	110	5
Cauliflower, 1 cup	25	105	110	1	15
Celery, diced, 1 cup	15	63	15	5	2
Cucumber, 1 medium	30	126	38	0	5
Green pepper, 1 medium	15	63	157	6	8
Lettuce, ½ head	15	63	15	22	5
Mushrooms, ½ cup	20	84	4	0	2
Onions, ½ cup	30	126	12	1	3
Radishes, 4	5	21	17	0	2
Spinach, raw chopped, 1 cup	14	59	45	90	24
Tomato, 1 medium	40	168	70	33	15
Soup, 1 cup					
Minestrone	105	441	†	47	‡
Onion (dry form)	150	630	10	†	‡
Tomato	90	378	20	20	‡
Tomato (with milk)	175	735	25	24	‡
Tomato, vegetable, and					
noodle (dry form)	245	1,029	30	34	‡
Tangerine juice, 1 cup					
Canned	120	504	90	20	‡
Frozen	110	462	110	20	‡

[a]Adapted from B. P. Perloff and R. R. Butrum, "Folacin in selected foods," *Journal of the American Dietetic Association* 70(1977):161–71.
*Sweetened varieties provide approximately 25 more Calories.
†None or less than 1 percent.
‡Data not available.

Cereal Group

Foods from this group make up a large part of the snack list for most people. These foods are frequently eaten at parties or while watching TV. However, their contribution to total energy intake quickly mounts, as you can see by scanning the energy values in Table 10-2.

For example, one large Dutch pretzel supplies as much energy as does an average slice of bread, but you may be more apt to eat several pretzels at a time than several pieces of bread. A roll or muffin has about twice as many Calories as do crackers in the amounts shown in the table. The protein and micronutrient content of a Danish pastry (the breakfast chosen by many snackers) is about the same as that of a piece of toast; however, the energy value of a Danish equals that of a piece of toast plus a bowl of cereal with one-half cup of milk, and a glass of juice, all of which provides a greater amount and variety of nutrients.

Cakes vary in energy content from about 120 Cal (500 kJ) for angel food or a thin slice of pound cake, to about 300 Cal (1,280 kJ) for plain cake—plus 30 to 50 percent more calories if it is iced. Pies also differ in energy value. If your energy intake might easily exceed your energy needs, you should choose the chiffon or custard types rather than those such as pecan, mince, or butterscotch that are very high in energy. Popcorn is a good snack for people who like to munch but want to keep energy intake down—as long as the popcorn is not doused with melted butter or margarine.

Milk Group

This group offers many snacks that are good sources of calcium, riboflavin, and protein. You can choose from Table 10-3 whatever foods fit your energy needs. Calcium values are included in this table to give an idea of how nutrient density varies within this group. For example, a cup of ice cream provides 110 more Calories (460 more kJ) than a cup of whole milk, but less calcium. A sundae may contain several hundred more Calories (depending upon how you make it) but very few additional vitamins or minerals. Powdered breakfast mix adds about 130 Calories and 10 percent of the U.S. RDA for calcium (plus other nutrients) to the nutritional value of milk.

The nutrient density of yogurt depends upon whether it is made from whole milk or from skim milk. The taste of plain yogurt can be varied by adding vanilla or maple extract and spices such as nutmeg or cinnamon. These additions do not increase energy value, as do flavorings made with fruit preserves. Foods you might add to cottage cheese to improve its taste range in energy value from fewer than 50 Calories (210 kJ) for tomatoes, carrots, cucumbers, or water-packed canned fruit to over 100 Calories (420 kJ) for a tablespoon of mayonnaise or one-half cup of fruit cocktail packed in syrup.

Meat Group

When kept at room temperature, many foods from the meat group are easily contaminated by disease-causing bacteria. These foods therefore cannot be kept for long in lockers, desk drawers, or vending machines. However, there are several ways for snackers to ensure an adequate intake of the foods from this group.

1. Schedule one meal a day that includes meat or a meat alternate. The amount you eat may supply a large portion of your total daily need for foods from this group. Remember that the basic four system calls for only two 3-ounce servings of meat per day.

2. Order a meat sandwich at a snack bar or delicatessen. If you need a more nutrient-dense diet, it may be worth paying a little extra for lean rather than regular meat (Table 10-4), or for a sliced chicken sandwich rather than a hot dog. If your diet already contains enough cereal products, ask for an open-face sandwich that uses only one slice of bread.

3. Choose a meat alternate. Hard-boiled eggs are not as temperature sensitive as are many meat products.

TABLE 10-2. Energy Value for Snacks from the Cereals Group

Food	Energy (Cal)	Energy (kJ)
Bread, 1 slice (25 g)	70	300
Crackers		
Round, 1⅞″, 4	60	250
Cheese, 1″ square, 10	45	190
Saltines, 4	50	210
Oyster, 10	35	150
Graham, 2½″, 2	60	250
Rye wafers, 2	45	190
Danish pastry (4″)	270	1,135
Muffins (2½″–3″)	100–130	420–545
Rolls		
Brown and serve	90	375
Hamburger or hot dog	120	500
Cake (1/12 of 8″, two-layer), plain	310	1,300
+White icing	+90	+375
+Chocolate icing	+140	+590
Fruitcake (1/15 of pound loaf)	120	500
Angel food (1/16 of 9″ tube pan)	120	500
Devil's food (2 x 2 x 4″)	280	1,180
+White icing	+100	+420
Devil's food cupcake (2¾″), iced	160	670
Gingerbread (3″ square)	200	840
Coffee cake (⅙ cake)	230	970
Popcorn, 1 pint, salted	50	210
+Butter, 1 tablespoon	+125	+525
+Sugar coated	+200	+840
Pretzel		
Dutch, twisted, 1	60	250
Thins, twisted, 1	25	105
Sticks, 10	25	105
Pie, ⅙ of 9″ pie		
Strawberry	250	1,050
Banana or plain custard, chocolate chiffon, pumpkin	300–350	1,260–1,470
Apple, blackberry, blueberry, chocolate or lemon meringue, coconut custard, rhubarb	360–400	1,510–1,680
Butterscotch, mince, peach, raisin	410–450	1,720–1,890
Pecan	580	2,520

SOURCE: C. F. Adams, *Nutritive Value of American Foods in Common Units,* Agriculture Handbook No. 456 (Washington, D.C.: U.S. Department of Agriculture, Agricultural Research Service, 1975).

TABLE 10-3. Nutritional Values for Snacks from the Milk Group
(with Common Additions)

Food	Energy		Percent U.S. RDA
	(Cal)	(kJ)	Calcium
Milk, whole, 1 cup	150	630	30
+Powdered breakfast mix	+130	+546	+10
+Chocolate syrup, 2 T.	+90	+378	—
Buttermilk, 1 cup	90	378	30
Half-and-half, 1 T.	15	63	6
Powdered creamer, 1 T.	30	126	*
Ice cream, regular, 1 cup	260	1,092	20
+Fudge sauce, 2 T.	+120	+504	—
+Whipping cream, ¼ cup	+220	+924	+5
+Whipped topping, pressurized, ¼ cup	+50	+210	*
+Peanuts, ⅛ cup	+100	+420	+2
+Coconut, ¼ cup	+110	+462	—
+Root beer, 1 cup	+100	+420	—
Ice milk, soft serve, 1 pint	540	2,268	50
Yogurt, plain, 1 cup			
Made from whole milk	150	630	25
Made from skim milk	120	504	30
+Preserves or jam, 1 T.	+60	+252	—
Cheese			
Cheddar, 1 oz. (on pie)	110	462	20
Parmesan (on spaghetti), 2 T.	150	630	40
American, 1 oz.†	110	462	20
Pizza, cheese	230	966	
Tapioca, 1 cup	220	924	15
Pudding (mix made with whole milk)	320	1,344	25
Pudding (home recipe), vanilla	280	1,176	30
Pudding (home recipe), chocolate	390	1,638	25
Cottage cheese, 1 cup			
Creamed	260	1,092	25*
Uncreamed	170	714	20*
+Pineapple, canned, ¼ cup			
Heavy syrup	+65	+273	—
Water packed	+25	+105	—
+Tomato, 1 medium	+40	+168	2
+Mayonnaise, 1 T.	+100	+420	—

*Check nutrition information panel on label; products vary.

†If a 2-pound package is 8 inches long, ¼-inch slice equals 1 ounce.

SOURCE: R. G. Hansen, A. W. Sorenson, and A. J. Wittmer, "Index of Nutritional Quality Food Profiles" (Logan, Utah: Utah State University, 1975). © 1975, Utah State University. Used by permission.

TABLE 10-4. Nutritional Values for Snacks from Meat Group

Food	Energy (Cal)	Energy (kJ)	Protein (grams)
Beef, roast, 1 oz.			
Lean	70	294	7.7
Regular	125	525	6.7
Hamburger, 3 oz.			
10% fat	186	781	
21% fat	235	987	19.8
Corned beef, 3 oz.	315	1,323	19.5
Tongue, beef, 3″ x 3″ x ⅛″	49	206	4.3
Chicken, sliced, 2 oz.	95	400	18.0
Chopped chicken livers, ½ cup	165	693	17.5
Clams			
4 cherrystones	56	236	7.8
1 pint	372	1,562	64.0
Crab, deviled, ½ cup	225	945	13.7
Oysters, 1 cup	158	664	20.2
Oyster stew, 1 cup	220	925	12.0
Salmon, smoked, 1 oz.	50	210	6.1
+Cream cheese, 1 T.	+52	+218	1.1
Sardines, solids and liquid, 1 oz.	88	370	5.8
Tuna salad, ½ cup	175	735	15.0
Ham, boiled, 1 oz.	66	277	5.4
Ham, deviled, 1 oz.	100	420	3.9
Bologna, 1 oz.	86	361	3.4
Frankfurter, 1 medium	135–170	567–714	6.0–7.5
Knockwurst, 1 link	189	794	9.6
Liverwurst, 1 oz.	87	366	4.6
Salami, 1 oz.	88	370	5.0
Pork and beans with tomato sauce, ½ cup	155	651	7.8
Egg, hard-boiled, medium to extra large	70–95	294–399	5.7–7.4
Omelet, plain, large egg	111	466	7.2
Peanuts, ½ cup	420	1,764	19.0
Peanut butter, 1 T.	95	399	4.0
Pecans, ½ cup	371	1,558	5.0
Sunflower seeds, ½ cup			
Hulled	406	1,705	17.4
Unhulled	128	538	5.5
Additions for sandwiches			
Bread, 2 slices	140	588	4.2
Butter, 1 t.	34	148	—
Lettuce, tomato, onion	25	105	—
Mayonnaise, 1 T.	101	424	—

SOURCE: C. F. Adams, *Nutritive Value of American Foods in Common Units,* Agriculture Handbook No. 456 (Washington, D.C.: U.S. Department of Agriculture, Agricultural Research Service, 1975).

TABLE 10-5. Sandwich Fillings from Various Food Groups

Fillings	Fruits and Vegetables	Milk Products	Meat or Meat Alternates
Avocado			
With lemon	X		
With bacon	X		X
Bean dip combined with celery, onion, tomato, bell pepper, or combinations of these	X		X
Carrot and celery, grated			
With dates or raisins	X		
With nuts or coconut	X		X
Cream or other soft cheese			
With chopped celery, green onion or chives, radishes, cucumbers, peppers, or other vegetables	X	X	
With chopped nuts and dates	X	X	X
With pineapple, coconut, and small marshmallows	X	X	
Egg (boiled) or egg salad			
With tomato and lettuce	X		X
With bacon			X
With cheese		X	X
Nuts diced or mashed with celery, tomatoes, carrots, onion, and mayonnaise	X		X
Peanut butter with crushed pineapple, mashed bananas, and dates or raisins	X		X
Radishes or cucumbers, sliced, with sour cream or yogurt	X	X	
Tomato and lettuce			
With avocado	X		
With bacon	X		X
With cheese	X	X	

Canned beans might be eaten if you have a can opener and a fork or spoon. In the long run, sunflower seeds, nuts, and peanut butter are probably the most convenient meat substitutes for snackers.

Food Group Combinations

Several snack options include foods from more than one group. Depending on the type of pizza you order, for example, its nutrient composition can be very similar to that of many vegetables. Soups are another disguise for vegetables. Cream soups made with milk supply calcium and riboflavin, as well as the nutrients found in vegetables.

There are many more sandwich options than just hamburgers, cheeseburgers, and hot dogs. Fillings can be selected to provide nutrients from one or more of the food groups, depending upon what is needed to balance out your total diet. The nutrient density of a sandwich depends upon what is put between the two slices of bread. Butter, mayonnaise, and jelly reduce the nutrient density, but the fillings shown in Table 10-5 may enhance the nutri-

TABLE 10-6. Energy and Several Nutrients Provided by Fast-Food Meals

Meal	Energy (Cal)	Energy (kJ)	Percentage of energy from fat	Percent U.S. RDA Protein	Iron	Riboflavin	Calcium
Hamburger (regular-small) and french fries							
With chocolate shake	780	3,276	31	42	21	57	47
With soft drink	572	2,402	32	24	16	24	6
With soft drink and apple pie	832	3,494	38	28	19	26	8
Cheeseburger (regular-small), french fries, and soft drink	624	2,621	35	29	15	32	15
Hamburger (super), french fries, and soft drink	858	3,604	44	45	23	40	17
Hamburger (¼ pound), french fries, and soft drink	728	3,058	36	45	24	39	8
Fish fillet, french fries, and soft drink	728	3,058	40	28	11	23	10

SOURCE: U.S. Department of Agriculture, Agricultural Research Service, NE-36, Consumer and Food Economic Institute, "Nutritive Value and Cost of Fast Food Meals," prepared by P. Isom, *Family Economics Review,* Highlights/Fall 1976. Nutritive values from "Nutritional Analysis of Food Served at McDonald's Restaurants," based on a nationwide study by the WARF Institute, Madison, Wis., January 1973, for McDonald's Corporation.

tional value of the sandwich and complement the nutrient contribution made by the bread.

Other snack food combinations are possible without bread. Fruit and cheese go together nicely. Some people like peanut butter spread between two halves of a banana or on chunks of apple. Celery might be stuffed with any of a variety of soft cheeses.

EATING OUT

Estimates of the percentage of American meals eaten out range from 30 to 50 percent, and there are indications that this trend will further increase. If you are one of the many people who frequently eat out, you need to think about how to order the most nutritionally appropriate meals.

Fast Foods

One of the major changes in the American diet during the last decade is the increase in popularity of hamburger carry-outs or fast-food establishments. Franchise food outlets now account for approximately 30,000 of the estimated 145,000 restaurants in this country.

The Nutritional Value. Table 10-6 shows the energy, percentage of energy from fat, and percentage of U.S. RDA for protein, iron, riboflavin, and calcium of several meals that are typically served at fast-food restaurants. The first four meals are basically regular (small) hamburgers or cheeseburgers plus french fries; beverages vary, and one meal includes apple pie. The energy value of these meals ranges from 572 to 832 Cal (2,400 to 3,490 kJ). They average about a fifth of the RDA for a man or an active teen-ager but about a third of the energy recommended daily for a woman or young child. Three of these meals provides about 28 percent of the U.S. RDA for protein (the meal with the shake provides more), and fat supplies 31 to 38 percent of the energy. Riboflavin and calcium are primarily provided by the milk of the shake. Iron content varies only slightly. The percentage U.S. RDA of other nutrients (not shown in Table 10-6) is approximately the same: thiamin, 19 to 25 percent; vitamin A, 3 to 6 percent; and vitamin C, 21 to 24 percent.

Three other types of meals are often featured at fast-food restaurants—a special hamburger, a quarter-pound hamburger, or fried fish—all shown in Table 10-6 with french fries and a soft drink. The first two meals supply more protein and energy than do small-hamburger-based meals; the percentage of energy from fat is also higher. The meal containing fried fish is of comparable energy value, but protein and iron are lower than in the meals including hamburgers; this meal is also relatively high in fat.

Making Appropriate Substitutions. A more detailed analysis of individual items offered at fast-food establishments is shown in Table 10-7. This information may help if you want to make some substitutions in the meals presented in Table 10-6.

To lower energy value, you might order a regular (small) hamburger or cheeseburger (approximately 250 fewer Calories) rather than the larger varieties, especially if your protein and iron needs are met by other foods. For the shake you might substitute a soft drink (less energy but no calcium), or a carton of milk.

The major general problems with fast-food meals seem to be:

1. Iron density is often low compared to the needs of women and teen-agers.
2. Calcium, riboflavin, and vitamin A are low unless milk or a shake is ordered.
3. Vitamin C is low without french fries.
4. There are few sources of folacin or fiber.
5. Percent of energy from fat is high in some meal combinations.

The identification of these potential problems suggests the nutrients that should be sought from foods eaten elsewhere during the day. Another possibility is to explore other side orders. Coleslaw can provide vitamin C, folacin, and fiber; its energy value largely depends upon how much mayonnaise it contains. Baked beans offer iron and some calcium, folacin, and fiber, but they also increase the energy value of your diet. Some fast-food establishments offer salad bars that may have the nutrients you want to complement your meal. Many carry-outs are beginning to serve breakfasts and therefore have tomato juice or fruit juice. Although you may not be used to these beverages in the middle of the day, why let old habits stand in the way of getting to your body the nutrients it needs?

Cafeterias

Cafeterias are usually not glamorous places to eat and the quality of their food varies, but they may make it easier to plan the type of diet you want. Many cafeterias offer a broad selection of vegetables, soups, and salads. Some offer fresh fruits, sliced cheese, a variety of breads, and margarine instead of butter—if you ask for it. Another advantage is that you have a chance to see portion sizes, which help you gauge what else to select. If the cafeteria is not crowded, you may be able to wait until you have finished the main part of your meal before deciding whether you want a dessert or not.

Restaurants

The major problem with most restaurant meals is lack of a variety of vegetables. Menus feature a meat course, and some form of potatoes almost automatically appears on your plate. The vegetable

TABLE 10-7. Energy and Nutrients Provided by Individual Foods Available from Fast-Food Establishments

Food[b]	Energy (Cal)	Energy (kJ)	Protein	Vitamin A	Thiamin	Riboflavin	Calcium	Iron	Vitamin C	Folacin[a]	Percentage of food energy from fat
Hamburger[b]											
Regular, small	260	1,092	20	3	12	21	5	14	6	6	36
¼ pound	410	1,722	41	5	15	37	7	21	5	10	41
Super	540	2,268	40	4	18	38	16	21	8	12	52
Cheeseburger[b]	310	1,302	25	6	13	30	14	13	6	8	41
Fish fillet[b]	410	1,722	24	2	15	21	9	9	2	8	49
French fries[b]	200	840	4	*	7	2	1	2	15	6	42
Apple pie[b]	260	1,092	3	*	*	2	2	3	3	2	51
Chocolate shake[b]	310	1,302	17	*	5	33	41	5	*	2	20
Soft drink[c]	100	420	*	0	0	0	0	0	0	0	0
Milk[c]	160	672	20	6	4	25	30	*	4	2	48
Orange juice,[c] (canned) 1 cup	130	546	2	10	10	2	2	6	170	25	0
Tomato juice,[c] 1 cup	45	189	4	40	8	4	2	10	70	12	0
Coleslaw,[c] 1 cup	120	504	2	4	2	2	6	4	50	15	80
Baked beans,[c] 1 cup	380	1,596	35	6	10	6	15	35	8	8	3

[a] Adapted from B. P. Perloff and R. R. Butrum, "Folacin in selected foods," *Journal of the American Dietetic Association* 70(1977):161–71.
[b] U.S. Department of Agriculture, Agricultural Research Service, NE-36, Consumer and Food Economic Institute, "Nutritive Value and Cost of Fast Food Meals," prepared by P. Isom, *Family Economics Review*, Highlights/Fall 1976. Nutritive values from "Nutritional Analysis of Food Served at McDonald's Restaurants," based on a nationwide study by the WARF Institute, Madison, Wis., January 1973, for McDonald's Corporation.
[c] U.S. Department of Agriculture, Agricultural Research Service, Consumer and Food Economic Institute, "Nutrition Labeling—Tools for Its Use" Agriculture Information Bulletin No. 382 (April 1975).
*Insignificant amount of nutrient present.

"du jour," if included, often seems to have been given little thought by the chef. Salads may or may not be included in the price of the meal and seldom do they include more than lettuce and a slice of tomato.

When looking for vegetables on menus, do not overlook items listed as soup courses or appetizers such as mushroom or cucumber dishes. Sometimes there are a variety of vegetables in the kitchen that are served with different entrees; you may request side orders of these although they are not listed on the menu. If the restaurant has a bar, you probably can get an order of tomato juice with or without the vodka. Restaurants that have a salad bar may be the answer to your vegetable needs—stack on the beans, tomatoes, beets, carrots, cucumbers, radishes, onions, and parmesan cheese. Sometimes there is a set price for the salad bar—as much as you want—plus beverage and bread. Fruits may also be part of appetizers, salads, or desserts—alone or in combination with assorted cheeses.

Women, as well as sedentary men, often find that portion sizes and number of servings in restaurants are so large that the total energy value of the meal exceeds their energy needs. This means that either they eat more food than they should, or they leave food on the plate. The first pattern leads to obesity;

the second means that food as well as money is needlessly wasted.

The waste of food can be reduced if you order a la carte and do not select more than you can eat. This, however, means that there are fewer types of food and less nutrient variety in your meal. A doggy bag may keep the food from being wasted if you have ready access to a refrigerator.

Another approach to the problem is to request smaller portions. This is possible for sliced meats, steaks, or chops and pieces of chicken, but not for dishes such as casseroles and many other items on the menu. Do not expect such substitutions to lower your bill; the special attention they require in the kitchen costs the restaurant more than is saved in the price of food.

Another way to cut back your total energy order is to omit the entree. Many meat or seafood appetizers as well as quiches are large enough to satisfy people with lower energy needs, especially if such a selection is combined with soup, salad, and bread. If the waiter or waitress raises an eyebrow, explain what you are doing and the nutritional reasons *why*. Application of nutrition knowledge may require some self-confidence when dining in fancy restaurants, but why perpetuate traditions that conflict with selection of a diet appropriate for you?

STUDY QUESTIONS

1. What are the health-related problems more common among snackers and how can they be dealt with?

2. What are the limitations on your snack food options, and how can you deal with them?

3. What snacks may be selected from each of the four food groups?

4. How might you add more vegetables to your snack choices?

5. What factors must you consider when snacking at fast-food establishments to ensure that your diet is appropriate for you?

6. What tactics can you use when eating at cafeterias and restaurants to ensure that your diet is appropriate for you?

SUGGESTED READING

1. P. Isom, "Nutritive value and cost of fast-food meals," *Family Economics Review*, Agricultural Research Service, U.S. Department of Agriculture (Fall 1976).
2. H. Appledorf, "Nutritional analysis of foods for fast-food chains," *Food Technology* 28(1974):50.
3. J. A. Thomas and D. L. Call, "Eating between meals: A nutrition problem among teenagers?" *Nutrition Reviews* 31(1973):137–40.
4. N. R. Beyer and P. M. Morris, "Food attitudes and snacking patterns of young children," *Journal of Nutrition Education* 6(1974):131–33.
5. J. A. Hruban, "Selection of snack foods from vending machines by high school students," *Journal of School Health* 47(1977):33.
6. J. Goldberg, "The fast-food phenomenon," *Family Health* 7(1975):38.
7. C. M. Young, L. F. Hutter, S. S. Scalan, C. E. Rand, L. Lutwak, and V. Simko, "Metabolic effects of meal frequency on normal young men," *Journal of the American Dietetic Association* 61(1972):391.
8. J. Mayer, "Snacks," *Family Health* 6(1974):32.

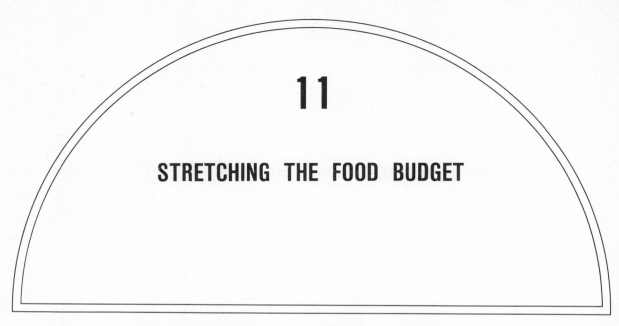

11

STRETCHING THE FOOD BUDGET

A chapter on stretching the food budget may initially seem out of place in a nutrition book. You might think it belongs only in a family life or money management course. This topic does, however, merit serious consideration here because price is often a primary factor in determining which foods we select to meet our nutrient needs. It is useless to know what we should eat, unless we know how to get these nutrients from a diet we can afford. This chapter discusses the most economical food choices—those that provide the most nutrients for a given level of expenditure.

WHERE THE DOLLAR GOES

Let's take a broad look at food budgets to see why they must be stretched by some people and what type of adjustments—dietary and nondietary—can be made either to make more money available for the purchase of nutrients or to make the money buy more nutrients.

Most Vulnerable Budgets

Despite inflation, average food expenditure as a percentage of average disposable income has de-

clined between 1950 and 1970. In 1976, the average consumer spent about 17 percent of disposable income on food. Nevertheless, the food budget of certain groups of people is being squeezed by increasing taxes as well as by the soaring cost of fuel, medical care, and other expenses. Inflation is seriously affecting (and in some cases, ruining) the diets of people such as the elderly who live on fixed incomes.

In spite of unemployment compensation, loss of a job by the family wage earner(s) can create a nutritionally hazardous situation—especially if the people involved are accustomed to purchasing expensive foods. Almost overnight, persons whose income is reduced need to know how to select less expensive foods and still maintain an adequate nutrient intake.

The number of people in a household is a factor in determining the types of food that can be afforded on a given income. The U.S. Department of Agriculture (USDA) prepares weekly and monthly food plans that are nutritionally adequate and may be purchased by people at four income levels—liberal, moderate-cost, low-cost, and thrifty (the least expensive). According to these food plans, two-person families can purchase the moderate-cost diet on an annual income of $5,000 to $10,000. If there are six people to feed, the same diet is affordable only on an income over $20,000. Although the total food bill increases with the size of the family, the cost of food per person decreases in larger households. According to the USDA food plans, a person living alone pays about 25 percent more for his or her food than does each person in a five-member household.

The family food budget increases as children grow from toddlers to teen-agers. Figure 11-1 shows that feeding a ten-year-old costs about twice as much as feeding a two-year-old. If a woman is pregnant or nursing an infant, or if a member of the family has special dietary needs that are medically indicated, the cost of feeding that person increases the total food budget. The School Lunch program has reduced the amount of money some parents must spend for their family's food, but the cost of feeding a family is generally greater if many snacks and meals are eaten away from home.

Adjustments to Inflation

The spiraling inflation of the 1970s has increased consumers' interest in how they can purchase the best possible diet with their food dollars. A 1974 government survey of Americans entering supermarkets showed that nourishment is the greatest concern regarding grocery shopping choices of 39 percent of those questioned, but almost as many people (37 percent) ranked saving money on food prices as most important. Another study regarding adjustments in lifestyle due to inflation showed that four of the sixteen ways consumers save money affect their diet patterns (Table 11-1). None of the food-related adjustments (italicized items) is necessarily detrimental. However, almost one-fifth of the people surveyed are postponing medical and dental checkups to save money. When such practices are coupled with dubious food choices and are carried on for a long time, they may spell significant health problems for some people.

Distribution of the Food Dollar

The nutritional adequacy of a diet depends upon both how much money is available for food and how the food dollar is spent. Although adequate diets can be selected on relatively small budgets, studies have shown that many people do not know how to plan these types of diets.

The Ideal. The USDA diet plans are based on the

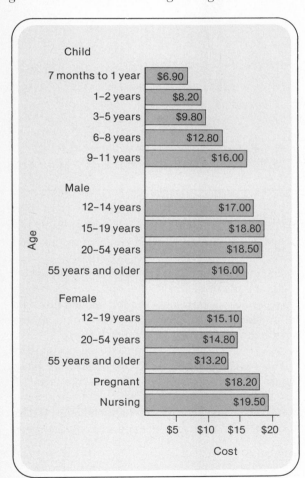

FIGURE 11-1. Weekly cost of feeding people of different ages.

TABLE 11-1. Adjustments in Lifestyle As a Result of Inflation

Behavior Change	Percentage of People Surveyed
Minimizing use of electricity	65
Spending free time at home instead of going out	54
Not buying clothes the way we used to	44
Shopping more at discount stores	44
Cutting back on gifts	43
Bargain hunting	38
Not eating out in restaurants	37
Repairing things normally thrown out	34
Cutting back on beauty parlor and barbershop	25
Using fewer prepared and frozen foods	24
Cutting out magazines and newspapers	21
Giving up hobbies and sports that cost money	21
Buying less liquor and beer	19
Doing without meat at some meals	19
Postponing medical and dental checkups	18
Looking for tips on money managing	17

SOURCE: "The General Mills American Family Report 1974–1975: A Study of the American Family and Money." Reproduced by permission of the Consumer Center of General Mills, Inc. © General Mills, Inc. 1975.

nutritional needs of people in all age/sex categories and the cost of foods that supply these nutrients. Figure 11-2 compares the amount of several types of food that would be purchased for an adult male according to the thrifty plan ($11.10 per week) and the liberal plan ($22.30 per week). The greatest differences are in milk, meat, vegetables, and accessories.

The less expensive plans provide 100 percent of the RDA for energy; between 100 and 140 percent of the RDA for calcium, vitamin A, riboflavin, thiamin, and magnesium; and 150 percent or more of the RDA for protein, iron, vitamin C, niacin, and vitamin B_{12}; but only about 95 percent of the RDA for pyridoxine. These values have been adjusted for vitamin losses from cooking and discarding meat drippings and half of the separable fat from meat. However, the thrifty food plan includes a much smaller allowance than do the more expensive plans for food that is discarded or allowed to spoil. Enriched cereal products must be used in all food plans.

The menu cycle shown in Appendix Table A11-1 is an example of the thrifty food plan for one week. If you are on an extremely limited budget, this type of guideline may be the safest way to ensure the nutritional adequacy of your diet.*

The Real. Our discussion of ideal diet plans shows that a nutritionally adequate diet can be purchased on a limited budget. In actuality, however, this does not always happen. The USDA household dietary survey (Chapter 13) conducted in

---

* Additional information regarding the food plans is available from the Consumer and Food Economics Institute, Agricultural Research Service, USDA, Hyattsville, Maryland 20702.

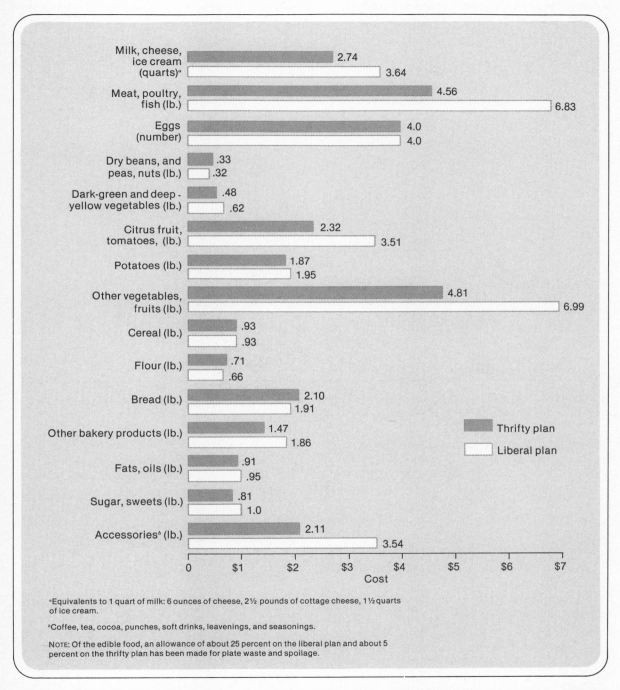

[a]Equivalents to 1 quart of milk: 6 ounces of cheese, 2½ pounds of cottage cheese, 1½ quarts of ice cream.

[b]Coffee, tea, cocoa, punches, soft drinks, leavenings, and seasonings.

NOTE: Of the edible food, an allowance of about 25 percent on the liberal plan and about 5 percent on the thrifty plan has been made for plate waste and spoilage.

FIGURE 11-2. Amounts of food suggested per week for an adult male in the USDA thrifty and liberal food plans (based on food prices in the spring of 1975).

Although the USDA thrifty food plan (the least expensive plan) meets most adult nutrient needs, the 1965 USDA dietary survey showed that, compared to families with higher incomes, poorer families more frequently select diets that fail to meet the RDA for the seven nutrients studied.

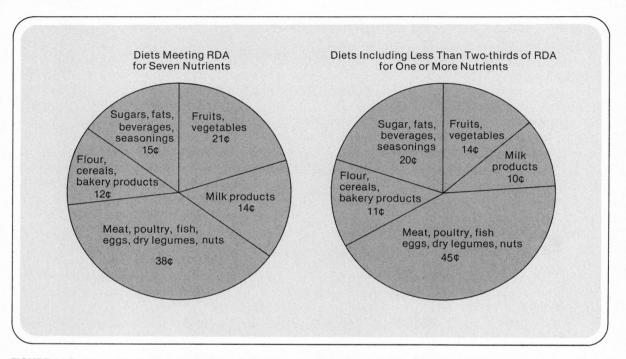

FIGURE 11-3. Use of the food dollar by households spending the same amount of money on food but purchasing diets of different quality. (Based on data from 1965 USDA survey for families spending slightly more than the U.S. average for food.)

1965 showed that the quality of diets decreases as family income declines. The intake of the seven nutrients tabulated in this survey met the RDA for 37 percent of the families with an annual income of less than $3,000; 53 percent of the families with an annual income of $5,000 to $7,000; and 63 percent of the families with an annual income of $10,000 or more.

The choice of foods by people at all income levels accounted in part for the quality of their diets. Some of the wealthier subjects in this study failed to use their diet dollars wisely. Figure 11-3 shows how the food budget was spent by two groups of people who spent the same total amount of money on food. The circle on the left shows the choices of families whose diets met the RDA for all seven nutrients tabulated; the circle on the right shows what was purchased with the same amount of money—result-

ing in diets that provided less than two-thirds of the RDA for one or more nutrients. Those who used their dollars more wisely purchased more fruits and vegetables; more dairy products; fewer sugars, fats, beverages, and seasonings; and less meat, poultry, fish, eggs, dry legumes, and nuts. The amounts spent on the cereal group were about the same.

Nonfood Purchases

When looking for ways to save money in the grocery store, it is worth taking a critical look at everything that goes into the shopping cart. Money saved on nonfood items might be used for purchasing sources of energy, protein, vitamins, and minerals. Table 11-2 shows that approximately 21 percent of the money spent by the average shopper in a grocery store is used for nonfood items, and another

TABLE 11-2. How the Average Family Spends a $4,000 Annual Food Bill

Food	Dollars	Percent of Total Food Bill
Baked goods, snacks	228	5.7
Dairy products	258	6.5
Frozen foods	212	5.3
Fresh meat, provisions	796	19.9
Fresh fish	28	.7
Fresh poultry	114	1.4
Produce	438	11.0
Baby foods (excluding cereals)	18	.5
Cereals, rice	54	1.4
Canned foods		
Fruits	36	.9
Juices, drinks	36	.9
Meat, poultry	44	1.1
Seafood	26	.7
Soups	24	.6
Vegetables	56	1.4
Milk	10	.3
Coffee, tea	104	2.6
Dried fruits, vegetables, milk	44	1.1
Jams, jellies, preserves	14	.4
Macaroni, spaghetti, noodles	18	.5
Puddings	6	.2
Sugar	30	.7
All other edibles	214	5.4
Beer	182	4.6
Wine, distilled spirits	26	.7
Candy	40	1.0
Soft drinks	90	2.3
Total	**3,146**	**79**
Nonfood		
Paper goods	84	2.1
Soaps, detergents, laundry	86	2.2
Other household products	74	1.9
Pet foods	54	1.4
Tobacco products	150	3.8
Groceries (not elsewhere classified)	28	.7
Health and beauty aids (nonprescription)	152	3.6
Prescriptions	16	.4
Housewares	38	1.0
All other general merchandise	172	4.3
Total	**854**	**21**

SOURCE: Calculated from U.S. Department of Agriculture, Agricultural Research Service, "This Is a Food Bill," 1975-690-659 (Washington, D.C.: Government Printing Office, 1975).

5 percent goes for beer, wine, or other alcoholic beverages. The percentages for many items seem small, but for a family of four that spends approximately $4,000 a year in grocery stores, some of the annual totals (such as for paper goods, soaps, pet food, soft drinks, and housewares) may suggest places to consider pinching pennies.

COST OF NUTRIENTS

We have already learned in Chapter 8 that it is short-sighted to evaluate the nutritional value of a food on the basis of its content of a single nutrient, but it can be helpful to compare the cost of nutrients provided by foods that vary in price. Once we have identified the most expensive nutrients, we can concentrate our economy efforts on foods that provide these nutrients.

The horizontal bars in Figure 11-4 show the amounts of energy and eight nutrients supplied by one dollar's worth of various foods. This information is based on 1969 food prices because more recent nationwide price comparisons of the cost of nutrients are not available, except for protein. Because of the increase in the consumer price index since 1969, the nutrient yield values are probably closer to the amount purchased for almost a dollar and a half rather than one dollar. The relative value of nutrients supplied by different types of food, however, has probably fluctuated very little.

The darker portion of the bars in Figure 11-4 corresponds with the amount of each nutrient that equals the U.S. RDA; for energy, the two darker areas correspond with the RDA for adult males and females. Therefore, comparing the dark portion of each bar to the entire length of that bar gives you an idea of the cost (as a fraction of approximately $1.50) of meeting your needs for each nutrient from various types of foods. The least expensive sources are those where the dark bar is short and the entire bar is long.

Although the cost of nutrients varies depending upon food sources, when all eight charts in Figure

11-4 are viewed, we can see that vitamin C and vitamin A are among the least expensive nutrients to purchase in the grocery store if we select the most economical sources of each. For vitamin C, the best buys are citrus fruit and tomatoes; for vitamin A, your least expensive sources are dark-green and deep-yellow vegetables. Calcium is relatively inexpensive from milk, but other foods are more costly sources of this mineral.

Meeting your needs for thiamin and riboflavin costs approximately the same fraction of a dollar, but the best buys among foods are different for these vitamins. Dairy products are the least expensive sources of riboflavin (followed by eggs and grain products); cereal products, beans, and potatoes are among the cheapest sources of thiamin.

Perhaps the most unexpected information in all the charts in Figure 11-4 relates to the cost of dietary sources of iron. Beans, peas, and legumes are your most economical choices—eggs and enriched or whole-grain cereal products are also good buys. Women and teen-agers on a budget should give particular attention to these foods because of their higher RDA for iron. In a similar manner, persons with high energy requirements might find their greatest savings among the cheaper sources of calories.

The cost of meeting protein needs is, perhaps surprisingly, not much more than meeting the U.S. RDA for minerals and vitamins if you select wisely. The three sources of protein at the top of the protein chart are all equally good buys since 45 grams of protein equal 100 percent of the U.S. RDA for milk products and eggs, whereas 65 grams equal 100 percent of the U.S. RDA for vegetable sources of protein such as beans, peas, or nuts.

BEST BUYS IN EACH FOOD GROUP

Since nutrients come packaged in combinations within foods, another place to look for bargains is within each food group. Three general guidelines might help identify where you will find savings:

186

SECTION III / ADJUSTING DIETS TO INDIVIDUAL LIFESTYLES

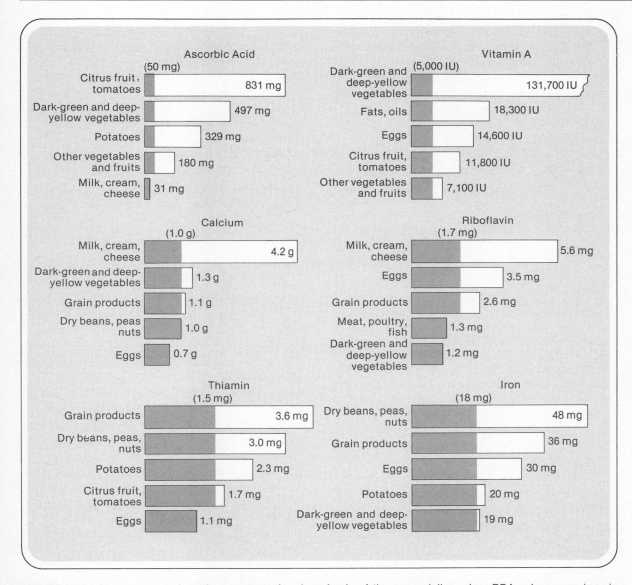

FIGURE 11-4. The energy and nutrient content of various foods of the same dollar value. RDA values are given in parentheses and indicated by the dark parts of the bars. The least expensive sources are those where the dark bar is short and the entire bar is long. (Based on 1965 survey data and 1969 prices.)

Money can be saved by shopping most carefully both for the foods eaten frequently and for the most expensive types of food as well as by being aware of which nutrients are generally provided by which foods.

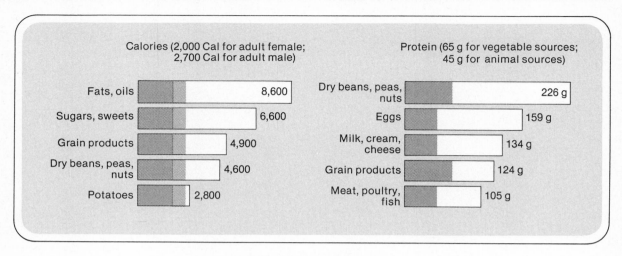

FIGURE 11-4. (*continued*)

1. Foods used frequently should be considered carefully because they often make up a large part of the food budget. For many people this means daily staples such as cereal products, bread, fruit juices, and dairy products.

2. Saving a small percentage on expensive foods (meats, some cheeses, out-of-season produce) may reduce the total budget more than saving a larger percentage on cheaper foods like beans, canned vegetables, or flour.

3. When making cost comparisons, keep in mind which nutrients are generally provided by certain foods and which are not. For instance, the cost of fruits should be compared to their content of vitamins A or C; it is faulty reasoning to select one fruit over another on the basis of its niacin content. Niacin content is more important when considering the price of beans, nuts, potatoes, and cereal products (review Figure 8-4).

Meat Group

Since foods in this group command a large portion of the food dollar, look carefully here for bargains. The most obvious approach is to compare your needs to how much you eat. Trimming the quantity of foods from this group may reveal easy savings if you learn to select only as much of these foods as you need. Many Americans could probably reduce their meat consumption by about one-third without doing harm to their nutritional status if other foods in the diet are wisely chosen.

Beans and peas are your best buys within the meat group for protein, iron, and thiamin. They contain riboflavin and calcium (which are low in meats) but no vitamin B_{12}. Beans and vegetable protein extenders can be used in combination with meat and/or grains or grain products as main dish extenders. The nutrition labels for these products show the relative amounts of nutrients in such products. Peanut butter should not be overlooked as a meat alternate. To stretch the food budget, one may find that a smaller hamburger plus some peanut butter fits both the budget and nutrient needs better than a large hamburger.

Although meat is almost synonymous with protein in the minds of many people, three other factors might be considered when buying meat: energy value, iron density, and fat content. Rather than trying to remember all three of these characteristics of every product, pick whichever of them concerns you most: energy value, if you want to alter your body weight; iron density, if you have trouble get-

The most economical and nutritionally appropriate selections within the meat group depend upon the importance to you of the protein content, energy value, iron density, and fat content of each product you might choose.

TABLE 11-3. Cost of 20 Grams of Protein from Various Sources

Food	Iron INQ[a]	Cost of 20 Grams of Protein (cents)
Dry beans	1.7–3.0	13
Peanut butter	0.4	16
Bread, white enriched	1.2	18
Beef liver	4.9	20
Hamburger	2.1	21
Chicken, whole, ready-to-cook	1.6	23
Eggs, large	1.8	23
Milk, whole fluid	0.1	24
Tuna, canned	1.2	28
Chicken breasts	1.6	29
Ham, whole	1.2	41
Frankfurters	.8	44
Pork loin roast	1.1	51
Haddock, fillet, frozen	.9	55
Ham, canned	1.2	55
Bologna	.8	59
Beef rib roast	1.8	60
Veal cutlets	1.9	65
Pork chops, center cut	1.1	67
Lamp chops, loin	.5	86
Bacon, sliced	.7	92

[a] Excerpted from R. G. Hansen, A. W. Sorenson, and A. J. Wittmer, "Index of Nutritional Quality Food Profiles" (Logan, Utah: Utah State University, 1975). © 1975, Utah State University. Used by permission.

SOURCE: U.S. Department of Agriculture, Agricultural Research Service; Department of Labor, Bureau of Labor Statistics, "Average Retail Prices in U.S. Cities," February 1976.

ting enough of this mineral in your diet; or fat, if you need to reduce intake of this macronutrient.

Table 11-3 ranks several foods within this group according to the cost of the protein they provide. The INQ for iron may be more interesting, however, to iron-seekers and weight-watchers. Organ meats are usually one of your best buys. They are generally higher in most micronutrients and lower in fat than muscle meats, but usually higher in cholesterol.

One way to stretch the meat budget is to prepare the less expensive cuts. Frugal cooks become expert at stews and rely less upon broiling. Prime beef is usually the most tender, juicy, and flavorful type, but the less expensive grades can be equally good sources of nutrients and just as appetizing if properly cooked.

Poultry is usually less expensive when purchased whole rather than cut in pieces. Baking a couple of chickens at the same time saves energy. The cooked meat taken off the bones can be frozen and combined with less expensive cereal products for main dish casseroles. To make the most of the nutrients you buy, do not discard the drippings or stock of poultry (as well as of meat). You may prefer to cool this liquid and remove the fat before using the remaining liquid for soups or sauces.

Fish prices vary depending upon the season and how close to the water you live. Often, however, fish are nutritional bargains. Most fish are lower in fat and cholesterol than is meat, and some types of seafood are an excellent source of trace elements. Fatty types of fish or fish oils also provide vitamin D, which is important in the diets of children.

Eggs are a better protein and iron buy than is meat. If you tire of having them fried or scrambled, try serving omelets, souffles, or eggs Benedict for a main dish; chopped hard-boiled eggs on a salad; spinach and egg combinations in sandwiches; or homemade eggnogs. When egg whites are used for an angel food cake or meringue, be sure to use the yolks for something like a custard; yolks can also be poached and crumbled over salads.

Milk Group

Nonfat dry milk costs about a third of the price of whole fluid milk. If the taste and texture of reconstituted milk do not suit your palate, try mixing equal parts of this with whole milk or using it in recipes. Cream cheese is the most expensive way to buy calcium; yogurt is four times more expensive than milk; cottage cheese almost three times more; and ice cream is double the price based on the calcium value of whole milk. Riboflavin costs vary in similar proportions. Higher-priced items sometimes provide more energy, as in the case of ice cream and sweetened yogurt, but they provide variety in texture, taste, and appearance. Choose what fits your preferences and your budget.

Cereal Group

Enrichment of milled products makes foods within this group among the best buys in the supermarket for iron, thiamin, niacin, and riboflavin.

Whole-grain products contain comparable amounts of these nutrients as well as more of several trace elements (see Chapter 12). Products that contain no preservatives are preferred by some people, but they may be more expensive. Because these foods become stale more quickly than do cereal products with preservatives, they should be purchased in smaller quantities but at more frequent intervals.

Cereal products can be a significant source of protein in the total diet because they are eaten so frequently. Even after one allows for differences in protein quality, they are a less expensive source of this nutrient than is meat. A high-protein product, however, may not be a wise investment. Paying 20 percent more for a high-protein bread or cereal is not making use of your nutrition knowledge if your diet is already adequate in protein (see Chapter 8).

Many diet breads have fewer calories per serving simply because they are sliced more thinly. The dieter may be paying more for a dieting convenience—not for a food with markedly less energy per pound of bread. Most specialty breads and rolls likewise cost more money than can be justified on nutritional grounds. Similarly, raisins are a good source of iron, but there are so few in raisin bread that it is hardly worth paying a higher price simply because of their nutritional value.

Breakfast cereals can consume a significant portion of the food budget if eaten frequently. The cheapest cereals are the kinds that must be cooked, such as oatmeal or cream of wheat. Instant-cooking cereals save time but not money. Dry cereals climb higher on the price-of-nutrients scale, and presweetened ones are about twice the price of nonsweetened ready-to-eat varieties. The content of most vitamins and iron (but not other trace elements) is approximately the same for enriched and whole-grain cereals; fortified cereals provide additional amounts of some nutrients. Differences in carbohydrate, protein, fat, and energy values are generally minor; presweetened cereals contain more sucrose and less complex carbohydrate.

Enriched macaroni, noodles, and spaghetti offer many money-saving opportunities. Used with meat, eggs, and cheese in casseroles and other recipes, they stretch main-dish serving sizes while helping to keep cost down.

Fruit and Vegetable Group

The comparative prices of frozen, canned, and fresh fruits and vegetables depend upon the season. Fresh vegetables, in season, are usually the best buy. Canned items are usually cheaper than frozen. Dieters should know that canned diet fruits generally are more expensive than fresh fruits, though both have the same nutrient densities. The cost of vegetable soups may vary depending upon market availability of fresh vegetables.

Within this group of foods, the potato ranks as well or better than most vegetables as an inexpensive source of vitamin C, niacin, riboflavin, iron, and thiamin. It is a fairly inexpensive source of protein, but other vegetables are better buys for vitamin A, calcium, and folacin, which is not shown in Figure 11-4. When you are shopping for vitamin A, the color intensity of green or yellow fruits and vegetables can be a general—though not always reliable—guide for comparing prices to nutrient content.

Fruit juices, like breakfast cereals, deserve special budgetary evaluation because they are a common item in many diets. Compare the energy and percent U.S. RDA values for juices shown in Table 10-1 to their prices. Juice substitutes may be cheaper but not necessarily more economical. If a juice substitute contains only ascorbic acid and sucrose, and if your total diet is lacking other nutrients provided in significant amounts by fruit juice, you probably should purchase the more expensive type of juice.

Fiber content is another factor to consider when shopping within this group. Many whole fruits, especially when they are in season, are as inexpensive as juices, and whole fruit is a much better source of fiber.

Other Energy Sources

After making sure that nutrient needs are met by foods from the basic four groups, persons with high energy needs need to look for additional sources of energy. You should shop, as well as eat, with these guidelines in mind.

Fats and oils are the least expensive form of energy (Figure 11-4), but this economy must be put into perspective depending upon the percent of fat in your total diet. Paying less for this source of energy today, but more for medical care in the future, is false economy. Cereals and breads, the third cheapest energy source, provide not only calories but some of the trace elements for which no RDA have been established.

The RDA for niacin and thiamin increase parallel to the RDA for energy, and therefore you should look for cheap energy sources that provide these nutrients as well. Of the inexpensive sources of energy in Figure 11-4, beans, whole-grain or enriched cereal products, and potatoes are better choices than fats and oils for thiamin; beans, peas, and nuts for niacin (not shown in Figure 11-4). Sweets and sugars are cheaper per calorie than potatoes, beans, and peas; but sugar provides no other nutrients, and pastries are very nutrient-dilute.

The cost of alcoholic beverages—a source of energy—should not be overlooked in the budget planning of persons who use them. Ranking these products is difficult because their energy values vary from light beer to sweet mixed drinks and cordials, and their costs vary from cheap wine to the best champagnes. Personal lifestyle and preferences, as well as culturally defined uses of these beverages, determine their role in the diet and in the budget. For example, an inexpensive wine is a rare treat to some people but an insult to the tastebuds of others. The health problems due to excessive use of this source of energy may seriously threaten the total budget, either now or later in life.

Soft drinks are an expensive way to purchase

Foods not found in any of the four food groups may be inexpensive sources of energy, but caution must be exercised lest this type of food displace from the budget foods that are important dietary sources of protein and micronutrients. Money can be saved on food by planning and analyzing your shopping patterns.

energy. The price per bottle should be compared to amounts of other foods such as 25 grams of sugar, which provide approximately 100 Cal (420 kJ) of energy. The difference between the cost of a soft drink and $\frac{1}{18}$ (25 grams of sugar/454 grams per pound of sugar) the price of a pound of sugar tells you how much you are paying for the other qualities of a soft drink.

Coffee and tea provide no energy or nutrients, but in 1974 they accounted for about 2.6 percent of the average supermarket bill (Table 11-2). Instant coffee may be either cheaper or more expensive depending upon how much of a pot of regular coffee gets stale and is poured down the drain. Presweetened instant tea yields fewer cups per container than nonsweetened because it contains sugar. It is cheaper, though less convenient, to add your own sugar.

MONEY-SAVING, NUTRIENT-SAVING GUIDELINES

Most people plan their clothing purchases and compare values when shopping for household appliances or a car. Food purchases, which annually add up to more than any of these expenditures for many families, should be considered just as carefully.

Saving While Shopping

The first place to look for savings is before and during your trip to the grocery store.

Preparation. Preparing a grocery list and menu plan takes time, but it may minimize return trips (thus saving gasoline) and improve the nutrient balance of your diet. Watch for advertised specials in the newspapers and unadvertised specials in the store; they may be savings, but only if such foods fit your meal plans before they spoil. Timing of shopping is important. If you are hungry when you shop, you may select foods to meet current appetite rather than the week's nutrient needs. If you are

hurried or tired when you shop, you may not take time to compare nutritional value and cost.

Plan Your Path. Going through the aisles first for the basic foods and then again for foods of lower nutrient density is time-consuming, but it helps make you more aware of the amount of foods of different nutrient value you are purchasing. A quicker way to make this comparison is to group these foods separately when you get to the check-out counter and ask the cashier to subtotal them for you. The figures may suggest some nutritional grounds for changes in your grocery buying patterns, as basic foods should probably account for most of your grocery bill.

Take Time to Read. Unit pricing and nutrition information may be in small print, but these two sets of values offer the best ways to combine nutrition knowledge and economy planning. The drained weight and the number of pieces per container can help you select the appropriate size container to minimize waste or insufficient serving sizes. Open dating (which states the last day that a food can be marketed) can help you select the freshest product. Because some vitamins, though generally not minerals and protein, gradually are destroyed over time, the freshness and storage conditions of unprocessed fruits and vegetables is an important nutritional consideration when shopping.

To ensure that your money is spent for what you think it is purchasing, read the ingredient information on food labels. The sequence of listing ingredients tells the relative amount of each ingredient in a product. The first item listed is the major or predominant component of the food; the last item listed is present in the least amount.

For example, the ingredients in a can of stew might be listed in any of various orders—such as gravy, meat, potatoes . . . ; meat, gravy, potatoes . . . ; potatoes, gravy, meat. . . . If you plan for this stew to provide a major source of meat in your diet, select the product that has meat listed first. If you prefer to cut down on fat intake and have other sources of meat in your diet that day, a predominance of potatoes might be preferable. If you have taken care of other nutrient needs during the day and are looking for inexpensive energy, the predominantly gravy product may be what you want. Check the price, however, since a stew that is mostly gravy should be significantly cheaper than those that are predominantly meat.

This principle of ingredient predominance also applies to frozen dinner entrees. The smart shopper knows that a meat and gravy dinner differs from a gravy and meat dinner.

Chapter 29 supplies further information concerning food labels.

Look Up, Look Down. The shopper whose vision is limited to eye level may miss the best bargains. The foods least essential to your diet and those often yielding the greatest profit margin to the grocer are often easiest to find; eye-level space is not wasted on things that the grocer assumes you will buy anyway.

Another precaution is to consider carefully the nutritional value of items placed within eye range when you stand in the check-out line. The penny-wise, nutrition-conscious shopper musters all defenses against impulse buying in this area of the store.

Quantity of Purchases. Unit pricing reveals that many, though not all (coffee is often an exception), products are cheaper when purchased in larger quantities. If the product maintains its nutritional value and other qualities from the time the package is opened until it is emptied, and if you have adequate and appropriate storage space, buying larger sizes is a good way to save money. However, purchasing larger containers may make it necessary to plan several, successive meals that repeat the same food. Foods that can be prepared in a variety of ways circumvent the boredom problem, but be sure that you do not rely so heavily on the same food that you compromise the nutrient variety of your diet.

Green beans, for example, are nutritionally stable in the refrigerator for several days, but do not let them completely displace from your diet leafy vegetables that are needed for vitamins A and C and folacin.

The Cost of Convenience. Figure 11-5 shows some of the results of a USDA study comparing the cost of several types of convenience foods to the cost of the ingredients for preparing the same food at home. Bars that extend beyond 100 percent indicate that you can save money by making this food at home or from fresh ingredients.

Some of the results of this USDA study have been summarized as follows:

Nearly all of the frozen, chilled, or ready-to-serve *baked goods* were more expensive than preparing them from recipes or mixes. Better than one-half the products made from a complete mix were less expensive than their home-prepared counterpart.

Frozen and chilled cheese *pizzas* were about 60 percent more expensive than both home-prepared and packaged combination cheese pizzas.

All forms of *margarine* were less expensive than butter in bulk or quarters, but margarine in a tub or in a squeeze bottle was higher in price than stick margarine.

Scrambled *eggs* prepared from a frozen "cholesterol-free" egg product were almost twice as expensive as scrambled fresh eggs.

All frozen *beef* entrees and dinners and two of three skillet main dishes made from mixes were more expensive than their respective home-prepared counterpart.

Eight of nine *chicken* convenience products were more costly than similar products prepared from fresh chicken.

Frozen *fish* sticks and crabcakes were less expensive, but frozen haddock dinner, tuna noodle casserole, and shrimp newburg in a pouch were considerably more expensive than these products prepared at home.

Of the 37 *vegetable* convenience products studied, 16 single ingredient items in the canned or frozen form were cheaper than their fresh or home-prepared counterpart. Still, 6 of these 16 processed vegetables were more expensive than their fresh form during the fresh vegetables's growing season.

Products prepared from dehydrated *potatoes* and frozen

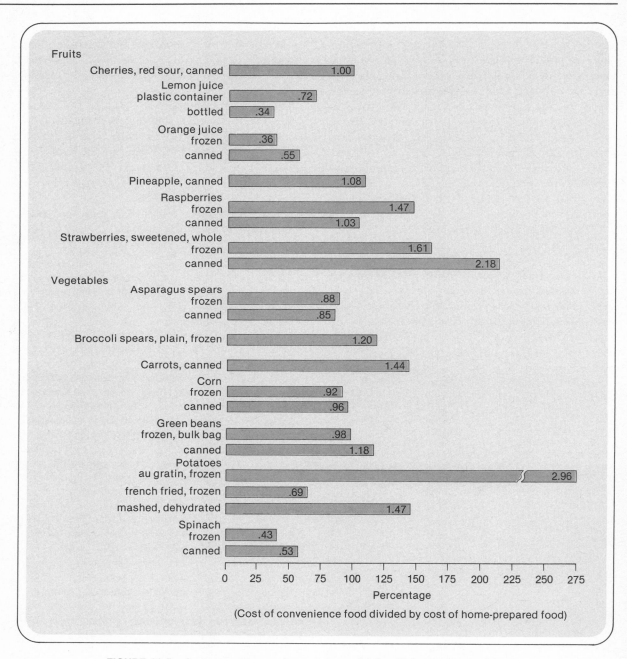

FIGURE 11-5. Cost comparisons of convenience foods with home-prepared foods.

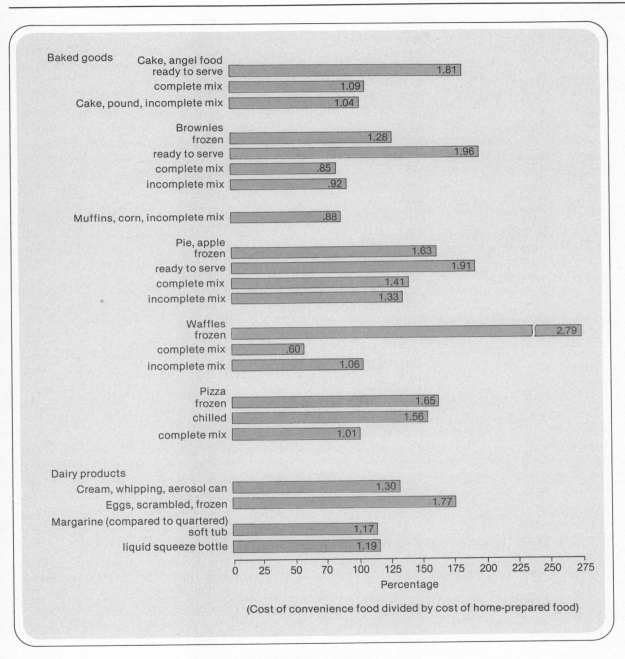

FIGURE 11-5. (*continued*)

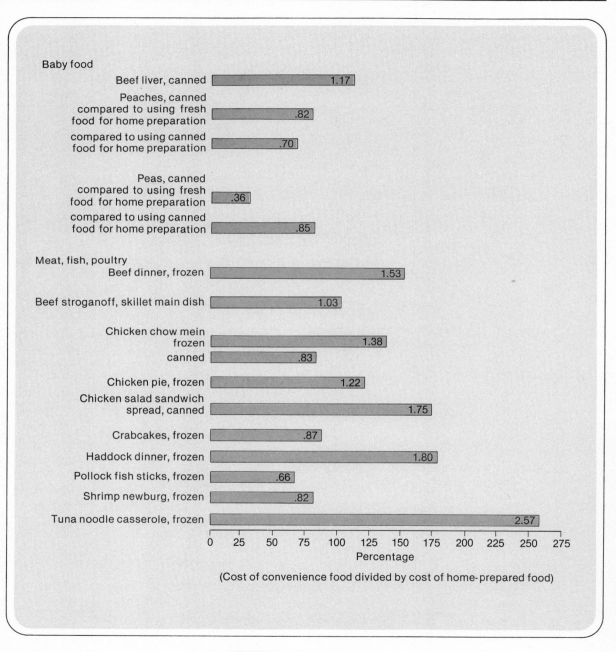

Baby food
Beef liver, canned — 1.17

Peaches, canned
compared to using fresh food for home preparation — .82
compared to using canned food for home preparation — .70

Peas, canned
compared to using fresh food for home preparation — .36
compared to using canned food for home preparation — .85

Meat, fish, poultry
Beef dinner, frozen — 1.53

Beef stroganoff, skillet main dish — 1.03

Chicken chow mein
frozen — 1.38
canned — .83

Chicken pie, frozen — 1.22

Chicken salad sandwich spread, canned — 1.75

Crabcakes, frozen — .87

Haddock dinner, frozen — 1.80

Pollock fish sticks, frozen — .66

Shrimp newburg, frozen — .82

Tuna noodle casserole, frozen — 2.57

Percentage

(Cost of convenience food divided by cost of home-prepared food)

FIGURE 11-5. (*continued*)

vegetable side dishes were more expensive than similar products prepared from scratch. Cut frozen french-fried potatoes were less expensive than french fries prepared from fresh potatoes.

Over 60 percent of the convenience *fruit* and *berry* products had a higher cost than their fresh counterpart. Frozen orange juice concentrate was the best orange juice buy.

Of the 162 convenience foods studied by the USDA, 36 percent had a cost per serving lower than their home-prepared or fresh counterpart. However, comparisons of convenience versus home-prepared foods involve other variables besides price alone—such as the energy used to prepare the food, leftover portions of ingredient packages that spoil before they are used, and the value of the time of the persons preparing the food. Singles may find TV dinners cheaper than purchasing small quantities of the items included, since the unit price of small containers is usually greater than for larger ones. The other option for people who eat alone—larger portions of fewer foods—makes it difficult to maintain adequate nutrient variety in the diet.

Elderly people or younger ones with physical handicaps or time limitations may find that convenience products offer a greater variety in both foods and nutrients than they would otherwise be able to prepare. Some people enjoy eating and appreciate their body's need for nutrients, but do not like to spend time cooking. Under these circumstances, access to the easier-to-prepare items may ultimately influence the amount and variety and therefore the nutritional value of their diet.

Unsatisfactory Purchase. Most defective merchandise—clothing, tools, toys, automobiles—is returnable to the merchant; food is no exception. Grocery stores and large companies have a reputation to maintain in a competitive market. Most of them are willing to refund your money if food products do not meet your expectations and you take the time to return the product.

Savings at Home

The time and effort that go into thoughtful shopping can be wasted if you fail to use nutrition knowledge in the kitchen and at the table. The nutrients that have been purchased can be diminished between the check-out counter and your mouth.

Unpacking the Groceries. Many fresh fruits and vegetables that are bruised by rough handling start to rot more quickly. Foods that require refrigeration, but are left in a warm car while other errands are run en route home, do not retain their usability nearly so long as those maintained at the proper temperature.

Since some of the nutrients in many foods gradually deteriorate, you should rotate them in storage areas. Newly purchased ones go on the bottom of the stack, to the back of the freezer, or behind older cans of food in the pantry.

Frozen foods should be stored in usable units. A 5-pound package of hamburger can be a bargain if it is thawed in amounts appropriate for meals or recipes. If bacon and sausage are used only occasionally, these packages should also be broken and rewrapped for freezing in the amounts that will be used each time you cook them.

Preparing Food. Nutrient value of fruits and vegetables is affected by food processing—both in the factory and in the home. The nutritional value of many foods can be protected by the careful cook. Boiling should be done for the shortest time possible to prevent the destruction of vitamins sensitive to moist heat—thiamin, folacin, and vitamin C. Because minerals and water-soluble vitamins dissolve in cooking water, boil foods in as little water as possible to minimize nutrient loss. During World War II many people used a food that is rarely part of the diet today except in soul food—pot liquor. The juices and cooking water from vegetables were

TABLE 11-4. Losses in Vitamins As a Result of Cooking Vegetables and Keeping Them Warm

Vegetable	Time (hours)		Vitamin Loss (%)			
	Cooking	Warming	Vitamin C	Thiamin	Riboflavin	Niacin
Cabbage, boiled	*	0	70	60	50	†
Carrots, boiled	*	0	70	50	30	50
Potatoes, boiled	*	0	10	15	†	15
	*	1	20	20	†	20
Potatoes, baked	*	4	60	20	†	‡
Spinach, boiled and drained	1/6	1	95	90	80	85

* Cooked until done.
† Data not available.
‡ Insignificant loss.

SOURCE: Combined from articles published by F. Streightoff, H. E. Munsell, M. L. Orr, et al., in *Journal of The American Dietetic Association* 22(1946):17, 511; 25(1949):420, 770.

served over corn bread or on potatoes, rice, or starchy vegetables. In those days potato skin, rich in B vitamins and nondigestible carbohydrate, was also buttered and eaten—not fed to the garbage can. The smart food preparer today drains cooking fluids into a cup or stock pot, not into the sink. Many Europeans, as well as soup-and-sauce makers in this country, save cooking water and vegetable scraps to add flavor and nutrients to various dishes.

Reheating leftovers and leaving them for several days in the refrigerator destroys some of the nutrients (Table 11-4). Therefore, cook only what is needed. To avoid reheating vegetables, remember that many packages of frozen foods can be sliced with a sharp knife, the unused portion rewrapped and returned to the freezer for later use. Large bags of frozen vegetables from which you can take out the amount you need are also helpful if you are preparing small quantities and want to avoid leftovers that will need to be reheated. Frozen vegetables should not be thawed but should go directly into boiling water.

Riboflavin is particularly sensitive to destruction by light. Many of the rich sources of this nutrient, such as milk and cheese, are packaged to protect this vitamin. These products should not be left out in the light for extended periods of time after packages are opened or milk poured.

Energy Savers. One-burner meals or meals that are completely cooked in the oven are ways to save energy and money, though they do not necessarily save nutrients.

Cool air is lost each time a refrigerator or freezer is opened because additional energy is necessary to restore the cold temperature. Keeping the refrigerator full minimizes the amount of air that must be cooled.

The Garbage Study. A nutritional anthropologist conducted a study that has challenged nutrition educators to impress on their audiences the importance of food waste. By examining the garbage from many homes the researchers estimated how much food had been used and how much discarded. Not all the food could be measured—some left no indication in the garbage. Taking into account bottles returned, food without containers, and food ground up by disposals, the researchers calculated the percentage of the food that entered the home as groceries but left the home as garbage. The cost of this food per household per year was more than sixty dollars.

Savings at the Table. The best way to reduce waste of the nutrients in food at the table is to match portions to appetites. Leftovers that would serve only one or two people in the family can masquerade as "choices," if those from several meals are all served on the same evening buffet-style.

Holidays and Company. The best laid plans regarding nutrition and budget are often thrown to the wind for holiday and company meals. Under such circumstances, we can see how diet is affected by tradition and what society defines as etiquette. In one meal, a food preparer can spend more money on extra touches than was saved during an entire week of careful planning. Food does indeed contribute many nonquantifiable pleasures to holiday occasions, but it is worth considering how far you must deviate from the basic guidelines of nutrition and economy in order to conform to socially defined menus appropriate for holidays and company meals.

STUDY QUESTIONS

1. What factors affect the amount of money a family has available for the purchase of food?

2. How do the food selections of poorer families compare to those of families with higher incomes?

3. What are the least expensive sources of vitamins A and C, riboflavin, thiamin, calcium, iron, protein, and energy?

4. Which foods should the careful food shopper concentrate attention on?

5. What nutritional factor(s) should guide your food selections in the meat group?

6. How should you select the most economical food buy from the milk group?

7. Which products are usually the best buys within the cereal group?

8. What factors must be considered when looking for economical choices within the fruit and vegetable group?

9. Where should foods not found in any of the four food groups fit in the food budget?

10. How can planning and analyzing your shopping patterns help you save money on food?

11. How do convenience foods generally compare in cost with fresh or homemade foods?

12. How can you avoid wasting nutrients in the preparation and serving of food?

SUGGESTED READING

1. B. Peterkin, "Food plans and family budgeting," *Family Economics Review*, Agricultural Research Service, U.S. Department of Agriculture (Spring 1975).
2. B. Peterkin, "The appropriate family food plan," *Family Economics Review*, Agricultural Research Service, U.S. Department of Agriculture (Fall 1976):20–21.
3. B. Peterkin, "Dietary guidance for food stamp families," *Family Economics Review*, Agricultural Research Service, U.S. Department of Agriculture (Winter 1976):18–24.
4. "Are Americans careful food shoppers?" *FDA Consumer* 10(1976):15–17.
5. N. J. Barrett and A. Driscoll, "The impact of inflation on families," *Family Economics Review*, Agricultural Research Service, U.S. Department of Agriculture (Spring 1976):20–23.
6. P. Isom, "Costs of milk and milk products as sources of calcium—an update," *Family Economics Review*, Agricultural Research Service, U.S. Department of Agriculture (Summer 1976):5–7.
7. D. Odland and C. Adams, "Textured soy protein as a ground beef extender," *Family Economics Review*, Agricultural Research Service, U.S. Department of Agriculture (Summer 1976):3–4.
8. M. K. Head and F. G. Giesbrecht, "Effects of storage and handling on vitamins in fresh lima beans,"

Journal of the American Dietetic Association 69(1976):640.

9. G. G. Harrison, W. L. Rathje, and W. W. Hughes, "Food waste behavior in an urban population," *Journal of Nutrition Education* 7(1975):13–16.

10. J. P. Ikeda, "Expressed nutrition information needs of low-income homemakers," *Journal of Nutrition Education* 7(1975):104–106.

11. J. P. Chassy and J. B. Nichols, "Food cost tables to help stretch your dollars," from *1974 Yearbook of Agriculture*, U.S. Department of Agriculture. Washington, D.C.: Government Printing Office, 1975.

12. J. E. Bryant, ed. (Money Management Institute), *Your Food Dollar.* Chicago and Toronto: Household Finance Corporation and Household Finance Corporation of Canada, 1972, reprinted 1974.

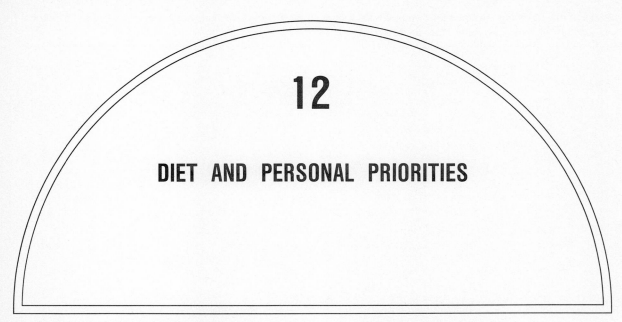

12

DIET AND PERSONAL PRIORITIES

Personal values influence the food choices of people regardless of their activity patterns or energy needs, their reliance upon snacks, or their financial means. Such food preferences usually do not take into consideration the nutritional value of preferred (or avoided) foods, but they do not necessarily conflict with selection of an appropriate diet. This chapter discusses the nutritional value of various diets when food preferences are affected by (1) ethnic influences; (2) religious instruction; (3) vegetarian guidelines; or (4) acceptance or rejection of food on the basis of the use of chemicals in agriculture, various methods of food processing, and the inclusion of additives. The selection or avoidance of any food or group of foods, regardless of the reasons, may affect the nutrient composition of your total diet. The effect can be beneficial or detrimental, depending upon your ability to use nutrition knowledge within your personal value system.

ETHNIC INFLUENCES

The American diet—no matter how much we enjoy it—is far from perfect nutritionally. Many of our diets have the following problems:

1. Provide more energy than we use
2. Have low nutrient density
3. Rely heavily upon foods that contain fat, cholesterol, sugar, or sodium
4. Fail to include sufficient amounts of fruits and vegetables
5. Neglect dairy products

Correcting these nutritional problems may be easier if you use more of some foods that you do not commonly eat.

Broadening your awareness of the diet patterns of other people offers several advantages that are of more importance than simply being cultural curiosities. Although some ethnic diets selected by other cultures often repeat the same mistakes made in the traditional American diet, some of these food patterns have nutritonal merits. If we identify the good points in other diets and adopt them in place of some of our poor diet habits, we may have—in nutritional terms—the best of all worlds.

Diets in Other Countries

People around the world select different foods to provide the same nutrients. Table 12-1 compares the

Some of the nutritional imperfections in traditional American diets may be minimized by learning about the foods more frequently chosen by people in other countries.

Nutrient	United States Diet	East African Masai Diet	Egyptian Diet
Carbo-hydrates	Bread, rice, potatoes, cereal, sugar	Milk	Dates, figs, bananas, egg-plant, baklava, halva, bread
Fats	Beef, salad dressing, margarine, fried foods, milk	Meat, milk	Lamb, cheese, chicken
Protein	Beef, poultry, milk, cheese	Milk, meat, blood	Fish, lamb, cheese, chicken, beans, chick-peas
Vitamins	Bread, green beans, potatoes, corn, peas, carrots, milk, tomatoes, orange juice	Milk, meat, wild fruits	Fish, limes, oranges, several green leafy vegetables, mangoes
Minerals	Bread, milk, cheese, beef, corn, lettuce, spinach	Milk, blood, meat	Helba (grain), cheese, grape leaves, yogurt, beans, dates

TABLE 12-1. Sources of Nutrients in Diets around the World

foods primarily used as sources of carbohydrates, fats, protein, vitamins, and minerals in six different countries to the foods selected by most Americans to meet these nutrient needs. Although some of the foods listed are available and are used in the United States, many (such as blood drunk by the Masai, seaweed eaten by the Japanese, and snails savored by the French) are so different from our usual foods that they would probably not be eaten even if they were widely available in our markets. Other foods shown in Table 12-1 (such as cashew fruit in the Brazilian diet and papaya eaten in Guatemala) cannot easily be added to our diet because they are not grown in our country and are therefore very expensive if available at all. On the other hand, some of the foods are part of the American diet, but could be used more frequently:

1. Fish (used by the Egyptians and Japanese) and chicken (eaten more often by the French and Guatemalans) are both lower in fat and cholesterol than beef.

2. Artichokes (a good source of vitamins and minerals for the French) is not one of our more popular vegetables.

3. Milk is used much more frequently by the Masai than by American adults (whose diets often fail to meet the RDAs for calcium).

4. Beans and peas combined with cereals such as corn and rice provide protein and other nutrients without also contributing fat to the diet of Brazilians and Guatemalans.

Diets in the United States

America, the melting pot, is expressed in our diet as much as it is in our family trees. Our various ethnic stocks give many of us food preferences that

The foods preferred by certain groups in the United States influence the variety of foods used by the broader American population.

Japanese Diet	Guatemalan Diet	Brazilian Diet	French Diet
Rice, oranges, broccoli, bean sprouts	Tortillas, black beans, pineapple, papaya, cornmeal	Rice, pumpkin, coconuts, bananas, manioc flour, pineapple	Bread, potatoes, artichokes, turnips, sauces, crepes
Raw and cooked fish, tempura	Cheese, chicken	Red palm oil, olive oil, butter	Cheeses, chicken, pâté de foie gras, sausages
Raw and cooked fish, shrimp, eggs, beef, eel	Chicken, black beans, cheese, tortillas	Dried beef (jerky), feijoada (beans, dried beef, tongue, and other ingredients), fish	Chicken, cheeses, snails, beef, ham
Seaweed, raw and cooked fish, rice, shrimp, oranges, strawberries, tofu	Black beans, tortillas, chicken, chard, papaya, carrots, cheese, pineapple, peppers	Cashew fruit, mangoes, oranges, tomatoes, several squashes, red palm oil	Beets, chard, snails, bread, cheeses, potatoes, artichokes, plums, grapes
Shrimp, raw and cooked fish, seaweed, green onions, tofu	Black beans, chard, tortillas, cheese, cornmeal	Dried beef (jerky), beans, cornmeal, fish	Artichokes, snails, bread, cheeses, beets, chard

are influenced by the country from which our ancestors emigrated.

Many of the dishes now considered characteristic of certain regions of the United States are actually specialties of the immigrants who congregated in those areas. Pennsylvania Dutch food includes many German (Deutsch) dishes. Most people from Pennsylvania are more familiar with sauerbraten and scrapple than are Californians or Texans. A salad served as the last course of a meal may startle many people, but not someone familiar with the Pennsylvania Dutch way of eating.

The cuisine for which tourists travel to New Orleans blends the delicate foods of the French, the herbs and wild game of the Indians, and the highly flavored foods of the Spanish. Gumbo and other Creole dishes are favorites of many people who grew up in Louisiana. In a similar way, the Scandinavians have enriched the food culture of Minnesota, and the Mexicans have contributed strongly to the diet of the Southwest.

Preferences for foods that are specialties of other countries are not, however, restricted to people of any one state. Chinese restaurants are located from Los Angeles to Boston. Irish pubs and English chips are found in many parts of the country. In some cities it is hard to find restaurants that serve certain ethnic dishes, but in New York or San Francisco the selection includes Thai, Polish, Indian, Russian, and many other kinds of food.

The impact of other cultures upon American eating patterns changes over time. When people leave an area of the country, or even broaden their circle of friends in their home town, they assimilate other foods into their diet. The person who has traveled or lived in another country sometimes comes home with different food preferences.

Political and social factors also affect food choices. Peanut soup appeared for the first time on many restaurant menus in 1976. Soul food has evolved from the diet of a segment of the Black population in the South to an interesting and nutritious part of the broader American diet. The increasing number of Cubans and Puerto Ricans in this country has had a rather recent impact upon the diet of their fellow Americans. The influx of Vietnamese and other Southeast Asians during the early 1970s will probably have an increasing influence on the American diet in years to come.

Nutritional Characteristics

Each ethnic diet offers some dishes that might complement the nutritional value of the more conventional American diet. For example, Chinese food is nutrient-dense because it is low in fat, vegetables are used frequently, and desserts are not emphasized. The sauces of French food are high in energy, but they add appeal to many vegetables often slighted by Americans. Mexican dishes that combine beans and cornmeal take advantage of the fact that the amino acids in the protein of these two foods complement each other and enhance the nutritional value of either eaten alone; the red peppers used in Mexican dishes are an excellent source of vitamin C. Most Europeans traditionally use more potatoes than Americans and many strongly flavored vegetables such as cabbage, parsnips, and several kinds of greens. These foods are excellent sources of micronutrients, but they are rejected by many people in the United States.

It is impossible in a few pages to discuss all the advantages and disadvantages of ethnic influences on the American diet. Table 12-2 summarizes the diet patterns (according to each food group) predominantly practiced by Chinese, Italian, Japanese, Jewish, Polish, Puerto Rican, and Spanish-American

people and by people living in the southern United States. Factors that might enhance the nutritional value of each diet pattern are included in parentheses of this table. Some items are common to several of these diet patterns and distinguish them from most American diets. The following might be worth considering as additions or substitutions in your current diet:

1. The fruits and vegetables column for all diets suggests some foods worth trying. Do you know whether you like watercress, figs, zucchini, artichokes, chard, or eggplant? How long has it been since you had a fresh pineapple, a tangerine, or apricot nectar?

2. Organ meats are used frequently by other cultures but are usually rejected by Americans. Maybe chitterlings is stretching your adventuresome spirit too much, but chopped chicken livers are worth trying as a dip or spread for crackers. You might like tongue if you tried it.

3. In ethnic diets where the people dislike or simply do not use milk, various cheeses contribute the nutrients provided by this group of foods. If you always reach for American, Swiss, or cheddar cheese, you have not given yourself a chance to enjoy some other tasty sources of calcium and riboflavin.

4. It would take several weeks to sample all the bread and cereal products from different cultures. If the foods you have been eating from this group seem bland and tasteless, try pumpernickel, then rye, then corn bread. You do not have to be Jewish to like bagels. Have you ever made a dumpling? Tortillas can be an interesting addition to your diet, and you can buy them ready for frying.

5. Many soups eaten often by other cultures are available in cans in this country. Table 12-2 and your own initiative may allow you to broaden the variety of these in your diet.

These suggestions are only a starting point. Since some people are more familiar with one type of national dish than are others, you may want to swap ideas with friends about other foods that would be interesting to try. The possibilities mainly depend upon personal preferences and perhaps also upon overcoming some ideas left from your childhood about what you do or do not like.

Religion influences diet patterns through specific dietary instructions and by heightening social awareness of nutrition problems.

RELIGIOUS INFLUENCES

Food is closely tied to many aspects of religion. Christians who observe communion are humbled by partaking of the Lord's Supper; many Hindus would starve rather than eat beef; strict Moslems and Jews will not eat pork.

Dietary Instruction

Many of the ties between religion and diet are not as extreme as the examples above, but they are pervasive. The Jewish dietary patterns are shown in Table 12-2. Abstinence from alcohol is taught by many religions. This diet pattern could increase the nutrient density of the diet, depending upon what other beverages, if any, are selected instead of beer, wine, and whiskey.

Although Catholics may now eat meat on Friday, the past instruction that they eat fish on that day has become so much a part of American food culture, that many menus continue to make Friday fish day.

Mormons go beyond many religions in providing dietary guidance for members of their faith. Alcohol, coffee, tea, and cola beverages are not used by strict Mormons. Members of this faith believe that gluttony—regardless of what is eaten—conflicts with the teachings of their church. Mormons are also instructed to maintain a year's supply of food in case of an emergency. Since many foods cannot be preserved indefinitely, the reserves must be cycled. Their diet therefore includes some foods (such as whole-grain cereals, canned fruits and vegetables, and dried milk) that are quite different from the daily fare of most people.

Social and Scientific Impact

The interrelationship between religion and food is broader than symbolism or dietary instruction. The social program of many religions revolves around the kitchen of their place of worship. These facilities are also used for many community feeding programs such as those for the elderly.

Often, weekly sermons delivered in various churches, synagogues, and interfaith centers address the question of how the membership should respond to the world food problem. This awareness may lead to decreased consumption of animal sources of protein and more careful consideration of how much food is needed by individuals. Such changes in diet patterns alter the nutritional status of some Americans although the changes are motivated by a concern for other people rather than for their own nutritional well-being.

Religious instruction regarding food use sometimes has repercussions that go beyond the lives of members of that faith. The Seventh Day Adventists teach their members to abstain from meat. Nutrition researchers who are members of this church have made significant contributions to scientific knowledge regarding the nutritional value of combinations of nonmeat foods. This church has supported the development of vegetarian products that are now used by many people who are not Seventh Day Adventists.

VEGETARIAN DIETS

Vegetarian diets have been practiced (primarily for religious reasons) in the United States for many years, but during the last decade they have become popular among a much larger group of people. On some college campuses, as many as 25 percent of the students observe a vegetarian diet to some degree. The reasons for choosing this pattern vary. They may be religious, philosophical, nutritional, ecological, financial, or other reasons.

All vegetarian diets cannot be lumped into one category. Foods that are acceptable differ among vegetarians:

1. A *pure, or strict, vegetarian diet* excludes all foods of animal origin—meat, poultry, fish, eggs, and dairy products.

2. A *lacto-vegetarian diet* includes dairy products, but excludes meat, poultry, fish, and eggs.

TABLE 12-2. Diet Patterns and Food Preferences of Ethnic Groups in the United States

Ethnic Group	Milk	Meat	Fruits and Vegetables	Cereal	Other Foods
Chinese[a]	Milk or milk products are rarely used beyond infancy due to traditional scarcity and expense. For some, milk is unacceptable and disliked. Cheese is rarely used. Ice cream is popular. Bean curd is high in calcium and protein, and can help meet needs for these nutrients, but not for vitamin A. (Mix milk into cereals. Use milk for making steamed eggs.)	Usually served in mixed dishes. Pork, fish, and eggs are popular; chicken and shellfish are used less frequently. Meat may not be served often to young children, since it is considered difficult to chew. (Baby food meat or minced and chopped meats may be acceptable for children.)	A wide variety of vegetables is used, such as spinach, broccoli, leek, various greens, bok choy (cabbage), carrot, pumpkin, sweet potato, mushroom, soybean, brussels sprout, turnip, radish, watercress, kohlrabi, white eggplant, bamboo shoot, and snowpea. Fruits considered to be a delicacy may be used as snack food, not as dessert. Some fruits are reserved for men. Fruits used in different regions include large dates, figs, winter melon, mango, red tangerine, papaya, pineapple litchee nut, and others more commonly used in American diets. (Encourage use of some source of vitamin C daily. Emphasize use of foods high in vitamin A, especially if milk is not used.)	Regional differences in consumption exist. Wheat products, including noodles, steamed bread, millet, and rice are eaten in the north; rice in the central regions; rice, rice flour, and "sticky rice" in the south. (Encourage use of enriched or brown rice.)	Soybean oil, peanut oil, and lard are used. Sweets include sugar, molasses, brown sugar, and, occasionally, preserves. Seasonings most often used are salt, ginger, garlic, scallion, parsley, red and green pepper, sugar, and vinegar. Sodium intake as MSG (monosodium glutamate) may be high. (Encourage substitution of vegetable oils for lard. Encourage use of seasonings that provide vitamin C.)

| Italian | Most adults drink very little milk, except in coffee. Children may or may not get recommended amounts of milk. Cheese is eaten frequently, and is used in the preparation of many cooked foods. (Encourage the use of milk.) | Veal, beef, pork, and chicken are the most popular meats. Meat is often fried. Sausages and salami are frequently served. Organ meats (liver, tripe, heart, lungs) are also used. Shrimp, lobster, squid, snail, and mussels are eaten. Fish may be fresh, canned (anchovies, tuna, sardines), or dried (cod). Eggs are used in omelets and in preparing other dishes.
Many varieties of dried beans and peas are used in soups, stews, pasta, and salads. (Encourage cooking methods other than frying.) | Large quantities of green vegetables (both cooked and raw) are used: escarole, Swiss chard, mustard greens, dandelion greens, broccoli, eggplant, zucchini, artichoke, and mushroom. Vegetables are often first boiled and then cooked in oil. Peppers and tomatoes are used in the preparation of many foods. Potatoes are seldom eaten, probably because pasta is considered the "starchy" part of the meal.
Many kinds of fruits are liked. Grapes, oranges, tangerines, and figs are among the most popular. Persimmons and pomegranates are holiday favorites. Raw fruit is often served for dessert. (Consider methods of cooking vegetables that require shorter cooking time and use less oil.) | Pasta is a staple of the Italian diet. Rice is also used by Italian families. Bread is eaten every day at each meal. The use of whole-grain and enriched cereals (such as oatmeal and farina) for breakfast has increased.
(Italian bread may not be made with milk and may not be enriched unless it is packaged and labeled as such.) | Olive oil is the preferred cooking oil. Lard may also be used in cooking, and salt pork for flavoring soups and tomato sauce. Butter may be preferred for baking. Olives are well-liked. Cakes, pastries, and frozen desserts (spumoni) are used on festive occasions. |

a Styles of cooking vary and are known as Mandarin (north), Shanghai (central), and Cantonese (south). Eating habits are influenced by the belief in the importance of balancing the intake of "hot" and "cold" foods. This classification is based on beliefs regarding the reaction a food has within the body; it is unrelated to temperature or seasoning. In general, the actual cooking time of most Chinese dishes is brief. Foods are steamed, boiled, or stir fried in a small amount of hot fat.

NOTE: Nutrition considerations are included in parentheses.
SOURCE: Adapted from *Cultural Food Patterns in the U.S.A.*, The American Dietetic Association, 1976. Copyright The American Dietetic Association. Reprinted by permission.

CHAPTER 12 / DIET AND PERSONAL PRIORITIES

TABLE 12-2. Diet Patterns and Food Preferences of Ethnic Groups in the United States (*continued*)

Ethnic Group	Milk	Meat	Fruits and Vegetables	Cereal	Other Foods
Japanese	Milk (fresh and canned) is used in small-to-moderate amounts. Milk desserts, such as ice cream, may be used. Cheese is used only in small amounts. (Consider use of milk in cooking, such as in simple milk puddings, and greater use of cheese.)	A variety of saltwater and freshwater fish is eaten. These are broiled, boiled, and used in soups. Raw fish is consumed on occasion. Smoked, dried, and canned fish are also eaten. The main dish often is a combination of meat and vegetables seasoned with soy sauce. Beef, pork, and poultry are preferred to lamb and veal. Eggs are frequently eaten raw, fried, boiled, scrambled, and in soups. Many dried beans and peas commonly used in Japan are rarely available in the United States. (See Chapter 20 regarding the safety of raw fish and raw eggs. Encourage the use of organ meats.)	A large variety of vegetables (both raw and cooked) is eaten: spinach, broccoli, carrot, green beans, pea, cauliflower, tomato, cucumber, eggplant, peppers, and squash. These may be prepared with meat, fish, and chicken. A large variety of fresh fruit is eaten: orange, tangerine, grapefruit, apple, pear, and melon. (Par cooking and draining of water causes loss of nutrients in food.)	Polished white rice is the staple; the short-grain, sticky variety is preferred. Consumption of wheat products (as in breads and cereals) has increased. (Washing restored or enriched rice prior to cooking removes some of the added nutrients. Suggest more frequent inclusion of potato cooked in the skin in place of rice.)	Butter is used in small amounts. Deep-fat frying of fish, shellfish, and vegetables for *tempura* is one of the few times when fat is used in food preparation. Simple cakes and cookies made of sugar and rice flour containing little or no fat are eaten. Soy sauce is used frequently. *Miso* sauce (a soybean product) is used as seasoning for these same dishes. Many varieties of pickles are eaten.[b] Tea is a much more popular beverage than milk or coffee.
Jewish[c]	Dietary laws prohibit using meat and milk at the same meal. Cottage cheese and pot cheese are eaten plain or in *blintzes* (pancakes) and noodle puddings. (Encourage use of milk at breakfast. Nondairy substitutes may sometimes be used with meat; their	Orthodox Jews use only meat that is *kosher*.[a] Meat is usually broiled, boiled, roasted, or stewed with vegetables added. Liver and tongue are used frequently. Fish that have fins and scales may be used, but shellfish (such as oysters, crab, and	Spinach or sorrell leaves are used for *schav*, a popular soup. Green peppers are often served stuffed with meat or a dairy mixture. Tomatoes are extensively used. Potato pancakes (*latkes*), potato pudding prepared with eggs, and noodles or noodle	Bagels, rye bread, and pumpernickel do not have milk or milk solids. *Matzoth* is the only bread product allowed during Passover, and is commonly used throughout the year. Whole grains such as oatmeal, barley, brown rice, buckwheat groats (*kasha*) are	Sweet (unsalted) butter, usually whipped, is preferred to salted butter. Chicken fat is often the choice for browning meats and frying potato pancakes. Pickled cucumbers and tomatoes, horseradish, and condiments are commonly used.

nutrient content should be compared to that of milk.)	lobster) and scavenger fish (such as sturgeon and catfish) are not allowed. Fish and eggs are considered *pareve* (neutral) and may be eaten with milk or meat. Eggs are used frequently. Dried beans, peas, and lentils are eaten often, especially as soup.	pudding, are popular. Beets are used in soup (*borscht*). Cooked, dried fruits (prunes, raisins, apples, peaches, pears, apricots) are commonly served. Fresh or stewed fruits are often eaten as dessert with the meat meal. (An average serving of cooked, dried fruit supplies much more energy than fresh fruit or juice).	used. Danish pastries, coffee cakes, homemade cakes, and cookies may be eaten in large quantities. Honey cakes are served for various holidays. (Matzoth, crackers, and saltines are not enriched.)	Soft drinks are served with meat meals because milk beverages are forbidden. (Encourage greater use of vegetable oils.)
Polish	Children drink fresh milk, while adults may prefer buttermilk. Sour cream is also popular and used in soup, salad dressings, with berries, and raw vegetables. Cheese is often used. Cottage cheese may be served with sour cream.	Beef and pork are the most popular meats. Pigs' knuckles, sausages, smoked and cured pork, chicken, goose, duck, and organ meats (liver, tripe, tongue, brains) are also eaten. Fish (fresh, smoked, dried, or pickled) is used. Eggs are used in the preparation of pancakes, noodles, dumplings, and soups. Legumes are used in soups.	Potatoes are used in soups, stews, pancakes, and dumplings. Other popular vegetables include carrot, beet, turnip, cauliflower, kohlrabi, broccoli, sorrel, green pepper, pea, spinach, and green beans. Fruits rich in vitamin C are not traditionally popular, but citrus fruits may be used more liberally today than previously. Dried fruits are well liked.	Bread probably will be eaten at each meal. Pumpernickel, sour rye bread, white bread, and sweet buns are commonly used. Oatmeal, rice, noodles, dumplings, cornmeal, porridge, and kasha are eaten frequently.	A wide variety of fats and oils is used. Candy, sweet cakes, and other sweets (such as honey) may be eaten frequently. Coffee with cream and sugar is a favorite beverage. Tea is infrequently consumed. (The use of fruits as desserts might be encouraged if energy intake exceeds energy needs and if fruits are used infrequently.)

[b] Seasonings and pickles are often high in sodium.

[c] Jewish dietary laws are observed in varying degrees by Orthodox, Conservative, and Reformed denominations. Orthodox families place great value on traditional and ceremonial rituals of their religion and observe the dietary laws under all conditions. Conservative and Reformed families often make individual decisions about which laws to follow.

[d] Animals and poultry must be slaughtered by a ritual slaughter (*shochet*) according to specified regulations. Before cooking, meat is koshered by one of two methods: (1) It is soaked in cold water for half an hour; salted with coarse salt (koshering salt); and drained to let blood run off. It is then thoroughly washed under cold running water and drained again before cooking. (2) It is quick-seared. Liver, for example, cannot be koshered by soaking and salting because of its high blood content.

TABLE 12-2. Diet Patterns and Food Preferences of Ethnic Groups in the United States (*continued*)

Ethnic Group	Milk	Meat	Fruits and Vegetables	Cereal	Other Foods
Puerto Rican	Although milk may not be consumed as such, a cup of *cafe con leche* (coffee with milk) may contain 2 to 5 ounces of milk. Domestic American cheese is used in limited quantities. Native white cheese (resembling farmer cheese, but firmer and saltier) is used. (Evaporated milk and nonfat dry milk might be used in cooking, puddings, and cereals.)	Chicken is often eaten in combination with other foods. Expensive cuts of pork and beef are frequently selected and are usually fried. Ham butts and sausage are used to flavor different dishes. The intestine of the pig is eaten either fried (*cuchifritos*) or stewed with native vegetables (*salcocho*) and chick-peas. Fish is used in limited amounts, but salt codfish is a common choice. Eggs are used often in cooking, and they are fried or scrambled. Beans are eaten almost every day. A sauce called *refrito* (green pepper, tomato, garlic, lard) is served with the beans and rice. Pigeon and chick-peas are very popular. (Salt codfish is a major source of sodium in many diets. The quality of protein in chick-peas is almost as good as that in soybeans.)	Yautia, apio, malanga, name, and plantain are frequently used. (These have fair amounts of B vitamins, iron, and vitamin C.) Pumpkin, carrot, green pepper, tomato, and sweet potato are well liked. Pumpkin is used to thicken and flavor foods. Head lettuce, cabbage, fresh tomato, and onion are often eaten in basic salad ingredients. Long cooking of vegetables (as in stews) is common. Chicken and vegetable soups are often served as the main dish. Bananas and fresh pineapple are quite popular and frequently eaten. Fruit cocktail, canned pears, peaches, and peach, apricot, and pear nectar are commonly used. (Diets may be low in leafy vegetables, or nutrients may be destroyed during long cooking.)	Plantain is often eaten in place of bread. French bread, rolls, and crackers are the most frequent choices. Breakfast cereals are cooked in milk instead of water.	Butter is used in small amounts; lard and salt pork are used for flavoring many dishes, often in large amounts. Olive oil is a favorite for vegetables and salads. Sugar is used liberally in beverages and desserts. Guava, orange, and mango pastes and boiled papaya preserves are often eaten between meals. Black malt beer is a favorite beverage. (Margarine and corn, cottonseed, or soybean oil may be substituted for lard and salt pork. Guava and mango pastes retain some of the vitamin C even after boiling.)

Spanish-American/Mexican[e]	Limited amounts of milk and cheese are used.	Chicken, pork chops, frankfurters, cold cuts, and hamburgers are the most commonly used meats, but even these may be eaten infrequently. Eggs are often used. In rural areas, people may have their own chickens. Beans are usually eaten with every meal. They are cooked, mashed, and refried with lard. (The protein value of beans and lentils is enhanced when eaten with animal proteins such as milk, meat, eggs, or cheese.)	Potatoes are usually fried. They may be used three times a day. Chilies from green and red peppers are good sources for vitamin A, even when dried. Green peppers are usually called "mangoes." Tomato, pumpkin, corn, field greens, onion, and carrot are used frequently. Banana, melon, peach, and canned fruit cocktail are the more popular fruits. Orange and apple are used occasionally as snacks. (Vitamin C in potatoes is destroyed more by frying than by baking or boiling. Melons, such as cantaloupe, are good sources of vitamin C, especially if citrus fruits are not used frequently.)	Bread (purchased or homemade) is a popular item. Tortillas from enriched wheat flour are made daily. Sweet rolls are purchased. Prepared breakfast cereals are common, but occasionally oatmeal is used. Fried macaroni is served with beans and potatoes. (Where corn tortillas are used, encourage use of dried skim milk.)	Lard, salt pork, and bacon fat are used liberally. Most foods are fried. Soft drinks, popsicles, and sweets of all kinds are eaten frequently. (Milk, ice cream, juices, and other foods discussed in Chapter 11 would improve nutrient density of the diet.)

[e]The southwestern part of the United States is a unique blending of several cultural backgrounds—Anglo, Indian, Mexican, and Spanish. A merging of food habits has resulted. The food pattern described refers primarily to the Spanish or Mexican cultures, but they are similar to the Indian.

TABLE 12-2. Diet Patterns and Food Preferences of Ethnic Groups in the United States (continued)

Ethnic Group	Milk	Meat	Fruits and Vegetables	Cereal	Other Foods
Southern United States	Limited amounts of milk are consumed. Buttermilk is often preferred. Cheese may be used in sandwiches or baked with macaroni.	Chicken and pork are very popular. Pigs' feet, hog jowls, and ham hocks are often stewed, boiled with vegetables. Spareribs are baked or barbecued. Chitterlings (intestines) are cut, dredged with cornmeal or flour, and fried crisp. Beef is used in hash or stewed with vegetables. Fresh catfish, fresh white buffalo, and canned fish are often eaten. Boiled shrimp, fried scallops, and oysters are popular in coastal regions. Rabbit, squirrel, opossum, and other small game are eaten, usually in a stew. Dried black-eyed peas and beans cooked with salt pork are popular. (Salt pork and bacon are high in fat. Stewing, baking, roasting, and boiling are preferable to frying if the diet is already high in fat.)	Few vegetables are eaten raw. Turnip greens, mustard greens, collards, cabbage, and green beans are cooked in water with bacon, ham hocks, or salt pork. The cooking liquid (pot liquor) may be eaten with corn bread. Tomato, white potato, and sweet potato are popular. Citrus fruit may be infrequently eaten. Fruits may be eaten between meals. Watermelon and lemonade are favorites in summer. (Quick-cooking vegetables in very little water would protect some vitamins. Addition of baking soda to the water in which vegetables are cooked to make them stay green destroys some vitamins.)	Few whole-grain cereals are used. Hominy grits with gravy, hot biscuits with molasses, and corn bread are eaten extensively. Rice cooked with ham fat, tomatoes, onion, and okra is especially popular. Dumplings, pancakes, and hoecakes are favorite foods. Cakes, cookies, pies, other pastries, and sweet breads of low nutrient density are very popular. (Baked goods should be made with enriched flour or enriched corn meal.)	Bacon and salt pork are liberally used in vegetable cookery. Lard is used for baking and frying. Gravies are used generously. Molasses and cane syrup are employed as sweeteners. Ice cream, jams, and jellies are frequently eaten. Large quantities of soft drinks are consumed, especially by children. (Bacon and salt pork are high in fat and sodium.)

The difficulty in designing a nutritionally adequate vegetarian diet varies directly with the number of restrictions on foods. Depending upon which foods are omitted from the diet and which are added to supply adequate energy, a vegetarian diet may be lower in fat and cholesterol and higher in fiber and certain micronutrients than a nonvegetarian diet.

3. An *ovo-lacto-vegetarian diet* includes eggs and dairy products, but excludes meat, poultry, and fish.

These distinctions are important because the complexity of designing a nutritionally adequate vegetarian diet depends upon the restrictiveness of that diet. For instance, the strict vegetarian must be careful to select foods that provide the nutrients supplied by eggs and dairy products as well as meat, whereas the ovo-lacto-vegetarian need be concerned only about including sources of the nutrients commonly found in meat.

Potential Advantages

Although vegetarian diets were at one time considered by many nutritionists to be faddist, some nutritionists today acknowledge that there are potential advantages to this diet if the vegetarian learns how to compensate for possible problems and uses nutrition knowledge. The crucial factor in determining the nutritional value of this (or any other) modification of the diet is the comparative nutrient composition of the foods not eaten versus those added to the diet.

Fat Intake. The major sources of fat in the average American diet are meat, dairy products, butter or margarine, and the oils used in cooking or on salads. Because many foods that are acceptable to vegetarians (such as vegetables, fruits, beans, and cereals) contain very little fat, a vegetarian diet may provide less fat than a nonvegetarian diet. On the other hand, some vegetarian foods (such as nuts, seeds, salad dressing, fried vegetables, and margarine) are as high or higher in fat than animal products. If these foods replace meat in the vegetarian diet, there may be no difference in total fat intake compared to a nonvegetarian diet.

Cholesterol Intake. Because cholesterol is found only in animal products, strict vegetarians have a very low cholesterol intake.° However, ovo-lacto-vegetarians, who rely heavily upon eggs to meet their needs for protein, iron, and vitamin B_{12} may have an even higher cholesterol intake than nonvegetarians. Eggs are a good source of many nutrients needed by people who do not eat meat, but one egg contains about three times as much cholesterol as 3 ounces of most meats (see Table 12-3).

Fiber. Another characteristic of meat and dairy products is that they contain very little fiber. Many of the plant foods usually eaten by vegetarians are good sources of fiber.

Micronutrients. The vitamin and mineral composition of a vegetarian diet depends upon the substitutions that are made for animal products. There are several general potential advantages and disadvantages related to micronutrients.

Cutting down on animal foods that supply fat may mean you reduce your total intake of certain fat-soluble vitamins, but well-chosen nonmeat products can provide ample vitamin A (as carotene), vitamin E, and vitamin K. However, milk products and fish are needed to provide vitamin D for children and teen-agers.

Vegetarian diets that substitute fruits and yellow and dark-green vegetables for meat supply more of some micronutrients (calcium, vitamin A, vitamin C, and some B vitamins) than nonvegetarian diets. Beans, cereals, and nuts provide protein and B vitamins, but no vitamin C or vitamin A, and relatively little calcium. This difference in micronutrient composition emphasizes the importance of including both of these categories of vegetable products—and milk, if possible—within the vegetarian diet.

° Mayonnaise, a source of cholesterol, may be used even by strict vegetarians.

TABLE 12-3. Energy, Fat, Protein, and Cholesterol Value of Foods Used by Vegetarians and Nonvegetarians

Food	Energy (Cal)	Fat (g)	Protein (g)	Protein INQ	Cholesterol[a] (mg)
Nonvegetarian					
Beef, chuck roast, 3 oz.					
Lean	150	4.4	26.3	4.0	77
Lean with fat	215	12.4	24.1	1.6	*
Chicken, half breast, fried	160	5.1	25.7	5.7	63
Haddock, fried, 3 oz.	190	7.3	22.2	4.3	60
Tuna, drained, 3 oz.	170	6.5	22.6	5.0	60
Ovo-lacto-vegetarian					
Cheddar cheese, 2 oz.	225	18.2	14.2	2.0	56
Cottage cheese (4% fat), ½ lb.	240	9.5	30.8	7.1	48
Eggs, 2 medium	140	10.2	11.4	2.7	500
Milk, 1 cup	160	8.5	8.5	2.0	34
Strict vegetarian					
Beans, 1 cup					
Kidney	218	0.9	14.4	2.3	0
Lima	189	0.9	12.9	2.2	0
Navy	224	1.1	14.8	2.4	0
Bread, 2 slices					
White	152	4.8	1.8	1.0	0
Whole-grain	122	5.2	1.6	1.5	0
Green peas, 1 cup	165	1.0	9.0	1.9	0
Oatmeal, cooked, 1 cup	132	2.4	4.8	1.4	0
Peanut butter, 2 T.	188	16.2	8.0	1.5	0
Peanuts, ¼ cup	210	18.0	9.4	1.6	0
Soybeans, 1 cup	234	10.3	19.8	3.0	0
Sunflower seeds, ¼ cup	203	17.2	8.6	1.5	0
Blended vegetable proteins					
Egg substitutes	Products vary; check the nutrition information on the packages.				
Sausage substitutes					

[a] R. M. Feeley, P. E. Criner, and B. K. Watt, "Cholesterol Content of Foods," *Journal of The American Dietetic Association* 61 (1972): 134–49.

* Data not available.

SOURCE: Excerpted from R. G. Hansen, A. W. Sorenson, and A. J. Wittmer, "Index of Nutritional Quality Food Profiles" (Logan, Utah: Utah State University, 1975). © 1975, Utah State University. Used by permission.

Avoiding Nutritional Problems

Several potential problems must be faced by vegetarians to avoid nutrient deficiencies or excessive energy intake.

Protein and Energy. The protein INQ for vegetable products is generally lower than the protein INQ for animal products. Therefore, vegetarians must allot a larger percentage of their daily energy intake to sources of protein than must nonvegetarians. This fact is shown by examining Table 12-3. The amounts of foods shown in this table are based on serving sizes that provide approximately 150 to 200 Cal (630 to 840 kJ). Note that the grams of protein provided by plant foods is consistently lower than the grams of protein provided by animal products that supply a comparable amount of energy. Also, since the amino acid pattern of vegetable proteins is not as well balanced as that of animal proteins (see Chapter 3), a larger quantity of vegetable proteins is required to meet the needs for this macronutrient.

Suppose, for example, that during one day you choose to eat the following foods:

	Energy (Cal)	Protein (grams)
Bean sprouts, 1 cup	35	4.0
Sunflower seeds, 1/4 cup	203	8.6
Navy beans, 1 cup	224	14.8
Oatmeal, 1 cup	132	4.8
Peanut butter, 4 tablespoons	376	16.0
Eggs, 2	140	11.4
	1,110 Cal	59.6 grams

These foods provide a protein intake approximately comparable to two servings of meat (see Table 12-3), but they supply a much larger amount of energy than do two servings of meat (approximately 500 Cal). This is not necessarily incompatible with a nutritionally balanced diet. It simply means that less energy can be allotted in the total diet of the vegetarian to foods of low nutrient density (such as fried foods and pastries) or to foods that supply only energy and no micronutrients (such as candy, soft drinks, and alcoholic beverages). If a vegetarian fails to realize this, there is an increased risk of the total daily energy intake exceeding energy needs.

One way to handle this problem is to select the vegetable products that have the highest protein INQ or to include eggs and low-fat dairy products. Many other vegetables (Table 12-4), such as green beans, asparagus, and even lettuce, have a high protein INQ, but they provide very little protein— generally 1 to 5 grams—in an average serving. It is difficult to consume enough of these foods to supply 65 grams of protein during one day.

Soybeans are one of the most concentrated vegetable sources of protein, and their amino acid pattern is better than that in other plant products. Some commercially blended vegetable protein products are formulated from several plant foods that have complementary amino acid patterns (see Chapter 3). The quality, or PER, of these products is therefore closer to the quality of animal products.[*] Table 12-5 shows the types of vegetable products that are high and low in several of the essential amino acids.

Omitting Meat. Since all vegetarians omit meat from the diet, they must give particular attention to certain micronutrients as well as protein. Vitamin B_{12} is of primary concern to vegetarians because it is found only in animal products. Table 12-6 shows that nonvegetarians can easily meet their RDA (3 micrograms for an adult) for this nutrient by eating two servings of lamb if this were their only source of vitamin B_{12}. Beef, chicken, and many seafoods are also good sources of this nutrient; liver is especially rich in vitamin B_{12}.

[*] The labels of many of these products show nutrition information. The percentage U.S. RDA for protein value (lower part of the labels) is calculated on the basis of protein quality as well as the grams of protein per serving (see Chapter 29).

TABLE 12-4. Protein Content and INQ of Selected Vegetables

Vegetable	Protein (g)	Protein INQ	Energy per Serving[a] (Cal)	(kJ)
Asparagus	3	3.5	30	125
Bean sprouts (mung)	4	4.0	35	145
Broccoli	5	4.4	40	170
Brussels sprouts	7	4.5	55	230
Carrots	0	0	10	42
Corn	3	3.5	30	125
Green beans	2	1.6	45	190
Lettuce, one head	3	3.5	30	125
Potatoes	2	0.9	80	335
Spinach	5	3.9	45	190
Squash, summer	2	2.4	30	125
Squash, winter	4	1.1	130	545
Tomatoes	2	1.8	40	170
Turnips	1	1.0	35	145

[a] Serving size is 1 cup unless otherwise stated.

SOURCE: Excerpted from R. G. Hansen, A. W. Sorenson, and A. J. Wittmer, "Index of Nutritional Quality Food Profiles" (Logan, Utah: Utah State University, 1975). © 1975, Utah State University. Used by permission.

TABLE 12-5. Complementary Amino Acid Composition of Protein Sources Acceptable to Vegetarians

Essential Amino Acid	Vegetable Protein Source	
	Relatively Low	Relatively High
Lysine[a]	Corn, cereals, sesame and sunflower seeds	Legumes, nuts, whole grain with germ, soybeans
Sulfur-containing amino acids (cystine and methionine)	Legumes, leafy vegetables, peanuts	Cereals,[b] whole grain with germ, sesame and sunflower seeds, yeast
Threonine[a]	Corn, cereals, whole grain with germ	Legumes, nuts, yeast
Tryptophan	Corn, legumes	Sesame and sunflower seeds

[a] Supplied in relatively high amounts by cheese, eggs, milk, and meat.
[b] High in methonine but low in cystine.

SOURCE: Adapted from D. Erhard, "Nutrition education for the 'now' generation," *Journal of Nutrition Education* 2 (Spring 1971):135. © 1971, Society for Nutrition Education. Used by permission.

TABLE 12-6. Vitamin B$_{12}$ Content of Foods

Food	Vitamin B$_{12}$ (mcg)[a]
Liver, 3 oz.	
Calf	54
Chicken	23
Lamb, 3 oz.	1.9
Beef, 3 oz.	1.3
Frankfurters, 3 oz.	1.2
Pork, 3 oz.	0.5
Chicken, 3 oz.	0.4
Oysters, 3 oz.	16
Mackerel, 3 oz.	8.0
Salmon, canned, 3 oz.	3.6
Egg, 1 medium	1.0
Milk, 1 cup	1.0
Cheese, 1 oz.	0.3–0.7
Yogurt, 1 cup	0.3
Breakfast cereals, vitamin-fortified, 1 oz.	1.5
Yeast	None
Beans	None
Vegetables	None
Fruits	None

[a] The adult RDA for vitamin B$_{12}$ is 3 micrograms (mcg).

SOURCE: Adapted from U.S., Department of Agriculture, Agricultural Research Service, "Pantothenic Acid, Vitamin B$_6$, and Vitamin B$_{12}$ in Foods," *Home Economics Research Report* No. 36 (August 1969).

The vegetarian who eats eggs and dairy products can avoid problems with this vitamin. A glass of milk and an egg each provide 1 microgram (one-third of the adult RDA) of vitamin B$_{12}$. Other dairy products can help supply this vitamin—but it would take 10 cups of yogurt or about half a pound of cheese to provide 3 micrograms of vitamin B$_{12}$ for a lacto-vegetarian.

The strict vegetarian does have a few ways of getting this nutrient. One option is taking a vitamin pill; another is eating vitamin B$_{12}$ fortified foods such as some cereals.° However, "natural" or additive-free cereals do not provide vitamin B$_{12}$.

The nerve damage caused by vitamin B$_{12}$ deficiency is a real possibility. Cases among vegetarians have often been reported in the medical literature. This need not happen, however, if the information discussed above is used.

Another nutrient that requires special attention is iron. Milk is a poor source of this mineral, and an egg supplies only 1 milligram of iron. Table 12-7 lists foods of plant origin from which a thoughtful vegetarian can select enough sources to meet his or her RDA for iron.

Enriched cereal products with added iron and whole-grain cereals can be very helpful in meeting iron needs. Vegetarians must be careful, however, not to rely too heavily upon foods such as grains that contain large amounts of phytate (see Chapter 24).

Table 12-7 shows that many other vegetables contain smaller amounts of iron. Several servings during one day can add up to 25 to 50 percent of the U.S. RDA. Other good sources of iron for the vegetarian are dried fruits and prune juice. Although these provide more energy per usual serving than do fresh fruits and other fruit juices, their higher iron content may mean they are better choices as snacks or breakfast beverages for the vegetarian.

Omitting Milk. The strict vegetarian eliminates from the diet an excellent source of calcium and vitamin D. Calcium needs may be met by regularly eating sufficient amounts of green leafy vegetables and other good sources of this mineral (see Table 2-5), but this takes careful planning. Teen-agers should be especially aware of this potential problem

° Fifty percent of the U.S. RDA equals the current adult RDA (3 micrograms). The adult RDA for vitamin B$_{12}$ is met by eating enough fortified cereal to supply 50 percent of the U.S. RDA value shown on the label of a product.

TABLE 12-7. Sources of Iron for Vegetarians

Food	Energy per Serving[a]		Iron INQ	Percent U.S. RDA per Serving[b]
	(Cal)	(kJ)		
Beans				
Kidney	230	966	2.6	26
Lima	260	1,090	2.9	33
Navy	225	945	2.9	28
Peas				
Black-eyed	190	800	2.2	18
Green	165	700	1.9	23
Split	290	1,220	1.9	23
Asparagus, canned	45	190	11.6	23
Beets, broccoli, brussels sprouts, carrots, corn, parsnips, potatoes, sauerkraut, tomatoes	25–75	105–315	Varies	4–8
Green beans	45	190	8.2	16
Lettuce, one-fourth head	8	34	18.2	4
Spinach	40	170	12.8	22
Prune juice	200	840	6.7	60
Bran flakes, 40% bran, 1 oz.	105	440	15.0	70
Bread, ¼ lb.[c]				
Enriched white	308	1,295	1.2	16
Whole-grain	275	1,155	1.6	18
Molasses, blackstrap (third extraction), 1 T.	45	190	9.0	18

[a] Serving size is 1 cup unless otherwise stated.
[b] Women and all teen-agers need 100 percent of the U.S. RDA for iron (18 milligrams); men need only 55 percent (10 milligrams).
[c] Serving size given is large for comparison purposes; differences per slice are quite small.
SOURCE: Excerpted from R. G. Hansen, A. W. Sorenson, and A. J. Wittmer, "Index of Nutritional Quality Food Profiles" (Logan, Utah: Utah State University, 1975). © 1975, Utah State University. Used by permission.

because of their higher needs for calcium.

Dietary sources of vitamin D are not needed by most adults, but vegetarians who do not drink milk should be aware of the importance of spending some time outside in the sunshine—not staying in the library or laboratory, or in front of the television all day. On the other hand, more vitamin D is needed by teen-agers and young children than can be synthesized from the sterol in skin; they need milk.

Severe nutritional deficiency diseases are rare in the United States today, but the danger of serious conditions developing in vegetarian children is so real that the American Academy of Pediatricians issued a formal statement urging parents to be especially cautious about vegetarian diets. It is impor-

The personal reasons for preferring natural or organic foods are important considerations in diet planning, but these preferences should not be confused with a careful evaluation of nutritional value.

tant for vegetarians to weigh carefully their reasons for omitting milk from their diet versus the risk of developing a deficiency of vitamin D and calcium that can impair the function of the nervous system and the development of bones and teeth.

Diet Awareness

A final point to consider is that vegetarian diets may benefit people simply by making them more conscious of the importance of their diet. If, as a nonvegetarian, a person was very nonchalant about food and nutrition, becoming a vegetarian may heighten that person's awareness of the fact that food (be it animal or plant) has an effect upon health. A greater interest in one's diet offers the possibility of improving one's nutritional status.

In the final analysis, a vegetarian diet might be compared to a high-powered motorcycle. The benefits or dangers of both depend upon the person using it, not only what that person knows, but also how this knowledge is used to maximize the benefits and minimize the dangers that might result—whether you are choosing a diet or a mode of transportation.

PROCESSED VERSUS NATURAL FOODS

In recent years, there has been a growing trend in America toward a lifestyle built around "natural" ingredients. This reaction to our supermechanized, "plastic" way of life is not restricted to food attitudes. The natural-is-good ethic makes some individuals prefer leather to polyester, straight hair to coiffures, sandals to high heels, as well as oatmeal to ready-to-eat cereals. Hundreds of products from dogfood to shampoo to adhesive creams for false teeth are advertised as "natural."

The nutritional value and safety of many foods can indeed be altered by how they are grown and processed. These changes are important considerations when you select foods, but terms such as *natural, processed,* and *refined* provide very little solid

nutrition information unless they are defined and unless the nutrient composition of such foods is compared in at least a semiquantitative framework.

Definition of Terms

Natural foods are difficult to define precisely. In general, they are foods that have not been processed in any way. Fresh fruits and vegetables clearly fall into this category, as do eggs and most meat products. The lines of classification are vague, however, when we consider the following foods:

1. Milk that is pasteurized to prevent growth of potentially harmful bacteria (such as those that cause diarrhea or tuberculosis)
2. Cheese and yogurt made in factories by processes quite similar to those used for centuries
3. Wine, other alcoholic beverages, and fermented foods such as sauerkraut
4. Dried beans and fruit
5. Peanuts and seeds that are roasted
6. Meats preserved with either sodium chloride or sodium nitrite
7. Sugar derived from beets or sugarcane (often referred to as refined) and molasses derived from sorghum and syrup from maple trees (often called natural)

The picture that emerges is that canning, freezing, dehydrating, and milling are considered by most people to be processes that destroy naturalness, whereas roasting, pasteurizing, fermenting, drying, salting, and smoking do not disqualify a food from the natural category. The use of additives (see the last section in this chapter) also means that a product is no longer considered a natural food.

Organic foods is a term often linked to *natural foods,* but these terms are not synonymous. Organic foods are commonly considered to be those grown without the use of chemical fertilizers and chemicals that kill or inhibit bacteria, fungi, insects, or rodents.

Processing may either enhance or reduce the acceptability of a food for you, depending upon changes in taste, texture, color, or shelf life. These are important personal considerations, but they should not be confused with an evaluation of nutrient composition of the food. Let's take a look at the specific effects of these processes upon the nutritional value of food.

Factors Affecting Growth

The logical place to begin an evaluation of the nutritive value of various items in the diet is the food as it is grown.

Genetics and Environments. The growth and metabolism of a plant, like that of an animal, is controlled by the genetic information inherent in its simplest form. A seed of a plant and a fertilized ovum of an animal both contain DNA (Chapter 5). This nucleic acid controls the synthesis of specific enzymes and determines what chemicals can be used and what nutrients can be made by metabolic reactions within each plant. Plant hormones, which respond to light, temperature, and other environmental stimuli, also influence the growth of a plant.

Among the genetically determined characteristics that distinguish one plant from another (tomatoes from wheat, cherries from carrots, and so on) is the enzymatic machinery for synthesizing vitamins. The capability to make certain vitamins as well as the inability to make others is inherent in each plant. The amount of vitamins made depends primarily upon weather conditions and the adequacy of water. Vitamins are synthesized by a long series of reactions starting basically from carbon dioxide in the air and water in the soil. Synthesis of some vitamins is also dependent upon the availability of sulfur or nitrogen in the soil.° Without going into the details of botanical syntheses, we can see that plants do not derive their vitamins directly from the soil.

° Cobalt must be provided in the diet of animals that synthesize vitamin B_{12}.

Minerals, on the other hand, are not synthesized. They are acquired from the soil along with the water taken in by the plant roots. The mineral content of a plant depends to a certain degree upon the mineral content of the soil, but beyond a certain range, this variable has an all-or-none effect. If the mineral content of the soil is below a critical level needed to keep the plant alive, the seed will not germinate—no growth will occur at all.

The micronutrient content of plant foods therefore depends upon the genetic material of a plant and the environmental conditions affecting the expression of its genetic potential. Genetically different strains of the same plant may vary as much as two fold in their vitamin or mineral content (Table 12-8). Water, temperature, and sunlight mainly affect the size and growth rate of a plant, but these

TABLE 12-8. Range of Nutrient Content of Different Varieties of Tomatoes and Carrots

| Nutrient | Range As a Percentage of the U.S. RDA | | | |
| | Tomatoes (1 medium, 150 g) | | Carrots (1 cup) | |
	Low	High	Low	High
Protein	1.3	2.4	Less than 1	
Vitamin A	24	40	256	330
Vitamin C	27	59	0	10
Thiamin	5	8	3.4	4.7
Riboflavin	3.5	7.0	1.5	2.2
Copper	4.5	9.9	2.1	3.2
Iron	3.8	6.4	1.4	2.0
Magnesium	3.2	5.0	1.7	2.2
Phosphorus	3.1	4.7	2.3	3.1
Zinc	0	0	1	1.5

SOURCE: Reprinted from G. A. Leveille et al., "Nutrient composition of carrots, tomatoes, and red tart cherries," *Federation Proceedings* 33 (1974): 2264–66. Used by permission of the publisher and author.

growing conditions can also influence vitamin synthesis to a certain degree.

Fertilizers. The primary purpose of fertilizers is to augment growth of plants by ensuring the availability of the elements necessary for botanical metabolism. The yield of crops per acre can be increased by fertilizers. They have little effect upon vitamin content of plants, but they can increase nitrogen and mineral content.

Chemical fertilizers add nitrogen and minerals to the soil; these are formulated from salts made primarily of nitrogen, carbon, oxygen, hydrogen, potassium, phosphorus, and sodium. (Soil can be tested by agricultural chemists to determine the most appropriate formulation needed.) The most commonly used organic fertilizers, excreta and compost, provide a broad array of chemicals. *Animal excreta* mainly contain the indigestible components of the animal's diet, cells that have been sloughed from the digestive tract, intestinal bacteria, and the metabolites of bacteria. *Compost* contains the chemical compounds present in leaves, garbage, and whatever else is put into the compost pile. When compost is aged, bacteria present in the ingredients and those in the soil use these chemicals for their own metabolism. (The higher temperature in the center of a compost pile than at the periphery is caused by bacterial metabolism and release of energy.) Most of the nitrogen originally present in compost is in a chemical form that cannot be used directly by the plants, but these complexes are transformed by bacterial metabolism into more utilizable nitrogen compounds similar to those present in formulated fertilizers. Thus, the nitrogen becomes available for synthesis of amino acids and protein by the plant.

Changes during Growth and Storage. The composition of plants varies to a certain degree as they grow.° During different stages of development, for

° This change in composition also takes place in humans and other animals. For instance, an infant's body contains a higher percentage of fat and water than the average adult's body.

instance, some plants convert sugars to starch and vice versa, or they gradually change their water and micronutrient content. The nutritive value of a food is therefore influenced to some degree by the stage of maturity when a food is harvested.

Botanical enzymatic reactions, including those that alter certain vitamins, continue after some plants have been harvested. Reduction of temperature slows these reactions; this is one reason why some food should be refrigerated. Heating for sufficient time at high enough temperature destroys enzymes and terminates metabolic reactions within plants. This is why many foods are blanched (heated in water or steam under various conditions) before they are packaged.

Certain vitamins in plants can be destroyed after harvesting by light, heat, or reaction with the oxygen in air. The extent of such changes largely depends upon how the food is stored. For example, since exposure to light gradually changes the chemical structure (destroying the biological activity) of riboflavin and pyridoxine, foods such as milk, cheese, and yogurt should be packaged in cardboard cartons, dark glass, or paper that does not transmit light rays. Vitamin C is destroyed by oxygen and heat; therefore, citrus fruits and tomatoes should be eaten or preserved as soon as possible after they are harvested.

Distance from Markets. The way to get the greatest nutritive value from most foods is to pick the food from your own garden, take it into the house, wash it, and eat it immediately. Though home gardening has increased tremendously during the 1970s, only a small percentage of Americans have such facilities. Therefore, most of us are dependent for many of our foods on farmers who live far from our homes. Even farmers can have fresh homegrown foods only about four to six months out of each year. Furthermore, some plants bear fruit all summer, but the growing season for others is short.

When food must be transported a considerable distance to reach people, the decision regarding at what stage of maturity it should be harvested must take many factors into consideration. If some fruits and vegetables were picked at their prime, enzymatic and chemical changes that would occur during transportation would unfavorably alter their taste, texture, and vitamin content by the time they reached the grocery store. These considerations mean that the maturity, or ripeness, as well as the vitamin content of foods at the time they are purchased is influenced by the time necessary for transporting from farm to processing plants (for canned or frozen food) or from farm to grocery store (for fresh foods).

Foods grown close to the processor or the market can be picked at a later stage of maturity. Foods that must be transported some distance are more often harvested prior to the attainment of maximal vitamin content. The nutritive value of fresh foods, therefore, largely depends upon whether they are grown locally and how they are stored in transit. The nutritive value of canned or frozen foods depends upon the distance between the farm and the processing plant and what measures are taken to preserve vitamin content en route and as part of the processing procedure.

EFFECTS OF PROCESSING

The effects of processing upon the nutritive value of food are generally considered more within the scientific domain of food technology than within the strict scope of nutrition. Although these changes can be only briefly discussed here, several general concepts are important in the broader context of nutrition and food choices.

General Concepts

Processing alters the nutrient composition of foods, but these changes do not affect all nutrients or all foods in the same way. A person who has nutrition knowledge should be able to identify the conditions that most often affect certain nutrients and thus be able to make informed comparisons of processed and fresh foods.

The general guidelines for predicting nutrient losses due to processing are:

1. Mineral content of foods is decreased primarily by processes that expose food to water. Minerals dissolve from the food into the water, which may be discarded in the factory or drained off in the kitchen. Minerals generally are not destroyed by heat, light, or oxidation.

2. Different vitamins are destroyed by different environmental conditions (see Chapter 11). The extent of vitamin destruction depends upon the type of process, conditions of storage before and after processing, and characteristics of the food. For example, vitamin C is partially protected from oxidation by the natural acidity of oranges and sauerkraut.

3. Food composition (content of macronutrients, micronutrients, and fiber) is altered by processes that separate and discard edible portions of foods. This occurs during milling, peeling, trimming, removing fat, or making juice.

4. The nutrient density of foods is reduced by adding sugar, syrups, and other sweeteners or fats.

Variable Micronutrient Changes

As an example of the general concepts discussed above, Table 12-9 shows the changes that occur in several fruits processed by different methods. Nutrient density or INQ helps us make comparisons. A reduction in the INQ (the ratio of micronutrient content to energy content) indicates that there has been a loss of micronutrients, if the process such as drying does not alter the macronutrients (energy value) of the food. However, in processes that increase energy value (such as when sugar is added to canned or frozen fruits or to juices) reduction of micronutrient INQ does not necessarily indicate destruction or loss of vitamins or minerals.

Drying. A comparison of the INQ for several micronutrients in raw fruits versus dried, uncooked fruits (Table 12-9) shows the variable effects of this type of processing:

The amount of each vitamin that is destroyed by processing varies in different foods and also depends upon the conditions of processing.

TABLE 12-9. Changes in Nutrient INQ of Fruits Processed by Different Methods

Fruit	Vitamin A INQ	Vitamin C INQ	Thiamin INQ	Riboflavin INQ	Iron INQ
Apricots					
Raw	24.2	7.0	0.84	0.98	1.16
Dried, uncooked	19.3	1.9	0.08	0.80	2.7
Dried, cooked	16.4	1.3	0.06	0.73	2.7
Canned, heavy syrup	9.4	1.7	0.35	0.37	0.46
Nectar	7.8	2.2	0.33	0.29	0.46
Peaches					
Raw	17.4	7.7	0.88	1.93	1.83
Dried, uncooked	6.8	2.6	0.07	1.0	2.9
Dried, cooked	6.9	1.1	0.07	0.92	2.9
Canned, water-packed	6.8	3.4	0.41	1.1	1.2
Canned, heavy syrup	2.5	1.3	0.15	0.4	0.5
Plums, raw	2.6	4.6	1.23	1.08	1.5
Prunes					
Uncooked	2.9	0.6	0.44	0.77	2.0
Cooked	2.9	0.3	0.42	0.83	2.0
Juice	0	1.0	0.23	0.20	6.7
Grapes	0.71	1.8	1.18	0.62	0.8
Raisins	0.03	0.2	0.58	0.37	1.5
Juice, sweetened	0.05	0	0.50	0.75	0.3
Apples					
Raw	0.33	1.6	0.88	0.39	0.7
Juice	0	0.6	0.26	0.56	1.6
Applesauce, unsweetened	0.46	0.8	0.77	0.27	1.5
Applesauce, sweetened	0.20	0.50	0.33	0.18	0.7

SOURCE: Excerpted from R. G. Hansen, A. W. Sorenson, and A. J. Wittmer, "Index of Nutritional Quality Food Profiles" (Logan, Utah: Utah State University, 1975). © 1975, Utah State University. Used by permission.

1. Vitamin A is almost completely destroyed in grapes when raisins are made, but less is lost by drying apricots and peaches. The vitamin A of plums is not destroyed when prunes are made.

2. Some vitamin C in apricots, peaches, plums, and grapes is destroyed by drying.

3. Most of the thiamin in apricots and peaches and a large percentage of the thiamin in plums and grapes is destroyed by drying.

4. Riboflavin is destroyed to a greater extent in peaches and grapes than in apricots and plums.

5. Iron INQ increases in dried fruits because the fresh fruits are dried on metal trays, and iron passes from the trays into the drying fruit.

This comparison therefore shows that vitamin sensitivity to drying differs for each vitamin and for various fruits. Minerals are not destroyed by drying.

Cooking. A comparison of the INQ values for dried, uncooked fruits versus dried, cooked fruits (Table 12-9) shows:

1. Vitamin C is destroyed by cooking apricots, peaches, and prunes.

2. Vitamin A is destroyed in apricots, but not in peaches or prunes.

3. There is little additional destruction of thiamin and riboflavin by cooking dried fruits.

It is difficult to tell from Table 12-9 what the effect is of cooking alone, since certain vitamins in these fruits had been previously destroyed to a great extent by drying. However, Table 12-10 shows that cooking reduces the vitamin C INQ of cabbage and green peppers but has little effect upon carrots.

Converting to Juice. Table 12-9 shows that the INQ of micronutrients is changed when juice is made from fruit. In this case, several factors have a bearing on the nutrient composition of the product:

1. Nutrients (micro- and macro-) are not always equally distributed in the peel and pulp (which are discarded) and the juice.

2. The fruit may be heated during the juice-extraction process, thus destroying certain vitamins.

3. Sugar may be added, thus diluting the nutrient density.

A detailed explanation of these changes in each type of juice goes beyond the scope of this discussion, but Table 12-9 helps to show how all four of the general guidelines may influence the nutritional value of foods that are considered to be both natural and processed.

Canning and Freezing

The major nutrient loss during canning and freezing is caused by heat. Food is sometimes cooked to improve texture and palatability, but the major advantage is the destruction of bacteria. Sterilization is important for foods that are eaten immediately, but it is even more crucial for preserved products (such as canned goods) that are stored at

TABLE 12-10. Changes in Vitamin C INQ of Certain Vegetables When Cooked	
Vegetable	Vitamin C INQ
Cabbage	
Raw	80.5
Cooked	61.3
Carrots	
Raw	7.8
Cooked	7.7
Green peppers	
Raw	240.0
Cooked	179.0

SOURCE: Excerpted from R. G. Hansen, A. W. Sorenson, and A. J. Wittmer, "Index of Nutritional Quality Food Profiles" (Logan, Utah: Utah State University, 1975). © 1975, Utah State University. Used by permission.

room temperature (see Chapter 18). In certain foods heat inactivates naturally occurring enzymes that destroy thiamin and vitamin C. It also destroys undesirable food components, such as factors in beans that interfere with the protein-digestive enzyme, trypsin.

Most foods are heated in the presence of water, or blanched, before canning or freezing. The method chosen depends upon the food and the desired effect. For example, tomatoes, sweet potatoes, and beets may be blanched in steam or steam under pressure to facilitate peeling. Spinach is often heated in water at 170°F; and peas and string beans are boiled. Since the time and temperature of blanching may differ among processing plants as well as among different foods, the nutrient loss is not always the same. Table 12-11 shows the average percentage of loss of five micronutrients in five canned foods. Although nutrient destruction varies in these foods, vitamin C and thiamin losses are generally greater than losses of carotene, riboflavin,

The practical significance of substituting whole-grain cereal for a milled-grain product depends upon the amount of nutrients gained compared to the amount needed in the diet and upon whether these nutrients are lacking in the diet.

TABLE 12-11. Average Percentage of Loss of Nutrients in Canning

Canned Food	Carotene	Thiamin	Riboflavin	Niacin	Vitamin C
Asparagus[a]	—	8	10	6	5
Corn[b]	3	66	3	14	—
Green beans[b]	13	29	4	8	45
Spinach[a]	—	15	12	17	33
Tomato juice[b]	33	11	3	2	33

[a] Reprinted from R. F. Cain, "Water-soluble vitamins: Changes during processing and storage of fruits and vegetables," *Food Technology* 21(1967): 998. Copyright © by Institute of Food Technologists.

[b] Adapted from E. J. Cameron, et al., *Retention of Nutrients during Canning* (Washington, D.C.: National Canners Association, 1955). © 1955, National Canners Association. Used by permission.

or niacin. Folic acid and pantothenic acid (not shown in this table) are also sensitive to heat.

Macronutrients are not greatly affected by extremes of temperature. Cooking increases the digestibility of some proteins, but heating protein in the presence of certain sugars degrades some of the amino acids (especially lysine and threonine). Extreme heat can produce undesirable degradation products of lipids, and to a lesser extent of carbohydrates.

Freezing is generally not destructive to vitamins, but nutrient loss does result from blanching prior to freezing. When you compare the nutritive value of canned and frozen foods, keep in mind that frozen foods are usually cooked longer and at a higher temperature in the kitchen than are canned foods.

Loss of vitamins during dehydration is not as great as during canning. The gaseous atmosphere inside containers of dehydrated foods results in increased retention of vitamin C, but causes considerable loss of thiamin.

Milling

Cereal products are preserved by milling rather than by canning or freezing. The major purpose of milling is to change grain into a form (such as meal or flour) that can be used in the preparation of breads, baked goods, and other foods for which whole grains cannot be used. Milling also helps to rid cereals of microscopic insect eggs that lodge in crevices of grain kernels and are difficult to remove even by thorough washing.

Degree of Milling. During the milling of wheat, the hard bran, coarse aleurone, and fat-containing germ are removed, leaving primarily the endosperm portion of the kernel. Milling reduces the fat content from about 2 percent to about 0.33 percent, but it also causes a loss of vitamins and minerals. The extent of nutrient loss depends upon the degree of milling necessary to produce different types of flour. The amount of each vitamin and mineral lost depends upon the distribution of that micronutrient in the part of the grain that is removed compared to its concentration in the flour that is left. Table 12-12 shows what happens to the concentration of zinc and iron, depending upon the type of milled product produced.

Enrichment. Some nutrient losses due to milling are compensated for by the addition of four micronutrients to cereal products, which are then said to be *enriched*. The iron, thiamin, and niacin content of these products are comparable to unmilled cereal (Table 12-13). Riboflavin content is actually slightly

TABLE 12-12. Zinc and Iron Content in Wheat Products		
Wheat Product	Zinc[a] (mg/100 g)	Iron[b] (mg/100 g)
Crude wheat bran	9.8	14.9
Crude wheat germ	14.3	9.4
Whole-grain cereal		
Dry form	3.6	3.7
Cooked form[c]	0.5	0.5
Whole-grain wheat		
Durum	2.7	4.3
Hard	3.4	3.1–3.4
Soft	2.7	3.5
White	2.2	3.0
Wheat flour		
Whole	2.4	3.3
80% extraction	1.5	1.3
All-purpose	0.7	0.8 (2.9)[d]
Bread flour	0.8	0.9 (2.9)[d]
Cake and pastry		
flour	0.3	0.5

[a] Reprinted from E. W. Murphy, B. W. Willis, and B. K. Watt, "Provisional Tables on the Zinc Content of Foods," *Journal of The American Dietetic Association* 66 (1975): 345.
[b] From B. K. Watt and A. L. Merrill, "Composition of Foods—Raw, Processed, Prepared," *Agriculture Handbook No. 8 Agricultural Research Service*, (Washington, D.C.: USDA, 1963).
[c] Changes reflect change in food composition due to higher water content of cooked cereal.
[d] Based on product with minimum level of enrichment in 1975.

greater in enriched products than in whole-grain cereal.

Major Nutrient Losses. The percentage of nutrients lost in the preparation of white flour ranges from 40 to 90 percent of the amount present in whole grain (Table 12-14). To identify the differences between whole-grain products and white flour that are most significant for making food choices, it is informative to compare the amount of micro- nutrient loss due to milling in an average daily diet of cereal products to the amount of micronutrients needed in an average daily diet. (We will use the U.S. RDA as a guide for purposes of discussion.)

First, let's calculate the micronutrient loss based on an average daily diet. Total cereal consumption in the United States averages about 150 grams of flour and cereal per person per day. Flour is used for many products other than bread, and it is impossible to substitute whole grain for flour in many recipes. To point out what might be the greatest possible differences, however, let's assume that 150 grams of whole grain are substituted for white flour in the total average daily diet. Table 12-14 lists the amount of nutrients that would be lost if a person ate 150 grams of white flour each day instead of 150 grams of whole wheat. The percentage of the U.S. RDA lost is also given for each of these nutrients. We can see that substituting 150 grams of whole grain in your diet would increase your intake of pyridoxine, folacin, pantothenic acid, vitamin E, and calcium by 4 to 10 percent of the U.S. RDA. The increase in phosphorus, magnesium, zinc, and copper would be much greater—between 25 and 60 percent of the U.S. RDA.

Other Trace Elements and Fiber. It is more difficult to evaluate the significance of losses of trace elements because there is no standard such as the U.S. RDA to use as a basis for estimating daily need. Table 12-14 compares the amounts of four trace elements lost during milling to estimates of average daily intakes. The relative loss of chromium and selenium is fairly small, but losses due to milling are much larger for manganese and molybdenum.

The loss of fiber during milling of 150 grams of wheat is about 3 grams. Chapter 24 discusses ways of evaluating the importance of this amount of fiber in the diet.

Significance of Differences. The final criterion for determining the importance of the differences pointed out above is whether or not other foods in

TABLE 12-13. Thiamin, Riboflavin, Niacin, and Iron Content
of Enriched and Whole Wheat Products

Wheat Product	Thiamin (mg/lb)	Riboflavin (mg/lb)	Niacin (mg/lb)	Iron[a] (mg/lb)
Enriched bread, rolls, or buns[b]	1.8	1.1	15	25
Enriched flour[b]	2.9	1.8	24	40
Whole wheat bread[c]	1.2	0.5	13	14
Whole wheat flour[c]	2.5	0.5	20	15

[a] Proposed levels; decision pending (as of July 1977).
[b] Standards for enrichment effective April 1974.
[c] Calculated from values in C. F. Adams, "Nutritive Value of American Foods in Common Units," *Agriculture Handbook* No. 456 (Washington, D.C.: USDA, Agricultural Research Service, 1975).

TABLE 12-14. Loss due to Milling of Nutrients Not Restored by Enrichment

Nutrient	Percentage of Nutrient Lost due to Milling	Amount of Nutrient Lost from 150 grams of Wheat (mg)	Amount of Nutrient Lost from 150 grams of Wheat As a Percentage of U.S. RDA		
Calcium	60	40	4		
Vitamin E	86	2.07	6		
Pantothenic acid	50	0.75	7.5		
Folacin	67	0.03	7.5		
Pyridoxine	72	0.18	9		
Copper	68	0.54	25		
Zinc	78	4.05	27		
Phosphorus	71	460	45		
Magnesium	85	233	57		
				Average Daily Intake[a] (mg)	Amount of Nutrient Lost As a Percentage of Average Daily Intake
Chromium	40	0.003		0.06	5
Selenium	16	0.015		0.10	15
Molybdenum	48	0.04		0.05–0.50	8–80
Manganese	86	4.5		2.5–7.0	64–180

[a] From Food and Nutrition Board, National Academy of Sciences—National Research Council, *Recommended Dietary Allowances,* 8th ed. (Washington, D.C.: 1974).

your diet provide adequate amounts of the nutrients lost during milling. If your diet already contains a sufficient amount of these nutrients, there is no advantage in consuming more. If your diet is currently lacking these nutrients, substitution of whole-grain cereal for foods made with white flour (such as bread, cake, crackers, cookies, hamburger and hot dog buns, and pancakes) would make an important difference in the adequacy of your diet.

EFFECTS OF ADDITIVES

The safety of chemicals added to foods is important to all of us. Our concerns result from personal, sociopolitical, scientific, and other factors. We must identify the basis of our concerns before we can objectively weigh the potential dangers of food additives. The fear of additives is magnified by the fact that few people have sufficient understanding of chemistry to comprehend the names of additives listed on food packages. To nonnutritionists the word *cyanocobalamin* might elicit ideas of *cyanide* poisoning or *cobalt* radiation beams. But this chemical sounds healthy and wholesome when you call it *vitamin B$_{12}$*.

The sociopolitical values that often go along with negative attitudes toward additives are derived in some cases from the early American ethic and the concept of self-reliance. Many of those who hold such views do not want the food industry, government, or anybody else directing their lives, much less tampering with what they put in their mouths.

These factors influence public policies on the use of additives. Nutritionists must keep them in mind when counselling individuals or advising groups of people on food-consumption alternatives.

Toxicity and Hazard

The scientific concern regarding additives focuses on their safety. The question of safety can be considered only if we use carefully defined terms:

Toxicity means the capacity of a chemical substance to harm living organisms.

Hazard is the capacity of a chemical to produce injury under conditions of use.

Many vitamins and naturally occurring components of food are toxic, but there is little hazard to consuming them in the quantities normally provided by a varied diet. Oxalic acid is a toxic, natural ingredient in spinach, but consumption of this food is not hazardous unless, like Popeye, you eat nothing else. Chapter 20 gives an example of how to put into perspective the potential harm of a toxic substance depending upon how much of it is consumed.

Additives is another term that causes confusion due to lack of definition. Technically, an additive is any minor substance or element put into a food to achieve a specific effect. An average American annually consumes about 10 pounds of additives other than sugar, cornstarch, and table salt. Approximately 9 of these 10 pounds are the same chemicals as occur naturally in foods (salts of calcium and sodium, fatty acids, monoglycerides) or spices (such as mustard and pepper). Vitamins and minerals in fortified and enriched foods are other additives frequently consumed.

Evaluation of Toxicity

Federal laws (made by Congress) and regulations (administered by the Food and Drug Administration, or FDA, of the Department of Health, Education and Welfare) determine whether chemicals may be added to foods. The criteria for deciding about the use of an additive depend upon whether the additive was used prior to 1958, when a law called the Delaney Amendment was passed by Congress.

New Additives. Since 1958, all petitions to the FDA for permission to use a food additive have been evaluated according to the following criteria established by the Delaney Amendment:

The FDA may not approve a petition by a manufacturer to add a chemical to food if that substance in any amount is known to cause cancer. Petitions are granted for use of other chemicals at a tolerance level well below the concentration that is safe for experimental animals. Additives used in food prior to 1958 are currently being reevaluated by FASEB scientists.

1. If the chemical causes cancer in experimental animals, it cannot be used as an additive. Even if it were to be used at a level a million fold lower than that which causes cancer, the petition is denied.

2. Additives that have harmful effects but do not cause cancer can be used in limited amounts. Extensive tests performed in the laboratories of the company petitioning to use the additive establish the amount of the substance that produces various physiological abnormalities. Then the FDA examines the records of these experiments and decides how much of the additive can be ingested with no ill effects. Finally, the FDA determines a *tolerance level*, usually about one-hundredth of the no-effect level, and this is the concentration at which the additive may be used.

Older Additives. In 1958, when the Delaney Amendment was passed, hundreds of chemicals were already commonly used as additives. The FDA requested the help and advice of the Federation of American Societies of Experimental Biology (FASEB). This federation is not a government agency; it is comprised of six professional groups that have rigid criteria for their membership regarding experience and training in pharmacology, physiology, nutrition, biochemistry, pathology, or immunology.

FASEB selected from their 20,000 members an expert panel of over 800 scientists to review the results of past experiments regarding the toxicity of additives that were being used in 1958. The additives that were considered acceptable by the FASEB review committee are referred to as *Generally Recognized As Safe*, or GRAS, additives. Those that produce no ill effects may be used in any amount; those that do produce harm are restricted by a tolerance level.

Consumer and scientific concerns regarding additives have provoked further reevaluation of the GRAS list, which began in 1970. This study is also being conducted under the auspices of FASEB. Because of the thoroughness of this review and the vast amount of work involved, the study spans several years. Periodic reports are released regarding groups of additives. The evaluation has resulted in banning a few additives and establishing new or lower tolerance levels for others.

Purpose of Additives

Because additives may have harmful effects when they are used in large amounts, it is logical to query why they are used at all. The substances that appear on the GRAS list are classified according to purpose. Table 12-15 states the functions of several classes of additives, examples of additives in each class, and some foods that contain each class of additives.

Benefits versus Risks

The dilemma regarding the use of additives requires that careful consideration be given to both the risks and the benefits of these substances. The experiments completed in 1977 that showed saccharin causes bladder cancer in laboratory rats is a classic example of the importance and complexity of benefit-risk evaluations. Some people, especially diabetics, benefit from the availability of saccharin; however, at the same time, there is a risk (which cannot currently be measured) that saccharin is dangerous to health.

If the urbanization of America were reversed and we again became an agricultural society, many methods of food preservation and many additives would not be necessary. Few people consider this solution a realistic option, but society can establish guidelines regarding the factors that do and do not justify the use of each additive. A committee of the National Academy of Sciences (NAS) has drafted such recommendations (Table 12-16). These guidelines need further expansion and clarification. They do not provide easy answers to questions about BHT or "XYZ"—any additive that may be used today or tomorrow. However, this long-range approach to the problem may be in the direction of the only

TABLE 12-15. Functions of Food Additives and Examples of Their Usage

Functions in Foods	Some Commonly Used Additives	Some Foods in Which Used
Preservatives		
Antioxidants—To prevent oxidation, which results in rancidity of fats or browning of fruits	Butylated hydroxyanisole (BHA), tocopherols (vitamin E), citric acid, ascorbic acid	Vegetable shortenings and oils, potato chips, pudding and pie filling mixes, whipped topping mix, canned and frozen fruits
Other—To control the growth of mold, bacteria, and yeast	Sodium benzoate, propionic acid, calcium propionate	Table syrup, bread, cookies, cheese, fruit juices, pie fillings
For consistency/texture		
Emulsifiers—To uniformly disperse tiny particles or globules of one liquid in another liquid	Monoglycerides, lecithin, polysorbate 60, propylene glycol monostearate	Salad dressing mixes, margarine, cake mixes, whipped topping mix, pudding and pie filling mixes, chocolate, bread
Stabilizers/thickeners—To maintain smooth and uniform texture and consistency; to provide desired thickness or gel	Algin derivative, carrageenan, cellulose gum, guar gum, gum arabic, pectin, gelatin	Instant pudding mixes, ice cream, cream cheese, frozen desserts, chocolate milk, baked goods, salad dressing mixes, frozen whipped toppings, jams, jellies, candies, sauces
Acids/bases—To control the acidity and alkalinity of many foods; may act as buffers or neutralizing agents	Citric acid, adipic acid, sodium bicarbonate, lactic acid, potassium acid tartrate	Gelatin desserts, baking powder, baked goods, process cheese, instant soft drink mixes
Nutrient supplements—To improve the nutritive value of foods	Potassium iodide (iodine), vitamin D, thiamin mononitrate (vitamin B_1), riboflavin (vitamin B_2), ascorbic acid (vitamin C), niacin (a B vitamin), vitamin A palmitate, ferrous sulfate (iron)	Iodized salt, milk, margarine, enriched or fortified breakfast cereals, enriched macaroni, enriched rice, enriched flour, instant breakfast drink
Flavors and flavoring agents (both natural and synthetic)—To give a wide variety of flavorful products without restrictions of season or geographic locale	Natural lemon and orange flavors, dried garlic, herbs, spices, hydrolyzed vegetable protein, vanillin and other artificial flavors (mainly fruit flavors)	Pudding and pie filling and gelatin dessert mixes, cake mixes, salad dressing mixes, candies, soft drinks, ice cream, barbecue sauce

SOURCE: *Today's Food and Additives* (White Plains, N.Y.: General Foods Consumer Center, 1976). © 1976, General Foods Corporation. Used by permission.

TABLE 12-15. Functions of Food Additives and Examples of Their Usage (*continued*)

Functions in Foods	Some Commonly Used Additives	Some Foods in Which Used
Colorings (both natural and synthetic)—To enhance the appearance of foods	Carotene, caramel color, beet powder, artificial colors[a]	Margarine, cheese, soft drink mixes, candies, jams, jellies, fruit flavored gelatins, pudding and pie filling mixes
Miscellaneous additives (include anticaking agents, antifoaming agents, flavor enhancers, humectants, curing agents, sequestrants, and firming, bleaching, and maturing agents, nonnutritive sweeteners)	Sodium silico aluminate, monosodium glutamate (MSG), glycerine, saccharin	Dessert mixes, soft drink mixes, seasoned coating mixes, salad dressing mixes, flaked coconut, special diet products

[a] Most colors used today are approved synthetic colors since there are not enough natural colors available.

TABLE 12-16. Guidelines for Determining Whether Additives Should Be Used

Situations in Which Food Additives Are Acceptable	Situations in Which Food Additives Should Not Be Used	Risk–Benefit Relation; Factors to Consider
Improving or maintaining nutritional value	Disguising faulty or inferior processes	Hazard to the consumer
Enhancing quality	Concealing damage, spoilage, or other inferiority	Consumer needs and wishes
Reducing wastage	Deceiving the consumer	Requirements of food supply and public health
Enhancing consumer acceptability	Achieving otherwise desirable results when it would entail substantial reduction in important nutrients	Needs of the food producer and processor
Improving keeping quality	Achieving effects that can be obtained by economical, good manufacturing practices	Economic factors
Making the food more readily available	Using more than the minimum necessary to achieve the desired effects	Availability of methods and mechanisms for regulatory control
Facilitating preparation of the food		Threat to the adequacy, wholesomeness, or availability of the food supply in the absence of protection afforded by the additive

SOURCE: Adapted from Subcommittee on Food Technology of the Food Protection Committee, National Academy of Sciences/National Research Council, *The Use of Chemicals in Food Production, Processing, Storage and Distribution* (Washington, D.C., 1973).

solution to controversies plagued by hysteria, politics, profit motives, and limitations of current scientific knowledge.

The people who are entrusted with making decisions that affect the lives of millions—indeed billions—of people must step back from the heated debates and clearly define the facts and issues. Nonscientists should have a seat in this decision-making forum, and they must be knowledgeable about and responsible for the consequences of their decisions. For example, thousands of people are starving around the world partly because of a lack of the food production and preservation technology we have in the United States. On the other hand, it would be foolish for us to ignore the risks inherent in our technological progress. The correct path for the future can only be charted by careful decisions based upon the relative benefits and risks to all segments of society, for today and tomorrow.

STUDY QUESTIONS

1. How may some of the nutritional imperfections in traditional American diets be corrected by learning about foods chosen by people in other countries?

2. How do the foods preferred by groups within the United States influence the variety of foods used by the broader American population?

3. In what ways can ethnic foods now rarely eaten add variety and nutrients to your diet?

4. What kind of dietary instructions do various religions give?

5. Why is it difficult to design a nutritionally adequate vegetarian diet?

6. Select two total daily diets, one vegetarian and one nonvegetarian, and compare their energy value, fat and cholesterol content, and the percent U.S. RDA of calcium, iron, and vitamins C, A, and B_{12}.

7. Upon what factors does the nutrient composition of a plant food depend?

8. How can nutrient composition change after food is harvested?

9. How can the nutrient composition of food change during processing?

10. Why is it difficult to make general statements about the loss of micronutrients in foods due to processing?

11. How might your nutritional status in terms of specific micronutrients be improved by using whole-grain products in place of enriched flour?

12. What are the FDA guidelines for banning an additive or allowing its use at a tolerance level?

13. How are additives used in food prior to 1958 being reevaluated?

14. What would be the benefits and the risks of allowing the inclusion of saccharin in the American food supply?

SUGGESTED READING

1. Food and Nutrition Board, National Academy of Sciences, "Soil fertility and the nutritive value of crops." Reprinted in *Nutrition Reviews* 34(1976): 316–17.
2. C. Cromwell, "Organic foods—an update," *Family Economics Review*, Agricultural Research Service, U.S. Department of Agriculture (Summer 1976):8–11.
3. R. L. Hall, "Food additives," *Nutrition Today* 8(1973):20–31.
4. R. L. Hall, "GRAS—Concept and application," *Food Technology* 29(1975):48–53.
5. "Patulin, a carcinogenic mycotoxin found in cider," *Nutrition Reviews* 32(1974):55–56.
6. F. Aylward, "From farm to consumer: The storage, preservation, processing, and distribution of food," *Nutrition* (London) 29(1975):265–74.
7. L. E. Grivetti and R. M. Pangborn, "Origin of selected Old Testament dietary prohibitions: An evaluative review," *Journal of the American Dietetic Association* 65(1974):634.

8. H. G. Schutz and O. A. Lorenz, "Consumer preferences for vegetables grown under 'commercial' and 'organic' conditions," *Journal of Food Science* 41(1976):70–73.

9. W. J. Darby and L. Hambraeus, "Proposed nutritional guidelines for utilization of industrially produced nutrients," *Nāringsforskning. Arg.* 19(1975): 113–20. (Available from The Nutrition Foundation, Washington, D.C.)

10. B. K. Armstrong et al, "Hematological, vitamin B_{12}, and folate studies on Seventh-day Adventist vegetarians," *American Journal of Clinical Nutrition* 27(1974):712–18.

11. "Problems in iron enrichment and fortification of foods," *Nutrition Reviews* 33(1975):46–47.

12. W. J. Darby, "The case for the proposed increase in iron enrichment of flour and wheat products," *Nutrition Reviews* 30(1972):98–102.

13. "Exploring food additives," *FDA Consumer* 10(1976):4–10.

14. *How Safe Is Safe? The Design of Policy on Drugs and Food Additives.* Academy Forum. Washington, D.C.: National Academy of Sciences, 1974.

15. W. W. Lowrance, *Of Acceptable Risk.* Los Altos, Calif.: William Kaufmann, Inc., 1976.

16. "The benefit-risk equation," *FDA Consumer* 8(1974):27–31.

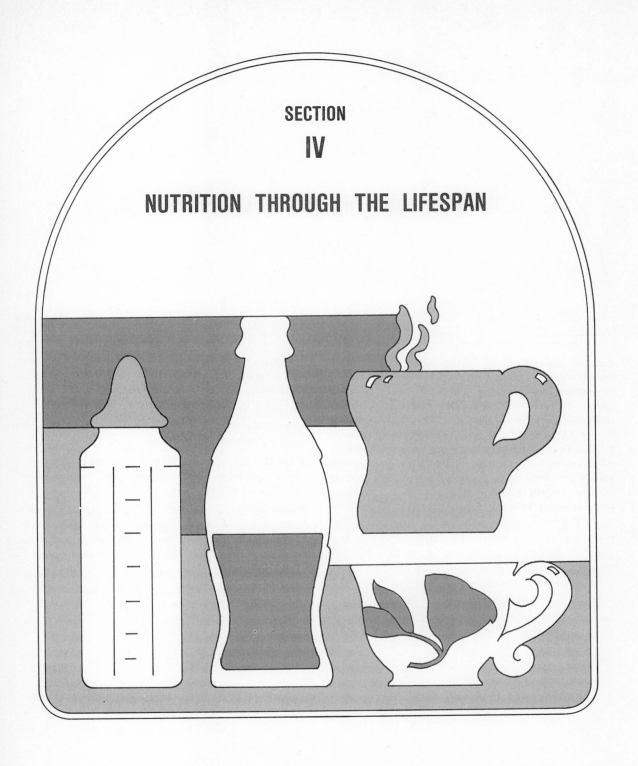

SECTION

IV

NUTRITION THROUGH THE LIFESPAN

NUTRITION THROUGH THE LIFESPAN

Both nutritional needs (which are physiologically determined) and diet patterns (which are influenced primarily by socioeconomic factors) vary during the lifespan. An understanding of how people of all ages can select a nutritionally appropriate diet is a part of being able to apply nutrition knowledge. The information in Chapters 13 through 19 may help you (1) answer questions about nutrition you may have at some time in your life, (2) advise friends or members of your family who are older or younger than yourself, and (3) modify your diet over the years because of physiological or socioeconomic changes.

CHAPTER 13 IDENTIFYING NUTRITION PROBLEMS gives an overview of the reports and surveys that help identify specific nutrition problems more common to people during each phase of the lifespan.

CHAPTER 14 FROM SINGLE CELL TO BABY discusses nutrient needs for women before and during pregnancy and suggests dietary modifications to meet these needs.

CHAPTER 15 FEEDING MOTHER AND BABY deals with how a mother should adjust her diet after her baby is born and how the nutrient needs of a baby can be met.

CHAPTER 16 THE FORMATIVE YEARS discusses the nutrient needs of children and factors to consider when planning diets for them.

CHAPTER 17 A CHANGING BODY compares the nutrient needs and diet patterns of teen-agers to those of young children and to those of adults.

CHAPTER 18 APPROPRIATE DIETS FOR MEN AND WOMEN explains the similarities and the differences in nutrient needs of adult males and females and how these needs can be met by modifying the food selections of each.

CHAPTER 19 MAXIMIZING THE SENIOR YEARS discusses the physiological and socioeconomic factors that influence the adequacy of diets of older people.

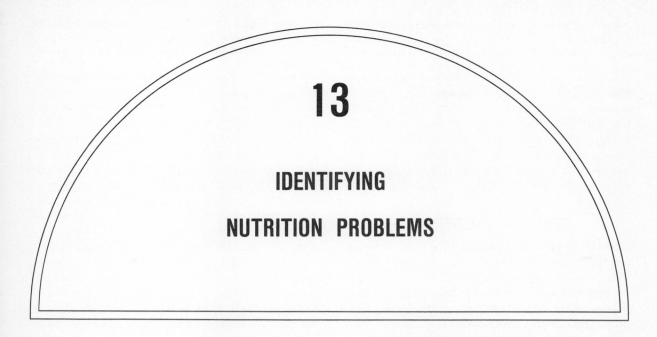

13

IDENTIFYING

NUTRITION PROBLEMS

The main purpose of this section, "Nutrition Through the Lifespan," is to explain how and why nutrients are needed in varying amounts by people of different ages, and to discuss how these needs can be met by gradually modifying food choices over the years. One way to identify the nutrient needs of people within a certain age group is to focus on the nutrients for which the RDA is higher during that phase of life. This method is used in the chapters that follow. Another way to identify potential problems in diet planning is to find out which nutrients are currently consumed in smaller amounts than they were in the past, and which nutrients are most often consumed in less than the amount recommended for people of various ages. This information can be gleaned from the reports and surveys that are discussed in this chapter. The numbers listed in tables and figures, such as those in this chapter, can be misleading unless you are aware of the following variables: (1) how each study was conducted, (2) what population of people was surveyed (and any socioeconomic factors influencing their food selections), and (3) the standards or criteria used for measuring the adequacy of the diets in each survey.

AVERAGES VERSUS INDIVIDUALS

Few people always eat exactly the same foods as others. Even those who live in institutions (such as nursing homes or prisons) or who eat communally (as in military facilities) usually have some options at mealtime. Their diet also can fluctuate, depending upon portion sizes and the amount of food left on the plate. Their nutrient intake can be further altered by adding food from other sources.

Since the nutritional value of even a tightly controlled diet can vary greatly, it is easy to appreciate the tremendous differences in energy and nutrient intake of people who have very few restrictions on what they eat. This variability makes it impossible to determine from surveys any specific problems that are applicable to all individuals. The best we can do is to look at average dietary intakes for large populations and general trends in food consumption. Then, using this knowledge and what we have learned in preceding chapters, we can try to identify characteristics of diet patterns that favor good nutrition and those that present problems for people of different ages.

One final precaution should be mentioned before going into the details of food and nutrition surveys. Average values can be misleading. They mask the fact that values for some people fall far below the average. For example, the average intake of niacin for a group of people may be adequate, but this does not prove that everyone within that population has an adequate niacin intake.

CHANGES IN DIET PATTERNS

One way to get a perspective on the current American diet is to analyze how it has changed over the years. During this century, some of the increases or decreases in consumption of different foods have improved the quality of the average diet, while others have been detrimental.

The trends shown in Figure 13-1 are derived from calculations of the amount of food available per person. These data, collected by the U.S. Department of Agriculture (USDA), are called *disappearance data*, as opposed to consumption data. Commodity specialists of the Economic Research Service of the USDA calculated these values from statistics on the nation's food production; imports and exports; net changes in stocks; military takings; and amounts used for feed, seed, and nonfood products. The remaining food is considered to have "disappeared" into civilian consumption. The disappearance data do not take into account food wastage and other losses, nor do they tell how much food was actually distributed to people on an individual basis. When we refer to this information, therefore, the term *consumption* actually means the amount of food per person that entered the human food supply system.

Food Consumption Trends

We can look at trends in food consumption in several ways. Comparing the number of pounds of food eaten can give us an idea of the relative amounts of food in the diet. But, measuring the differences in the amount of food eaten per person today as a percentage of the amount eaten per person in the past is more informative when we are trying to identify changes in diet patterns. The bar graphs in Figure 13-1 show the percentage increase or decrease in consumption of different types of food. The impression we get from trend data depends upon the time period used for comparison. Figure 13-1 gives us a broad perspective by comparing the average 1975 diet to the average diet in 1909–1913; it also shows more recent changes by comparing the 1975 diet to the 1965 diet.

Since the basic four food groups are organized according to the nutrient contribution of foods, changes in food consumption among and within these classifications provide a clue to fluctuations in the nutritional value of the diet. We can see from the graphs that:

1. There has been an increase in consumption of foods from the meat and milk groups.
2. There has been a decrease in total consumption of foods from the fruit/vegetable group and the cereal group (largely due to lower consumption of potatoes and fruits other than citrus).
3. Of the foods that provide only small amounts of micronutrients, use of oils and sugar and other sweeteners has increased while use of butter, tea, and coffee has decreased.

Let's now take a closer look at changes within each group. The increased consumption of foods in the meat group in the 1975 diet is due mainly to increased use of poultry (31 more pounds per person annually) and meat (16 more pounds per person) compared to the diet in 1909–1913. There has been little change in consumption of fish, eggs, nuts, and legumes such as beans and peas. Consumption of dairy products has decreased 10 percent since 1965, but it is still greater than the average intake in 1909–1913.

Consumption of citrus fruits has increased tremendously (57 more pounds per person compared to 1909–1913), but consumption of other fruits has

Food *disappearance data* (prepared by the USDA) show changes that have occurred during this century in the types of foods available in the United States, and provide estimates of energy, macronutrient, and micronutrient consumption per person.

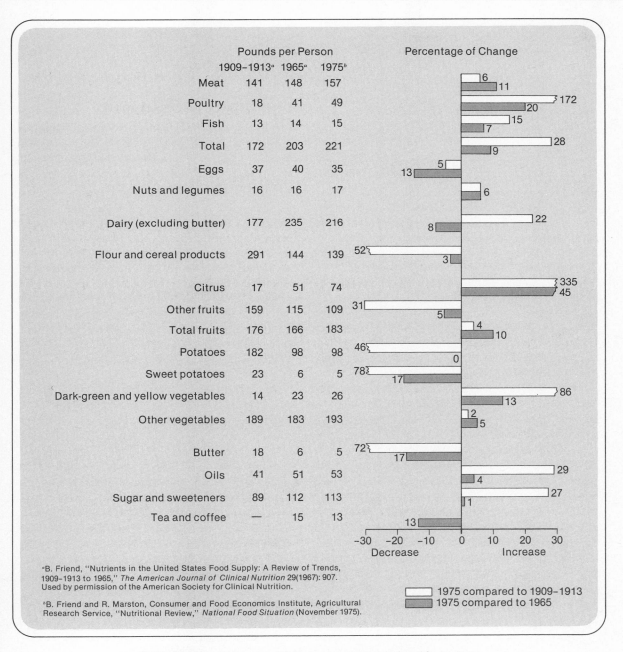

[a]B. Friend, "Nutrients in the United States Food Supply: A Review of Trends, 1909–1913 to 1965," *The American Journal of Clinical Nutrition* 29(1967): 907. Used by permission of the American Society for Clinical Nutrition.

[b]B. Friend and R. Marston, Consumer and Food Economics Institute, Agricultural Research Service, "Nutritional Review," *National Food Situation* (November 1975).

FIGURE 13-1. Changes in food disappearance during this century.

declined by an almost equal amount. The major change within the vegetable group is the large reduction (84 pounds) in the use of potatoes. Consumption of dark-green and yellow vegetables has almost doubled in the last sixty years, but total intake is only about 26 pounds per person annually.

Use of flour and cereal products has dropped to a level (139 pounds) less than half of what it was early in this century.

The consumption of foods that provide energy but little or no micronutrients has increased. Use of sugar and other sweeteners has increased by 23 pounds per person between 1909–1913 and 1965; use of oils has increased by 10 pounds per person during the same interval. Consumption of these foods did not change much, however, between 1965 and 1975.

The USDA does not tabulate alcohol consumption, but in 1971 the average annual consumption of absolute alcohol from distilled spirits, wine, and beer among the drinking-age U.S. population was 2.6 gallons per person. This was a 32 percent increase since 1958. The energy value of this amount

of alcohol (excluding the energy from other macronutrients in some alcoholic beverages) equals an average intake of approximately 210 Cal (880 kJ) per person each day.

Macronutrient Consumption Trends

The next step in evaluating dietary trends is to see how changes in food consumption have affected nutrient intake and energy value of the diet. These calculations are made by the Agricultural Research Service of the USDA on the basis of the food disappearance data of the Economic Research Service. The trends in consumption of protein, fats, carbohydrates, and total energy intake are shown in Figure 13-2. A major change since 1909–1913 has been the increased consumption of fats. This trend partly reflects the greater total intake of vegetable oils (margarine and salad and cooking oils). Since about two-thirds of our dietary fat comes from animal products, this change is also due to the increased consumption of poultry, beef, and dairy products.

Protein intake has remained relatively constant

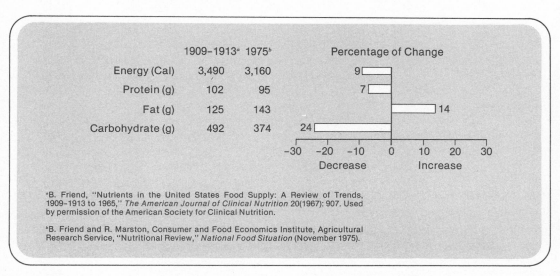

FIGURE 13-2. Changes in food energy and macronutrients available per person per day in 1975 compared to 1909–1913.

since about 1910, but the dietary sources of protein have changed. The increased intake of poultry, beef, and dairy products has been offset by the decline in the use of potatoes and cereal products.

Carbohydrate intake has declined. The increased use of sugar is not nearly as large as the decreased intake of cereals. Fiber intake (not shown in the figure) has decreased from 6 grams a day at the turn of the century to about 4 grams a day in 1975.

In the 1970s the total energy intake of Americans who have a rather sedentary lifestyle is only about 9 percent less than the amount consumed by active, mainly rural Americans around the turn of the century. The major change in regard to energy intake is that sixty-five years ago about 32 percent of calories came from fats and 56 percent came from carbohydrates. Currently, approximately 41 percent of energy comes from fats, and carbohydrates account for only about 47 percent.

Micronutrient Consumption Trends

Consumption of all micronutrients calculated by the USDA, except magnesium, has increased compared to 1909–1913 (Table 13-1). During the last ten years, the largest improvements have been in vitamin C, niacin, and iron availability. However, in this same period, intake of calcium has declined.

It should be emphasized again that all the data discussed here refer to the nutrients available in the food supply; they are not necessarily the amounts eaten. Keep in mind that a great deal of food is wasted in the United States, and that some people eat more, while others eat less of the foods that supply these nutrients. Perhaps the most informative comparisons using these data are those shown in the lower portion of Table 13-1. The nutrients available in the food supply are compared here to the adult male RDA, the adult female RDA, and the teen-age male RDA. We can see that the nutrients in shortest supply are magnesium (for everyone), calcium (for teen-agers), and iron (for women and teen-agers). If 20 percent of the available food sup-

ply were dumped in the garbage or fed to pets as table scraps, the amounts of thiamin, riboflavin, niacin, and vitamin B_6 available for each person would be close to or fall below the adult RDA. Table 13-1 also shows that there is little reason, in terms of food availability, for American diets to be low in vitamin A, vitamin C, or vitamin B_{12}. When these deficiencies do occur, they are probably due to individual factors (such as those discussed in the preceding section) or to lack of nutrition knowledge.

SURVEYS

The main purpose of a nutrition survey is to assess the nutritional status of a population, but the information obtained can be used for several purposes. Basic researchers use surveys to correlate specific nutrient inadequacies with signs of deficiency or the incidence of certain diseases. Health planners use the same data to evaluate the need for nutrition intervention and to design responsive health programs. The food industry applies findings to product development and to programs to fortify frequently consumed foods with nutrients that are commonly lacking. Educators use the information to identify needs and motivate people to improve their diets nutritionally.

The three major nutrition surveys in the United States are the USDA Household Survey, the Ten-State Nutrition Survey, and the Health and Nutrition Examination Survey (HANES). The combined applications of all three surveys have a vast potential for improving the nutritional status of our population. Each study has a different design and provides a different type of information—this must be kept in mind at all times during any discussion of these surveys.

USDA Household Survey

Food consumption surveys have a long history in the United States. Some of the earliest nutrition

TABLE 13-1. Micronutrients in the U.S. Food Supply[a] and Comparison of Amounts Available in 1975 to the RDA

Year	Calcium (mg)	Magnesium (mg)	Iron (mg)	Thiamin (mg)	Ribo-flavin (mg)	Niacin (mg)	Vitamin A (IU)	Vitamin C (mg)	Vitamin B6 (mg)	Vitamin B12 (mcg)
1909–1913	816	410	15.2	1.64	1.84	19.0	7,600	104	—	—
1965	961	340	16.5	1.80	2.26	21.4	7,800	102	2.18	9.5
1975	910	339	18.3	1.87	2.29	23.3	8,200	116	2.25	9.5
1975 Availability										
Percentage of adult male RDA	113	96	183	133	143	129	164	257	112	316
Percentage of adult female RDA	113	113	101	187	190	179	205	257	112	316
Percentage of 15–18-year-old male RDA	75	84	101	124	127	116	164	257	112	316

[a]Amounts disappearing into the food supply per person per day.

SOURCE: U.S., Department of Agriculture, Agricultural Research Service, Consumer and Food Economics Institute, "National Food Situation" prepared by B. Friend and R. Marston in *Nutritional Review* (November 1975). B. Friend, "Nutrients in the United States food supply. A review of trends, 1909–1913 to 1965," *The American Journal of Clinical Nutrition* 20(1967):907. © 1967. The American Society for Clinical Nutrition. Used by permission.

surveys were conducted around the turn of the century by W. O. Atwater, a leader in the development of the study of nutrition by the USDA. Though the scope of these studies seems rather limited today, at the time they were made they provided important information and ultimately contributed to current nutrition knowledge. The first comprehensive national nutrition survey in this country was conducted in 1936–1937. This survey identified several problems in the American diet. It stimulated an awareness of the need for a cereal enrichment program which subsequently significantly increased the amounts of niacin, riboflavin, thiamin, and iron in American diets. The 1936 survey also contributed to the development of the nutrition education program within the USDA and similar efforts by other health education groups. The National School Lunch Program was also largely an outgrowth of the needs identified by this study.

Surveys were repeated in 1942, 1948, 1955, and 1965–1966. Another survey, which is budgeted to cost between three and four million dollars, began in 1977. The following discussion is based on the results of the 1965 survey.

Survey Design. The 1965 survey by the USDA was a study of a random sample of the U.S. population. It included people from all regions of the country and at all income levels. The surveyors questioned each interviewee about the food consumed by all members of the household during a 24-hour period. Food consumption within 14,500 households was recorded, and the results were summarized in terms of average quantities of foods eaten, percentage of persons using those foods, average quantities of nutrients in all foods eaten, and the percentage of the total nutrients contributed by each major group of foods. Kinds and amounts of food eaten were tabulated in eleven food groups— milk and milk products; eggs, meat, poultry, and fish; legumes and nuts; fats and oils; grain products; tomatoes and citrus fruit; potatoes; dark-green and yellow vegetables; other vegetables and fruit; sugars

and sweets; and beverages other than milk and juices.

Results. The problems identified during the survey as being most common among each population group are discussed in detail in the following chapters. Table 13-2 provides an overview of the nutrients consumed in amounts less than the 1968 RDA. The average protein intake met the RDA for all groups. Average vitamin C intake fell below the RDA only for men age 75 and over. Vitamin A intake was a problem primarily for teen-age girls and older women and men. Average intakes of thiamin and riboflavin met the RDA for most males, but thiamin was below the RDA for all females 12 years old and over. Intakes of riboflavin fell below the RDA with increasing frequency as women advanced in years.

The main deficiencies shown in Table 13-2 are in calcium and iron. Females above the age of 9 had low average intakes compared to the RDA for both of these minerals. Children primarily had trouble meeting their RDA for iron. The average intake of both minerals was below the RDA for teen-age males. In later years, men had less of a problem with iron, but had inadequate intakes of calcium after age 35.

Implications. There are many ways of applying and interpreting the results of the USDA Household Survey—the reports alone fill several volumes. For example, when compared to the results of the 1955 survey, these data can tell us how diets changed during that decade.

Figure 13-3a compares the percentage of households surveyed in 1955 and 1965 on the basis of meeting the RDA for the seven nutrients evaluated. The decline in diet quality, despite a coincidental improvement in average income and increased availability of most vitamins and minerals in the food supply (Table 13-1), emphasizes the importance of programs such as nutrition education. The greater prevalence among poorer people (Figure

TABLE 13-2. USDA Household Survey, 1965—Average Intakes below the RDA

Age (years)	Sex	Calcium	Iron	Vitamin A	Thiamin	Riboflavin	Vitamin C	Protein
Under 1	Both		****					
1–2	Both		****					
3–5	Both		**					
6–8	Both							
9–11	F	***	****		*			
	M	*						
12–14	F	***	****	*	*			
	M	**	***		*			
15–17	F	****	****		**			
	M	*	*					
18–19	F	***	****	*	*			
	M							
20–34	F	***	****		*	*		
	M							
35–54	F	****	****		*	**		
	M	*						
55–64	F	****			*	*		
	M	**						
65–74	F	****	*	*	**	**		
	M	**						
75 and over	F	****	*	**	**	***		
	M	***		*		**	*	

KEY: * 1 to 10 percent below the RDA; ** 11 to 20 percent below the RDA; *** 21 to 29 percent below the RDA; **** 30 percent or more below the RDA.

SOURCE: U.S., Department of Agriculture, Agricultural Research Service, "Household Food Consumption Survey 1965–66."

13-3b) of diets that failed to meet the RDA points to the importance of identifying those in need, making available to them either supplemental food or food stamps, and developing programs to help them purchase foods and plan diets to meet their nutrient needs.

Ten-State Nutrition Survey

The 1965 USDA Household Survey, like those conducted earlier, stimulated efforts to improve the nutritional status of Americans. Along with other social and political forces, the findings of this survey

The Ten-State Nutrition Survey primarily selected people from the low-income segment of the U.S. population. It included biochemical and physical examinations as well as a dietary questionnaire.

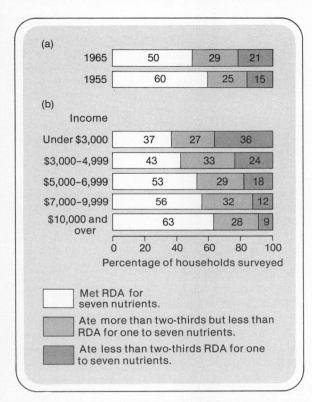

FIGURE 13-3. Comparison of the adequacy of diets in the 1955 and 1965 USDA Household Surveys (a) and of the adequacy of diets in relation to income as learned from the 1965 USDA Household Survey (b). SOURCE: Agricultural Research Service, Household Food Consumption Survey 1965–66; Report Nos. 1 to 18 (Washington, D.C.: U.S. Department of Agriculture, 1968–1974).

contributed to a heightened interest in nutrition among health workers, legislators, and the general public. Congressional hearings early in 1967 called attention to the probability that serious hunger and malnutrition existed among some population groups in the United States. Later that year Congress directed the Department of Health, Education, and Welfare (DHEW) to determine the magnitude and location of malnutrition and related health prob-

lems in the United States. The study that resulted is called the *Ten-State Nutrition Survey*.

Survey Design. A series of ad hoc committees developed an overall plan for conducting a survey that would fulfill the Congressional mandate. The major differences between this study (conducted between 1968 and 1970) and the 1965 USDA survey are the following.

1. Information was obtained primarily with regard to the nutritional status of the low-income segment of the population, because malnutrition was expected to be most prevalent in that group.
2. The criteria used for determining the extent of nutrition problems included examination of the subjects for physical and biochemical signs of deficiency. This type of information cannot be provided by dietary intake surveys. It is determined by measurement of height, weight, and skinfold thickness; physical examination for signs of nutritional deficiency (Chapter 27); and biochemical analyses of blood and urine samples.
3. Information was collected so that cultural and socioeconomic factors that might influence the prevalence of nutrition and health problems could be determined.

The Ten-State Nutrition Survey collected demographic data (such as age, income level, and size of household) on over 86,000 persons. All of these subjects lived in the census districts within each of the ten states that had the lowest average income. Of the total number initially included in the study group, 40,000 individuals were invited to participate in a more detailed clinical evaluation, which included a medical history, physical examination, and collection of blood to check for anemia. Selected subgroups (high-risk populations such as infants, young children, adolescents, pregnant or lactating women, and persons over 60 years of age) received more detailed biochemical and dietary evaluation.

Because the 1965 USDA Household Survey had

245

shown that poorer people more often consume diets that do not meet the RDA, the correlation between financial means and nutritional status was carefully evaluated. A large proportion of the families included in the survey were living below or only slightly above the poverty level. To differentiate the degree of poverty within this population, income level was expressed in terms of a *poverty income ratio* (PIR) for each family. This ratio was determined on the basis of specific characteristics that affect family income, such as family size, sex of head of household, and place of residence (farm or nonfarm). The ten states were then divided into two large subsamples based on PIR—*low-income-ratio* states and *high-income-ratio* states. Care must be taken not to misinterpret these terms. The classification simply means that in the low-income-ratio states, more than half of the families were living below the poverty level, whereas in the high-income-ratio states, more than half of the families were living above the poverty level.

Results. The results of the Ten-State Nutrition Survey indicated that a significant proportion of the population studied was malnourished or had a high risk of developing nutritional problems. Table 13-3 provides an overview of the relative importance of nutritional problems among blacks, whites, and Spanish-Americans throughout the lifespan. Impaired growth and development were found in a substantial number of children and adolescents, while obesity was identified as a prevalent problem among adolescents, adult white males and females, and adult black females. Adolescents between the ages of 10 and 16 had the highest prevalence of unsatisfactory nutritional status. Elderly persons showed evidence of general undernutrition, which was not restricted to the very poor or to any single ethnic group. Poor dental health associated with low levels of dental care was encountered in many segments of the population. The combined findings of the survey regarding each nutrient are:

1. Iron—A high prevalence of low hemoglobin and hematocrit values (a measure of anemia) was found throughout all segments of the population. This appears to be due to iron deficiency.

2. Protein—Biochemical blood tests suggested that a relatively large proportion of pregnant and lactating women had marginal protein nutriture. Nutritional problems related to protein were also noted in low-income-ratio states among some groups of blacks and Spanish-Americans.

3. Vitamin A—Spanish-Americans in the low-income-ratio states had a major problem in regard to vitamin A nutriture. Young people in all subgroups, except Spanish-Americans in high-income-ratio states, had low vitamin A values.

4. Vitamin C—The prevalence of poor vitamin C status increased with age, but vitamin C nutrition was not a major problem among children or teen-agers.

5. Riboflavin—Riboflavin status was poor among blacks of all ages, Spanish-Americans of all ages in the low-income-ratio states, and white children in the low-income-ratio states.

6. Thiamin—Nutritional status in relation to thiamin did not appear to be a problem, except in adolescents between the ages of 10 and 16 years.

7. Iodine—Goiter was found to be more prevalent than expected, but there was no evidence of poor iodine status in the population surveyed. (This finding suggests that the goiters resulted from causes other than iodine deficiency; see Chapter 27.)

Implications. The final report of the Ten-State Nutrition Survey emphasized that the findings of this study are limited to an evaluation of only a few of the nutrients known to be essential for good health. The investigators could not evaluate all possible problems because little is known about the human requirements of many nutrients (such as trace elements), and adequate information on the distribution of these and other nutrients in the food supply is not available.

Several lessons can be learned, however, by looking carefully at the results of this survey. An example of the variation in severity of specific nutritional problems is the high prevalence of low vitamin A values among Mexican-Americans in the low-income-ratio states compared to the absence of vitamin A problems in Puerto Ricans in the high-income-ratio states. This type of analysis points out that efforts to correct nutrition problems must be tailored to the different social, cultural, and economic characteristics of each group.

The survey also showed that the number of years of school completed by the person responsible for buying and preparing the family's food was related to the nutritional status of children under the age of seventeen. It is not possible, however, to conclude that lack of education alone caused lower nutritional levels, since the number of years of school completed is also associated with other factors that affect nutrition (such as income status).

Another possible explanation for nutrition problems is that many persons included in this survey made poor use of the money available for food. For example, they did not often buy foods rich in vitamin A. The study found that many households that emphasized meat in their diets would benefit from learning to use less expensive protein sources such as fish, poultry, or beans.

HANES

The results of the Ten-State Nutrition Survey pointed out the need for DHEW to develop a program of continuing surveillance of the nutritional status of Americans. The ongoing program that was developed is called the Health and Nutrition Examination Survey (HANES).

Survey design. The first HANES, conducted in 1971–1972, examined 30,000 individuals who were a representative sample of the U.S. population aged 1 to 74. The design of this survey allowed for more detailed evaluation of population groups where malnutrition is most common—preschool children, women of childbearing age, the elderly, and the poor. The evaluation of nutritional status was based on dietary intake, several measures of obesity, blood analyses for signs of anemia, and physical examination for signs of deficiencies of several nutrients.

One important feature in the design (and therefore in the interpretation) of the HANES is that the RDA was not used as the standard for evaluation of dietary intake. Table 13-4 shows that the vitamin C and iron standards were approximately equal to the RDA for each population group, but that the HANES standard of adequacy for calcium was much lower—roughly 50 percent of the RDA for children, adolescents, and adult men, and 75 percent of the RDA for women. Vitamin A standards also were lower—about 70 percent of the RDA for children and men and about 90 percent of the RDA for women.

These lower standards mean that in some instances intakes of calcium and vitamin A that would have been considered inadequate by the criteria used for the USDA Household Survey are considered adequate by the standards used for the HANES. Therefore, the design of this study helped to identify population groups with intakes of calcium and vitamin A well below the RDA. On the other hand, when we review the HANES results, we must keep in mind that the standards do not always correlate with the RDA.

Results. We can look at the results of the HANES in several different ways. By concentrating on different bars in the graphs shown in Figure 13-4, we can compare differences that correspond with income level, race, or age and sex for each of the two vitamins and two minerals.

First, focus on the bars to the far left for both income below and above poverty level for the total population of males and females. We can see that iron is the nutrient that most frequently failed to meet 100 percent of standard value. This was especially true for women. Mean calcium intakes were lower, compared to the standard, for women than

TABLE 13-3. Relative Severity of Nutritional Problems Found in the Ten-State Nutrition Survey, 1968–1970

Low-Income-Ratio States[a]

Ethnic Group	Age (years)	Sex	Iron	Protein	Vitamin A	Vitamin C	Riboflavin	Thiamin	Iodine	Growth and Development	Obesity
Black	0-5	Both	▲	○	●	○	●	○	○	●	—
	6-9	Both	▲	•	•	○	●	○	○	●	—
	10-16	F	▲	•	•	○	●	•	○	•	•
		M	▲	○	•	○	●	•	○	•	•
	17-59	F	▲	•	○	•	●	○	○	—	▲
		M	▲	○	○	●	●	○	○	—	○
	Over 60	F	▲	•	○	○	●	○	○	—	●
		M	▲	•	○	●	●	○	○	—	○
White	0-5	Both	●	○	•	○	•	○	○	●	—
	6-9	Both	●	○	•	○	•	○	○	●	—
	10-16	F	●	○	•	○	•	•	○	•	•
		M	●	○	•	○	•	•	○	•	●
	17-59	F	●	○	○	○	○	○	○	—	●
		M	●	○	○	●	○	○	○	—	•
	Over 60	F	●	○	○	○	○	○	○	—	●
		M	●	○	○	●	○	○	○	—	○
Spanish-American	0-5	Both	●	○	▲	○	●	○	○	●	—
	6-9	Both	●	○	▲	○	●	○	○	●	—
	10-16	F	●	•	▲	○	●	○	○	•	—
		M	●	○	▲	○	●	○	○	•	—
	17-59	F	●	•	▲	○	•	○	○	—	—
		M	●	•	▲	○	•	○	○	—	—
	Over 60	F	●	•	▲	○	•	○	○	—	—
		M	●	•	▲	●	○	○	○	—	—
Pregnant and lactating women			▲	●	—	—	—	—	—	—	—

KEY: ▲ High prevalence of deficient values; ● medium prevalence of deficient values; • low prevalence of deficient values; ○ minimal deficiencies; — data not available.

Iron	Protein	Vitamin A	Vitamin C	Riboflavin	Thiamin	Iodine	Growth and Development	Obesity	Sex	Age (years)	Ethnic Group
●	○	•	○	•	○	○	●	—	Both	0–5	Black
●	○	•	○	•	○	○	●	—	Both	6–9	Black
●	○	•	○	•	•	○	•	•	F	10–16	Black
●	○	•	○	•	•	○	•	○	M	10–16	Black
●	○	○	○	•	○	○	—	▲	F	17–59	Black
●	○	○	○	•	○	○	—	○	M	17–59	Black
●	○	○	○	•	○	○	—	●	F	Over 60	Black
●	○	○	•	○	○	○	—	○	M	Over 60	Black
•	○	•	○	•	○	○	●	—	Both	0–5	White
•	○	○	○	○	○	○	●	—	Both	6–9	White
•	○	•	○	○	○	○	•	•	F	10–16	White
•	○	•	○	○	○	○	•	•	M	10–16	White
•	○	○	○	○	○	○	—	●	F	17–59	White
•	○	○	○	○	○	○	—	○	M	17–59	White
•	○	○	○	○	○	○	—	●	F	Over 60	White
•	○	○	•	○	○	○	—	○	M	Over 60	White
●	○	○	○	○	○	○	●	—	Both	0–5	Spanish-American
●	○	○	○	○	○	○	●	—	Both	6–9	Spanish-American
●	○	○	○	○	○	○	•	—	F	10–16	Spanish-American
●	○	○	○	○	○	○	•	—	M	10–16	Spanish-American
●	○	○	○	○	○	○	—	—	F	17–59	Spanish-American
●	○	○	○	○	○	○	—	—	M	17–59	Spanish-American
●	○	○	○	○	○	○	—	—	F	Over 60	Spanish-American
●	○	○	○	○	○	○	—	—	M	Over 60	Spanish-American
▲	●	—	—	—	—	—	—	—	Pregnant and lactating women		

[a] Kentucky, Louisiana, South Carolina, Texas, West Virginia—more than half of the families were living below the poverty level.
[b] California, Massachusetts, Michigan, New York (and New York City), Washington—more than half of the families were living above the poverty level.

SOURCE: U.S., Department of Health, Education, and Welfare, Center for Disease Control, "Ten-State Nutrition Survey, 1968–1970," Publication Nos. (HSM) 72–8130 and 72–8131.

TABLE 13-4. HANES Standards of Dietary Adequacy and HANES Standards Expressed As an Approximate Percentage of the RDA

Population Group		Comparison RDA Group	HANES Standards of Dietary Adequacy				HANES Standards As an Approximate Percentage of RDA			
Age (years)	Sex	Age (years)	Calcium (mg)	Iron (mg)	Vitamin A (IU)	Vitamin C (mg)	Calcium	Iron	Vitamin A	Vitamin C
1–5	Both	1–6	450	15[a]	2,000	40	55	100	100[b]	100
6–9	Both	7–10	450	10	2,500	40	55	100	75	100
10–12	Both	11–14	650	18[c]	2,500	40	50	100	50	90
13–19	Both	15–18	650[d]	18	3,500	50[e]	50	100	70[b]	110
20–69	F	23–50	600	18[f]	3,500	55	75	100	90	120
	M		400	10	3,500	60	50	100	70	130
70 and over	F	Over 51	600	10	3,500	55	75	100	90	120
	M		400	10	3,500	60	50	100	70	130

[a] HANES standard for 4–5 year olds and RDA for 4–6 year olds use 10 milligrams (mg).
[b] Slight variation within age groups as summarized here.
[c] 10 milligrams for females.
[d] 550 milligrams for 17–19 year olds.
[e] 55 milligrams for male 17–19 year olds.
[f] 10 milligrams after age 50.

SOURCE: Adapted from S. Abraham, F. W. Lowenstein, and C. L. Johnson, "Preliminary Findings of the First Health and Nutrition Examination Survey, United States 1971–72: Dietary Intake and Biochemical Findings," Publication No. (HRA) 74–1219–1 (Washington, D.C.: U.S. Department of Health, Education, and Welfare, 1974).

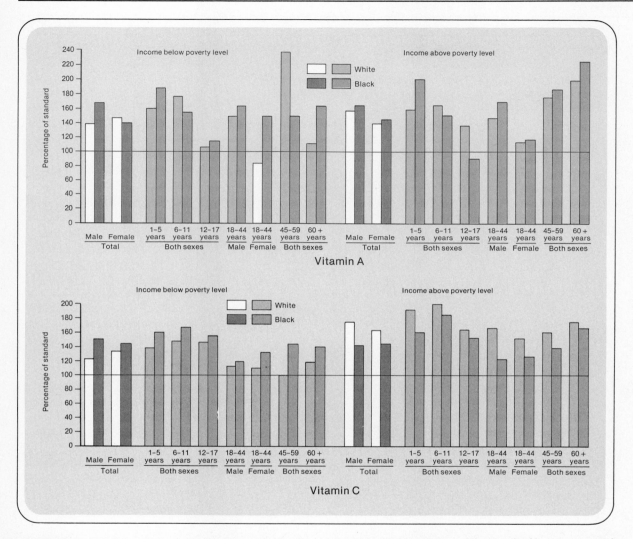

FIGURE 13-4. HANES preliminary results. Mean intakes of micronutrients as a percentage of the standard by age, sex, and race for different income levels, 1971–1972. SOURCE: S. Abraham, F. W. Lowenstein, and C. L. Johnson, *Preliminary Findings of the First Health and Nutrition Examination Survey, United States, 1971–72: Dietary Intake and Biochemical Findings,* Publication No. (HRA) 74-1219-1 (Washington, D.C.: U.S. Department of Health, Education, and Welfare, 1974).

for men; but keep in mind that the standard for women was higher—600 milligrams compared to a standard of only 400 milligrams for men. For vitamins A and C, there appeared to be little difference between adequacy of the diets of males compared to females.

Comparing the income below and above poverty levels yields another perspective on how nutrition problems vary among groups. Income level had little effect upon the dietary adequacy of vitamin A and calcium (except for people 45 years old and over), but iron intakes were lower in the poorer

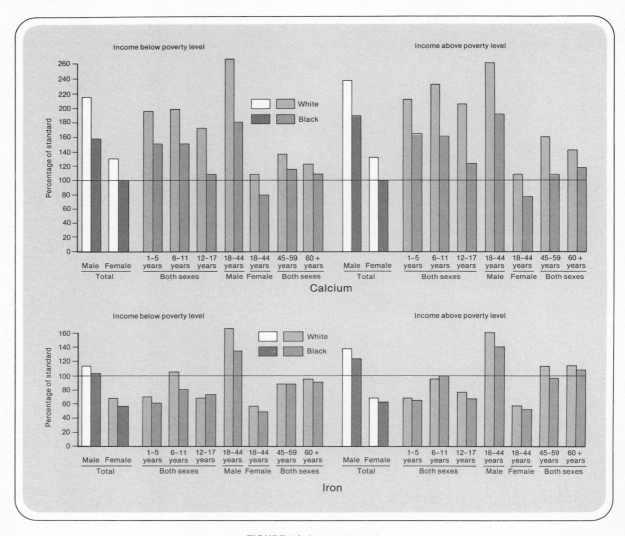

FIGURE 13-4. (*continued*)

population. The vitamin C graph suggests an interesting difference—increase in income had little effect on vitamin C intake among blacks, but definitely increased intake of this nutrient among whites. The nutrient that differed most between racial groups was calcium. (This finding might be attributed to a lower intake of milk among blacks.)

Figure 13-4 can also help us focus on problems that vary in severity according to age.

1. Vitamin A—Intakes were lowest compared to the standard for adolescents and adult women.
2. Vitamin C—Intakes were better for the population 17 years old and under.

TABLE 13-5. Mean Nutrient Intakes of Women As a Percentage of the Standard and the Percentage of These Women with Intakes Less Than the Standard		
Nutrient	Mean Intakes As Percentage of Standard	Percentage of Women with Intakes Less Than Standard
Calcium	110	55.59
Iron	59	92.13
Vitamin A	114	64.90
Vitamin C	150	49.04

SOURCE: S. Abraham, F. W. Lowenstein, and C. L. Johnson, "Preliminary Findings of the First Health and Nutrition Examination Survey, United States 1971–72: Dietary Intake and Biochemical Findings," Publication No. (HRA) 74-1219-1 (Washington, D.C.: U.S. Department of Health, Education, and Welfare, 1974).

3. Calcium—Intakes were lower for older people and adult women.

4. Iron—Intakes were rarely above 100 percent of the standard except for adult males.

Many other comparisons can be drawn from the figures. The few examples above may help you focus on other differences that are of specific interest to you.

Implications. The HANES reinforces many observations made in earlier studies. It shows again that nutrition problems vary among males and females of different ages, and that income (and associated socioeconomic factors) influence the dietary adequacy of some—but not all—nutrients.

Table 13-5 is included as a final precaution against misinterpreting the significance of mean intakes. This table shows that even though mean intakes of calcium, vitamin A, and vitamin C are above 100 percent of the standard for adult females, between 49 and 65 percent of the women surveyed

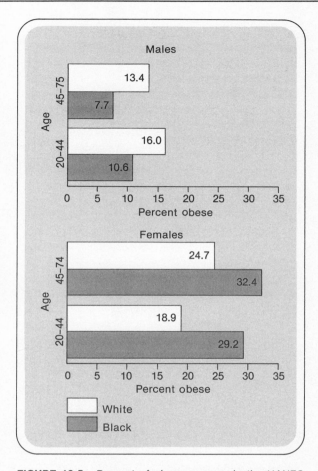

FIGURE 13-5. Percent of obese persons in the HANES survey. SOURCE: S. Abraham, *Preliminary Findings of the First Health and Nutrition Examination Survey, United States, 1971–72: Anthropometric and Clinical Findings,* Publication No. (HRA) 75-1229 (Washington, D.C.: U.S. Department of Health, Education, and Welfare, 1975).

had diets that fell below the standard for these three nutrients.

The HANES findings showed that the incidence of obesity varied among different groups (Figure 13-5). The population with the highest percentage of obese persons was older black women; the lowest percentage was found among older black men.

The findings of the physical examinations for signs of deficiencies of several nutrients are discussed in Chapter 27.

CRITICAL QUESTIONS

The information in this chapter has provided an overview of existing nutrition problems in the United States. The discussions of the details of survey design and interpretation of results should help you to ask critical questions when you read about or hear people discuss the results of nutrition studies or the incidence of malnutrition. Such questions might be:

What nutrients were considered?

What standards were used and what is the significance of that standard?

Did the survey measure changes in food patterns, food intake, results of physical examinations, or results of biochemical analyses?

How were the subjects in the survey selected and what segments of the overall population do they represent?

These factors are often overlooked by people who lack a basic understanding of nutrition. Accurate interpretation of surveys requires thoughtful application of nutrition knowledge.

In the next chapters we will use this information as we examine potential problems and nutrient needs among people in specific age groups.

STUDY QUESTIONS

1. How should we view average nutrient intake values calculated from nutrition surveys?

2. What are disappearance data?

3. What are the three major surveys regarding nutrition that have been conducted in the United States?

4. How was the USDA Household Survey designed?

5. How was the Ten-State Nutrition Survey conducted?

6. How was the HANES carried out?

7. What information must be available so that you can evaluate reports regarding the nutritional status of Americans?

SUGGESTED READING

1. "Highlights of the Ten-State Nutrition Survey," *Nutrition Today* 7(1972):4–11.
2. F. Clark, "Recent food consumption surveys and their uses," *Federation Proceedings*, 33(1974): 2270–74.
3. D. M. Youland and A. Engle, "Practices and problems in HANES," *Journal of the American Dietetic Association* 68(1976):22–24.
4. J. P. Madden, S. J. Goedman, and H. A. Guthrie, "Validity of the 24-hour recall," *Journal of the American Dietetic Association* 68(1976):143–47.
5. "Standard values in nutrition," (Symposium issue) *Nutrition* (London) 29(1975):69–100.
6. H. A. Guthrie, "Nutritional status measures as predictors of nutritional risk in preschool children," *American Journal of Clinical Nutrition* 29(1976): 1048–50.
7. M. Z. Nichaman, "Developing a nutrition surveillance system," *Journal of the American Dietetic Association* 65(1974):15.
8. S. M. Garn and D.C. Clark, "Problems in the nutritional assessment of black individuals," *American Journal of Public Health* 66(1976):262–66.
9. B. Friend, "Nutritive value of the United States per capita food supply," *American Journal of Clinical Nutrition* 27(1974):1.
10. *Ten-State Nutrition Survey, 1968–1970.* Center for Disease Control, U.S. Department of Health, Education and Welfare Pub. No.'s (HSM) 72-1830, 31, 32, 33, 34. Washington, D.C.: Government Printing Office.

11. *Preliminary Findings of the First Health and Nutrition Examination Survey, United States 1971–1972: Dietary Intake and Biochemical Findings.* U.S. Department of Health, Education and Welfare Pub. No. (HRA) 74-1219-1. Washington, D.C.: Government Printing Office, 1974.

12. *Preliminary Findings of the First Health and Nutrition Examination Survey, United States, 1971–1972: Anthropometric and Clinical Findings.* U.S. Department of Health, Education and Welfare Pub. No. (HRA) 75-1229. Washington, D.C.: Government Printing Office, 1975.

13. *Dietary Levels of Households in the United States, Spring 1965.* Household Food Consumption Survey 1965–66, Report Numbers 1–18. Consumer and Food Economics Research Division, Agricultural Research Service, U.S. Department of Agriculture. Washington, D.C.: Government Printing Office, 1968.

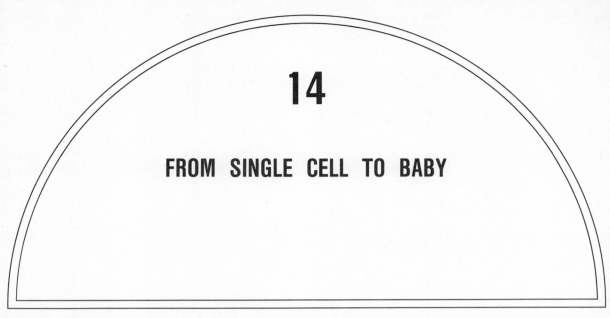

14

FROM SINGLE CELL TO BABY

The growth and development of a single fertilized cell into a 7-pound, 4-ounce cuddly, crying, hungry, wetting human being in only 280 days is the most impressive example of the synthesis of body cells and tissues from the nutrients provided by food. A successful pregnancy is dependent not only upon an adequate supply of nutrients but upon other health-related factors as well. This chapter focuses on how fetal growth and development are affected by:

1. The nutritional status of the mother before pregnancy
2. Physiological changes in the mother's body that influence, and are influenced by, the availability of nutrients
3. The ability of the mother to select foods that provide sufficient amounts of the nutrients needed for both herself and her unborn child

PREPARING FOR PREGNANCY

Many couples begin preparing for parenthood long before the woman is pregnant. They move into an apartment or house that will accommodate a growing family; they juggle budget priorities to allow enough money for medical expenses and an additional family member; they try out the sounds of different names for their baby. Another item on this list of preparations should be nutrition planning.

Prepregnancy

Diet is important during pregnancy, but the nutritional status of a woman at the time she becomes pregnant also has a bearing on her baby's health. The importance of the nutritional status of women before pregnancy is due to two factors.

1. Adequate maternal stores of nutrients at conception are necessary to maintain a normal pregnancy.
2. The birth weight of an infant is more often related to the mother's weight at conception than to her weight gain during the following nine months.

The First Months

Nutritional preparedness is especially important during the early weeks of pregnancy. Changes in a woman's body begin even when the fetus is very small. These physiological adjustments to pregnancy create an increased need for energy and nutrients, although the woman may not even know she is pregnant.

Adequate nutrient stores are needed especially by women who have *morning sickness* (nausea and vomiting) early in pregnancy. If the woman stops eating or restricts her food intake to avoid feeling ill, her body and the fetus become dependent upon her nutrient reserves.

Benefits for Both

Many women are aware that their diet during pregnancy affects the well-being of their baby, but fewer women realize that it affects their own health also. Complications of pregnancy occur most often among mothers who give birth to infants who are very small or very large. Cesarean sections, an additional risk to the mother, are more common among women whose health was poor at the time of conception.

The strongest evidence that maternal diet affects the health of the baby is that low birth weight of the infant (which closely correlates with neonatal mortality) is associated with poor nutritional status, low prepregnancy weight, and low weight gain during pregnancy. Giving birth to a premature baby is also linked to factors not directly related to nutrition, such as socioeconomic status, biological maturity of the mother, short stature, certain infectious and chronic diseases, and smoking.

It is important to note that newborns with birth weights 1 to 2 pounds above average fare as poorly as infants born 1 to 2 pounds underweight. Larger than ideal babies are most frequently born to women who have diabetes, and pregnancy complicates the management of their existing disease.

The correlation between the quality of a mother's diet and the quality of her baby's health is not as strong as the correlation between maternal nutrition status and infant birth weight. Some studies indicate that the physical condition of infants correlates with maternal diet during pregnancy, but other studies indicate that the baby's health is measurably im-

paired only if the mother's diet is far below recommended levels. Analysis of the results of the latter studies emphasized the importance of taking into consideration maternal nutrition stores and the severity of dietary inadequacies. Maternal intakes of protein below 45 grams, calcium below 600 milligrams, iron below 10 milligrams, and vitamin A below 2,000 IU seem to create an increased risk of impairment to the health of the newborn.

It is difficult to prove a direct effect of maternal diet upon a baby's health because so many other factors are involved in the success of pregnancy. Figure 14-1 shows the interlocking relationship between nutrition and genetic, social, psychological, and physiological forces. The success of the pregnancy is also influenced by the mother's interest in health matters, access to medical care, and intellectual capability and willingness to follow medical advice. Nutrition during pregnancy is just one part of maintaining overall health status—an adequate diet alone will not guarantee good health for mother or baby.

PHYSIOLOGICAL CHANGES

The physiological changes that occur during pregnancy support the idea that pregnancy is a normal state. Many biological adaptations occur in response to the retention within the uterus of a fertilized ovum. These increase the probability that a fetus will develop and survive as a healthy infant.

Use of Nutrients

During pregnancy the mother's body makes better use of some dietary nutrients. Food moves more slowly through the intestines, thus increasing the exposure of nutrients to absorptive cells. This decreased motility contributes to constipation (which is an annoyance to some pregnant women), but it also enables iron and other nutrients to be more efficiently absorbed. On the other hand, there is an increased flow of blood through the kidneys, and a

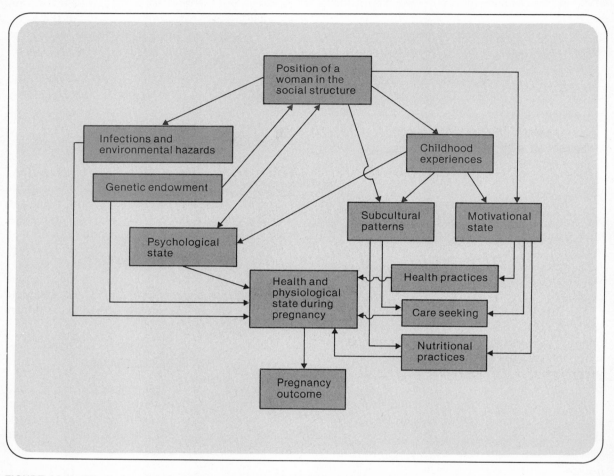

FIGURE 14-1. Effect of social structure on women's physiological state and pregnancy outcome. SOURCE: J. R. Udry, *Maternal Nutrition and the Course of Pregnancy,* National Academy of Sciences, Food and Nutrition Board, Committee on Maternal Nutrition (Washington, D.C.: 1970).

greater loss of amino acids, glucose, and possibly micronutrients in urine.

The secretion of acid and pepsin by the stomach cells decreases during pregnancy. Although gastric motility is reduced, the slower emptying of the stomach may allow for better digestion.

Another change that enhances fetal development is the increased activity of several enzymes, includ-

ing those involved in phosphorus metabolism and the pyridoxine-containing enzymes necessary for the addition or removal of amino groups on amino acids that are used for protein synthesis. Also, hormonal changes during pregnancy direct reactions within the body toward synthetic processes rather than tissue degradation.

Additional nutrients are needed during pregnancy because maternal blood volume increases, energy needs are greater, and additional maternal and fetal tissue must be synthesized and maintained.

Blood Volume

One of the most remarkable changes during pregnancy is the increase in blood volume. The circulatory system of a pregnant woman contains approximately one-third more blood than that of a nonpregnant woman. The fluid part of the blood increases more than the red blood cells (see Chapter 22), so the concentration of red blood cells (and therefore of hemoglobin) is diluted. This synthesis of about 5 cups of additional blood accounts for a large portion of the increased nutrient needs during pregnancy. Protein and iron are part of the hemoglobin molecule; energy sources are needed for the synthetic reactions; folacin and vitamin B_{12} are needed for red blood cell division; and other vitamins and minerals have cofactor roles and maintain the integrity of the cells.

Energy Needs

The daily RDA for energy increases by approximately 300 Cal (1,260 kJ) throughout the nine months of pregnancy. Metabolism increases in several body systems, and more energy is needed because the heart must work harder to pump a larger volume of blood. A woman accumulates fat stores early in pregnancy, but during the last weeks (when the fetus is growing rapidly) some of these stores are utilized. During the latter months of pregnancy many women reduce their physical activity, thus making available more energy for the biological processes necessary for the growth and life support of the baby. This reduction in activity is not necessary, however, if the mother increases her energy intake proportionally.

Tissue Synthesis

The fetus is considered by most people to be the only product of pregnancy, but a baby that weighs 7 pounds represents only about one-fourth of the 28 pounds gained by an average woman during pregnancy. The other 21 pounds are added in maternal tissue needed to support the life of the baby during and after birth. Enlargement of a pregnant woman's breasts accounts for about 1 pound of this weight gain, newly formed blood weighs about 3 pounds, the uterus weighs about 2 pounds, the placenta weighs about $1\frac{1}{2}$ pounds, and the fluid that serves as a protective cushion around the fetus weighs another 2 pounds. During the early months of pregnancy, other parts of the mother's body (nonreproductive tissues) build up about 12 pounds of nutrient stores that provide a reserve of energy for the latter months and after the baby is born.

Tissue Maintenance

The tissues that account for weight gain during pregnancy are quite different from those formed by a nonpregnant woman who gains 28 pounds of fat from overeating. Many metabolic reactions occur within the cells of the placenta, uterus, breasts, and fetus. Since oxygen is used in the final phase of energy release from nutrients (Chapter 5), the amount of oxygen consumed in a tissue provides an estimate of the degree of energy utilization by that tissue. Figure 14-2 shows that during the first two-thirds of pregnancy most of the energy is needed for the tissues and processes that support fetal development. During the latter months a larger percentage of energy is needed for actual fetal growth and metabolism.

The growth and maintenance of the tissues formed during pregnancy may not seem as interesting as the growth and development of the fetus, but the latter is actually dependent upon the former. The placenta is much more than just an extension of the sack that surrounds the fetus during development. It determines the total environment for life in utero, and the umbilical cord from the placenta is the lifeline for the fetus (Figure 14-3). The placenta controls the passage from the maternal circulation

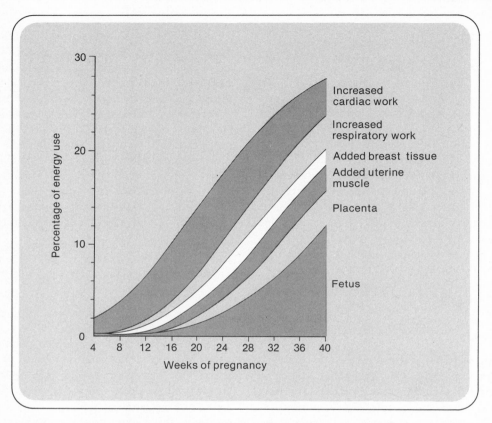

FIGURE 14-2. Components of increased oxygen consumption during pregnancy. SOURCE: F. E. Hytten and I. Leitch, *The Physiology of Human Pregnancy,* 2d ed. (Oxford, England: Blackwell Scientific Pubs., Ltd., 1963). Distributed in the United States by F. A. Davis Co. Used by permission.

into the fetus of nutrients, oxygen, hormones, antibodies, and other vital substances. It also guarantees the removal of metabolic waste and carbon dioxide from the fetal circulation.

Feeding the Fetus

The maternal blood supply reaches the placenta via arteries that branch off the major arteries going to her legs. Within the walls of the placenta (Figure 14-3) these vessels branch out into smaller vessels that end in lakes. Components of the maternal blood cross over through special filters from the lakes into the umbilical blood to nourish the fetus. Waste products from the fetal blood pass in the opposite direction and are carried away from the placenta by veins into the liver of the mother.

The fetal and maternal circulatory systems both draw on the same pool of nutrients. In the competition between mother and fetus for nutrients, the fetus has the advantage due to the way its blood circulatory system is arranged. Vitamins C and B_{12},

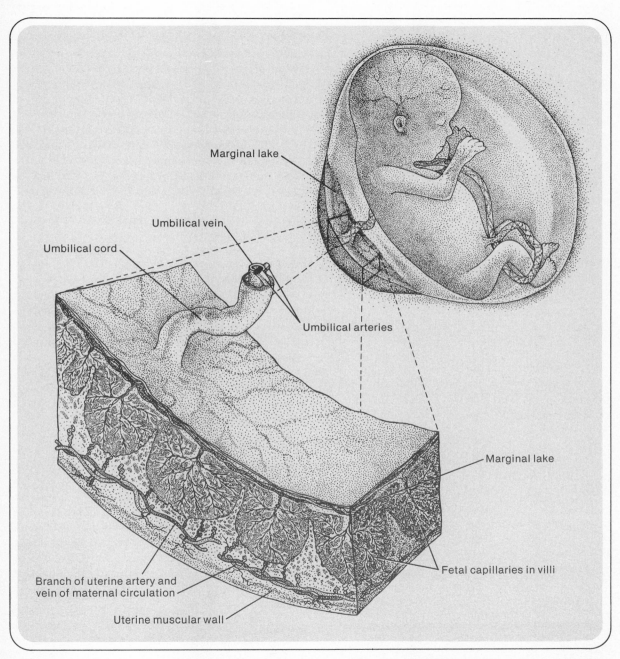

Marginal lake

Umbilical vein

Umbilical cord

Umbilical arteries

Marginal lake

Fetal capillaries in villi

Branch of uterine artery and
vein of maternal circulation

Uterine muscular wall

FIGURE 14-3. Placental circulation. (Redrawn from Placental Circulation, Ross Clinical Education Aid No. 2. © 1960, Ross Laboratories. Used by permission.)

iron, folacin, and pyridoxine pass to the fetus from the maternal circulation even if this transfer depletes the mother's reserves. The concentrations of other nutrients are maintained at approximately equal levels in the two circulatory systems. The fetus that is well nourished in utero can store enough iron to last three to six months, but its reserves of most other nutrients are relatively low. Since much of the iron reserve is built up during the last weeks of pregnancy, premature infants must be given foods that contain iron or iron supplements earlier in life than is necessary for full-term babies.

Weight Gain

The recommended weight gain during pregnancy is about 3 to 4 pounds during the first four months and about 0.8 pound per week thereafter. This totals about 23 pounds. The range of recommended weight gain is between 20 and 28 pounds, depending upon many factors. Increasing numbers of obstetricians are not recommending rigid weight-gain restrictions for their patients.

The rate of weight gain is an important index of the progress of a pregnancy. A gain of less than 2 pounds or more than 7 pounds during any of the last six months is a signal to the doctor that something may be wrong.

The pregnant body normally retains more water, but a sudden gain in weight (especially after the twentieth week) may indicate excessive retention of water. This is a complication of pregnancy that often goes hand-in-hand with hypertension and other problems that require special supervision by the physician. An increased incidence of prenatal death and prematurity occurs in pregnancies when the rate of weight gain is either too low or too high.

Pregnancy is not the time for a woman to adjust her own body weight unless her doctor advises this. Ideally, such changes are made before she becomes pregnant; otherwise, they should be started shortly after delivery and definitely before another pregnancy.

DIETARY CHANGES

The responsibility of pregnancy motivates many women who have been rather careless about their diet to become more interested in developing better eating patterns. Since the same general principles of nutrient needs and nutrient density govern diet selection before and after conception, the woman who is awakened to the importance of nutrition during her first pregnancy may improve her nutrition status for the rest of her life. She also may be better prepared nutritionally if she plans to have a second child.

Increased RDA

During pregnancy a woman's RDA for energy increases only about 15 percent, but her RDA increases by approximately 25 to 35 percent for vitamin C, vitamin A, vitamin B_{12}, thiamin, riboflavin, pyridoxine, zinc, vitamin E and iodine (Table 14-1). The RDA for protein, calcium, phosphorus, and magnesium are about 50 to 65 percent higher than those of a nonpregnant woman over 22 years old. The greatest increases are for vitamin D (which is not required in the diet of adults) and folacin (which doubles during pregnancy).

Since mothers-to-be eat many meals with fathers-to-be, let's compare their nutrient needs (Figure 14-4). The energy needs of pregnant women are about 400 Cal (1,320 kJ) less than those of a man, but their RDA are quite similar for thiamin, iodine, vitamin A, vitamin E, and riboflavin. The RDA is greater for pyridoxine, magnesium, vitamin C, zinc, vitamin B_{12}, protein, calcium, phosphorus, and, of course, iron. These comparisons make it clear that a pregnant woman needs to know the best sources of certain nutrients, and they must be emphasized in her diet at all times.

Increased Nutrient Density

Unless energy expenditure (due to exercise) increases during pregnancy, the increased nutrient

Women who continue to exercise during pregnancy have greater flexibility of food choices than do women who are inactive.

TABLE 14-1. Percentage of Increase in the RDA of Women during Pregnancy

Nutrient	Amount Required during Pregnancy	Percent Increase[a]
Energy	2,300 Cal	15
Iodine	125 mcg	25
Riboflavin	1.5 mg	25
Vitamin A	5,000 IU	25
Pyridoxine	2.5 mg	25
Vitamin E	15 IU	25
Thiamin	1.3 mg	30
Vitamin C	60 mg	33
Zinc	20 mg	33
Vitamin B$_{12}$	4 mcg	33
Calcium	1,200 mg	50
Phosphorus	1,200 mg	50
Magnesium	450 mg	50
Protein	76 g	65
Folacin	800 mcg	100
Vitamin D	400 IU	No RDA

[a]Based on the RDA for a woman 23 years old or older.

NOTE: Iron supplements are definitely needed by a pregnant woman.

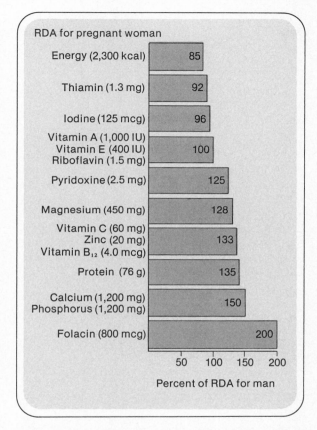

FIGURE 14-4. Comparison of the RDA for a pregnant woman and the RDA for a man (based on RDA for both aged 23 to 50 years old).

needs shown in Table 14-1 must be met without adding more than about 300 Cal (1,320 kJ) to the total diet. Therefore, during pregnancy the woman's diet must be considerably more nutrient-dense and requires a great deal of attention. A pregnant woman cannot simply eat more of the same foods. She must place greater emphasis on sources of specific nutrients (see Table 14-1) while carefully monitoring her intake of foods (such as those high in sugars and fats) that dilute the overall nutrient density of her diet. The woman who continues to be active and to exercise during her pregnancy increases her energy needs, and therefore has more flexibility in food selection. She does not have to limit her food selections to only the most nutrient-dense foods as does the inactive pregnant woman.

Protein. The RDA for protein during pregnancy is 76 grams, or 30 grams more than a nonpregnant woman needs. A major change in protein intake may not be necessary since surveys have shown that many Americans consume more protein than their RDA. On the other hand, the Ten-State Survey found that many pregnant women in the population studied failed to meet their RDA for protein.

A woman who is preparing for pregnancy should evaluate the protein content of her present diet and plan how much of which foods is needed to provide

The greatest increases in nutrient density needed by pregnant women are for protein, calcium, magnesium, phosphorus, folic acid, and vitamin D.

Although doctors may prescribe iron supplements, iron-rich foods continue to be important sources of other nutrients for pregnant women.

76 grams of protein. Two 3-ounce servings of most meats furnish about 50 grams; a quart of milk provides another 35 grams; and cereals and beans add a bit more.

Folacin. The RDA for folacin and iron are the most difficult for women to meet. Since the folacin RDA doubles from 400 to 800 micrograms during pregnancy, this vitamin merits thoughtful attention. Folacin has many metabolic functions, but its role in the synthesis of DNA (which is necessary for cell division) makes it especially important for a woman whose body is making additional blood as well as forming fetal, placental, and uterine tissue.

Table 14-2 shows that few foods supply more than 100 micrograms of folacin (one-eighth the pregnant woman's RDA) per serving. Therefore, even the better sources of this nutrient must be eaten frequently. If a woman does not usually eat good sources of folacin, the months during her pregnancy may be a good time to try some innovative ways of preparing these foods to make them more appealing to her.

Raw spinach can be used in mixed green salads or simply combined with mushrooms, Parmesan cheese, and a spicy dressing. Chicken livers can be browned and served as a main course or chopped and combined with various seasonings to spread on crackers. Cereals fortified with folic acid (perhaps sprinkled with wheat germ) can also help meet her RDA.

Calcium and Vitamin D. The formation of approximately one-quarter pound of bone in a newborn baby depends on an adequate supply of calcium and vitamin D. Calcium is also important for maintaining the nervous system and for helping the blood to clot if small vessels break in either the maternal or the fetal circulation.

Four glasses of milk provide enough calcium, vitamin D, and riboflavin to meet the pregnant woman's RDA for these nutrients, as well as substantial amounts of vitamin B_{12}, vitamin A, niacin, and protein. If a woman had not previously included milk in her diet, addition of this much whole milk would increase her total energy intake by 600 Cal (2,520 kJ). One way to help avoid exceeding her energy needs is to add skim milk to the diet instead of whole milk. Skim milk provides the same amounts of protein and micronutrients, but only about 400 Cal (1,680 kJ) of energy in four glasses.

There are several ways, depending upon individual food preferences and diet patterns, to meet the RDA for calcium and vitamin D. A glass of milk with every meal (you do not have to give up coffee after the meal) plus another glass as a snack is the simplest approach for the woman who prefers to develop habits and not waste time planning different sources every day. After several months of this routine, however, some women may seek variety. Powdered milk can slip into many recipes without making much difference in taste or texture. Fortified skim milk can be prepared at double strength to double the nutrient content and increase the energy value by only about 20 percent compared to whole milk.

Cheeses with high nutrient density and plain yogurt can be eaten as snacks or combined with other foods. Cheese sauces or condensed cheese soups add extra calories to the diet, but they provide calcium and vitamin D and may add appeal to vegetables such as broccoli, brussels sprouts, or asparagus (which are also helpful in meeting her higher RDA for folacin).

Iron. Many physicians prescribe supplemental iron during the earliest prenatal evaluation because it is so difficult to meet this requirement during pregnancy. However, even when supplemental iron is taken, dietary sources of this nutrient should not be overlooked. Iron-rich foods such as liver and dark-green leafy vegetables provide other minerals and vitamins needed in larger amounts by pregnant women and trace elements, most of which are not available in vitamin-mineral supplements.

TABLE 14-2. Approximate Folacin Content of Foods[a]

Food Group	Food Serving[b]			
	100–150 mcg per Serving	50–100 mcg per Serving	20–50 mcg per Serving	Less Than 20 mcg per Serving
Fruits	Cantaloupe (1 medium), orange juice	Avocado (½ medium), orange (1 medium)	Banana, dates, strawberries, watermelon	Most other fruits
Vegetables	Beets, broccoli (1 medium stalk), romaine lettuce, spinach	Asparagus, brussels sprouts, collards, kale, parsnips, green peas, tomatoes, tomato juice	Green beans, cabbage, carrots, cauliflower, corn, eggplant, peppers, potatoes, squash, sweet potatoes, turnip greens	Bean sprouts, celery, cucumber, leaf lettuce, radishes, turnips
Cereals	Cereal (folic acid-fortified, ready-to-eat), wheat germ (1 oz.)			Cereal (cooked, unfortified, 1 oz.), cake (1 piece), bread (1 slice), cookie
Eggs and dairy products			Egg (1), cottage cheese, yogurt	Other dairy products
Legumes		Beans (cooked), peanuts (½ cup), sesame seeds (½ cup)		Peanut butter (1 T.)
Meats	Beef liver (3 oz.), chicken liver (3 oz.)			Most other meats, fish, and poultry (3 oz.)

[a] Total folacin rather than free folacin.
[b] 1 cup unless otherwise specified.

Source: Adapted from B. P. Perloff and R. R. Butrum, "Folacin in Selected Foods," *Journal of the American Dietetic Association* 70 (1977): 161–72.

Salt and Fluids

Salt restriction is not recommended during pregnancy unless a problem arises that in the opinion of a doctor indicates a need for this change. Although salt has a role in the pregnant woman's diet, this should certainly not be interpreted as license to increase its use. The increase in the RDA for iodine (Table 14-1) during pregnancy means it is important to use iodized salt.

Fluids are also important in the diet during pregnancy. Part of the increased need can be met if milk is used as the source of calcium, vitamin D, and riboflavin. Juices or tomatoes used as sources of vitamin C and folic acid also provide fluids. Since water with meals may make a pregnant woman feel full but still hungry, it is better to try to increase water intake between meals. A glass next to the kitchen sink or on the desk at work can serve as a reminder of the importance of fluids during pregnancy.

NUTRITIONAL RISKS DURING PREGNANCY

During pregnancy the potential benefit of nutrition on health is influenced by several socioeconomic factors. For example, the age of the woman and her role in society may be closely linked with her nutritional status and the success or failure of her pregnancy. Under certain circumstances, pregnant women have particular difficulty with diet planning.

Mothers in Their Teens

The most vulnerable mother-and-fetus combination results from teen-age pregnancies. Compared to mature women, teen-age mothers have a higher percentage of babies with low birth weights, these women have more complications of pregnancy, and more of their babies die during or shortly after delivery (Table 14-3).

A teen-age girl matures sexually several years before she attains an adult skeleton. The pelvic structure of an adult woman is tailored to pregnancy, but when fetal development starts before skeletal growth is complete, the female body is not equipped to carry and deliver the baby with the greatest possible protection.

The pregnant woman who is still growing herself has three nutritional challenges:

1. Meeting her own needs for growth
2. Meeting the needs of a fetus
3. Meeting her needs for pregnancy

Pregnant teen-agers need to have a thorough knowledge of nutrition in order to manage a diet that meets all these needs.

Physiological changes and concomitant increases in the RDA do not explain the total nutrition problem for pregnant teen-agers. Few teen-agers have financial security, many are still in school, and those who work bring home small paychecks. The pregnant teen-ager who lives with her family will probably have better food and medical care than if she lives away from home. If she is on her own, it may be very difficult to obtain the care and the diet she knows she needs.

Mothers Who Have Small Children

Multiple pregnancies in close succession can be a tremendous drain on a woman's nutrient stores. The iron stores of women in the United States are rarely sufficient to supply all the iron needed for a single pregnancy. The toll of calcium, magnesium, and other nutrients is also high. A woman who allows enough time between giving birth and again becoming pregnant has a better chance of replenishing her nutrient stores. Family spacing offers benefits for both the mother and her children.

Mothers on a Budget

Pregnant women who must plan diets to meet their increased nutrient needs but have limited food

TABLE 14-3. Birth Weight and Mortality Rate of Infants

Age of Mother (years)	Median Weight of Infant (kg)	Percentage of Infants of Low Birth Weight (under 2,500 kg)	Mortality of Infants (death rate per 1,000 live births)		
			Neonatal (under 28 days)	Postnatal (28 days to 11 months)	Infant (under 1 year)
Under 15	3.02	18.7	41.2	17.6	58.7
15–19	3.21	10.5	22.7	10.1	32.8
25–29	3.31	7.3	16.6	5.8	22.4

SOURCE: U.S. Department of Health, Education, and Welfare, Public Health Service, *Vital Statistics of the United States, 1965: Natality,* vol. 1 (Washington, D.C.: Government Printing Office, 1967). Cited by Committee on Maternal Nutrition Board, Food and Nutrition Board, National Academy of Sciences in "Maternal Nutrition and the Course of Pregnancy" (1970), pp. 43–44.

budgets should give special attention to the information in Chapter 11. Many of the best sources of folacin and calcium are the dark-green leafy vegetables, which are cheaper than many high-energy desserts or snacks that have low nutrient density. Baked beans and navy beans are relatively inexpensive sources of folacin, protein, B vitamins, iron, and other nutrients. Iodized salt is the same price as plain salt. Enriched bread is cheaper than most specialty types. Potatoes are not as rich in vitamin C as the more expensive citrus fruits, but they can contribute to meeting the needs for this nutrient as well as several others.

Mothers with Health Problems

A discussion of the dietary needs of pregnant women who have preexisting health problems is beyond the scope of this book. Women who are overweight or underweight, or those who have hypertension, a family history of diabetes, paleness, and/or other signs of anemia should be aware that they need early medical attention and special diet counseling.

STUDY QUESTIONS

1. How should a woman prepare herself for pregnancy?

2. Why are additional nutrients needed during pregnancy?

3. What does the rate of weight gain during pregnancy indicate?

4. How does the increase in the energy RDA during pregnancy compare to the increases in protein and micronutrient RDA?

5. What are the greatest increases in nutrient density needed during pregnancy?

6. How can a pregnant woman meet her need for iron?

7. Why must some women be especially careful about their diets during pregnancy?

SUGGESTED READING

1. J. R. Mahalko and M. Bennion, "The effect of parity and time between pregnancies on maternal hair chromium concentrations," *American Journal of Clinical Nutrition* 29(1976):1069–75.
2. "Nutrition needs during pregnancy," *Dairy Council Digest* 45(July-August 1974).
3. Committee on Maternal Nutrition, Food and Nutrition Board, *Maternal Nutrition and the Course of Pregnancy*. Washington, D.C.: National Academy of Sciences/National Research Council, 1970.
4. M. W. Blackburn and D. H. Calloway, "Energy expenditure and consumption of mature, pregnant and lactating women," *Journal of the American Dietetic Association* 69(1976):29–36.
5. C. Phillips and N. E. Johnson, "The impact of quality of diet and other factors on birth weight of infants," *American Journal of Clinical Nutrition* 30(1977):215–25.
6. "Iron supplementation for gestational anemia," *Nutrition Reviews* 33(1975):332–33.
7. L. Lumeng et al, "Adequacy of vitamin B_6 supplementation during pregnancy: A prospective study," *American Journal of Clinical Nutrition* 29(1976):1376–83.
8. M. F. Thompson, E. H. Morse, and S. B. Merrow, "Nutrient intake of pregnant women receiving vitamin-mineral supplements," *Journal of the American Dietetic Association* 64(1974):382.
9. A. Lechting et al, "Influence of maternal nutrition on birth weight," *American Journal of Clinical Nutrition* 28(1975):1223–33.
10. E. H. Morse et al, "Comparison of the nutritional status of pregnant adolescents with adult pregnant women: I. Biochemical findings," *American Journal of Clinical Nutrition* 28(1975):1000–13.
11. E. S. Weigley, "The pregnant adolescent: A review of nutritional research and programs," *Journal of the American Dietetic Association* 66(1975):588–91.
12. L. F. Moscovitch and B. A. Cooper, "Folate content of diets in pregnancy," *American Journal of Clinical Nutrition* 26(1973):707–14.
13. D. B. Coursin, "Maternal nutrition and the offspring's development," *Nutrition Today* 7(1973):12–19.

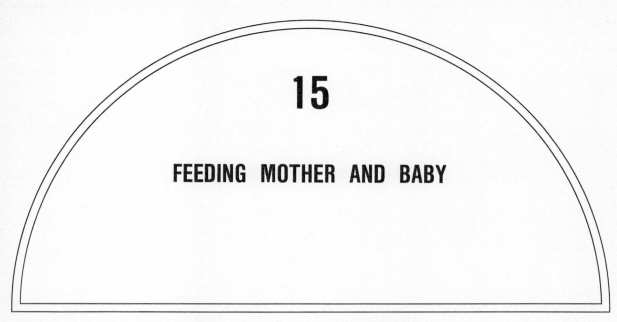

15

FEEDING MOTHER AND BABY

The interdependence of nutritional status for the mother and infant does not cease when the baby is born. Although the linkage between their circulatory systems is broken at delivery, the daily pattern of activity of the mother and her nutrient needs are affected by the baby. On the other hand, the infant continues to be dependent upon the mother (and to some degree upon other members of the family) for the foods that furnish the nutrients necessary for its growth and development.

This chapter compares the nutrient needs of a mother who breastfeeds her baby to those of a mother who bottlefeeds her baby. It also explains the differences and similarities among the types of milk fed to infants and what foods or nutrient supplements are needed, depending upon whether the baby is breastfed or bottlefed.

FEEDING MOTHERS

The postpartum diet of a mother depends upon how her baby is fed, her pace of life, her health, and her own nutrient needs. A new mother leads a very busy life and has little time to learn about nutrition while caring for her baby. This kind of planning should be made well in advance.

Nursing Mothers

The mother who chooses to breastfeed her infant assumes the responsibility for ensuring that the milk produced by her mammary glands contains the nutrients needed by her baby. These needs cannot be met simply by increasing the amount of cow's milk that she drinks. Maintenance of her health as well as production and secretion of milk are dependent upon increasing nutrient intake by the amounts shown in Table 15-1. Many of these nutrients are not transferred directly to the mother's milk, but they are needed for synthesizing the types of protein found primarily in human milk and for maintaining the metabolic activity of her body cells, especially those in breast tissue.

Nutrient Density. The diet of a lactating woman should be slightly different from the diet she needed during pregnancy. Her energy needs increase by another 200 Cal (840 kJ); this is about 25 percent more energy than she needed before she became pregnant.

The RDA for protein and all micronutrients (except iron, vitamin E, and pyridoxine) are more than 25 percent greater for a lactating woman than those

During lactation nutrients are needed for the synthesis of the components of milk and for the maintenance of maternal cells, especially those in breast tissue.
The diet of a woman during lactation must have a higher nutrient density than at any other time during her life.

TABLE 15-1. Percentage of Increase in RDA for a Lactating Woman Compared to a Nonlactating Woman

Nutrient	Amount Required	Percent Increase
Iron	18 mg	0
Energy	2,500 Cal	25
Pyridoxine	2.5 mg	25
Vitamin E	15 IU	25
Thiamin	1.3 mg	30
Niacin	17 mg	31
Vitamin B$_{12}$	4.0 mcg	33
Riboflavin	1.7 mg	38
Protein	66 g	43
Vitamin A	6,000 IU	50
Folacin	600 mcg	50
Calcium	1,200 mg	50
Phosphorus	1,200 mg	50
Magnesium	450 mg	50
Iodine	150 mcg	50
Zinc	25 mg	63
Vitamin C	80 mg	78
Vitamin D	400 IU	*

*No RDA for nonpregnant woman.
NOTE: Comparison based on the RDA for women 23 to 50 years old.

for a nonpregnant woman. The largest relative increases are for vitamin C, vitamin A, vitamin D, folacin, calcium, phosphorus, iodine, magnesium, and zinc. All of these are needed at levels 50 percent or more greater than the RDA for a nonpregnant woman.

The needs for protein and folacin are not as great as they were during pregnancy, but the needs for vitamin A, niacin, riboflavin, iodine, and zinc increase after the baby is born if the woman breastfeeds her baby.

Dietary Modification. We have seen in Chapter 8 that by carefully selecting the most nutrient-dense foods from all four food groups, a woman can meet most of her known nutrient needs by consuming about 1,400 Cal (5,880 kJ) and still have about 600 Cal (2,520 kJ) or about 30 percent of her total energy intake to use for nutrient-dilute substitutions. However, to meet her higher RDA, a lactating woman needs additional foods:

Fruits or vegetables,	
3 servings	150 Cal
Cereals, 1 serving	100 Cal
Milk, 2 cups	300 Cal
Meat, 2 ounces	150 Cal
Total	700 Cal (2,940 kJ)

This means that while she is nursing, the woman must consume about 2,100 Cal (1,400 for her basic diet plus 700 for the needs of lactation) of nutrient-dense foods to maintain herself and her baby. Since her total energy needs are 2,500 Cal, she has only 400 Cal or 12 percent of her total energy intake to distribute within her diet for nutrient-dilute foods such as desserts, fried foods, soft drinks, cream sauces, and similar sources of energy. Although her total energy intake increases, she has much less flexibility regarding her selection of nutrient-dilute foods.

To meet her nutrient needs without exceeding her energy needs, a lactating mother must select a diet of higher nutrient density than at any other time in her life. The sample menu in Table 15-2 shows that needs for protein, calcium, iron, and folacin can be met with less than 2,100 Calories of food. However, this diet has been carefully selected on the basis of nutrient composition data rather than the general guideline of additional servings of various types of foods.

Nonnursing Mothers

The nutrient needs of nonnursing mothers are quite different from their RDA before they became pregnant. These needs cannot be estimated as precisely as those for nursing mothers because each

TABLE 15-2. Sample Menu for Lactating Woman and the Contribution Made by Each Food to Meeting the RDA for Energy, Protein, Calcium, Iron, and Folacin

Food and Amount	Energy		Protein	Calcium	Iron	Folacin
	(Cal)	(kJ)	(g)	(mg)	(mg)	(mcg)
Milk, whole, 3 glasses	480	2,016	25.5	864	0.3	36
Cheese, cheddar, 1 oz.	113	475	7.1	213	0.2	5
Broccoli,[a] medium stalk	47	197	5.6	158	1.4	101
Potato,[a] baked, 1 medium	145	609	4.0	14	1.1	20
Spinach, raw, 1 cup	14	59	1.8	51	1.7	106
With oil and vinegar, 1 T.	90	378	—	—	—	—
Tomato juice, 6 oz.	35	147	1.6	13	1.6	47
Chicken, ½ breast	160	672	25.7	9	1.3	4
Liver, calf, 1 slice	222	932	25.1	11	12.1	123
Bread,[a] 1 slice						
Whole wheat	66	277	2.2	32	0.3	16
Enriched white	76	319	2.4	24	0.7	10
Rice,[a] ½ cup	112	470	2.1	11	0.9	9
Wheat flakes,[a] fortified, 1 oz.	106	445	3.1	12	4.5[b]	100[b]
Total	1,666[c]	6,996[c]	106.2	1,412	26.1	577
RDA	2,500	10,500	66.0	1,200	18.0	600

[a] Foods usually consumed with butter, sugar, or other foods that supply energy but few micronutrients.
[b] Products vary; check the labels.
[c] The remaining energy need may be met with other foods.

NOTE: This menu supplies slightly less than the RDA for folacin.
SOURCE: Nutrient composition values excerpted from C. F. Adams, "Nutritive Value of American Foods in Common Units," *Agriculture Handbook* No. 456 (Washington, D.C.: USDA, Agricultural Research Service, 1975); B. P. Perloff and R. R. Butrum, "Folacin in Selected Foods," *Journal of the American Dietetic Association* 70 (1977): 161–72.

woman's requirements for energy and nutrients depend upon factors that vary greatly.

Energy Intake. The new mother should determine her energy intake by balancing her increased energy need (due to the activity necessary when caring for the baby) and her decreased need (because of weight gain during pregnancy).

During delivery and the following week, women lose about two-thirds of the weight they gained during pregnancy. Most doctors feel that it is unwise to begin a strenuous diet immediately, but weight reduction should not be postponed indefi-

nitely. Many women who are overweight in their late thirties and forties realize that their gradual accumulation of excessive body fat began during their childbearing years. This problem can be avoided by beginning a moderate weight-reduction diet (see Chapter 9) a few weeks after delivery. An energy deficit of 250 Cal (1,050 kJ) per day should take off about 6 or 8 pounds in three months. A regular routine of exercises can help use up energy and strengthen abdominal muscles. A physician should be consulted about which exercises are recommended, when to start an exercise routine, and how vigorous it should be. Nursing mothers should consult their doctor about when and how to lose weight when they stop breastfeeding.

Nutrient Needs. The mother's nutrient needs depend upon the degree of depletion of her reserves during pregnancy. This consideration is especially important if the woman plans to have another child during the next few years. The mother must replenish her nutrient stores at the same time she is decreasing her energy intake (to reestablish her prepregnancy weight). Therefore, she must be as concerned about selecting a nutrient-dense diet for herself as she is about planning an appropriate diet for her baby.

FEEDING BABIES

The person who selects a diet for a baby must keep in mind several physiological and anatomical differences between infants and older people.

1. The rate of weight gain as a percentage of body weight is greater for infants than for older children. A larger percentage of the total food intake is therefore required for building body tissues than for maintaining the body.
2. The composition of the human body changes during the first year of life. The body of a one-year-old child contains a greater percentage of proteins and lipids and a smaller percentage of water than a newborn baby's body.

3. The secretions of the digestive system (Chapter 4) and the functional capacity of the kidneys (Chapter 7) are not yet fully developed in the newborn infant. Most of the growth and development of the brain and nervous system occurs during the first four years of life.
4. The ratio of body surface (the area covered by skin) to body weight is higher for an infant than for an adult. Since the total amount of water in the body is so small, babies are easily dehydrated by the heavy perspiration that accompanies fever. Diarrhea and vomiting also cause rapid loss of body water and so are much more life-threatening to babies than to adults. It is therefore extremely important to avoid contamination of a baby's diet with organisms that cause fever, diarrhea, or vomiting (see Chapter 20).
5. A baby relies upon only one food for most of its nutrients. Any nutrients needed for the growth and development of the infant that are not contained in milk must be furnished by careful selection of other foods.

All these factors have important implications when planning a diet to meet the nutrient needs of an infant.

Nutrient Needs

The RDA for vitamin D, vitamin C, vitamin B_{12}, and folacin are the same throughout the first year of life, but the RDA for all other micronutrients increase with age (Table 15-3). The recommendations

TABLE 15-3. Changes in RDA during the First Year of an Infant's Life

| Age (years) | Weight (lbs) | Energy[a] (Cal) | Protein[a] (g) | Fat-Soluble Vitamins | | |
				Vitamin A (IU)	Vitamin D (IU)	Vitamin E (IU)
0.0–0.5	14	kg × 117	kg × 2.2	1,400	400	4
0.5–1.0	20	kg × 108	kg × 2.0	2,000	400	5

[a]Energy and protein values are based on the weight of the infant. The weight in kilograms is multiplied by the factor shown.

SOURCE: U.S., Food and Nutrition Board, National Academy of Sciences–National Research Council, *Recommended Dietary Allowances,* 8th ed. (Washington, D.C.: Government Printing Office, 1974).

for energy and protein are based on the weight of the infant because these needs increase as more body tissue is made and as cellular metabolism within the body increases. The numerical factors used for calculating energy and protein needs are slightly smaller for older infants, but the absolute amount needed increases as the baby grows. Although the RDA is a useful guideline, do not forget that the energy needs of infants, like adults, must be adjusted to energy expenditure. A placid baby who sleeps most of the time needs less dietary energy than the infant who is awake and active for many hours during each day.

Breast or Bottle?

Selection of an appropriate diet for an infant, like that of an adult, depends upon many factors. A major consideration is the nutritional difference between breast milk, cow's milk, and prepared formula. However, infant feeding involves many aspects of life—and all must be considered. The best method of feeding for any one baby is determined by careful evaluation of nutritional, physiological, psychological, economic, and social considerations.

Clarification of all the factors involved can be beneficial, regardless of which decision is finally made. More women might elect breastfeeding or continue it longer if they were convinced it was best

for them. But women who decide to bottlefeed their children need not feel guilty or inadequate if they have made a careful decision. Each method of feeding has merits and limitations. Let's sort them out.

Physiological Factors. One advantage of breastfeeding is that the nervous stimulation of the breast by the baby's sucking causes the release of hormones within the mother's body that accelerate the involution of her uterus and its restoration to normal size. Another advantage is that colostrum, the fluid secreted by the mammary glands during the first few days after birth, contains antibodies (see Chapter 21). When these antibodies are ingested, they improve the infant's resistance to certain infections. Although these antibodies are proteins, their special structure and the decreased acidity in the stomach of the newborn infant protect the antibodies from digestion. Biologically active antibodies are absorbed across the baby's intestinal mucosa into the blood.

The concentration of antibodies in the fluid consumed by the baby falls by the end of the first week, but some nutritionists think that enough antibodies are produced during the following weeks to provide additional benefits to the baby. The presence of these antibodies in the colostrum suggests that even if it is impossible for a mother to breastfeed for several months, there are decided immunological advan-

	Water-Soluble Vitamins						Minerals					
Vitamin C (mg)	Folacin (mcg)	Niacin (mg)	Riboflavin (mg)	Thiamin (mg)	Vitamin B$_6$ (mg)	Vitamin B$_{12}$ (mcg)	Calcium (mg)	Phosphorus (mg)	Iodine (mcg)	Iron (mg)	Magnesium (mg)	Zinc (mg)
35	50	5	0.4	0.3	0.3	0.3	360	240	35	10	60	3
35	50	8	0.6	0.5	0.4	0.3	540	400	45	15	70	5

tages to nursing the baby for the first few days or weeks.

Psychological Factors. The factors that are most difficult to measure are psychological. They vary more among mothers and babies than any other considerations. The psychological advantages or disadvantages depend upon how comfortable the mother and baby feel during feeding. A lactating mother and her baby can experience a close physical relationship that is satisfying to them both. The bottlefed infant does not touch its mother's body as intimately, but it is caressed, spoken to softly, and held near a warm body. Either relationship can be impaired if the mother is impatient or tired, or if the baby is uncomfortable or unhappy.

Many doctors feel that breastfeeding usually fosters a strong emotional bond between a mother and her baby and provides other psychological benefits for both, but the effects upon other members of the family should also be considered. The birth of a baby has broad ramifications upon the entire family. The husband who becomes a father for the first time must adjust to his own new feelings, his wife who is changing, and a third party within a relationship that had previously involved only two people. Since most of the waking hours of a baby (especially during the first weeks of life) are spent eating, bottlefeeding may be one of the few opportunities the father has to interact with his baby.

The choice between breastfeeding and bottlefeeding should be made by the mother and father together, keeping in mind their feelings and possible psychological effects upon other children in the family. The couple that makes this mutual commitment can more readily accept the minor adjustments in routine (who gets up for night feedings and who takes care of the house while the other person catches up on sleep) and interpersonal relations (who gets the most attention—baby, spouse, or other children) that vary depending on how the infant is fed and upon the unique characteristics of each family.

Social Factors. The decision about infant feeding is also influenced by society. In some circles breastfeeding is in vogue, but in others it is not encouraged. The feelings of people outside the family should not discourage a couple from doing what they feel is best for themselves and their baby. If breastfeeding in public makes your friends uncomfortable, plan your visits with them between feedings or postpone being with them for a few months. If your mother-in-law thinks that all good mothers breastfeed and you do not agree, abide by your own choice.

Economic Factors. The difference in the cost of bottlefeeding compared to breastfeeding is not great. Table 15-4 shows that it is slightly cheaper to buy formula, bottles, and nipples than it is to purchase foods to meet the nutrient needs of a lactating woman. These calculations do not take into consideration the value of the time spent preparing bottles for the baby or additional food for the mother. The actual difference in cost is mainly dependent upon which foods are selected for mother and baby.

Another economic consideration depends upon whether the mother has a job outside the home. If the family is not dependent upon her salary, this is of no concern. But if the food budget for the entire family is influenced by the mother's paycheck, the advantages of breastfeeding must be weighed against the possibility that her nutrient needs and the needs of other children may not be met if she does not have paid maternity leave or if she stays home longer than the leave time allowed.

Convenience. When mother and baby are both at home, breastfeeding is undoubtedly more convenient than bottlefeeding. When they are away from home together, breastfeeding is much simpler than carrying bottles and worrying about preparation. Many social situations present no problem for breastfeeding, but sometimes the mother (and possibly the baby) cannot be comfortable enough outside the home to enjoy the feeding. Under such circum-

TABLE 15-4. Comparison of Costs per Day of Breastfeeding and Bottlefeeding

Cost per Day of Meeting Additional Nutritional Requirements of Lactating Woman		Cost per Day of Using Commercially Prepared Formulas, Basic Equipment, and Fuel	
Suggested Additional Foods[a] and Amounts	Cost	Item	Cost
Milk, 2 cups	$0.21	All formulas, double	
Meat, 2 oz.	0.16	strength, 13 oz. can	$0.51
Vegetable, dark-green or deep-yellow, 1 serving	0.10	Unbreakable bottles with nipples (13	0.04
Citrus fruit or other good source of vitamin C, 1 serving	0.09	@ $0.49 each = $5.88)	
		Nipples (12 @ 3 for	
Other fruit or vegetable, 1 serving	0.15	$0.51 = $2.04)	0.01
Enriched bread or cereal, 1 serving	0.06	Energy, electricity	0.02
Total	$0.77	Total	$0.58

[a]The amounts of these nutrients are in addition to those recommended for nonpregnant women. Most of these figures represent an increase of 20 to 50 percent in needs for one day.

NOTE: Costs are approximate as of July 1974 in central Pennsylvania.

SOURCE: *Nutrition Newsletter,* Division of Nutrition Services, Pennsylvania Department of Health, 1975.

stances, the baby could be left at home and bottle-fed by a babysitter. If the normal time between feedings is prolonged extensively, the mother's breasts will become uncomfortable, but she can learn from the doctor or nurse how to express the milk from her breasts to avoid this problem. Occasional interruptions do not impair the continuation of the breastfeeding routine.

Bottlefeeding is sometimes more convenient than breastfeeding because other people can help the mother with feeding. If the mother chooses to work or to maintain outside activities that require her being away from home, bottlefeeding allows her more flexibility for scheduling her life.

Safety and Hygiene. The serious consequences of contamination of infant food have been mentioned earlier. Although breastfeeding generally avoids most sources of contamination, lactating mothers must be careful to wash their breasts carefully before each feeding. They must not become nonchalant about the convenience of breastfeeding and forget that bacteria on their skin may be transmitted to the baby. Mothers who bottlefeed their infants should carefully follow instructions regarding sterilization of bottles, nipples, and milk or formula.

Although the safety of bottlefeeding or breastfeeding usually depends upon the degree of precaution taken by the mother, there are mothers in the United States who do not have the refrigeration and cooking facilities to prepare and store milk or formula properly. Some mothers simply do not have the intellectual capacity to understand how to make up formulas or why it is important to do so carefully. In these situations, breastfeeding, along with maternal training in personal hygiene, may favor a better diet for the baby.

In developing countries breastfeeding offers advantages because of lack of facilities for maintaining milk in a safe condition. Whole milk is often not pasteurized, and powdered milk is reconstituted with water contaminated by disease-causing organisms (Chapter 26). These problems have been almost completely eliminated in the United States today, but were not uncommon earlier in this century.

Nutritional Differences

The nutrient composition of human milk and cow's milk must be considered in relation to the infant's nutrient needs.

Macronutrient Composition. The energy value and fat content of cow's milk and human milk are approximately the same (Figure 15-1). Human milk contains more carbohydrate (in the form of lactose) and therefore has a sweeter taste. Cow's milk contains more protein, primarily due to the presence of casein (which is less easily digested) rather than whey proteins (lactalbumin and lactoglobulin, which are more easily digested).

A quick calculation shows that the lower protein content of human milk is not necessarily a nutritional disadvantage. Human milk provides approximately 1 gram of protein per 60 Cal. The RDA (based on the baby's weight) is 2.2 grams of protein per 117 Cal, or approximately 1 gram of protein per 52 Cal. The protein density of human milk is therefore adequate to meet the baby's RDA if other foods of lower protein density are not added to the diet. However, adding large amounts of other low-protein foods, such as fruit juices, may mean that the protein density of the diet will drop below that recommended by the RDA (Table 15-3).

Micronutrient Composition. Figure 15-1 shows that human milk has a higher concentration of vitamin A, niacin, vitamin C, vitamin E, and copper. The other vitamins (except vitamin D, which is almost equal in concentration) are more concentrated in cow's milk. The mineral content is higher in cow's milk, but the concentration of these nutrients (except for iron and copper) in human milk is sufficient

to meet the needs of a growing infant. Minerals that are consumed in excess of nutrient needs are excreted by the kidneys. Under most circumstances, the kidneys of an infant can handle the amount of minerals in cow's milk, but when a baby loses large amounts of water due to perspiration in warm weather or because of fever it may not be able to excrete these minerals as well. The mineral content of many commercial infant formulas is therefore designed to simulate human milk rather than cow's milk.

OTHER SOURCES OF NUTRIENTS

The need of a baby for nutrient supplements and foods other than milk depends upon the infant's stage of maturity at birth and the type of milk or formula it is fed.

Dietary Supplements

Milk, regardless of its source, is not high in iron. A baby who has been well-fed by the mother through the placenta should have adequate iron stores to meet its needs for growth and development during at least the first three months of life. After this, iron-rich foods or supplements are needed.

The breastfed infant requires supplemental vitamin D; the need for this nutrient by bottlefed infants depends upon whether the milk or formula is fortified with this nutrient. It is very important that vitamin D supplements be given only in the amounts recommended by a pediatrician. Excessive intakes of vitamin D are toxic and can cause serious damage to the health of a baby. Since fat-free milk lacks the essential fatty acids, prolonged reliance upon this type of feeding may cause a deficiency of these nutrients unless other fat-containing foods supplement the infant diet. Good sources of vitamin C such as fruit juices can help meet the need for this nutrient of babies fed cow's milk.

Premature infants have special dietary needs that must be supervised by a pediatrician.

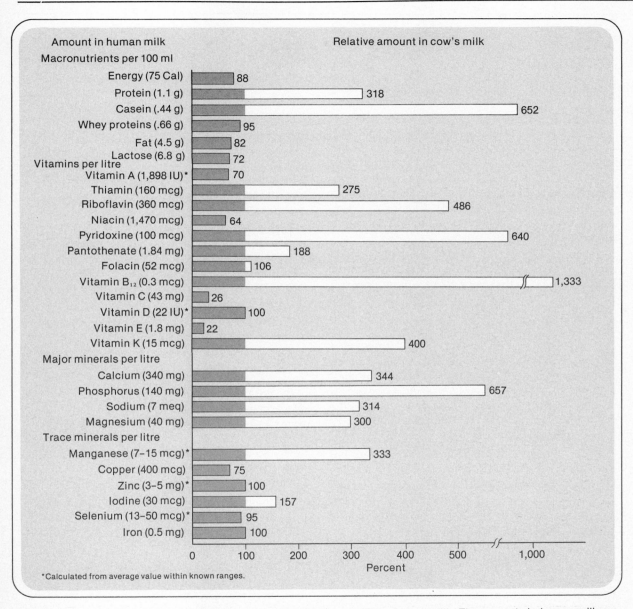

FIGURE 15-1. Percentage of various nutrients in cow's milk compared to human milk. The amounts in human milk are represented as 100 percent; those in cow's milk are represented by the bars. Absolute values for human milk are shown in parentheses. (Adapted from *Infant Nutrition,* 2d ed., by S. J. Fomon. © 1974, W. B. Saunders Company. Also used by permission of the author.)

Solid Foods

There is little consensus regarding when it is necessary to add solid foods to the infant diet. During the first three to four months of life there appear to be neither nutritional advantages nor disadvantages to supplementing milk diets with solid foods. Digestion, absorption, and utilization of solid foods appear to be adequate in the newborn, but it is difficult for most young infants to curl their tongue around food in their mouths. Until this mechanism is developed (at about three months), an infant's reaction to food is to push it out of the mouth unless it is placed far back on the tongue.

When solid foods are added to the diet, attention should be given to their nutrient density compared to that of milk, so that these foods will not displace the nutrients provided by milk. Table 15-5 lists the nutritive value of several baby foods prepared both at home and commercially. Fruits and vegetables that might be introduced early into a baby's diet have a low protein density, but they provide micronutrients that are needed by the baby, and their energy value per serving is so low that they do not greatly dilute the density of other nutrients in the total diet.

Table 15-6 gives a suggested schedule for introduction of juices and solid foods into the diet, but this regimen is flexible. Since some infants develop allergies to certain foods, it is suggested that foods be introduced one at a time. Then, if problems occur, the source of irritation is easier to identify and it can be withdrawn from the diet.

Fruit juices can be diluted at first and gradually given with less and less water. When solids are introduced, they should be offered to the baby at the time when the baby is most receptive—usually before the milk feeding. Fortified cereals and egg yolks can supplement the infant's stores of iron when they begin to be depleted. At first the baby may want only a small amount—perhaps no more than a teaspoon—of a new food. During the baby's second six months, however, several tablespoons of each food within the meal should probably be consumed.

The taste of fruits may be more appealing to infants than the taste of vegetables. Although there are similarities in the nutrient composition of these foods, most vegetables are better sources of iron, folacin, calcium, and several other nutrients. Babies therefore should be encouraged to accept vegetables as they expand their diet. The attitude of the person feeding the baby may influence the infant's reaction to the food.

Food Safety

Baby food (like adult food) should be protected from nutrient losses, and care is necessary to make certain it remains safe. Leftover baby food should be refrigerated, and discarded if not eaten after a few days. Packages that are opened should be carefully closed and protected from insects.

The Second Year

By the infant's first birthday the diet has broadened enough so that it can be planned around the general nutritional guidelines applicable to older people. At this age about 30 percent of the energy intake is supplied by milk. The remainder comes from baby food or the same foods as are prepared for other members of the family.

Planning an infant diet is facilitated by the nutrition labeling on commercially prepared baby foods. The U.S. RDA values used for these labels are especially designed for infants under 12 months old or children aged one to four years.

If the mother wishes to, she can prepare baby foods in the home. Table 15-5 compares the cost of several foods made at home to those purchased. Baby foods can be prepared at home by mashing and straining foods or using grinders marketed especially for this purpose. The primary consideration when making baby food is to maintain its safety and

Special considerations regarding infant and toddler feeding include avoiding obesity, reducing sodium intake, providing adequate nutrients for those with diet-related problems, and being aware of individual variation.

nutritional value. Care should be taken to make only the amount that can be preserved safely and that will retain its nutritive value. Utensils for preparing infant foods should be cleaned thoroughly between uses.

SPECIAL CONSIDERATIONS

Before closing this chapter, we should discuss two new areas of research and two related to situations where psychosocial factors may influence the nutritional status of an infant.

Infant Obesity

Nutritionists are currently studying more intensively the cumulative effects of diet upon health. The nutritional status of infants may have long-lasting effects that have not previously been appreciated. Research suggests that excessive weight gain during infancy may make it more difficult to maintain appropriate body weight later in life. During infancy fat cells of the body continue to divide and form new cells, but for most of the remaining years excessive energy is stored by increasing the size, rather than the number, of fat cells. Researchers have seen that overweight babies have a greater number of fat cells than other infants, and that adults who were fat when they were babies also have more fat cells than people who were not overweight at that stage of life.

This finding places great significance on the importance of infant feeding, but many other socioeconomic and genetic factors also influence body weight. The diet of infants, like that of adults, should balance energy intake with energy expenditure. Obesity can result from inactivity or consumption of an excessive amount of food. The lifestyle of the infant who spends most of its time in a crib or a small playpen may contribute to obesity as much as the lifestyle of the adult who spends most of his or her time behind a desk or in front of a television.

Sodium Intake

Sodium intake is one of several factors related to hypertension in many people (see Chapter 25). This disease is a major health problem in the United States, but its cause and treatment are not completely understood.

Many nutritionists think it is prudent to avoid excessive intake of sodium during infancy. This recommendation is based on the theory that many food preferences established early in life are maintained throughout the adult years. The infant who becomes accustomed to the taste of salty food may have difficulty reducing sodium intake in later life if this is recommended by a doctor.

For many years sodium was added as table salt to baby foods. This was done mainly to please the taste buds of the mother, who would test the food primarily to check its temperature before giving it to the infant. When researchers began to question the long-range effects of sodium, manufacturers reduced the amount of salt added to baby food. Between 1969 and 1972 this change in manufacturing practices reduced sodium intake by 22 percent for two-month-old infants and 30 percent for four-month-old and six-month-old infants. Surveys have shown that about half the average sodium intake of a six-month-old infant comes from baby foods and half from milk. Beyond this age sodium intake increases (as does energy intake), but a larger amount of sodium is derived from table foods. Milk has a relatively high sodium concentration (125 milligrams per cup), but this does not mean that milk should be avoided in the infant diet.

Because of the growing popularity of home-prepared baby foods, parents should be cautioned not to add salt to foods they chop or blend for their infants. Parents must also realize that the sodium content of canned and frozen foods (Table 15-5) is often higher than that of fresh foods or commercially prepared baby foods.

TABLE 15-5. Cost and Nutritive Value of Selected Baby Foods[a]

| Food[b] | Cost[c] (cents) | Percentage of U.S. Recommended Daily Allowance[d] | | | | | | | | Food energy (Cal) | Carbohydrate (g) | Fat (g) | Sodium[e] (mg) |
		Protein (g)	Vitamin A (IU)	Vitamin C (mg)	Thiamin (mg)	Riboflavin (mg)	Niacin (mg)	Calcium (mg)	Iron (mg)				
Milk, fluid, whole, 8 fl. oz.	5.1	47	23	6	14	68	2	48	1	159	12.0	8.5	122
Formula, commercially prepared without iron added, ready-to-use, 8 fl. oz.	24.8	20	33	36	28	32	23	22	1[f]	160	16.8	8.6	*
Instant cereal, mixed, dry, 1/2 oz.	2.2	8	*	*	72	58	36	24	77	52	4.4	.2	10
Teething biscuits, 1/2 oz.	5.3	6	*	*	11	10	4	11	2	54	9.1	.6	66
Strained baby foods, prepared commercially and at home													
Orange Juice													
Commercial	12.9	2	7	111	10	3	3	2	3	52	11.8	0.3	1
At home (from fresh)	8.8	4	13	140	18	5	5	2	2	47	10.5	.3	1
At home (from frozen concentrate)	3.2	3	13	129	18	2	4	2	1	45	10.7	.1	1
Beef													
Commercial (with broth)	39.0	74	*	8	4	28	32	2	11	112	*	6.5	166
At home (lean only)	36.3	167	1	†	10	38	58	2	25	214	0	9.5	60
Chicken													
Commercial (with broth)	39.0	73	‡	5	4	27	42	5	8	123	.1	7.8	156
At home (flesh only)	23.1	166	7	†	12	27	108	2	10	171	0	4.8	75
Carrots													
Commercial	14.8	3	564	15	4	5	5	4	3	35	7.6	.1	140
At home (from fresh)	7.9	4	700	17	10	8	6	6	4	31	7.1	.2	33
At home (from canned)	9.8	3	1,000	6	4	5	5	5	5	30	6.7	.3	236
Green beans													
Commercial	14.8	5	18	14	8	13	4	6	5	29	5.3	.2	105
At home (from fresh)	15.5	6	36	34	14	15	6	8	4	25	5.4	.2	4
At home (from canned)	14.0	6	31	11	6	8	4	8	10	24	5.2	.2	236
At home (from frozen)	14.5	6	39	14	14	15	5	7	5	25	5.7	.1	1

Food											
Pears											
Commercial	14.1	2	33[e]	33[g]	3	2	2	72	17.2	.2	6
At home (from fresh)	13.8	3	3	4	7	1	2	61	15.3	.4	2
Applesauce											
Commercial	14.1	1	8	2	3	1	2	82	20.0	.1	8
At home (from fresh)	8.3	1	*	6	3	1	2	54	14.1	.3	1
At home (from canned applesauce)	6.5	1	3	4	2	0	1	41	10.8	.2	2
Other strained baby foods, commercially prepared											
Mixed cereal with apples and bananas	14.1	5	33[e]	33[g]	33[g]	33[g]	1	84	18.9	.4	70
Beef with vegetables (high meat)	23.4	32	59	7	12	27	2	89	5.7	4.8	127
Chicken with vegetables (high meat)	23.4	34	50	9	8	24	6	88	5.8	4.5	130
Chicken noodle dinner	14.8	12	32	5	8	8	3	50	7.4	1.3	111
Macaroni, tomatoes, beef	14.8	14	32	4	22	12	3	71	8.8	2.9	155
Apple dessert	14.1	1	1	17	2	1	3	100	23.0	.8	16
Fruit dessert	14.1	1	11	10	4	1	1	97	23.6	.2	36
Vanilla custard	14.8	6	7	6	15	1	2	94	17.9	1.7	95

[a] For commercially prepared foods (except milk) the costs and nutritive values are averages for foods from three major baby food manufacturers; for home-prepared foods and for milk the nutritive values are derived from B. K. Watt and A. L. Merrill, "Composition of Foods—Raw, Processed, Prepared," Agriculture Handbook No. 8 (Washington, D.C.: USDA, Agricultural Research Service, 1963).

[b] Unless otherwise specified, values are for 100 grams (approximately 3½ oz.) of food. Cans of fruit juice contain 4.2 fluid ounces; jars of strained meat contain 3½ ounces; and jars of other strained foods contain 4½ to 4¾ ounces.

[c] Prices in Washington, D.C., July 1976.

[d] Allowance specified for use in nutritional labeling of foods for infants by the Food and Drug Administration. Title 21. Code of Federal Regulations CF2 (10–199), 125.1 b. Percentages in this table have not been rounded as required for use in food labels.

[e] Sodium content varies depending on the amount of salt added.

[f] Commercially prepared formula with iron added provides about 19 percent of U.S. RDA.

[g] Products vary widely in content depending on the amount, if any, of the nutrient added. Value is for product with nutrient added.

* Value judged to be insignificant or was not determined by manufacturers.

† Insufficient data available to provide a reliable value.

‡ Only one of three manufacturers gave a value. It represented 19 percent of U.S. RDA.

SOURCE: B. Peterkin and S. Walker, "Food for the Baby—Cost and Nutritive Value Considerations," Family Economics Review (Fall 1976). USDA, Agricultural Research Service, Consumer Food and Economics Institute.

Age (months)	Food	Primary Nutrients Provided
TABLE 15-6.	Possible Schedule for Introduction of Foods to an Infant's Diet	
½–1	Orange juice, grapefruit juice, tomato juice	Vitamin C
2–3	Enriched or fortified cereal	Iron, B vitamins
3–5	Mashed fruits such as banana, applesauce, pears (strained), apricots, prunes, peaches; mashed vegetables such as green beans, carrots, peas, broccoli flowers, spinach, squash, tomatoes	Most vitamins and minerals
4–6	Egg yolk	Iron, vitamin A, thiamin, protein
5–8	Meats (strained) and meat-vegetable combination dinners; enriched toast, crackers, and teething biscuits	Protein, iron, B vitamins
8–10	Vegetables (chopped), fruits (chopped), potato (mashed)	Most vitamins and minerals
10–12	Egg (whole), puddings, soft cheeses, yogurt	Most vitamins and minerals

Infants with Diet-Related Problems

The nutrition surveys discussed in Chapter 13 pointed out that the diets of many infants and their mothers did not meet the RDA. In September 1972, the United States Congress amended the Child Nutrition Act to include funding for a supplemental food program for *Women, Infants, and Children* (the *WIC program*).°

Pregnant or lactating women are eligible to participate in this program if they have shown inadequate nutritional patterns, high incidence of anemia, high rates of prematurity or miscarriage, or inadequate patterns of growth (underweight, obesity, or stunting). Infants and children up to five years of age are eligible if they have deficient growth patterns, nutritional anemia, or known inadequate nutritional patterns. Several other circumstances may also qualify a person for participation.

°New legislation regarding the WIC program is being developed during 1978.

The WIC program provides the foods shown in Table 15-7. These foods were selected because they are good sources of protein, iron, calcium, and vitamins A, D, and C—the nutrients often consumed in inadequate amounts according to survey results. Efforts are underway to expand the scope of the nutrition education component of the WIC program to increase the likelihood that these and other foods will be used most effectively by persons in the program.

Competitive Development

The final consideration that might influence the nutritional status and health of an infant involves the family's reaction to how quickly an infant develops eating skills, accepts new foods, and grows.

Families and friends are fascinated by each new development in a baby. When two grandchildren arrive in a family at nearly the same time or neighbors have babies of about the same age, there is a tendency to measure one's progress against the oth-

TABLE 15-7. Foods and Nutrients Provided Daily by the WIC Program

Food	Nutrient Specifications
Infants	
Infant formula, concentrated, 1 can (14 oz.)	Iron, 4 mg
Cereal, packaged, ⅚ oz.	Iron, 13 mg
Fruit juice, 3 oz.	Vitamin C, 30 mg
Women and Children	
Egg, 1	Iron, 1 mg; protein, 6 g; vitamin A, 500 IU
Milk, 1 qt.	Vitamin D, 400 IU; vitamin A, 1,500–2,000 IU; calcium, 1,200 mg; protein, 34 g
Cereal, packaged, 1⅕ oz.	Iron, 9 mg
Fruit juice, 9 oz.	Vitamin C, 90 mg

er's. This competition can influence the parents' expectations regarding their infant's growth and acceptance of solid foods.

The development of one child is a poor criterion to use to measure the development of another, and this is especially true in terms of diet patterns. Parents who are tempted to make such comparisons should remember that although nutrient needs govern when certain foods should be added to the infant diet, this schedule is flexible. There is little need to be concerned about differences between two children. Learning to eat is a developmental skill, but it requires patience. This personal quality is hardly an attribute of babies, and it often wears thin in parents.

Wise parents learn the nutrient and food needs of their infant, and they discuss their baby's growth and development with a pediatrician. They do not enter their baby into a competition with other children in the family or neighborhood. The baby who is forced to eat foods too early may develop aversions to foods that will last a lifetime. Also, the infant who is out front in the weight race may well be the loser in the long run.

STUDY QUESTIONS

1. Why are extra nutrients needed during lactation?

2. How should the nutrient density of a lactating woman's diet compare to that of her diet at other times?

3. What should be the major diet and nutrition consideration of women after pregnancy or lactation?

4. What are the physiological and anatomical differences between infants and adults that affect diet planning for infants?

5. What are some of the advantages and disadvantages of bottlefeeding and breastfeeding?

6. What are the nutrient differences between human milk and cow's milk?

7. What supplements and solid foods should be added to the infant's diet during its first year?

SUGGESTED READING

1. Committee on Nutrition, American Academy of Pediatrics, "Commentary on breast-feeding and proposed standards for formulas," *Pediatrics* 57(1976):278–85. Reprinted in *Nutrition Reviews* 34(1976):248–56.

2. "Current concepts in infant nutrition," *Dairy Council Digest* 47(March-April 1976).

3. B. Peterkin and S. Walker, "Food for the baby—cost and nutritive value considerations," *Family Economics Review*, Agricultural Research Service, U.S. Department of Agriculture (Fall 1976):3–8.

4. E. Maslansky et al, "Survey of infant feeding practices," *American Journal of Public Health* 64(1975):780–85.

5. H. E. Nizel, "Nursing bottle syndrome," *Nutrition News*, National Dairy Council, 38(February 1975).

6. Council on Foods and Nutrition, *Feeding Your Baby at Your Breast* (12 pages). Chicago: American Medical Association, 1972.

7. Council on Foods and Nutrition, *When Your Baby Is Bottle Fed* (4 pages). Chicago: American Medical Association, 1972.

8. G. A. Purvis, "What nutrients do our infants really get?" *Nutrition Today* 8(1973):28–34.

9. "Overfeeding in the first year of life," *Nutrition Reviews* 31(1973):116–18.

10. J. M. Potter and P. J. Nestle, "The effects of dietary fatty acids and cholesterol on the milk lipids of lactating women and the plasma cholesterol of breast-fed infants," *American Journal of Clinical Nutrition* 29(1976):54–60.

11. R. L. Huenemann, "Environmental factors associated with preschool obesity. I. Obesity in six-month-old children," *Journal of the American Dietetic Association* 64(1974)580.

12. American Academy of Pediatrics, Committee on Nutrition, "Salt intake and eating patterns of infants and children in relation to blood pressure," *Pediatrics* 53(1974):115–21.

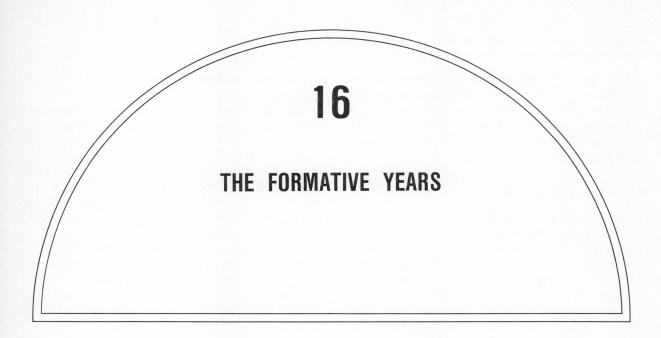

16

THE FORMATIVE YEARS

The diets of children affect their health during their entire lifespan. Therefore, we will now discuss the nutrient needs of children, the changes in food patterns characteristic of this age group, and how the nutrients needed for various body functions can be met by planning food choices on the basis of physiological needs, acceptability of foods, and lifestyle of children. We will also discuss the importance of developing constructive attitudes about food and nutrition during childhood.

FOUNDATIONS OF NUTRITION KNOWLEDGE

The food preferences and habits that influence nutritional status throughout life begin to be formed early in life. Toddlers learn a great deal about food from their parents and older children in the family. As their social world broadens, they learn from adults outside the family, television, and other children their own age.

Attitudes toward Food

During early childhood we develop attitudes toward food that will influence our diet patterns—and therefore our nutritional status—for the rest of our lives. Parents should be aware of the importance of a child's first encounters with food. They can improve the probability of their child's selecting an appropriate diet by being conscious of their own behavior in regard to food. Their example will influence the child's food choices long before the parents consciously try to teach their child about nutrition.

The parent who has a positive attitude toward food, expresses pleasure when eating a variety of foods, and tries to make mealtime a relaxed, enjoyable experience is starting to build a foundation upon which nutrition knowledge can later be added. The simple ideas that food is good and that eating is a pleasant experience are conveyed to children by actions—not by words. On the other hand, the child who learns by parental example to associate food with scowls, to correlate mealtime with teasing by older children or with parental harangues, or to leave food on his or her plate is being led toward a course of rejecting new foods, skipping meals, and wasting food.

Progressive Concepts

Fundamental concepts regarding diet and health are acquired long before the child starts going to school. The infant begins to understand the idea that food does something to the body when he or she is fed—a type of physical discomfort, hunger, is relieved. As children grow older, they may begin to correlate eating with other changes in the way they feel. They may notice that after eating they experience the disappearance of what adults call fatigue and irritability.

Beyond these basics, however, there are few ways for children to learn on their own the effects of appropriate or inappropriate food choices upon their bodies. It becomes the responsibility of older people to guide children in their food selection and to teach them that the type of food eaten is as important as eating enough food in order to maintain good health.

Although a young child is not capable of appreciating complex nutrition concepts, older people can help a child gradually build upon the ideas that "food is pleasing" and "food makes me feel better." A slightly more sophisticated concept is that "food helps me grow." As children mature, they can also be presented with the idea that different foods help in different ways. This concept provides the groundwork for teaching the child the basic four system and how much of each type of food is needed. The nutrients needed by the body and dietary sources of these nutrients are more difficult to master, but the child who has mastered earlier lessons and is convinced of the value of food should be more highly motivated and enthusiastic about learning the finer points of diet planning.

Importance of Home Training

The influence of the family on the nutrition knowledge of children has been documented in several ways. Recent surveys designed to find out how adults learn about nutrition show that approximately one-third of the people questioned cited mothers or grandmothers as their primary source of nutrition information. Probably, as fathers assume greater responsibility in parenting, their influence upon the diet of children will increase.

Other surveys have shown that the nutritional status of children increases parallel to the education level of their mothers. This observation must be evaluated carefully, however, before assuming a causal relationship. Other variables such as low family income, larger families, and less access to medical care also correlate with poorer nutritional status of children and less education of the mother (Table 16-1).

NUTRIENT NEEDS

The RDA changes considerably during the first decade of life. These changes help us identify how nutrient needs and appropriate food choices vary from early childhood through the onset of puberty (Chapter 17). Surveys have shown which nutrients are most frequently consumed in less than the recommended amounts during this stage of life.

RDA and Nutrient Density

The amounts of nutrients recommended for children as they grow do not always increase to the same degree as the need for energy. Table 16-2 shows that the energy needs of children 7 to 10 years old are almost double those of children aged 1 to 3. There is a comparable increase in the RDA for thiamin, pyridoxine, and vitamin B_{12}, and almost as great an increase for iodine and niacin. During this same span of years, the RDA for protein, vitamin A, riboflavin, and magnesium increase by only about

SECTION IV / NUTRITION THROUGH THE LIFESPAN

TABLE 16-1. Differences among Mothers and Children from Groups Surveyed in the Study of Nutritional Status of Preschool Children in the United States, 1968–1970

	Warner Rank Group			
	I	II	III	IV
Children with signs of malnutrition, %	14	17	6	2
Mothers with more than 12 years of education, %	3	15	45	70
Median annual income	$3,500	$6,500	$9,500	$13,000
Median annual income per person	$750	$1,500	$2,125	$2,827
Children examined by a dentist, %[a]	21	43	55	74
Children seen by a physician within 6 months, %[a]	45	61	66	71
Children born in a hospital, %	87	98	99	99
Infants with birth weight of less than 2.5 kg, %	16	11	4	5
Mothers with more than four pregnancies, %	40	24	18	18
Mothers younger than twenty at time of first pregnancy, %	72	42	24	8
Mothers younger than twenty-five, %	35	29	20	3
Mothers shorter than 155 cm, %	17	13	9	4
Mothers who cater to food preferences of children, %[a]	27	22	20	7
allow free meals and snacks, %	29	14	7	5
use food as a reward, %	64	54	52	39
withhold food when child misbehaves, %	40	31	32	25

[a] Results for children 48 to 71 months old only.

SOURCE: G. M. Owen, K. M. Kram, P. J. Garry, J. E. Lowe, and A. H. Lubin, "A Study of Nutritional Status of Preschool Children in the United States, 1968–1970," *Pediatrics* 53, no. 4 (April 1974): 597–646. Copyright 1974 American Academy of Pediatrics.

50 to 67 percent. The greatest change during these years is that the folacin RDA triples.

This type of analysis of the RDA suggests that as children grow older and have larger appetites, special attention should be given to sources of folacin (such as beans, leafy vegetables, and cereals fortified with folacin). The need for most other nutrients can be met by starting a toddler on a diet of sufficient nutrient density and simply maintaining that nutrient density while increasing the amount of food eaten.

The ratio of nutrient-to-energy needs of children for the nutrients listed at the bottom of Table 16-2 is quite different. The table shows the importance of emphasizing calcium, phosphorus, vitamin C, vitamin D, zinc, and iron in the diets of younger children. The RDA for these two vitamins and four minerals are as great (or greater, in the case of iron) for children 1 to 3 years old as they are for children 7 to 10 years old. Since the younger age group needs only about half a much energy, the density of these six micronutrients in the total diet must be twice that needed by the older age group.

In the real world of food this means that small

Nutrition surveys show that many children in all socioeconomic groups consume diets below the RDA in iron, vitamin A, and calcium, and, to a lesser extent, in vitamin C.

Nutrient	Age (years)			Percent Increase for Oldest Group Compared to Youngest Group
	1–3	4–6	7–10	
Gradual increases				
Riboflavin (mg)	0.8	1.1	1.2	50
Protein (g)	23	30	36	56
Vitamin A (IU)	2,000	2,500	3,300	65
Magnesium (mg)	150	200	250	67
Niacin (mg)	9	12	16	77
Iodine (mcg)	60	80	110	83
Energy (Cal)	**1,300**	**1,800**	**2,400**	**85**
Thiamin (mg)	0.6	0.9	1.2	100
Pyridoxine (mg)	0.6	0.9	1.2	100
Vitamin B_{12} (mcg)	1.0	1.5	2.0	100
Folacin (mcg)	100	200	300	300
As high or higher for youngest children				
Calcium (mg)	800	800	800	0
Phosphorus (mg)	800	800	800	0
Vitamin C (mg)	40	40	40	0
Vitamin D (IU)	400	400	400	0
Zinc (mg)	10	10	10	0
Iron (mg)	15	10	10	33 lower

TABLE 16-2. Changes in the RDA for Children

children have far less energy to allot to nutrient-dilute or energy-only foods. Table 16-3 shows that ½ cup of orange juice, 3 cups of milk, and 1 ounce of iron-fortified cereal each contribute substantial amounts of the nutrients needed in relatively large amounts. These food servings alone, however, total 642 Cal (2,696 kJ)—approximately half the RDA for energy of children aged 1 to 3. These three foods do provide some other nutrients as well; but, in general, the remaining nutrient needs of a 1- to 3-year-old child must be met with only approximately 650 Cal (2,730 kJ) of food. An average 8-year-old, on the other hand, has approximately 1,750 Cal (7,350 kJ) above those provided by the three foods shown in Table 16-3 to use on dietary sources of the remainder of the RDA.

Survey Findings

The Ten-State Nutrition Survey and the HANES help identify the nutrients most commonly lacking in the diets of children. The findings of these surveys cannot be compared directly because they studied different populations, they used different standards of dietary adequacy (Table 13-4), and their results were summarized according to different age groups. However, Table 16-4 shows the combined range of the percentage of preschool children in these two surveys whose diets failed to meet two-thirds of the RDA for several nutrients. The fact that a large percentage of this population had low intakes of iron correlates with the finding that approximately 35 percent of these children in the Ten-State Nutrition

TABLE 16-3. Energy and Nutrient Contribution of Three Basic Foods to the Diets of Children

Food	Energy (Cal)	(kJ)	Iron (mg)	Vitamin C (mg)	Calcium (mg)	Phosphorus (mg)	Vitamin D (IU)	Zinc (mg)
Orange juice, ½ cup	56	235	.3	62	14	41	0	.1
Milk, 3 cups	480	2016	.3	6	864	861	300	2.7
Wheat flakes, vitamin-mineral-fortified, 1 oz.	106	445	4.5	11	12	83	0	.6
Total	642	2696	5.1	79	890	985	300	3.4

Age (years)	Percent of the RDA Provided by These Foods							
1–3		49	34	197	111	123	75	34
4–6		35	51	197	111	123	75	34
7–9		26	51	197	111	123	75	34

Survey and about 10 percent of these children in the HANES had hemoglobin levels that were considered to be low (an indicator of anemia). Low hemoglobin levels were less prevalent among older children (about 16 percent of the 6- to 9-year-olds in the Ten-State Nutrition Survey and 7 percent of the 6- to 11-year-olds in the HANES), but these findings

TABLE 16-4. Percentage of Preschool Children with Nutrient Intakes Below Two-Thirds RDA in the Ten-State Nutrition Survey and the HANES

Nutrient	Percent
Protein	1–5
Calcium	12–40
Iron	75–85
Thiamin	17–31
Vitamin C	30–55
Vitamin A	7–42

definitely point to the need for cildren to consume more iron-rich foods.

Additional information regarding the nutritional status of American children is provided by a survey of approximately 3,000 preschool children conducted between 1968 and 1970. The results of this survey (the Study of Nutritional Status of Preschool Children in the United States) were tabulated after dividing the children into four groups according to socioeconomic criteria (including occupation, source of income of parents, dwelling type, and dwelling area). Group I had the lowest socioeconomic (Warner Rank) rating; Group IV had the highest.

Table 16-5 shows that based on the standards used for this survey, a large percentage of children in Group I had low daily dietary intakes of energy and nutrients. Groups II, III, and IV also had low intakes for iron, energy, calcium, and vitamin C. Since the standards used in this survey were consistently lower than those used by other nutrition surveys, it is necessary to use Table 16-6 to clarify the quality of the diets of these children.

TABLE 16-5. Percentage of Children with Low Daily Dietary Intakes*

Nutrient	Warner Rank Group			
	I	II	III	IV
Energy (Cal/kg)	34	19	15	15
Protein (g/kg)	3	1	0	0
Calcium (mg)	21	9	8	5
Iron (mg)	55	49	52	50
Vitamin A (IU)	5	0	0	0
Thiamin (mg)	9	2	2	2
Riboflavin (mg)	8	1	1	1
Vitamin C (mg)	16	7	2	2

*Based on standards used in a pilot study; values are considerably lower than the RDA for most nutrients.

SOURCE: G. M. Owen, K. M. Kram, P. J. Garry, J. E. Lowe, and A. H. Lubin, "A Study of Nutritional Status of Preschool Children in the United States, 1968–1970," *Pediatrics* 53, no. 4 (April 1974): 597–646. Copyright 1974 American Academy of Pediatrics.

Table 16-6 presents the range of mean nutrient intakes for children of different ages. Group I was the lowest, and usually, but not always, Group IV was the highest. A comparison of these values with the RDA (Table 16-2) confirms the finding that mean intakes were approximately equal to or greater than the RDA for vitamin C, riboflavin, thiamin, and protein. The nutrient intakes furthest below the RDA were for iron, vitamin A, calcium, and energy.

The frequency of low energy intakes has important implications for diet planning. Since protein intake was usually adequate but energy needs were low in one-sixth of the wealthiest and one-third of the poorest children, knowledge regarding appropriate selection of foods appears to be a part of the nutritional deficiency problem among this age group. Since iron, vitamin A, and calcium intakes were also often below standard, the foods selected to increase the energy intake of children not meeting their energy RDA should contain these nutrients

TABLE 16-6. Range of Mean Nutrient Intakes Reported in the Study of Nutritional Status of Preschool Children in the United States, 1968–1970

Nutrient	Age (months)		
	12–23	24–47	48–71
Protein (g)	41–52	48–52	54–61
Energy (Cal)	**1,001–1,167**	**1,230–1,371**	**1,417–1,653**
Iron (mg)	**5.4–7.5**	**7.2–7.7**	**8.5–9.0**
Calcium (mg)	**688–965**	**592–796**	**638–910**
Thiamin	0.7–1.8	0.8–1.7	0.9–1.5
Riboflavin	1.5–2.8	1.4–2.5	1.3–2.3
Vitamin C (mg)	40–104	42–108	49–109
Vitamin A (IU)	**334–559**	**300–499**	**310–506**

NOTE: Range of the 50th percentile values for Warner Rank Groups I, II, III, and IV.

SOURCE: Extracted from tables in G. M. Owen, K. M. Kram, P. J. Garry, J. E. Lowe, and A. H. Lubin, "A Study of Nutritional Status of Preschool Children in the United States, 1968–1970," *Pediatrics* 53, no. 4 (April 1974): 597–646. Copyright 1974 American Academy of Pediatrics.

if possible. Dairy products, potatoes, enriched flour, beans, and vegetables that would help supply both energy and these necessary micronutrients usually need more attention than do dietary sources of protein.

PLANNING DIETS

Translation of this nutrition knowledge into action must include consideration of the factors that determine the acceptability and availability of food for children.

Planning for Nutrients

The findings of the Study of Nutritional Status of Preschool Children show that one major problem is that parents and others responsible for feeding children need to know more about nutrition and, in particular, about dietary sources of specific nutrients. Low energy intakes suggest that many children—regardless of their socioeconomic rating—simply need to eat more food. The other low values for specific micronutrient intakes suggest which foods should be added to their diet—primarily sources of iron, calcium, and vitamin A. Since the average diets in all groups contain sufficient protein, the parents need to know the amounts of protein-rich foods (Table 16-7) that are needed to meet the protein RDA (30 grams for 4- to 6-year-olds and 36 grams for 7- to 10-year-olds) for their children. Then, they will know at what point in meal planning and budgeting it is wiser to include more sources of iron, calcium, and vitamin A such as carrots, squash, beans, green leafy vegetables, and cereal products rather than more meat and other protein-rich foods.

Planning for Appetites

The difficulty of feeding small children is sometimes further complicated by their capricious appetites. Fluctuations in appetite naturally accom-

TABLE 16-7. Amounts of Protein in Selected Foods

Food[a]	Protein (g)
Hamburger, cooked	27
Cheddar cheese	26
Ham	21
Hamburger, raw	21
Chicken, fried	19
Chicken, raw	19
Corned beef	16
Polish sausage	16
Steak	16
Cottage cheese, cream style	14
Bologna	12
Salmon, broiled or baked	7
Milk, cup	9

[a] Serving size is 100 grams (approximately 3 ounces) except for milk.

SOURCE: B. K. Watt and A. L. Merrill, "Composition of Foods—Raw, Processed, Prepared," *Agriculture Handbook* No. 8 (Washington, D.C.: USDA, Agricultural Research Service, 1963).

pany different activity levels; from day to day, the amount of energy used—and the amount needed—by a child vary. However, changes in a child's appetite do not always have a physiological basis.

Psychosocial factors also have a greater impact upon diet patterns as children grow older. They learn to use food and eating behavior to get attention from adults. The appropriate parental reaction to a child's acceptance or rejection of food should be consistent with the parent-child relationship, whether it be permissive or disciplined. The time and place that a child eats are not crucial determinants of the nutritional quality of the diet but, as discussed in Chapter 10, these factors do often affect the types of food that comprise the total diet. For children who consume a relatively large amount of food away from the table, special attention is

New foods may be more acceptable to small children if they are easy to handle and if their color, appearance, texture, and flavor are interesting.

Developing broad food preferences during early childhood makes it easier to modify the diet later in life.

needed to ensure that snacks are not limited to one type of food. A diet composed primarily of cereal products such as cookies, crackers, and ready-to-eat cereals without milk, or of nursing bottle beverages such as milk and juices is lacking in many of the nutrients needed by growing children. Parents who do not insist that their children eat at the table should make accessible fruits, vegetables, and dairy products; they should also encourage their children to enjoy a nutritionally varied selection of foods between family mealtimes.

Maintaining a varied nutrient intake becomes difficult when a child discovers a new favorite-food and that food temporarily becomes the primary energy source for the child. Parents need to consider the nutritive value of that food—both what it provides and what it lacks—and pay particular attention to adding to the diet sources of the other needed nutrients. Since food favorites change rather quickly for children, the remainder of the diet that is directed primarily by the parents needs frequent evaluation and modification.

Most children go through periods of eating very little. Rejection of food is often a part of normal psychological growth when the child is learning to assert his or her independence. Nutrition knowledge is helpful to parents during such periods. They should carefully observe what the child is eating, both in front of the parents and when the parents are supposedly not watching. If the child has been well fed previously, an occasional few days of reduced food intake has little detrimental effect, except perhaps reduced energy for the child. However, if these periods are prolonged and especially if weight gain plateaus, a pediatrician should be consulted.

Planning for Acceptability

Efforts to broaden the nutrient sources in a child's diet should take into consideration the youngster's manual dexterity. Children who have fun learning to use their fingers can practice with small pieces of chopped fruits, vegetables, or cheeses. As a child learns to use a spoon and then a fork, the types of foods that can be eaten without parental assistance will expand. However, if practicing such skills is forced on a child, negative attitudes toward the food may develop and persist long after the child has mastered use of the utensils.

Attention to the color of food can increase the pleasure of eating. Alert parents who wish to instill in their child an enjoyment of food for a lifetime might add to family meals colorful foods, even some that they themselves had overlooked in the past. For example, purple cabbage mixed with orange carrots and red radishes offers the same eye appeal—though different nutrients and flavors—as some colored breakfast cereals.

Interest in food may also be increased if parents include their children in grocery shopping, giving time and thought to these food encounters. The size, shape, and texture of produce such as eggplant, asparagus, artichokes, and various squashes may be fascinating to a child, as may also the colors and aromas of some cheeses. Seeing the various types of peas, beans, breads, and pastas may also help children realize that eating need not be a boring routine.

The preparation of foods influences their acceptability to a child. Boiling for a short time in a small amount of water helps maintain the color, texture, and delicate flavor (as well as the nutritive value) of vegetables such as green beans, celery, and carrots. If a child dislikes the stronger smell of foods such as cabbage or brussels sprouts, longer cooking in more water is justified in order to enhance their acceptability.

Planning for the Future

There are many merits of teaching children early in life to appreciate a wide variety of foods. Chapters 17, 18, and 19 discuss some of the changes in nutrient needs that in turn necessitate changes in diet patterns throughout the lifespan. These modifications are easier for persons who have broad food preferences. For example, the child who learns to know and appreciate the unique flavor of different foods can more easily forgo the pleasure of high-energy, sweet foods later in life when energy needs decline. In a similar manner, knowing the pleasant taste of spices such as dill, rosemary, or caraway helps a person realize that salt is not the only condiment that enhances the flavor of other foods. Other modifications such as reducing one's cholesterol intake, increasing one's folacin intake, or complying with a diet prescribed for a specific medical disorder are less difficult for the person who as a child became acquainted with a wide world of foods.

STUDY QUESTIONS

1. When and how do attitudes toward food develop?

2. How do children's nutrient needs change between the ages of one and ten?

3. Which nutrients are most often deficient in children's diets?

4. List three foods from each of the four basic food groups that might be eaten away from the table by a four-year-old child.

5. How can new foods be made more acceptable to a preschool child?

6. Name three foods that you have disliked since you were a preschooler, and explain why you do not like them.

SUGGESTED READING

1. N. R. Beyer and P. M. Morris, "Food attitudes and snacking patterns of young children," *Journal of Nutrition Education* 6(1974):131.

2. "Child nutrition programs," *Dairy Council Digest* 45(January-February 1974).

3. C. W. Woodruff, "Milk intolerances," Chapter 47 in *Present Knowledge in Nutrition.* 4th ed. New York and Washington, D.C.: The Nutrition Foundation, 1976.

4. R. L. Huenemann, "Environmental factors associated with preschool obesity: II. Obesity and food practices of children at successive age levels," *Journal of the American Dietetic Association* 64(1974): 588.

5. L. Juhas, "Nutrition education in day-care programs: A new challenge to our profession," *Journal of the American Dietetic Association* 63(1973):134.

6. G. M. Owen et al, "A Study of nutritional status of preschool children in the United States, 1968–1970," *Pediatric Supplement* 53(April 1974, Part II).

7. S. J. Fomon, *Prevention of Iron-Deficiency Anemia in Infants and Children of Preschool Age.* Public Health Service Pub. No. 2085. Washington, D.C.: Maternal and Child Health Services, Department of Health, Education and Welfare, 1970.

8. Committee on Nutrition, American Academy on Pediatrics, "Childhood diet and coronary heart disease," *Pediatrics* 49(1972):305–307.

9. L. S. Sims and P. M. Morris, "Nutritional status of preschoolers: An ecologic perspective," *Journal of the American Dietetic Association* 64(1974):592.

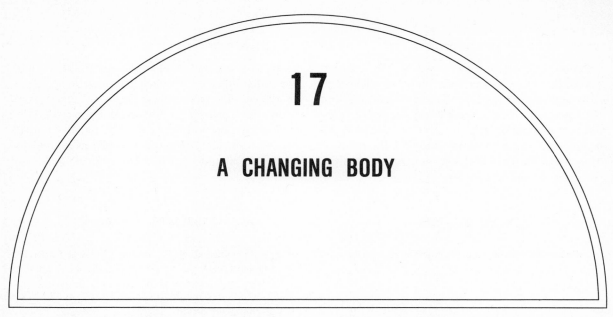

17

A CHANGING BODY

During the time when a young person's body begins to develop sexually, profound physiological changes occur that alter individual requirements for energy and nutrients. The benefits from choosing a diet wisely during these years spread over a lifetime. This chapter discusses how the body changes as it grows, why nutrient requirements fluctuate, and ways of ensuring that the foods selected are nutritionally appropriate.

WHAT NUTRITION KNOWLEDGE OFFERS

Too often efforts are made to convince people of the importance of good nutrition by warning them of the hazards of improper diet patterns. This approach motivates some people to change what they eat, especially if they are in situations where they are keenly aware of the vulnerability of their own health (such as after a heart attack). Under most circumstances, however, the threat of ill health is difficult for people to appreciate. Teen-agers are probably the least receptive audience to this approach because they generally think of themselves as healthy.

Failure to inform teen-agers of the real consequences of improper nutrition is a disservice to them. They should be given the opportunity to appreciate some of the more positive reasons for keeping their diet in tune with their changing nutrient needs.

Today

If nutritional information is presented in a meaningful way, there is a greater possibility that teen-agers will heed advice about the importance of their diet. A recent health behavior study queried students about their interest in various topics. Many expressed an interest in health-related topics (sex education; drugs, smoking, and alcohol ranked first and second), but nutrition ranked low (tenth) among their priorities. This finding may be discouraging to people who are convinced of the importance of diet and nutrition, but it also may provide a clue regarding the most effective way to present nutrition information to people of this age.

The study showed what many people thought was true—teen-agers are interested in their own health.

Teen-agers can best be motivated to learn about nutrition if the benefits of wise food choices are presented in a positive manner, but without exaggeration.

If we keep in mind that teen-agers have many interests regarding health, as well as an interest in nutrition, we might conclude that it is best to present the nutrition message as part of broader health education efforts.

Even the most well-adjusted, emotionally secure teen-ager lives in a world tinged with uncertainties. Caution must be taken that nutrition is not presented as one more thing to worry about. It should be offered as a relatively simple matter compared to other problems and as an opportunity to dispel minor uncomfortable feelings about how and why the body is changing. The teen-ager who knows what foods are needed by his or her body and who has the self-assurance of knowing that these needs are met, has one less thing to worry about. This may sound like flimsy reasoning to an adult; but to the fellow whose feet are three sizes larger than those of his friends, or to the girl who has not started menstruating when all her friends have, some confidence that his or her body is getting the nutrients it needs to grow and develop normally can bolster the teen-ager's feelings of well-being.

A second line of reasoning that may be convincing with teen-agers is that improving the quality of their diet can help them have more energy to enjoy life. Selecting adequate amounts of iron-rich foods helps to avoid the tired feeling due to anemia (which exists in many teen-agers); and wise food choices may improve their resistance to infections that make them miss out on social events as well as school. On the other hand, teen-agers can quickly see through grandiose claims that good nutrition alone will ensure a glowing complexion and bright and shining eyes. If any part of the message told them concerning nutrition is misleading, the credibility of the remainder of the message will be questioned. Good nutrition, complemented by other sound health practices, can indeed improve the possibility of feeling better, maturing normally, and protecting health—teen-agers need to know this but they should be promised nothing more.

Within a Decade

If nutrition concepts are mastered during the teen years, the person is better prepared to modify diet patterns later in life when nutrient needs change.

Changing Activity Patterns. Within a decade, if not sooner, the energy needs of almost all adolescents drop considerably. The young person who is not overweight and who takes care of nutrient needs can safely eat several hundred more Calories of nutrient-dilute foods than an adult. However, when growth tapers off and lifestyle slows down, the person who has become accustomed to eating frequently and never had to worry about energy-rich foods must know how to decrease energy intake and increase the protein and micronutrient density of the diet. Some foresight regarding this potential problem and knowledge about the varying nutritive value of foods can help prepare a teen-ager for the future.

Preparing for Parenthood. A teen-age girl may be more interested in nutrition when she learns that her diet today determines her nutrient stores, which may be needed in the future to support the growth and development of a baby. This awareness may motivate improved diet patterns now regardless of if and when she becomes pregnant.

Building sound nutrition knowledge during the high school years has other advantages for both boys and girls. Several years may pass before they assume the responsibilities of parenthood, but many people become more aware of the importance of nutrition when they need to know how to feed their children. By this time, they are far from the classroom and, unless they have previously studied nutrition, few of them know how to find the books or persons to help them. They have little access to nutrition information except what they read in newspapers, magazines, and paperback books, and often these publications are written by persons with little or no training in nutrition.

Years Ahead

A teen-ager may think that he or she is many years away from having to face health problems due to poor nutrition. Studies have shown, however, that the effects of dietary imbalance begin quite early in life. Autopsies of young American soldiers killed in Korea and Vietnam showed signs of atherosclerosis (Chapter 25). The disease was not obvious, but examination of the artery walls proved that its beginnings were there.

One of the warning signs of potential cardiovascular disease is the presence of large amounts of cholesterol in the blood. The higher the cholesterol level is above normal, the greater is the risk of heart attack. As a person ages, this measure usually increases unless special attention is given to the diet. A study of 15-year-old boys in Boston suggests that this cardiovascular-disease risk factor should be given serious consideration even by teen-agers. Researchers found that cholesterol levels of the teen-agers studied were similar to those found among 40- and 50-year-old men living in areas of the world where coronary heart disease is rare.

A teen-ager may have difficulty seeing the importance in these findings, but the information should be made available for their consideration. Other long-range benefits of developing sound diet practices during the teen years are discussed in Chapter 19.

CHANGING NUTRIENT NEEDS

Teen-agers may be motivated to have an interest in nutrition if we explain to them:

1. Why their nutrient needs are different
2. How these needs can be met by foods
3. What nutrients deserve their particular attention.

When They Change

We speak of the nutrient needs of teen-agers as if they were distinct from those of younger children or of adults, but this can be misleading. The change in a young person's requirements for energy and nutrients does not occur dramatically on the thirteenth birthday or on the twentieth. Fluctuations begin during pubescence, the period of life beginning with the development of secondary sexual characteristics and ending with the emergence of the capacity for sexual reproduction. On the average, pubescence ends at about age 13 for girls and age 15 for boys. An increased need for many nutrients continues through adolescence, the period of growth following pubescence. On the average, the growth for most females has leveled off by age $15\frac{1}{2}$ and for most males by age $17\frac{1}{2}$. A very slight amount of average growth continues for about another two or three years.

Averages such as those cited above help one estimate when nutrient needs change for groups of young people, but the ages at which sexual development begins and growth ceases vary greatly among individuals. A 10-year-old girl who begins menstruating has a greater need for foods that supply iron than her girlfriends who are not developing as rapidly. In a similar vein, the boy who is still growing taller at age 18 has a greater need for protein, calcium, and many other nutrients than a classmate who completed most of his growth at age 16. Awareness of the correlation between nutrient needs and individual development can help a young person make appropriate food choices as their nutrient needs change during pubescence and adolescence.

Why They Change

The body of a 17-year-old boy may weigh 175 pounds—perhaps twice as much as it did only six years before. This visible increase in body size is paralleled by an unseen accumulation of nutrients. The calcium content of a male's body, for instance, increases from 400 grams at age 10 to more than 1,000 grams at age 18—a gain of over 1 pound of this mineral alone. Other minerals, such as phosphorus and magnesium, also are incorporated into growing bones. Vitamin D, though not retained in the body, is needed for calcium absorption and utilization.

Dietary protein is especially important during these years for the synthesis of muscle tissues, enzymes, hormones, and other specialized proteins. The protein in food must be broken down and resynthesized into body protein, and so teen-agers also have increased needs for several vitamins, especially pyridoxine, which is necessary for many steps in amino acid metabolism. The requirements for both macronutrients and micronutrients increase not only because of growth but also because the larger body requires more energy and nutrients for maintenance.

Foods that supply iron are needed in greater amounts during pubescence and adolescence. Both sexes need about the same amount of iron during these years, but the reasons for the increased requirement differ between boys and girls. Boys gain more weight during their growth spurt than do girls, and a larger proportion of their weight gain is due to an increase in muscle. Synthesis of the muscle protein, myoglobin, is dependent upon an adequate supply of iron, which is present at the core of this protein molecule. Iron is also needed for the synthesis of hemoglobin, the oxygen-transporting protein of blood. A 180-pound teen-age boy has about a half gallon more blood in his body than he had when he weighed only 100 pounds at age 10.

Girls usually do not increase their blood volume or muscle mass as much as boys; a greater percentage of their weight gain is due to growth of fat cells (which contain little iron) in breast tissue and around their hips. Their increased iron need is for replacement of the blood lost during menstruation.

How Much They Change

The nutrient needs of many young people increase before they literally reach the teen years. Although the RDA values for boys and girls are the same through the first decade of life, after age 10 the RDA for many nutrients are different for males and females.

Child or Adult? The RDA values for ages 11–14 and 15–18 are compared to those of younger and older males and females in Figure 17-1. This figure shows that during the teen years the needs for some nutrients are the same as children's; in other cases, they are the same as adults'; and sometimes, they fit neither category.

A teen-ager has the same need for vitamin D as a child. The need for dietary sources of this nutrient continues as long as a person is growing. On the other hand, the RDA for vitamin A, vitamin E, vitamin C, folacin, vitamin B_{12}, zinc, and pyridoxine for boys and girls at age 11 are the same as the amount needed by men or women up to 50 years of age. It is especially important to note that the RDA for calcium, phosphorus, and iodine are higher for teen-agers than during either childhood or adulthood. The RDA for riboflavin is greatest between the ages of 15 and 22.

Postpuberty Difference. In the next chapter we will discuss differences in the nutrient needs of men and women. Some of these differences become apparent during the teen years. For example, boys need about 20 percent more vitamin A, vitamin E, riboflavin, and iodine than girls need. Boys should have little difficulty meeting their higher need for these micronutrients, however, because their RDA for energy is greater than girls—by 16 percent at ages 11–14 and by 33 percent at ages 15–22. On the other hand, the RDA for many micronutrients are as high for girls as for boys. This fact points to a special nutrition problem for girls that begins in their teens and remains with them throughout life. In order to meet their RDA for micronutrients and not exceed energy needs, they must select a diet with an overall vitamin and mineral density greater than that needed by boys.

This difference in appropriate nutrient density for

For some nutrients, the RDAs for teen-agers resemble those of younger children; for others, the RDAs are comparable to those of adults; and for a few, the RDAs are uniquely high during adolescence.

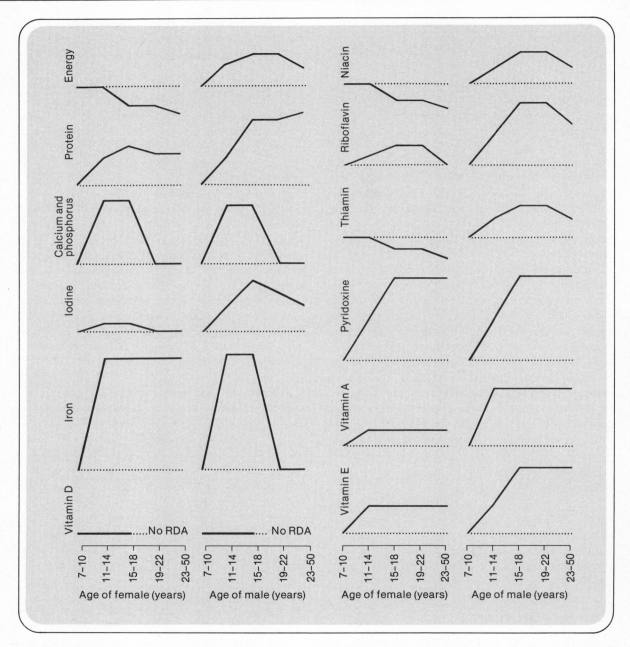

FIGURE 17-1. Relative changes in RDA for males and females. (Quarter-inch equals 10 percent change compared to RDA for children aged 7–10.)

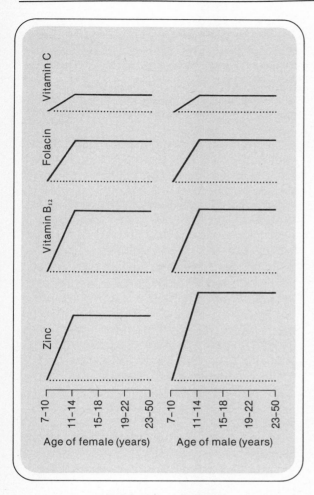

FIGURE 17-1. *(continued)*

boys versus girls does not apply to protein. Since teen-age males need both more energy and more protein than females, the appropriate protein density of their diet is similar for boys and girls.

MEETING NUTRIENT NEEDS

The logical steps in planning a nutritionally appropriate diet for teen-agers are to identify the most common problems, focus on the types of foods that would alleviate these problems, and then suggest ways to modify eating patterns to enhance the nutritional value of the overall diet.

Defining Possible Problems

The three surveys discussed in Chapter 13 differ in methodology and population sampling, but their general findings (Table 17-1) reveal that iron and calcium are the nutrients most often consumed in inadequate amounts by teen-agers. The low intake of calcium is not surprising, since the USDA Household Survey results (tabulated according to food intake rather than as nutrient intake) show that boys between the ages of 9 and 19 drink only about $2\frac{1}{2}$ glasses of milk rather than the 4 glasses needed to provide the RDA (1,200 milligrams) of calcium. Milk consumption for girls is even less—it drops from a little more than 2 cups a day at ages 9–11 to about $1\frac{1}{2}$ cups a day by ages 18–19. Over this same age span, use of beverages other than milk and juices (such as soft drinks, coffee, and tea) more than doubles (Figure 17-2).

Average vitamin A and thiamin intakes are also frequently well below the RDA. Getting enough riboflavin appears to be a greater problem among the low-income population studied in the Ten-State Nutrition Survey than among the USDA Household Survey population, which covered all groups. Low protein intakes are reported only among black and Spanish-American girls in the Ten-State Nutrition Survey.

Vitamin C seems to be the nutrient most often eaten in adequate quantities by teen-agers. However, Table 17-1 shows average findings, which do not tell the entire story. Closer examination of the results of the Ten-State Nutrition Survey, for instance, shows that although average intake of vitamin C was greater than the RDA, about 35 percent of the adolescents in this study consumed less than two-thirds of the RDA for this nutrient.

The surveys summarized in Table 17-1 do not provide information regarding all vitamins and

TABLE 17-1. General Evaluation of Adequacy of Diets of Teen-agers
Based on Three Nutrition Surveys

Survey	No Problem	Mild Problem[a]	Moderate Problem[a]	Severe Problem[a]	Very Severe Problem[a]
USDA Household Survey Females	Protein, vitamin C, riboflavin	Vitamin A, thiamin		Calcium	Iron
Males	Protein, vitamins A and C, riboflavin	Thiamin	Calcium	Iron	
Ten-State Nutrition Survey	Vitamin C	Protein,[b] vitamin A, thiamin, riboflavin, growth and development, obesity		Iron	
HANES	Vitamin C		Vitamin A	Iron, calcium	

[a] Based on average intakes.
[b] Found to be low among black and Spanish-American girls in low-income-ratio states.

minerals. We might predict (though we cannot prove) that vitamin D intakes parallel the low values for calcium, since milk is a major source of both these nutrients. We also may question the adequacy of zinc, magnesium, and copper in the diet, since these minerals are found in many, though not all, foods that are rich in iron. These two examples of how the intake of one nutrient might indicate the adequacy of another nutrient show that an understanding of nutrient distribution in foods allows you to raise important questions. The person who thinks critically about nutriton keeps these possibilities in mind but is careful not to assume they are true until proof is available.

The types of food most frequently overlooked by teen-agers are dairy products and vegetables.

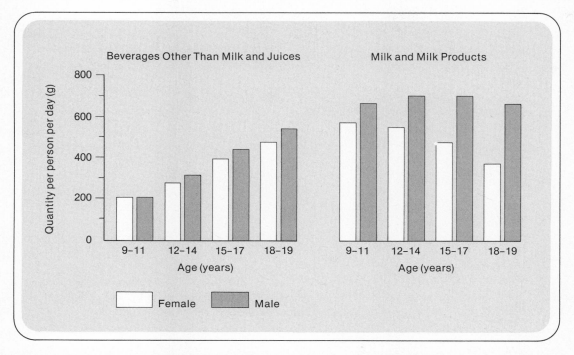

FIGURE 17-2. Increased intake of beverages other than milk and juices and decreased intake of milk. SOURCE: Agricultural Research Service, Household Food Consumption Survey 1965–66; Report Nos. 1 to 18 (Washington, D.C.: U.S. Department of Agriculture, 1968–1974).

Avoiding Problems

To improve the nutritional status of teen-agers, we must translate the findings regarding the nutrients most commonly lacking in diets into food equivalents. This information must then be combined with an awareness of food habits and preferences.

One study of about 125 students in New York (Table 17-2) provides an idea of the food preferences of a group of seventh to twelfth graders. Although food preferences do not always correlate with food intakes, the findings of this small survey help explain some of the dietary inadequacies shown in Table 17-1. Most teen-agers seem to like hamburgers, chicken, and other foods from the meat group. Therefore, they usually manage to eat enough protein (and probably enough vitamin B_{12}). The recommended four servings from the cereal group are easy to get if a person has cereal for breakfast, a hamburger or sandwich for lunch, and bread with dinner or a pastry made with enriched flour sometime during the day. Vitamin C intake can be met with a glass of fruit juice in the morning. The nutritional problem for most teen-agers therefore generally boils down to getting enough nutrients from dairy products and vegetables. What can they do about them?

Dairy Products. Although many teen-agers say they like milk, they simply like soft drinks better (Table 17-2). The result of this difference in prefer-

301

TABLE 17-2. Food Preferences of 125 Students

Foods Most Liked	Number of Students	Foods Most Disliked	Number of Students
*Soda pop	78	Liver	44
*Milk	70	*Fish	18
*Steak	65	Squash	17
*Hamburger	52	Clams	13
*Pizza	43	*Coffee	13
*Chicken	38	Spinach	12
*French fries	37	Cabbage	12
*Ice cream	34	Beets	12
*Spaghetti	31		
*Orange juice	29		
*Corn	29		
Turkey	27		
Lobster	24		
*Candy	21		
*Roast beef	21		
*Egg	20		
*Ham	19		
Shrimp	19		
Beer	19		
*Pie	18		
Milk shake	18		
*Pork chop	17		
*Apple	16		
*Bread	15		
*Frankfurter	15		
*Orange	15		
Lasagna	14		
Tuna	14		
*Cake	13		
*Peas	13		
Wine	13		
*Cheese	12		
Clams	12		
*Cereal	12		

*Item was reported eaten by 10 percent or more of the subjects during the three-day study.

SOURCE: B. C. Schorr, D. Sanjur, and E. C. Erickson, "Teen-age food habits: A multidimensional analysis," *Journal of the American Dietetic Association* 61(1972):415–20. Copyright The American Dietetic Association. Reprinted by permission.

ence is shown in Figure 17-2—use of milk decreases while use of other beverages increases during the teen years.

If energy needs are sufficiently high, there should be room in a well-planned diet for both soft drinks and milk. There is no ironclad rule about when—at meals, as a snack, with coffee—the milk should be included in the diet. The fact teen-agers should know, however, is that their bodies need 1,200 milligrams of calcium, and it is difficult to meet this need with fewer than 4 glasses of milk a day.

If energy needs are low, some diet substitutions may be necessary to meet calcium needs. One approach is to substitute milk for the foods consumed in amounts more than are really needed—for instance, a smaller hamburger plus a carton of milk instead of a superburger. Another approach is to substitute yogurt for a handful of cookies after school, or slice off some cheese for a snack instead of nibbling potato chips and pretzels. Fractions of servings of dairy products can add up over the day if the teen-ager remembers to eat cheeseburgers, sprinkle Parmesan cheese over foods, ask for cheddar cheese on hot apple pie, order pizza instead of fried chicken, or choose ice cream or cream pie for dessert instead of cake.

Vegetables. Many of the teen-ager's nutrient inadequacies can be overcome by giving more thought to including vegetables in their diet. Increased use of dark-green, leafy vegetables would provide needed iron, calcium, and folacin. Yellow and orange vegetables could correct the lesser, but still significant vitamin A problem. The lack of vegetables in the teen-ager's diet is compounded by their frequent snacking practice, which generally omits vegetables (Chapter 10).

The results of a nationwide survey of consumer preferences for different vegetables helps to explain why diets are often low for certain nutrients such as vitamin A or iron. Figure 17-3 ranks 26 vegetables according to the order of the percentage of people aged 10 to 14 who stated they liked these foods.

Only one item that is high on this list (carrots) is an excellent source of vitamin A. Corn and tomatoes are fair sources (about 25 percent of the U.S. RDA per serving), but most of the foods highest in vitamin A (sweet potatoes, spinach, squash, broccoli, and brussels sprouts) were low on the list. This survey also shows one reason for the low intake of iron by teen-agers—most of the better sources of this mineral are liked by less than 40 percent of the children surveyed.

There are two approaches to helping teen-agers increase their vegetable intake. First, they might be encouraged to eat more of the vegetables they like most. Corn and potatoes every day will not solve the problem, but a daily diet including one of these vegetables plus at least two more servings of the other preferred vegetables will help meet their needs for calcium, iron, and vitamin A.

A second approach is to help teen-agers expand their vegetable preferences. Special emphasis should be given to leafy vegetables that provide iron and folacin. Figure 17-3 suggests that this approach may be more effective with older adolescents (asterisks indicate the vegetables preferred by a greater percentage of people 15–19 years old than by people 10–14 years old). Although the change in preference patterns is not great, older adolescents show a trend toward liking the better sources of vitamin A and a few sources of iron and folacin.

Diet Patterns

An understanding of the diet patterns of teenagers provides clues to improving their nutrient intake.

Breakfast. Skipping breakfast is a common practice for people of all ages. Approximately 10 percent of all Americans eat no breakfast and another 4 percent have only coffee. Teen-agers neglect breakfast more than any other group in the population.

Breakfast is important because the body's ready reserves of energy, the blood glucose and liver gly-

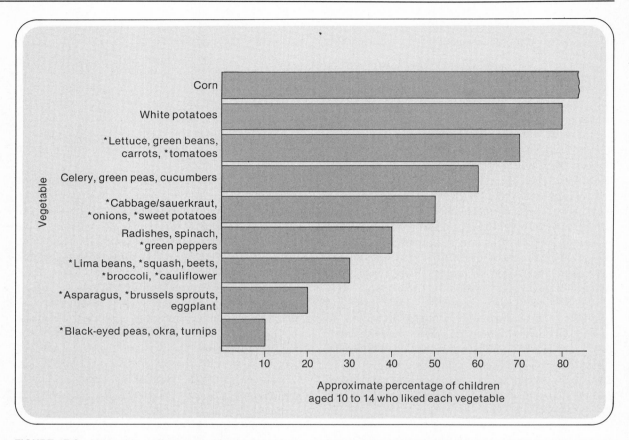

FIGURE 17-3. Vegetable preferences of boys and girls aged 10 to 14. Asterisks (*) indicate that a higher percentage of boys and girls aged 15 to 19 liked these vegetables than younger children. SOURCE: Adapted from *Consumers' Preferences, Uses, and Buying Practices for Selected Vegetables,* Marketing Research Report No. 1019, USDA, Economic Research Service.

cogen, become greatly depleted during the overnight fast. Ideally, breakfast should do more than just increase blood glucose levels. It should provide vitamins, minerals, protein, and some fat, as well as carbohydrates. A breakfast of varied macronutrient composition helps maintain more of a feeling of satiety or fullness during the morning than does a breakfast of only simple sugars and micronutrients. For example, Figure 17-4 shows that a sweet roll and a cup of black coffee with sugar will temporarily satisfy the need for energy, but such a break-

fast will leave you feeling hungry by midmorning. This situation might lead to further dilution of the nutrient density of the diet unless foods that provide protein and micronutrients are available when you become hungry at ten o'clock.

Studies have shown that people work better (especially during the late morning) if they eat an adequate breakfast, but there are no nutritional grounds for specifically defining which foods are acceptable for breakfast. This meal might become more popular among teen-agers if they could over-

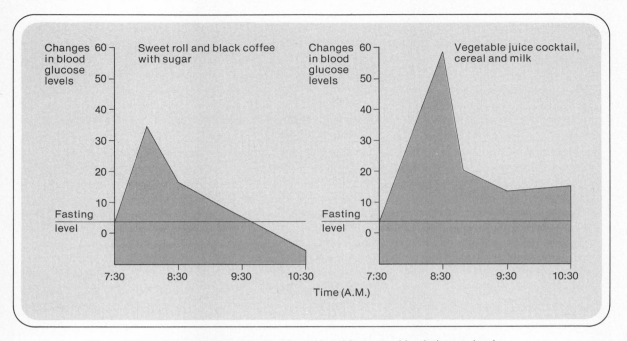

FIGURE 17-4. Effect of composition of breakfast upon blood glucose levels.

come the idea that their only choices are cereal or eggs. Sandwiches, soup, raw vegetables, or leftovers from dinner the night before could all replenish body stores of energy and at the same time help meet nutrient needs for the day. Fruit juice is not mandatory, but it should be kept in mind as a source of vitamin C (which is not provided in large amounts by most foods traditionally eaten later in the day).

Powdered breakfast foods stirred with milk may fit the lifestyle of some people. The major nutritional limitation of this combination is that it provides no fiber. This problem may be overcome by eating more vegetables, fruits, beans, and whole-grain products at other times during the day.

The person who does not care to eat early in the morning might try to drink some fruit juice (for energy and vitamin C) and then give careful thought to a midmorning snack that will fit into an overall diet plan for the day.

Snacking. To most teen-agers in America, snacking is a way of life. Teen-agers need to be conscientious about dental care but the potential hazards of snacking discussed in Chapter 10—stressful lifestyle and exceeding energy needs—probably are less relevant for people in this age range. Without snacking, an active teen-ager who may use up 3,500 to 4,000 Cal would have to eat very large meals to support growth and exercise.

The Ten-State Nutrition Survey showed that teen-age snacks are not as nutritionally imbalanced as had previously been feared (Table 17-3). Although the nutrient density of foods eaten as snacks was less than that consumed for meals, snacks made a significant contribution to meeting total daily

TABLE 17-3. Comparison of Snack Foods and Total Nutrient Intakes of Teen-agers

Nutrient	Males[a]			Females[a]		
		Mean Intake per 100 Cal			Mean Intake per 100 Cal	
	RDA per 100 Cal	Snack Foods	24-Hour Total	RDA per 100 Cal	Snack Foods	24-Hour Total
Protein (g)	2.0	2.3	3.8	2.2	2.2	3.7
Calcium (mg)	50.0	39.1	44.6	55.3	34.3	41.0
Iron (mg)	0.64	0.33	0.55	0.77	0.34	0.53
Vitamin A (IU)	178.0	128.0	193.5	212.0	117.4	196.0
Thiamin (mg)	0.05	0.03	0.05	0.05	0.03	0.06
Riboflavin (mg)	0.05	0.07	0.09	0.06	0.06	0.09
Vitamin C (mg)	1.7	2.6	2.8	2.0	3.9	2.9

[a] Aged 12 to 16 years.

NOTE: Based on data from Ten-State Nutrition Survey.

SOURCE: J. A. Thomas and D. L. Call, "Eating between Meals—A Nutrition Problem among Teen-agers?" *Nutrition Reviews* 31(1973):138. © 1973, The Nutrition Foundation, Inc. Also used by permission of the authors.

nutrient needs, especially for vitamin C. Suggestions in Chapter 10 may help teen-agers plan snacks to fit their lifestyle and their nutrient needs.

Alcohol. A source of energy that assumes a greater role in the diet during the teen years is alcohol. In the food preference study (Table 17-2) both beer and wine were cited. By the twelfth grade about 40 percent of boys and 15 percent of girls drink beer at least once a week (Figure 17-5). Use of wine and hard liquor is much lower. Average values for alcoholic beverage intake do not represent a large percentage of total energy intake, but in a national survey of students in seventh through twelfth grades 5 percent of those polled reported drinking enough alcohol to get "high" at least once a week. Approximately 23 percent drank this much at least four times a year.

The use of alcoholic beverages varies greatly among individuals and different regions of the country. The survey found that young people who customarily drink wine with their families or on special occasions do not exhibit a dramatic change during the teen years, but use of alcoholic beverages at parties and while sitting or riding around with friends at night does increase over this age range. Although many young people do not drink wine, beer, or liquor, the average statistics are sufficiently high that the effect of alcoholic beverages on the total diet should be considered seriously for those who do drink. Alcoholic beverages dilute the nutrient density of the diet. If they displace from the diet beverages that provide calcium, protein, and vitamin C, additional food sources of these nutrients are needed.

SPECIAL CONSIDERATIONS

Certain nutrition concepts that are not of particular interest to people of all ages are more relevant to teen-agers.

Teen-agers who participate in sports and those who are overweight or underweight need to know more about nutrition than others in order to plan appropriate diets.

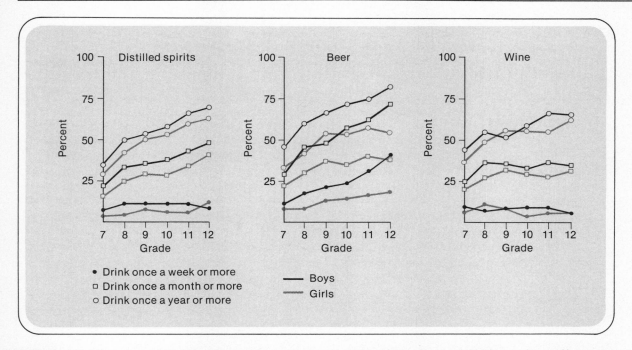

FIGURE 17-5. Percentage of drinkers among teen-agers by sex, school grade, frequency of drinking, and type of beverage. Source: N. E. Chafetz, *Second Special Report to the U.S. Congress on Alchohol and Health,* DHEW, Public Health Service; Alcohol, Drug Abuse, and Mental Health Administration, Rockville, Md., DHEW Publication No. (ADM) 75–212 (June 1974).

Sports

Athletes are often very interested in nutrition, but because of their enthusiasm for body building they are vulnerable to misinformation. Many teen-age sports enthusiasts are misled into believing promises regarding the benefits of protein, vitamin, and mineral supplements. Vitamin supplements are effective in correcting a deficiency of a vitamin, but once the body's need for these nutrients is met, extra supplements are pointless.

The need of athletes for nutrition knowledge is documented by Table 17-4. When a group of 140 physical education majors (over a third were females) was given a list of foods and asked which they recommended for different situations, more than 70 percent recommended wheat germ and supplementary vitamins to improve overall performance during the training season. A smaller percentage checked other types of supplements. Many of the students recommended these products for a pregame meal or to increase muscle mass.

Protein supplements for athletes are probably the greatest hoax of all. Table 17-5 shows that most athletes probably meet a large portion of their needs for this nutrient at the pregame meal alone. Athletes who buy protein supplements are paying a ridiculous price for a macronutrient that will be deaminated by the body and metabolized just like sugar in their soft drinks (Chapter 5).

Energy. One of the most important, nutritionally valid considerations in diet planning for athletes is the adequacy of energy intake. For many sports, a

307

TABLE 17-4. Percentages of Physical Education Students Who Recommended Food Supplements for Different Situations

Food Supplement	Eat in a Pregame Meal of an Endurance Sport	Omit in a Pregame Meal	Eat to Increase Muscle Mass	Eat during Entire Training Season to Improve Overall Performance	Eat to Increase Resistance to Colds, Infections, and so on	Omit in a Weight-Reducing Plan
Wheat germ	41	12	57	74	44	9
Gatorade	46	12	3	36	22	8
Gelatin	46	9	14	54	25	6
Calcium tablets	12	20	28	44	25	9
High-protein supplements	38	9	65	54	22	18
Iron supplements	34	13	56	69	45	7
Vitamin A	39	8	41	77	56	5
Vitamin B$_{12}$	41	7	41	75	57	7
B vitamins	33	9	39	72	53	3
Vitamin C	45	6	37	80	89	3
Vitamin D	37	9	40	76	49	4
Vitamin E	36	9	38	72	50	4

SOURCE: M. Cho and B. A. Fryer, "What foods do physical education majors and basic nutrition students recommend for athletes?" *Journal of the American Dietetic Association* 65(1974):540. Copyright The American Dietetic Association. Reprinted by permission.

person uses between 5,000 and 6,000 Cal (21,000 and 25,200 kJ) every day during training and game season.

Energy stores at the time of an event can affect endurance, and therefore performance, of an athlete. For events that last only a few minutes (such as racing sprints or short swimming races), glucose in the blood is the primary source of energy. Fruit juice and noncarbonated beverages are generally recommended for maintaining blood glucose reserves for such sports.

Other nutrient reserves are the major source of energy used in sports of longer duration. The Swedish physiologist Per-Olof Astrand has shown that during mild exercise, muscles rely mainly upon fat for energy. As exercise becomes more intensive, glycogen (the storage form of carbohydrate) becomes more important as the energy source. Astrand recommends a diet pattern that optimizes the body's capacity to store glycogen. One week in advance of a game the athlete should exercise to exhaustion the same muscles that will be used in the game. For the next three days a diet high in fat and protein (but low in carbohydrate) is eaten to deplete glycogen content. Then, for the next three days large quantities of carbohydrates are added to the basic diet. This pattern of eating provides maximal stores of glycogen in preparation for prolonged, severe exercise such as marathon races or mountain climbing. However, some athletes find that the glycogen-

TABLE 17-5. Sample Menus for Pregame Meals

Sample Menu	Plan 1 (approximately 500 Cal)	Plan 2 (approximately 900 Cal)
1	Milk, skim, 1 cup	Milk, skim, 2 cups
	Lean ham or other meat, 2 oz.	Hamburger patty, 2 oz.
	Bread or toast, 2 slices	Bread, 2 slices or 1 bun
	Fat spread, 1 t.	Fat spread, 1 t.
	Orange or other fruit, $\frac{1}{2}$ cup	Potatoes, mashed, 1 cup
		Tomato juice, 1 cup
		Peach or other fruit, $\frac{1}{2}$ cup or 1 whole
		Plain cookies, 2
2	Milk, skim, 1 cup	Milk, skim, 1$\frac{1}{2}$ cups
	Cheese (American or Swiss) in sandwich, 2 slices	Creamed chicken, $\frac{1}{4}$ cup diced chicken
	Bread, 2 slices	Bread, 2 slices
	Fat spread, 1 t.	Fat spread, 1 t.
	Tomato juice, 1 cup	Potatoes, mashed, 1 cup
		Green beans, $\frac{1}{2}$ cup
		Orange or other fruit, $\frac{1}{2}$ cup or 1 whole
		Angel food cake, 1 piece

SOURCE: *Nutrition for Athletes.* © 1971, The American Alliance for Health, Physical Education, and Recreation. Used by permission.

depleting diet recommended early in the week leaves them fatigued and unable to perform well during pregame practices. For many people, it is better to omit this phase and simply rely on a diet that provides adequate protein plus additional carbohydrate to build up glycogen reserves.

Some nutritionists and physiologists have serious reservations about the Astrand diet. Glycogen retains water, and both glycogen and water may be deposited in the muscle to such an extent that the athlete experiences a feeling of heaviness and stiffness. Carbohydrate loading has also been reported to produce cardiac pain and electrocardiographic abnormalities in an older marathon runner. Because of the effect of this practice on heart function, athletes should use this diet only with expert advice from competent physicians.

Water Deprivation. Water deprivation is a hazard for the athlete or anyone who exercises strenuously. This condition may result from attempts to lose weight prior to weighing in for certain categories of competition in boxing, rowing, or swimming. It can also occur during a game or practice in other sports.

Body heat production is much greater during physical exercise than when the body is at rest. The main way of dissipating this heat is the evaporation of water as perspiration. Unless adequate body water is available to rid the body of excess heat, the body temperature increases above normal. Physical exertion coupled with inadequate fluid intake can cause heat stroke, sudden collapse, and loss of consciousness.

Such tragedies have occurred to athletes because

of high temperatures, high humidity, and water deprivation preceding intense physical activity. Physiological changes that impair performance are detectable with losses as small as 3 percent of body water—a 2½ pound loss for a person weighing 140 pounds. When losses are 5 percent, evidence of heat exhaustion becomes apparent, and at 7 percent, hallucinations occur—a dangerous sign! Losses totaling 10 percent are extremely hazardous and lead to heat stroke. If this condition is not treated immediately, death will result.

Anyone who exercises strenuously should be certain to include beverages (milk, juice, soft drinks, coffee, tea, and plain water) in all meal and snack plans.° The best safety and performance is achieved on the field or court by replacing the water as it is lost in sweat, hour-by-hour. A record of water loss (measured by weighing in and out at games and practice) will help an athlete maintain sufficient body fluid—the natural thirst mechanism is not sensitive enough to stimulate adequate fluid replacement. A decrease in weight of 2 pounds represents a loss of 1 quart of sweat that must be replaced. If a game or practice lasts several hours, water or slightly sweetened beverages should be accessible and used during this time. The injury and loss of life due to heat stroke is avoidable if the body's need for water—the most important nutrient—is understood.

Underweight

The incidence of underweight among Americans has not received as much attention as the more pervasive weight problem, obesity. The Ten-State Nutrition Survey, however, reported a disturbing prevalence of impaired growth and development among people aged 10 to 16 years. This problem might have been anticipated among girls because of societal pressures that emphasize slimness for

women, but the survey found a comparable impairment of growth and development among teen-age boys.

Lack of energy or any nutrient can ultimately result in reduced growth of an experimental animal in a laboratory. In the real world of people, short stature and low body weight probably most often result from moderate deficiencies of several micronutrients and macronutrients. Very severe dietary deprivation during critical periods of development early in life (Chapter 27) can also prevent a person from attaining as great an adult height as is genetically possible.

The hazards of being underweight are difficult to measure. They usually depend upon the specific nutrient(s) lacking in the diet. Anemia (Chapter 22) and increased susceptibility to certain infections (Chapter 21) are often associated with poor growth and development in children.

Underweight teen-agers (see appendix Table A17-1) need not spend hours worrying about their condition, but they should examine their diet patterns to be certain that all nutrient needs are met. They should also discuss the appropriateness of their body weight with their doctor to be certain that their slimness is not due to a disease or other problem that is medically correctable. Reliance upon nutrient supplements or special foods advertised as body builders is a pointless waste of money. Furthermore, they may cause real health problems with serious, long-range effects to become even worse if medical supervision is not sought.

Overweight

The problem of overweight was discussed in Chapter 9, but the special situation of obese teen-agers merits some further discussion. The incidence of obesity among teen-agers is difficult to measure precisely. The reliability of weight charts as a measure of body fatness is decreased because we are dealing with a time of life when the growth spurt occurs, and it may start at different ages. However,

° Caffeine-containing beverages, such as colas, coffee, and tea, stimulate the nervous system and can increase nervous tension and agitation. They should be avoided in the pregame diet.

we can estimate that about 13 percent of all girls and 9 percent of boys between ages 12 and 19 are sufficiently overweight to be classed as obese. These percentages may seem trivial, but they mean that about three million teen-agers in the United States have a serious health problem—obesity.

The obese teen-ager is under constant social pressure. Specialists in adolescent medicine and nutritionists working with overweight teen-agers have found that the burden of self-blame and inferiority imposed by society on the obese adolescent is usually most intense among their own families. Ironically, the family may actually contribute to the obesity problem. Parental genes and family food habits appear to have much to do with the cause of obesity in children. For instance, if both parents are overweight, there is a high probability that their children will be overweight.

The psychological interaction between the obese child and the parents (especially the mother) can worsen the weight problem. The predisposition to obesity in the teen-ager might be traceable to early rejection or hostility in the mother–child relationship. This frequently leads to emotional depression, generalized slowing down by the child, and consequently to reduced activity and energy expenditure.

Weight reduction for a child is usually more successful when the parents make an effort to understand the fundamentals—both physiological and psychological—of obesity and when they accept their child's problem as their own. Obesity must be treated as a psychological and social, as well as dietary, problem. The interaction of these influences upon food choices is even more complex for teen-agers than for adults.

STUDY QUESTIONS

1. How might teen-agers be motivated to appreciate the benefits of good nutrition?

2. How can knowledge regarding nutrition help a teen-ager?

3. Why do nutrient needs increase during the teen years?

4. How do the RDA values for teen-agers compare to those of younger children and adults?

5. What nutrients were most commonly consumed in amounts smaller than the RDA by teen-agers studied in nutrition surveys?

6. What types of food are most frequently overlooked by teen-agers?

7. What are the three most common problem areas in diet planning among teen-agers?

8. Why do teen-age athletes need to know more about nutrition?

SUGGESTED READING

1. M. A. Walker and L. Page, "Nutritive Content of College Meals: I. Proximate composition and vitamins," *Journal of the American Dietetic Association* 66(1976):146–51; "II. Lipids," *Journal of the American Dietetic Association* 68(1976):34.

2. R. T. Frankle and F. K. Heussenstamm, "Food zealotry and youth: New dilemmas for professionals," *American Journal of Public Health* 64(1974):11–18.

3. Committee on Nutritional Misinformation, Food and Nutrition Board, *Water Deprivation and Performance of Athletes.* Washington, D.C.: National Academy of Sciences. (Reprinted in *Nutrition Reviews* 32(1974):314–15.)

4. M. A. Walker, M. M. Hill, and F. D. Millman, "Fruit and vegetable acceptance by students: Factors in acceptance and preference," *Journal of the American Dietetic Association* 62(1973):268.

5. E. E. Wein and E. B. Wilcox, "Serum cholesterol from pre-adolescence through young adulthood,"

Journal of the American Dietetic Association 61(1972):155.

6. "Young people and alcohol," *Alcohol Health and Research World,* National Institute of Alcohol Abuse and Alcoholism, U.S. Department of Health, Education and Welfare (Summer 1975).

7. J. I. McKigney and H. N. Munro, *Nutrient Requirements in Adolescence,* National Institute of Child Health and Human Development (DHEW Pub. No. NIH-76-771). Washington, D.C.: U.S. Department of Health, Education and Welfare, 1975.

8. R. H. Kirk, M. Hamrick, and D. C. McAfee, "Nutrition in health instruction: The Tennessee Health Project," *Journal of Nutrition Education* 7(1975): 68–71.

9. R. L. Huenemann, "A Review of teenage nutrition in the United States," *Health Services Reports* 87(1972):823–29.

10. J. A. Spargo, F. Heald, and P. S. Peckos, "Adolescent obesity," *Nutrition Today* 1(1966):2–10.

11. "Nutrition and athletic performance," *Dairy Council Digest* 46(March-April 1975).

12. N. J. Smith, *Food for Sport.* Palo Alto, Calif.: Bull Publishing Company, 1976.

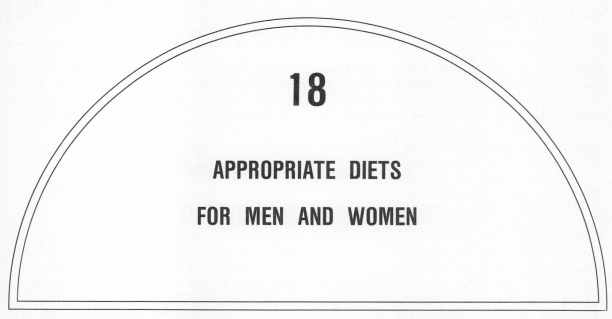

18

APPROPRIATE DIETS

FOR MEN AND WOMEN

Jack Spratt could eat no fat,
His wife could eat no lean,
So betwixt them both,
They licked the platter clean.

This nursery rhyme does not provide adequate guidelines for selecting diets appropriate to the nutrient needs of men and women, but it does call to mind a practical nutrition problem. Men and women need the same nutrients, but their diets must include different amounts of foods of varying nutrient density to enable them to meet their RDA and maintain their health.

This chapter explains why men and women should choose diets that emphasize different foods. It points out the dietary imbalances that are most common among women and those that are most common among men. Finally, it suggests ways that men and women can meet their nutrient needs without having to eat at separate tables.

DIFFERENCES BETWEEN MEN AND WOMEN

The selection of appropriate diets for men and for women must be based on an understanding of how the two sexes differ in anatomy and diet patterns.

The pace of life and the psychosocial factors that influence what we eat may have a role in determining which foods are appropriate for people of each sex.

Body Size and Composition

The interrelationship between body size and nutrient requirements is a fundamental nutrition concept. Therefore, it is logical that the RDA for a 5-foot 4-inch, 128-pound woman are, in many instances, lower than the RDA for a 5-foot 9-inch, 154-pound man. Height and weight do not, however, explain all the differences among the nutrient needs of males compared to females.

A comparison of the body composition of men and women who are not obese reveals that men normally have proportionally more muscle and less fat depots than women. The metabolic activity, and hence the energy and nutrient needs, of muscle cells is greater than that of fat cells. Hormonal differences also affect how the body uses nutrients.

Life Expectancy

The fact that women control a large portion of the money in this country is not because of women's

The differences between appropriate diets for men and women are based in part upon differences in body size and composition, different disease patterns, and different attitudes toward body weight and health.

liberation. It is simply because women outlive men and therefore inherit control of family investments.

Women outlive men by about seven years, but this phenomenon is not thoroughly understood. One major difference between the sexes is the occurrence of cardiovascular disease, the major cause of death among Americans. Cardiovascular disease affects men at a younger age than it does women. The dietary risk factors associated with this condition should be known and respected by both sexes, but the greater loss of life due to heart attacks and strokes among younger men suggests that they should give particular attention to the cholesterol content of their diet, the amount and type of fat they eat, and other dietary modifications discussed in Chapter 25. Elevation of serum cholesterol, a cardiovascular risk factor, increases with age in men. High serum cholesterol levels are much less common in women until after the menopause. This seems to indicate that hormonal differences lend some protection to women during the phase of life when so many men die of cardiovascular disease.

The difference in life expectancy may also be indirectly linked to the faster growth rate of children today and the greater heights they attain compared to their grandparents. This change is often largely attributed to improved diet and nutritional status, but parallel to this "progress" has been an increased incidence of cardiovascular disease. The significance of and correlation between these changes are difficult to evaluate because many other factors have changed at the same time—smoking, pace of life, lack of exercise, and advances in medicine—but they raise important questions. The coincidence between increased growth and increased incidence of heart disease suggests that there is a distinction between *maximal growth* and *optimal growth*. What has been considered a benefit may actually be a risk to some people. The greater gain in life expectancy during this century for females (27 years longer than in 1900) compared to males (21 years longer than in 1900) may indicate that the female body structure benefits from increased

growth. On the other hand, some males may currently be exceeding optimal body size. Men may be growing to heights that exceed the dimensions that the cardiovascular and other body systems are designed to serve.

Incidence of Obesity

The incidence of obesity among males and females differs in the white and black populations (review Figure 13-5). The HANES reported that a higher percentage of women are obese than men. Black women are more frequently obese than white women, but black men are less frequently obese than white men. In the older age group studied (45 to 74 years old), the incidence of obesity increases among women, but it decreases among men.

Obese people have a shorter life expectancy than nonobese people. However, the consequences of obesity are greater for men than for women. Comparison of the incidence of cardiovascular disease for men and women who are equally obese shows that increasing degrees of obesity have a much more harmful effect on men than on women (Figure 18-1).

Awareness of Body Weight

Although obesity seems to present a greater threat to health for males than for females, men seem to be less concerned about overweight than women are. Weight-reduction diets are a fairly common topic of conversation among women, but men talk about this subject less frequently.

A study among high school seniors revealed differences between males and females regarding their perceived and desired images of themselves. These teen-agers were shown line drawings of a series of body silhouettes (Figure 18-2) and were asked to choose which looked most like themselves and which they would most like to resemble. Although this group included a fairly typical distribution of obese, average, and lean students, 80 percent of the girls said they wanted to weigh less than they did.

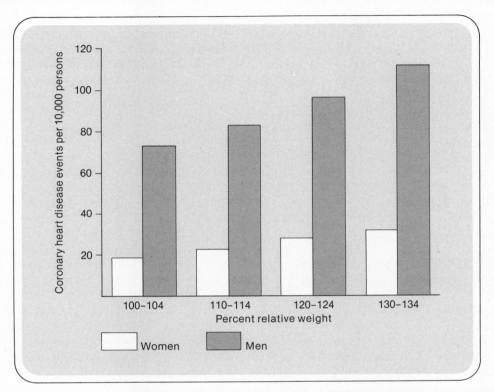

FIGURE 18-1. Average annual rate of coronary heart disease for men and women (ages 45 to 54) of increasing body weights. Source: Adapted from W. B. Kannel and T. Gordon, *The Framingham Study,* Section 30, DHEW Publication No. (NIH) 74-599 (February 1974).

Most of the boys, except those who were obese, wanted to weigh more.

Interest in and awareness of body weight also differed: girls weighed themselves more frequently, but boys reported their weight more accurately. These teen-agers had different opinions about which figures were most feminine and most masculine. More girls than boys selected the thinnest silhouette as most feminine. More boys than girls selected the broad-chested silhouette as most masculine.

Another study among the parents of obviously overweight adolescents shed some light on adult attitudes and awareness of overweight, which differ between males and females. The mothers were eager to have their overweight children of either sex in a weight-reduction program. The fathers usually agreed that their daughters should lose weight, but many strenuously disagreed that their sons should be considered overweight. Although this study did not probe the question, we might expect that the fathers probably held similar attitudes about the appropriateness of their own body weight and whether they would benefit from losing weight.

Menstruation

Most people are aware of a woman's extra need for iron. However, the high incidence of iron defi-

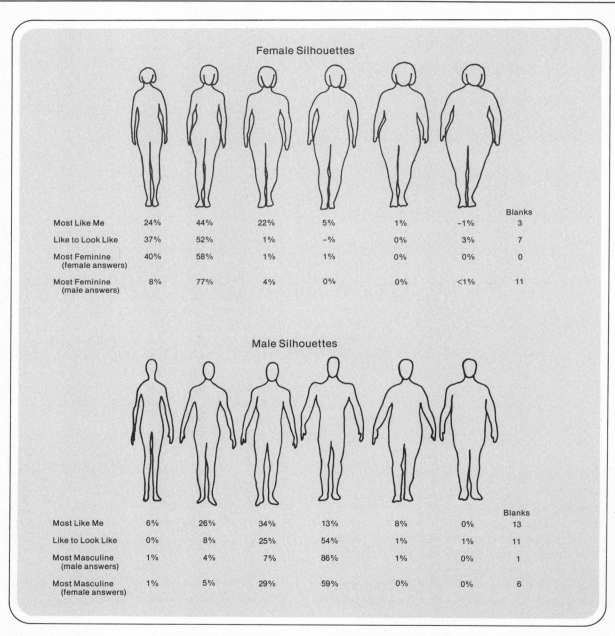

FIGURE 18-2. Evaluation of silhouettes by high school seniors. (Reprinted from "Adolescent attitudes toward weight and appearance" by J. T. Dwyer, J. J. Feldman, C. C. Seltzer, and J. Mayer, in *Journal of Nutrition Education* 1 (Fall 1969):14–19. © 1969, Society for Nutrition Education. Used by permission.)

ciency anemia among the female population indicates that women are unable or unmotivated to adjust their diets to meet their need for iron.

Women's RDA for iron—18 milligrams each day—may seem high considering that an average of only about 15 milligrams of iron is lost during each monthly period. Every day a woman should consume 8 milligrams of iron more than a man. This totals 240 milligrams (8×30) extra in one month. Why must a woman consume 240 milligrams if she loses only about 15 milligrams in menstrual blood? This can be explained by using two nutrition concepts.

1. Absorption of iron varies depending upon a person's iron stores and the type of food that supplies the iron. In an average mixed diet only about 10 percent of the dietary iron reaches the bloodstream. Therefore, only about 24 milligrams of the extra 240 milligrams needed each month in the diet of women are actually absorbed.

2. Chapter 8 explained that the RDA are designed to meet the needs of practically all healthy people. The recommendations must therefore be high enough to cover the iron loss of women who have a greater-than-average blood loss.

Although, on the average, only about 150 milligrams of dietary iron are needed each month to replace menstrual loss of iron, the RDA is based on replacing 240 milligrams in order to compensate for individual variation.

Oral Contraceptive Drugs

We learned in Chapter 14 that women who plan to become pregnant need to plan their diet carefully to ensure adequate nutrient stores. On the other hand, women who wish to avoid becoming pregnant and who use oral contraceptive drugs (OCD) also need to give special attention to their diets. The OCD that contain estrogens alter the absorption, metabolism, transport, or excretion of several nutrients.

Researchers are currently trying to determine whether the observed changes mean that different amounts of vitamins and minerals are required by women who are taking OCD. Unraveling the answer to this question is complicated by the fact that several laboratory tests are used to detect each micronutrient deficiency. In some instances, one of the measures for a particular vitamin is low for women who are taking OCD, but other tests for the same vitamin are normal. For example, women taking OCD excrete an increased amount of xanthurenic acid; this compound made from tryptophan is excreted by people whose diet is deficient in pyridoxine. Other tests for pyridoxine deficiency remain normal, however, in women taking OCD.

Low blood levels of several micronutrients have been found among OCD users.

1. Low folic acid levels in some but not all women. (This finding may be due either to impaired absorption or to more rapid transfer of folic acid from the blood to the tissues.)

2. Low vitamin C levels. (The hormones in OCD increase the activity of the enzyme that oxidizes vitamin C.)

3. Low vitamin B_{12} levels in about half the users. (Tissue levels of this vitamin do not appear to be affected.)

On the other hand, blood levels of three other micronutrients are higher in OCD users than in other women.

1. High vitamin A levels. (The hormones in OCD cause an increase in the concentration of the lipoprotein that links with this vitamin in the blood.)

2. Higher iron levels. (This finding may be related to the decreased amount of menstrual blood loss when women take OCD.)

3. High copper levels. (Levels of the protein that binds and transports copper are elevated.)

The significance of these changes in terms of health and the need for dietary modification or use of micronutrient supplements comprise a major area

317

of nutrition research. Until these questions are resolved, it is wise to remember that a little knowledge is a dangerous thing. For example, some doctors fear that women taking OCD who self-prescribe pyridoxine may create a nutritional problem for themselves. High intakes of pyridoxine can alter riboflavin metabolism and may cause a deficiency of riboflavin. The "cure" may be worse than the original problem, unless the vitamin-supplement regimen is supervised by a physician.

Alcohol Consumption

Certain foods are more often a part of the diet of men or of women. One of the greatest differences between the sexes is in the consumption of alcoholic beverages. Figure 18-3 shows that the percentage of men who drink alcohol is greater than the percentage of women who drink. Heavy drinking is much more common among men than among women.°

Both men and women drinkers should be aware of the energy value of the various types of alcoholic beverages. Men, who usually have fewer problems meeting their micronutrient RDA, should realize how much alcohol adds to their total energy intake, thus possibly contributing to obesity and associated health problems. Women need to be more keenly aware that alcohol reduces the nutrient density of their diet. The energy value of the alcoholic beverages a women drinks must be deducted from the relatively small amount of energy that can be alloted to nutrient-dilute foods or foods that provide only energy.

IDENTIFYING POTENTIAL PROBLEMS

Some nutrition problems are common to both sexes, but others occur more frequently among males or

° The disease alcoholism is usually accompanied by changes in the way the body absorbs, metabolizes, and excretes several nutrients. The food intake of people with this disease is often reduced. Further details of this medical condition go beyond the scope of this book.

among females. The nutrients, and therefore the foods, that should be emphasized by each sex can be identified by examining the RDA table and survey findings.

Nutrient Density

At first glance, the RDA table suggests that it is much easier for women than men to select a nutritionally adequate diet. Women have a lower RDA for protein, vitamin A, vitamin E, niacin, riboflavin, thiamin, iodine, and magnesium. The major reason that women have more difficulty meeting their RDA is that they need only about 75 percent as much energy as do men. When we compare the RDA per 1,000 Cal (4,200 kJ), we can see that women need a much more nutrient-dense diet for the nutrients shown in Table 18-1. The RDA per 1,000 Cal (4,200 kJ) is approximately the same for men and women for thiamin, riboflavin, vitamin E, niacin, and iodine.

Iron. The RDA for iron for women (18 milligrams) is almost double the RDA for men (10 milligrams). It is important therefore that women familiarize themselves with, and eat, foods that are good sources of this mineral. Many people equate red meat with iron. However, other foods, such as enriched and whole-grain cereals, vegetables, some dried fruits, and beans, also provide a great deal of iron (Table 18-2). Foods with a high iron INQ help women meet their iron RDA without exceeding their energy RDA.

Women who cut down on bread because they erroneously think it is fattening, fail to appreciate the potential contribution of cereal products to meeting their need for iron. They are, in fact, acting counter to the major program in this country developed to improve iron status—enrichment of bread and cereal products.

The program of enrichment with iron is an example of how the application of science must be based on a comparison of potential benefits and risks.

SECTION IV / NUTRITION THROUGH THE LIFESPAN

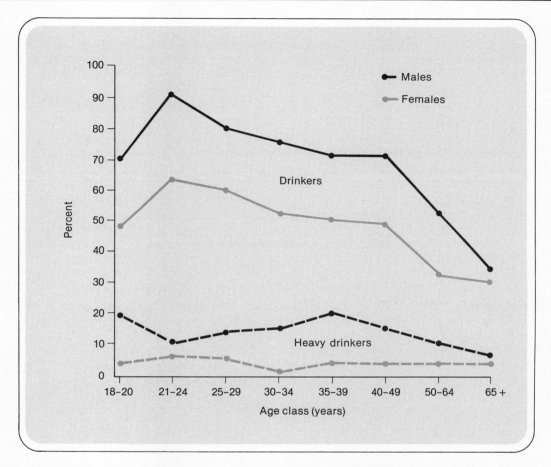

FIGURE 18-3. Percentage of drinkers and heavy drinkers among men and women. SOURCE: M. E. Chafetz, *Second Special Report to the U.S. Congress on Alcohol and Health,* DHEW, Public Health Service; Alcohol, Drug Abuse, and Mental Health Administration, Rockville, Md., DHEW Publication No. (ADM) 75-212 (June 1974).

When the Food and Drug Administration (FDA) proposed in the early 1970s to raise the amount of iron added to enriched foods, there was both opposition and encouragement from different groups of scientists. The philosophy behind any enrichment program is to add a nutrient that is low in the average diet to a food that is commonly used by most people. Breads and cereals were chosen as the foods to carry more iron into the American diet because they are inexpensive and therefore available to low-income groups who often have deficient diets.° Also, since they pass through factories between farm and table, the nutrient can be added during processing.

However, iron, like most other nutrients, can

°Fortification of salt with iodine was based on a similar philosophy.

TABLE 18-1. RDA per 1,000 Cal for Males and Females

Sex	Protein (g)	Vitamin A (IU)	Vitamin D (IU)	Vitamin C (mg)	Pyridoxine (mg)	Vitamin B$_{12}$ (mcg)	Folacin (mcg)	Calcium (mg)	Iron (mg)	Magnesium (mg)	Zinc (mg)
Male	20.7	1,850	147	17	0.7	1.1	150	296	3.7	130	5.6
Female	23.0	2,000	200	23	1.0	1.5	200	400	9.0	150	7.5

NOTE: Calculated by dividing the RDA for each nutrient by the RDA for energy.

TABLE 18-2. Selected Sources of Dietary Iron

Food	Serving Size	Energy (Cal)	Energy (kJ)	Iron INQ	Percentage of U.S. RDA per Serving
Beef, pot roast					
lean and fat	3 oz.	245	1,029	1.51	16
lean only	2½ oz.	140	588	2.46	15
Beef and vegetable stew	1 cup	210	882	1.70	16
Chili con carne with beans	1 cup	335	1,407	1.60	23
Liver, beef, fried	2 oz.	130	546	4.91	28
Oysters, raw	1 cup	160	672	10.54	73
Beans, most varieties	1 cup	200–350	840–1,470	1.7–3.0	26–33
Asparagus, canned	1 cup	45	190	11.64	23
Beans, green or yellow wax	1 cup	45	190	8.23	16
Spinach, cooked	1 cup	40	168	12.78	22
Apricots, dried uncooked	1 cup	390	1,638	2.69	46
cooked, unsweetened,					
fruit and liquid	1 cup	240	1,008	2.72	28
Prune juice	1 cup	200	840	6.71	58
Raisins	1 cup	480	2,016	1.54	32
Bran flakes, 40%, fortified	1 cup	105	441	14.97	68
Bread, whole-grain	¼ lb.	275	1,155	1.58	19
Spaghetti with meat balls					
and tomato sauce, canned	1 cup	260	1,095	1.62	18
Blackstrap molasses	1 T.	45	190	9.09	18

SOURCE: Excerpted from R. G. Hansen, A. W. Sorenson, and A. J. Wittmer, *Index of Nutritional Quality Food Profiles*, (Logan, Utah: Utah State University, 1975). © 1975, Utah State University. Used by permission.

have ill effects if it is consumed in excessive amounts. Iron is largely retained by the body. Very little is excreted in the urine, so over a period of years even a moderately excessive intake may result in considerable iron stores, especially in the liver and other organs. In the average varied diet, there is little likelihood that adding more iron to enriched foods will cause excessive iron stores and impairment to health. But some scientists opposed the increase in the iron enrichment level because they felt that a problem might arise for people with extremely high energy intakes who rely heavily upon enriched cereal products to furnish this energy. The scientists who favored the increase in the iron enrichment level thought that this possibility was rare and that the low intake of iron, especially among women and children, was a more serious problem.

The FDA has held public hearings to listen to both viewpoints. At the time of this writing, it has not yet decided whether the benefits of the higher enrichment level to iron deficient people outweigh the risks to others. This dilemma, like the saccharin issue mentioned in Chapter 12, is only one of many benefit-risk questions that arise with increasing frequency

Calcium. Although the RDA for calcium is lower for adults (800 milligrams) than for teen-agers (1,200 milligrams), intake of this mineral deserves more attention from adults than it usually receives. In this case, social influences conflict with nutrition wisdom. One of the best sources of calcium—milk—is not considered an appropriate beverage for adults on many occasions. For example, cabin attendants on airlines rarely offer (though they do provide) milk to adults; coffee or wine usually accompanies social luncheons or dinners.

An adult who does not drink milk will have trouble devising a diet that contains 800 milligrams of calcium unless particular attention is given to eating cheeses, other dairy products, and dark-green, leafy vegtables. Meat, cereals, and fruits cannot provide enough of this mineral. The U.S. RDA for calcium (1,000 milligrams) can be supplied by either 1 quart of milk or 5 ounces of cheddar cheese; but it takes 4 pounds of celery, 5 pounds of cabbage, 17 pounds of beef, or 25 pounds of potatoes to supply the same amount of this mineral.

Other Micronutrients. A woman must keep in mind all the nutrients she needs in a greater nutrient density (Table 18-1) as she plans her basic diet. Women can adapt their diets most easily by being broadly conscious of the nutrient density of their overall diet, rather than trying to give special attention to each nutrient. Those who are relatively sedentary, and especially those who are small, cannot nutritionally afford to eat many foods that supply only energy (Figure 18-4). Nutrient-dilute foods such as pastries and fried foods make it difficult for a woman to get adequate amounts of vitamins and minerals and still not exceed her energy needs. A nutritionally adequate diet for a small, inactive

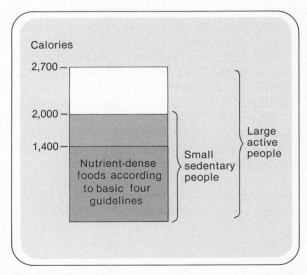

FIGURE 18-4. Distribution of energy for basic foods and nutrient-dilute foods for small sedentary people versus large active people.

321

woman is similar to a weight-reduction diet for a larger, more active person (Chapter 9).

Survey Findings

The three surveys discussed in Chapter 13 show that the type and degree of nutritional problems for men and women differ. Table 13-2, which summarizes the USDA Household Survey, indicates intakes below the RDA for women for all nutrients except vitamin C and protein. Their most severe dietary inadequacies are for iron and calcium. Adult males had a much better record. The average dietary intakes for men over age 35 showed a problem with calcium that worsened as the men grew older, but the average intakes for all other nutrients met the RDA for men between the ages of 18 and 74.

The Ten-State Nutrition Survey (Table 13-3) found that in the low-income and vulnerable groups studied, iron was as much a problem for men as for women. Obesity was much more prevalent among women in this population, and men had lower intakes of vitamin C than women. Minimal deficiencies of protein were found in black women and in Spanish-Americans of both sexes in the low-income-ratio states.

The HANES reported that mean dietary intakes of calcium, iron, and vitamin A were lower (compared to its standards) for women than for men.° This correlation held true regardless of ethnic group or income level. Vitamin C intakes, however, were approximately the same for males and females.

The results of blood analyses performed during the HANES suggest a problem that had not been anticipated by nutritionists. The survey found that men, as well as women, had low values for the two simple tests for anemia, hemoglobin and hematocrit determinations (Figure 18-5). These findings are surprising since the average dietary intake of iron for men was above the RDA, while that for women

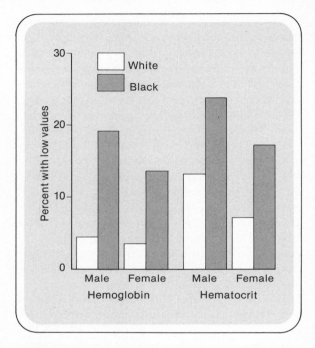

FIGURE 18-5. Indexes of anemia for males and females obtained from the HANES, 1971–1972. SOURCE: S. Abraham, F. W. Lowenstein, and C. L. Johnson, *Preliminary Findings of the First Health and Nutrition Examination Survey, United States, 1971–72: Dietary Intake and Biochemical Findings,* Publication No. (HRA) 74-1219-1 (Washington, D.C.: U.S. Department of Health, Education, and Welfare, 1974).

was below the RDA. Physicians in this country are accustomed to treating iron deficiency in women, but the extent of low hemoglobins and hematocrits —indexes of iron deficiency—among males is unexpected.

Several of the possible explanations for the differences between biochemical and dietary data involve concepts discussed in earlier chapters.

1. We might question the appropriateness of the standards for each measure.
2. Averages mask individual differences in dietary intakes.

° This difference between intakes for men and women is also apparent when the data are compared to the RDA as a standard.

On the basis of the USDA Household Survey it can be estimated that women should consume one more serving per day of foods from the cereal, milk, and fruits/vegetables group. The same survey shows that the average diets of men provide more than 130 grams of animal fat per day.

TABLE 18-3. Comparison of the Amounts of Foods Eaten by Men and Women

Food	Approximate Weight of One Serving (g)	Consumption by Males (g)	Consumption by Males (Approximate Servings)*	Consumption by Females (g)	Consumption by Females (Approximate Servings)*	Basic Four Guidelines (Servings)
Meat, poultry, and fish	100 (about 3 oz.)	340	3½	200	2	2
Cereal and grain products	30 (1 oz. cereal)	125	4	80	2⅔	4
Fruits and vegetables	100	425	4¼	300	3	4
Milk and milk products	240 (1 cup)	400	1⅔	290	1¼	2
Beverages other than milk and juices	240 (1 cup)	950	4	730	3	—

*Calculated by dividing consumption in grams by approximate weight of one serving of each type of food.

NOTE: Values for males and females 20 to 34 years old from the USDA Household Survey.

3. The indicators of anemia may be low due to something other than iron deficiency (such as the lack of another nutrient or some other problem to be discussed in Chapter 22).

4. The absorption of dietary iron may differ between men and women due to composition of the diet or other factors.

Whatever the reason for the incidence of anemia, men should not ignore the importance of iron in their diet simply because their RDA is lower than women's.

Food Patterns

The consistent finding of nutrition surveys that women more frequently fail to meet their RDA for certain nutrients than men can be explained in part by reviewing the types and average amounts of foods eaten by males versus females. This information can be estimated from the results of the USDA Household Survey, which reported the consumption in grams of different categories of food (Table 18-3). If we make some assumptions regarding the weight of an average serving of food in each group, we can compare the results of this survey to the basic four guidelines.

Table 18-3 suggests that the diets of men almost meet the minimum guidelines. The average milk consumption of men is slightly lower than recommended, but the slightly higher than recommended use of fruits and vegetables helps avoid inadequate intakes of calcium and other B vitamins.

On the other hand, women meet the basic four guidelines only for the meat group. They should consume approximately one more serving per day from each of the other three food groups. It is no wonder, therefore, that their nutrient intakes frequently fall below the RDA. Since the average energy intake of women is not below the RDA, it is reasonable to assume from Table 18-3 that nutrient-dilute foods and those that supply only energy are displacing nutrient-dense foods from their diets.

Although men do a better job of meeting their nutrient needs than do women, Table 18-3 suggests that they may have another type of dietary problem. An average consumption of 340 grams of foods from the meat group means that men consume more protein than they need and more fat (and cholesterol) than is advisable. This possibility is based on the following assumptions and calculations:

1. If meat averages 35 percent fat, men consume about 119 grams (340 grams × 0.35) of fat from foods in the meat group.
2. If milk is 3.5 percent fat, men consume another 14 grams (400 grams × 0.035) of fat from this group.
3. These two values show that men average an intake of 133 grams (119 + 14) of fat from these two groups alone. This does not include the fat that enters their diet as salad dressing, margarine, butter, or cooking oils.
4. The energy value of the 133 grams of fat from the meat and milk groups alone is 1,200 Cal (5,040 kJ). This equals about 40 percent of the energy from a 3,200 Cal diet (the average—and excessive—energy intake of Americans).

These analyses of food patterns lead to a practical understanding of survey findings, which are reported in terms of nutrients rather than foods consumed. The next step in our line of reasoning is to discuss how men and women can plan more appropriate diets based on the problems we have identified.

PLANNING APPROPRIATE DIETS

Food selections are largely determined by where we eat. Let's consider the options for modifying the diets of men and women when they eat out, snack, or eat at home.

Meals Away from Home

Planning diets that meet individual needs is easier when a couple eats out than when they eat at home, because each person can order the type of food that fits his or her particular nutritional needs. We have already seen (Chapter 10) that the appropriateness of fast-food meals depends upon the combined nutrient composition of the items selected compared to individual nutrient needs.

When a man looks at a menu, he should consider how much high-fat food he has already eaten or plans to eat that day. A medium-size hamburger may be a more appropriate choice than a large steak. A chicken sandwich (lightly spread with mayonnaise) supplies less fat than fried chicken. Broiled fish may be a wiser choice than pork chops. If a man is watching his weight and is certain that his diet contains enough meat, eating out may be a good time to omit meat and add vegetables to his diet. He can order several side dishes of vegetables or a large salad.

Women are often confronted with excessively large portions of food when they eat out. To avoid eating too much, they may choose to completely by-pass the list of entrees on the menu and order an appetizer, salad, vegetable(s), and beverage. The amount of quiche, seafood, or chopped chicken liver served as an appetizer in some restaurants is sufficient to meet the needs of many women, especially those who are inactive. This will prevent the meat portion of the meal from taking the place of vegetables and dairy products that are needed to balance nutrient intake. Women who have trouble including enough dairy products in their diet should scan a menu for salads made with cottage cheese or dishes containing other types of cheese.

Alcoholic beverages are consumed more frequently by most people when they eat out than when they eat at home. The alcohol in a Bloody Mary dilutes the nutrient density of tomato juice, but if a diet is frequently lacking in fruits and vegetables, this drink is preferable to a straight alcoholic beverage or one combined with a soft drink.

Desserts generally dilute the nutrient density of the diet, but some selections provide enough nutrients to compensate for their energy value. The appropriateness of custards, certain types of pies, ice cream, or fruit dishes in a diet depends upon their energy and nutrient content and other foods eaten during the day. If a woman wants to keep energy intake down, she should learn to enjoy a cup of coffee or tea after a meal without a dessert.

Snacking

Selecting appropriate snacks is a simple way to adjust an individual diet without complicating food preparation for a whole family. The amount of food eaten between meals, if properly chosen, may be enough to take care of differences in nutrient needs between men and women. The information in Chapter 10 should help men find snacks that keep their total intake of fat and cholesterol to a minimum while providing a sufficient amount of other nutrients. Women can best snack on nutrient-dense sources of iron, folacin, and calcium, such as raw, leafy vegetables or vegetable juice.

Meals at Home

When a man and woman eat together at home, planning appropriate diets for both need not be complicated or cumbersome (Table 18-4). One sim-

ple guideline is that the addition of nutrient-dilute foods and those that supply only energy should take place at the table—not in the kitchen. Let each person add to foods whatever sugar, salad dressing, sauces, and butter he or she may want, rather than mixing these in before serving. Women who are aware of their need for a nutrient-dense diet can then add only small amounts, while men can use more if they wish. A woman may also keep her iron and calcium needs in mind and reach for seconds of vegetables rather than meat. At the end of the meal, she can cut herself a smaller piece of pie for dessert to avoid excess energy intake.

Other maneuvers in the kitchen can improve the nutritional appropriateness of the diet for either a man or a woman. A mixed green salad prepared for a woman might have extra amounts of carrots (vitamin A), peppers (vitamin C), and tomatoes (vitamins A and C). Her cottage cheese and fruit salad can have more cottage cheese and less sweetened canned fruit than his. Fat content of the diet can be reduced for a man and nutrient density increased for a woman by removing the skin from chicken before cooking, trimming visible fat from meat, and buying

TABLE 18-4. Examples of Diet Modifications for Women and Men

Food	Women	Men
Hamburger	Half a bun with lettuce and tomatoes	Imitation mayonnaise (lower in fat and cholesterol) or spread lightly with regular mayonnaise
Mixed green salad	More carrots, peppers, tomatoes; perhaps use raw spinach (extra folacin)	Use low-calorie dressing or vinegar and spices
Coffee	Add whole milk (calcium and riboflavin)	Add nondairy substitute (low in fat and cholesterol)
Breakfast juice	Prune juice (iron); tomato juice (vitamin A) or vegetable juice cocktail (vitamins A and C)	Choice depends on other foods eaten that day
Snacks	Raisins, milk, cheese, yogurt, raw vegetables, fruit	Popcorn (without butter); cottage cheese; crackers, fruit

lean cuts of meat rather than those marbled with fat.

Breakfast is often prepared and eaten separately by each member of the family; therefore, it is fairly easy to tailor this meal to different nutrient needs. A woman should recognize that breakfast provides an opportunity to increase the nutrient density of her diet. Fortified cereal may be the best breakfast choice for a woman, whereas a man may have greater flexibility of choice. If a woman's diet later in the day will provide ample vitamin C, she should consider the folacin, iron, and vitamin A content of food options other than orange or grapefruit juice. Prune juice, tomato juice, or vegetable juice cocktail might better fit her diet plans.

Although it is unrealistic and unnecessary to pre-pare a different menu for each person in the family, beverages can be individually selected without causing much additional work. A woman may drink a glass of milk with her meal and add milk to her coffee to help meet her needs for calcium and riboflavin. A man who is concerned about fat and cholesterol, as well as calcium and riboflavin, might prefer skim milk with his meal and a nondairy substitute creamer in his coffee.

There are no ironclad rules about foods that are "right" or "wrong" for men and women. Each item must be considered in the context of a total diet. The suggestions above and those in Table 18-4 hopefully can stimulate your thoughts and lead you to choose the most appropriate total diet.

STUDY QUESTIONS

1. Why are there differences between appropriate diets for men and women?

2. How does menstruation affect the nutrient needs of women?

3. What nutrients are affected by the use of oral contraceptive drugs?

4. How does alcohol consumption affect energy intake and nutrient density of the diet?

5. What are the two main dietary considerations for women?

6. Why do women fail to meet their RDA more frequently than men?

7. How does the incidence of obesity among women compare to that among men?

8. What did the USDA Household Survey show about the approximate number of servings of food from each food group chosen by men and by women?

9. Plan a dinner menu that might be easily modified by a man and a woman to increase its nutritional appropriateness.

SUGGESTED READING

1. J. C. King, "Nutrition during oral contraceptive treatment," *Contemporary Nutrition* 2, No. 1 (1976).
2. M. A. Ohlson and L. J. Harper, "Longitudinal studies of food intake and weight of women from ages 18 to 56," *Journal of the American Dietetic Association* 69(1976):629–31.
3. M. Mead, "Comments on the division of labor in occupations concerned with food," *Journal of the American Dietetic Association* 68(1976):321–25.
4. B. Villet, "Heart attack: Not for men only," *Today's Health* 53(1975):24–27, 51–53.
5. E. R. Monsen, I. N. Kuhn, and C. A. Finch, "Iron status of menstruating women," *American Journal of Clinical Nutrition* 20(1967):842.
6. N. Nordquest and E. Medved, "A nutrition counseling session for college women on the pill," *Journal of Nutrition Education* 7(1975):29–31.
7. A. A. Rimm et al, "Relationship of obesity and disease in 73,532 weight-conscious women," *Public Health Reports* 90(1975):44–51.
8. "Effects of oral contraceptive hormones on nutrient metabolism: Symposium," *American Journal of Clinical Nutrition* 28(1975):333–413.
9. J. G. Chopra et al, "Maternal nutrition and family planning," *American Journal of Clinical Nutrition* 23(1970):1043.

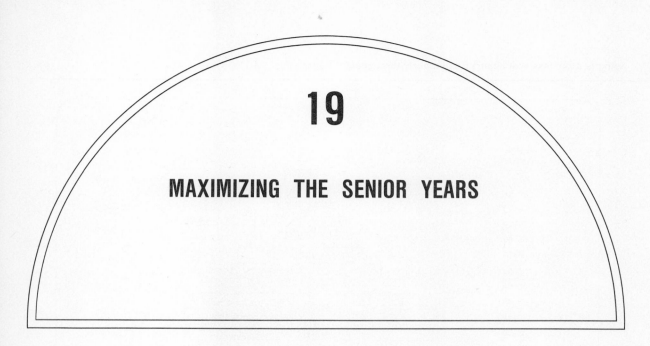

19

MAXIMIZING THE SENIOR YEARS

Aging begins at the moment of conception. It is a continuum, defined as the progression of changes in biochemical processes that determine structural and functional alterations with age in the entire body. These changes happen to everyone at varying rates and in slightly different sequences. In this chapter we discuss the alterations that occur in our bodies as we age and other factors that influence food choices among the elderly.

YOUNG PEOPLE AND ELDERS

Many young people find it difficult to relate to the elderly, especially those outside their own family or circle of friends. However, there are several reasons why the young should acquaint themselves with the nutritional needs of older people and the difficulties encountered in meeting these needs.

Social Concerns

During the years when the Peace Corps flourished, the youth of America began to participate more actively in international health and development programs than previously. This interest has continued and expanded to include involvement in efforts to improve the quality of life for many of the disadvantaged in our own country. All young people do not feel this concern and still fewer express it with an investment of time and energy, but many young volunteers help in programs for those less fortunate than themselves.

A large portion of the over-60 population in the United States might well be considered among the disadvantaged. Almost 7 million of the 30 million Americans in this age group live at or below 125 percent of the poverty level. Of the several million who are too frail to leave their residences, less than 30,000 received home-delivered meals in 1975.

The special nutritional problems and other needs of the elderly will become much more important to society during the lifetime of today's youth. Figure 19-1 shows that in 1970 there was an extremely large proportion of young people in the world compared to older people, but medicine and science are increasingly able to control many causes of death and to extend life expectancy. These advances, combined with the possible success of international efforts to control birth rates, mean that older people will make up a larger percentage of the total world

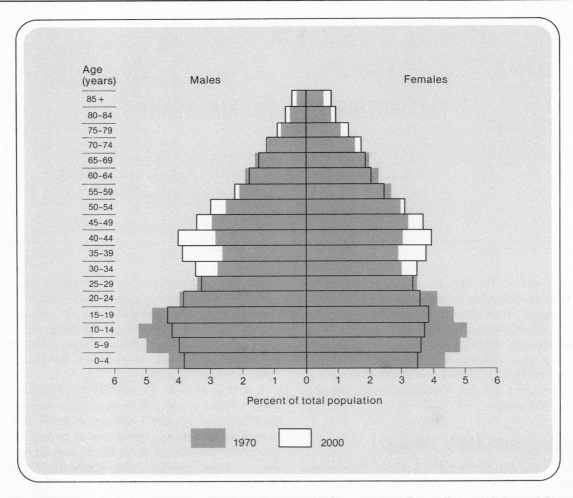

FIGURE 19-1. Predicted change in age distribution of the U.S. population. (From ''The populations of the developed countries'' by Charles F. Westoff, in *Scientific American* 114 (September 1974). Copyright © 1974 by Scientific American, Inc. All rights reserved.)

population as we approach the year 2000 (Figure 19-1). People who are young today have the opportunity of heightening society's awareness of the importance of improving the lot of this growing segment of society. Perhaps this can be accomplished before they themselves are numbered among the elderly.

Similarities Related to Diet

The socioeconomic position of youth today is similar in certain ways to that of the elderly. Many of the nutrition problems linked to lifestyle are therefore held in common.

One similarity is that both the young and the old

suffer most when unemployment rates rise. Reduction in income has obvious effects upon diet for people of all ages.

Another similarity is due to the erosion of the extended family concept in the United States during this century. The elderly are no longer maintained within the family unit and the youth are moving beyond the family unit at earlier ages. People who live alone—regardless of their age—tend to have less regular eating patterns than families who combine consuming food with communicating with each other.

Perhaps surprisingly, there is also a developmental similarity between the young and the old. We have learned in Chapter 17 that children enter pubescence at different ages and maturation does not occur at the same pace for all teen-agers. Physiological age does not parallel calendar age for older people either. Although the population over age 65 is generally classified as elderly for statistical purposes, this definition is incongruous with the health of many older people. It is more biologically accurate to define the aged as people who have experienced 65 percent of the alterations identified by gerontologists as being associated with aging—whether this happens at 40 or 80 years of age.

Shaping the Future

The period from age 20 to 40 is the time when nutrition may exert its maximal effect in the prevention of disease during the remaining adult life. It is important for people to accept this unrefutable fact as early in life as possible, because many nutrition-related problems that surface during later years are irreversible once they occur.

Preparations for old age are part of living. Many middle-aged adults try to plan some financial security and develop hobbies to enjoy after retirement. They acquire recommended medical supervision and some cope with the psychological problems that arise as they see more and more friends their own age die. Despite all these rational preparations for their later years, few people learn in advance how to modify their diet to adapt to the inevitable physiological and socioeconomic changes. The last week before retirement is not the time to make a quick change to new diet patterns. For many people, dietary problems have begun long before this date.

To avoid problems in later life, young adults should remind themselves that the chances of achieving the best possible nutritional status during the elder years are greatest if they master information about nutrition early and reinforce this knowledge with an awareness of physiological and socioeconomic variables that affect diet patterns.

INTERDEPENDENT PROBLEMS

It is misleading to discuss the food patterns and problems of the elderly in isolation from the physiological and socioeconomic changes that so often occur at the same time. These problems are interwoven and, together, they comprise the health of older people.

Physiological Changes

At any point in life, each individual body represents the cumulative effects of its physical, psychological, and social environment as well as its genetically determined characteristics. The changes that constitute aging are affected by the life a person leads. In general, however, similar changes in overall metabolism° occur in everyone.

The cellular changes that accompany aging are thought to be the result of a combination of two processes.

° Anabolism and catabolism occur in people of all ages. Most anabolic processes dominate during growth and decrease after biological maturity has been attained.

Cell death and decrease in cellular function contribute to the aging process.
The functioning of many body systems gradually declines during the later years of life, and changes in one system affect other systems.

1. Cell death—the actual amount of actively metabolizing body tissues declines with age.

2. Decrease in function—the rate of many, though not all, metabolic reactions is slower in older people.

Many theories have been proposed to explain why these alterations occur. Several theories involve various steps within the protein synthesizing mechanisms of the body. Others relate to the accumulation of waste products from normal cellular breakdown. Even more intricate theories suggest that aging is related to alterations in the stability of cellular membranes. Some changes have been attributed to viruses and others to the effects of radiation. How much the processes associated with aging can be slowed down is currently unknown, but this question remains a major challenge to physicians and basic science researchers.

The ultimate result of cellular changes is that the functioning of many body systems gradually declines (with varying severity) during the elder years. A few of the physiological changes are cited below. Note how each alteration affects another.

Alterations in Body Composition. Some examples of changes in body composition that are part of the aging process are (1) decreased total body water, (2) decreased calcium content in bones, and (3) partial replacement of the lean body mass of active muscles by fat.

Reduction in Energy Needs. As a consequence of the smaller amount of metabolizing body tissue and reduction in activity, energy needs are decreased. Basal metabolism of an average person over 70 is only 80 percent of that of a 22-year-old.

Skeletal System. The sedentary life of many older people complicates several nutrient-dependent processes in the body. Most adults do not require dietary vitamin D, but if an older person is rarely exposed to sunlight, he or she must obtain more of this nutrient from food. The skeletal system

of elderly people is also jeopardized because inactivity causes bone tissue to be dissolved faster than it is deposited. This principle of nutrition was noted years ago in bedridden hospital patients, and it was confirmed by studies on the early astronauts who had little exercise during their voyages into space.

Circulatory System. The optimal performance of many body functions is dependent upon an adequate blood flow, which brings oxygen, nutrients, and other substances to the cells, carries away wastes, and transports hormones and other specialized proteins from one organ to another. Functioning of the circulatory system of the elderly is often complicated by a reduction in the inner diameter of blood vessels. Arteries of older people also become less flexible and therefore fail to enlarge and constrict normally. Consequently, their circulatory system is less efficient in distributing blood to the heart and other muscles when exercising, or to the intestines and liver after eating. When the heart does not have maximal contractile power, blood also circulates more slowly through the kidneys, lungs, and other parts of the body.

Gastrointestinal Tract. Many of the nutrition problems of the elderly are related to changes in the gastrointestinal tract—from mouth to anus. By age 65, 53 percent of the elderly have lost all their teeth through decay and periodontal disease; 6 percent of the elderly need false teeth but do not have them. Saliva production is diminished, and this makes lubrication of food more difficult. A decreased sensitivity to taste and smell reduces the pleasure of eating and also interferes with stimulation of hydrochloric acid secretion by the stomach cells. The secretion of many digestive enzymes declines with age. Digestion is further impaired by a decreased flow of bile (necessary for fat digestion) and reduced flow of blood through the intestinal cells. A reduction in intestinal secretion of mucus combined with lack of exercise contribute to constipation, which plagues many older people.

Adjusting the diet to physiological changes is further complicated for the elderly by socioeconomic factors such as reduced income and political forces that increase social isolation.

Socioeconomic Determinants

In the United States, few of the elderly are cared for within the family. Many people over age 65 are widowed (14 percent of males and 52 percent of females) and a large percentage of them live alone. Widowers are especially vulnerable to poor diets, because most of them have always relied on their wives to purchase and prepare food. Late in life, they must learn to plan their own diets, and they rarely understand even the most fundamental concepts about nutrition.

Limited Income. The diet options of the elderly are often restricted by limited income. This situation is especially difficult for people who may have been accustomed to an unlimited food budget before retirement.

Many older people move into smaller living quarters after their children leave home, and sometimes they no longer have appliances (such as freezers or ovens) that allow greater flexibility in food choices or dishwashers that lighten the chores associated with food preparation.

Political Factors. The adequacy of diets may also be affected by politics. The nutrition problems of children and mothers are more visible to society than those of the elderly, who are tucked away in nursing homes, or unable to stray far from their boarding houses into the pathway of the rest of society. Older people have only recently begun to develop an effective political lobby and to impress upon society their unique needs. Their dependent position and lesser numbers in the past have permitted society to neglect them, but this situation is changing.

Some existing health and welfare policies make solving the problems related to the isolation of the elderly difficult. Although people tend to eat more regularly when they eat with others, elderly couples receive less benefits from the government than elderly individuals who live alone. Another impedi-

ment is that the existing health delivery system provides assistance for institutionalization of the elderly, but offers little help if those same people are cared for and fed within their own families.

These problems are compounded because research regarding health and social problems of the elderly and programs to implement this knowledge can only be funded by tax dollars. Younger people generate these moneys through their income tax and they primarily decide how the monies will be spent.

COMBINED EFFECTS UPON DIET

All of these factors—and more—affect the diets of older people by limiting their acquisition and enjoyment of food, as well as restricting the maximal utilization of nutrients that are eaten.

Acquisition and Preparation of Food

Acquisition of food is complicated by physical limitations. Carrying groceries is difficult, especially if one hand is needed for a cane. Something as simple as a grocery cart with a malfunctioning wheel creates an annoyance to a healthy person but an impasse to someone with the limitations of aging.

Elderly people with impaired vision have food problems that rarely occur to others. If they cannot drive a car, they can only buy the small amount of groceries they can carry on each shopping trip. Some elderly people have difficulty reading instructions on food packages and are discouraged from trying new foods. The fine print of the nutrition information panel of food labels is of limited value to many older people. Furthermore, impaired vision may cause a person unknowingly to consume food that is moldy (especially if taste perception is poor also), and the consequences of food poisoning are more severe for the elderly than for younger adults.

Weakness is a result of poor nutrition, but it can also cause dietary problems. Many elderly people are not strong enough to operate a can opener or open a jar. Frozen food packages are easier to open, but are often more expensive. Preparing a meal and cleaning up the kitchen may seem to be exhausting chores, and eventually an elderly person may feel that eating is not worth the effort.

Enjoyment of Food

The elderly person who assumes new activities and interests does not experience a significant change in his or her attitude toward food, but the person who retires in front of a television set or cannot even afford this entertainment may find that much of life revolves around meals. For the person who lives alone, being invited out to dinner or having someone bring food to the home may be a social interaction that greatly increases the pleasure of the day.

Although the significance of food in the daily routine may increase for older people, the enjoyment of eating may decline. Loss of taste and appetite, and the frustrations of food preparation are common problems. To make matters worse, eating causes upset digestion, pain to the mouth, and constipation—hardly pleasant experiences—for some elderly people.

Restricted taste sensitivity may have far-reaching consequences, especially when combined with a restricted budget and poor health. Condiments and spices are expensive, but salt is cheap. The elderly person may use large amounts of salt in hopes of attaining the desired taste sensation. If the person has hypertension, excessive intakes of sodium complicate control of this condition. If an individual has some degree of heart failure, high salt intake may lead to water retention. (This may be recognized as puffiness of the skin, edema, which also reflects the water load of the inner tissues.) A cycle ensues as more salt and water are retained, thus worsening the heart failure. This is accompanied by decreased blood flow to the kidneys, decreased urine output, and further swelling and incapacitation.

Use of Food by the Body

Socioeconomic factors and physiological changes alter nutrient requirements and utilization.

Energy Balance. The activity level of older people can lead to energy intakes that are either inadequate or excessive. Decreased income and the social situation of the elderly limit their activity. Many older people, especially women, have low back pain and other bone discomforts that restrict their exercise. Some people have physical handicaps that totally confine them to their homes, wheelchairs, or beds. Many of the elderly voluntarily reduce their activity, especially in bad weather, because they are afraid of having an accident. They know that people their age recover more slowly from broken bones.

If any of these circumstances impair acquisition and preparation of food, energy and nutrient deficiencies are likely. On the other hand, if food continues to be accessible and activity is minimal, the result may be obesity. The HANES identified both these nutrition problems—underweight and overweight—among the older Americans surveyed. This finding emphasizes the importance of tailoring a diet to individual energy and nutrient needs.

Absorption. The inability of many elderly people to absorb maximally the nutrients in their food is partly due to inevitable physiological changes. The most consistent problem is reduction of iron absorption due to decreased secretion of acid by the stomach. However, some problems occur because of improper selection of foods. Both folacin and vitamin B_{12} have primary roles in maintaining the absorptive surface of the gastrointestinal tract. People who reduce their intake of leafy vegetables (sources of folacin) or meat and dairy products (sources of vitamin B_{12}) lack the nutrients needed to ensure that other nutrients in food gain access to body cells. These foods are sometimes avoided by the elderly because they are difficult to prepare, uncomfortable to chew, expensive, or cause other problems.

Common Ailments. The multitude of physical problems common among the elderly vastly complicate their nutritional needs and diets. A physician may not be able to prescribe the ideal dietary modification to control or cure one disease because of another abnormal condition. For example, a low-cholesterol diet may be advisable for an elderly person and therefore he or she should reduce the intake of eggs. However, if this same person has difficulty chewing meat and also gets an upset stomach from drinking milk, eggs are one of the few sources of protein and vitamin B_{12} available.

The dynamics of diet planning and disease therapy become even more complex when a person has difficulty following prescribed diets. Failing vision restricts the usefulness of printed diet instructions and poor hearing may frustrate both the patient and the diet counselor. Advancing age is also often associated with loss of recent memory, which complicates learning about foods that should or should not be eaten.

IDENTIFYING PROBLEMS

The specific nutrients and diet patterns most frequently associated with malnutrition in the elderly have been identified by nutrition surveys. Health may also be impaired by beliefs in misinformation about the nutritional benefits of certain types of food.

Survey Findings

The results of the surveys discussed in Chapter 13 are a guide to the nutrition problems of the elderly. According to the Ten-State Nutrition Survey, dietary inadequacies of iron, riboflavin, and vitamin C, and obesity were the most common problems.

The USDA Household Survey reported low average intakes for energy, calcium, and thiamin, but average intakes of vitamin C, vitamin A, and riboflavin met the RDA. Although the iron RDA for postmenopausal women is only 10 milligrams, the average intake (8.8 milligrams) of this mineral was still below the recommended level.

The HANES results for people over 60 years old were not tabulated separately for men and women, but this survey shows how greatly nutrient intakes vary within population groups. Although the mean intake for protein and three of the four micronutrients studied exceeded the RDA, a large percentage of the people over 60 consumed less than the RDA for iron (50 percent), calcium (71 percent), vitamin A (62 percent), and vitamin C (36 percent). Protein intake was less than 50 grams for 34 percent of this population. The energy consumption values from the HANES give a clue to potential problems of overweight and underweight. Although half of the people over 60 years old had quite low energy intakes (less than 1,500 Cal), 18 percent consumed what was probably an excessive amount of energy (over 2,250 Cal), unless they were relatively active people. This observation is interesting in light of the finding that the incidence of obesity is higher among women over age 45 than among younger women, but lower among males over age 45 (Figure 13-5). Obesity in both age groups was more prevalent among women with incomes below poverty level than among those with incomes above the poverty level.

Quest for Health

Another source of possible nutrition problems among older people is due to food purchasing patterns. Some elderly people hope that certain products advertised as "health foods" can slow down their aging process. Their intense desire to cling to youth outweighs their powers of reason, making them vulnerable to unfounded claims.

Young people, who are also often attracted to

these products, might benefit from nutrition facts commonly directed to the elderly. Health foods are not necessarily dangerous, but two major types of problems can result from their misuse. First, if a person tries to solve health problems by relying on these foods (or the dietary supplements and tonics sold in "health food" stores) and does not seek medical attention, the problems will continue and probably worsen. The bodies of young people may be able to tolerate this abuse for some time, but eventually the health of young and old people may deteriorate past the point where it is possible to correct the health problem, even with competent medical care.

Second, products purchased in health food stores are often more expensive than foods bought elsewhere, although the nutritional value is no better (Table 19-1). If money is not a factor, then an older person can afford to pay these prices and the food may benefit him or her psychologically. However, if money is limited, the higher price of health food will probably mean that less food and nutrients are purchased. Wealthier, healthier people can afford to play this game with their psyche, but the elderly person with little money and failing health bears the brunt of unfounded claims for such products.

AVOIDING PROBLEMS

Although many physiological changes are an inevitable part of aging, the consequences of these changes can be altered to a certain degree by wise food choices and adjustments in lifestyle.

Dietary Approaches

Although the RDA of people over age 50 (Table 8-1) decreases for niacin, riboflavin, and iodine by an amount comparable to the decrease in the RDA for energy, the elderly generally need to learn to select the more nutrient-dense options for certain nutrients (Table 8-7). They should keep their consumption of low-nutrient-density foods in line with the exercise they are willing or able to do.

Energy Needs. A simple solution to the nutrient-density problem might be to say that desserts should be omitted—but this is traditionally the fun part of a meal. If possible, the pleasure of desserts should not be withheld from the elderly. Giving up candy between meals to increase the nutrient density of the diet may be tolerable if there is occasionally a custard or chiffon pie at the end of a meal. Smaller portions of sweets also decrease the dilution of the diet. Some desserts, such as fruit combinations and dairy products, can supply vitamins, minerals, and protein, as well as energy.

On the other hand, surveys have shown that many older people simply consume too little food and, therefore, not enough energy, protein, or micronutrients. Under these circumstances, the barrier to eating must be corrected, whether it is lack of money, inability to shop for and prepare food, or simply lack of motivation to eat.

Whether the goal is to increase nutrient density or total food intake, several nutrients merit special attention.

Protein. Protein problems are more common among the elderly than among any other group except pregnant and lactating women. Meat may be avoided because it is expensive or difficult to cut and chew, but poultry may be more acceptable to older people. Baked fish is simpler to flake than either of these other two protein sources. Cold cuts and frankfurters are high in fat, but they are easy to prepare. This choice is better than doing without protein, especially if other foods do not contribute much additional fat to the total diet.

Meat alternates may be more appropriate sources of protein for older persons. Beans are a possible substitute, but they may increase intestinal gas production and discomfort. Eggs, cheese, and dairy products require some culinary creativity to be

TABLE 19-1. Cost of Groceries from a Health Food Store as a Percentage of the Cost of Groceries at a Small Grocery Store

Food	Percentage	Food	Percentage
Produce		Cereal products	
Asparagus[a]	106	Barley	151
Bananas[b]	172	Cornmeal	172
Carrots[a]	132	Popcorn	150
Mushrooms[a]	97	Ready-to-eat cereals	
Oranges[a]	184	Raisin bran	137
Pears[a]	120	Granola[a]	141
Prunes	204	Rolled oats	65
Raisins	109	Buttermilk pancake mix	198
Zucchini[a]	102	Corn chips	187
Juices		Tortilla chips	154
Apple[a]	168	Condiments and oils	
Grape[a]	130	Corn oil	133
Orange[a]	218	Peanut oil	150
Tomato[a]	451	Salad dressing	126
Vegetable cocktail[a]	237	Salad dressing mix	121
Legumes		Mayonnaise	135
Beans		Imitation	243
Baby lima	118	Olive	125
Navy	156	Pickle, kosher dill	200
Red kidney	155	Salt[a]	426
Cashews, roasted	105	Tomato catsup	176
Peanuts		Vinegar	197
In shell	97	Apple butter[a]	254
Without shell	65	Blackstrap molasses	104
Pecans	70	Honey[a]	124
Sunflower seeds	58	Maple syrup	158
Walnuts	106	Orange marmalade[a]	257
Dairy products		Peanut butter[a]	149
Brie cheese	93	Strawberry preserves[a]	311
Gouda cheese	138		
Ice cream	204		
Milk	138		
Monterey jack cheese	161		

[a] Labeled "natural" or "organic."
[b] Labeled "ungassed."

NOTE: Based on prices in May 1977; both stores were in the same block in downtown Washington, D.C.

interesting foods if they are frequently repeated in the diet, but they overcome some impediments to food consumption that hinder many elderly people.

Cheese soup makes an easy-to-prepare sauce for vegetables rich in micronutrients that may otherwise not be eaten by the elderly.

Iron. Intake of iron suffers when meat consumption declines. The meat alternates mentioned above (except dairy products) also provide iron, but their lower iron density points to the benefits of vegetable sources of this mineral.

Prune juice is a good source of iron, and its laxative effect benefits some older people. But if prune juice displaces a citrus juice that had been a primary source of vitamin C, sources of this vitamin (such as tomatoes, potatoes, and other vegetables) become even more important in the diet.

Calcium. The amount of vegetables, dairy products, and other foods needed to supply the calcium RDA are the same for a person over 50 as for a 19 year-old who uses 15 percent (female) to 20 percent (male) more energy. Many calcium sources dwindle from the diets of adults long before cellular aging accelerates, but regardless of past diet patterns, these foods should be emphasized by the elderly.

Fiber. Lack of dietary sources of fiber, which normally stimulate intestinal motility, worsens the already existing tendency among some older people toward constipation. Dentures or lack of teeth may cause people to avoid fibrous foods (such as celery). Fresh fruits and vegetables, which provide bulk in the diet, may be omitted because of cost. Under these circumstances, beans and whole-grain cereals, rather than more highly milled products, should be emphasized in the diet.

Water. Water is important in the diet of the elderly. If fluids are slighted, it will be more difficult for the kidneys (which do not function optimally) to rid the body of metabolic wastes and toxins.

Because both calcium and water are needed, milk makes an excellent contribution to the diet of the elderly. Juices and other beverages, or just plain water, drunk with or between meals can help, too. If a person has hypertension, the mineral composition (primarily the sodium and potassium content) of the beverage may determine the type of fluids that are recommended. The high water content of fruits and vegetables is yet another reason—besides their fiber and nutrient content—to include them in the diet.

Activity Patterns and Lifestyle

Solution to the nutrition problems of the elderly requires a broad perspective. For example, increasing the opportunities to socialize can improve nutritional status. The older person who is motivated to prepare a simple meal to share with a friend is on the road to better nutrition. The city government that provides reduced bus fares for senior citizens eases their grocery shopping, and thereby improves their nutrition. The grocery clerk who handles food stamps graciously lessens the trauma of acquisition of food for older people.

Another approach to solving nutrition problems is to find ways of increasing energy expenditure, thus allowing greater flexibility in food choices. The older person who uses leisure time for walks, jogging, or active hobbies (such as carpentry or crafts) has less difficulty with diet planning than the person whose view of the world is limited to a television screen. Gardening (even on a small scale) provides an opportunity to exercise and greatly augments a person's interest in eating.

The merits of these suggestions depend upon individual interests, physical condition, and specific nutrition problems. However, they are examples of how both the diets and lifestyles of older people—those you know today and yourself in the future—might be designed for better health and more enjoyment.

Feeding Programs

Most government funded food programs are designed to meet the needs of elderly people with limited incomes. Some community programs, however, reach a broader group of senior citizens. Adequate, appropriate food is part of improving the quality of life, but the only true solution combines this with social and medical assistance. Two types of programs currently offer both food and social contact for the elderly: The Meals-on-Wheels Program provides a hot meal that is brought to the elderly person at home. The Congregate Meal Program brings the elderly to a central place where they eat together.

The implementation of these programs varies among communities. A variety of facilities (senior citizens centers, community centers, homes for the aged, public housing, churches, and schools) with kitchens are used. In some instances, food is prepared elsewhere and brought into the community. Nutrition education and economy shopping are part of many programs for both the staff and the participants. In some programs, the elderly help with the implementation of the program—they prepare and serve food, organize the social functions that accompany meals, and take meals to people in their homes.

Many factors determine the effectiveness of these programs. Proximity to the elderly in need must be considered. Transportation obstacles must be overcome. Often, locating the elderly, informing them of the program, and enlisting their participation are as important in the success of a program as is the menu and the way food is served.

Meals-on-Wheels and the Congregate Meal Program are major steps toward reintegrating the elderly into the community and improving their nutrition. The programs provide social contact and the people who provide the services are made aware of problems that had previously been appreciated by very few people. The success of these programs can be shown by comparing nutrient intakes of the participants to their RDA. The broader accomplishments of these measures, however, are largely accredited to the fact that the programs integrate an awareness of both nutrition needs and the role of food in life.

STUDY QUESTIONS

1. When does aging begin?

2. Why should young people be interested in the nutrition of the elderly?

3. What physiological changes contribute to the aging process?

4. What socioeconomic factors influence the diets of older people?

5. How do physiological and socioeconomic changes interact to affect the acquisition and preparation of food?

6. Why are nutrient needs of the elderly altered?

7. What do surveys show about the dietary intakes of people over age 60?

8. What are the potential problems that may result from misuse of health foods?

9. Which nutrients must older people pay closest attention to when they plan their diets?

10. What approach may be taken to improve the nutritional status of elderly people?

SUGGESTED READING

1. J. Weinberg, "Psychologic aspects of aging," J. Pelcovits, "Nutrition for older Americans," and D. Holmes, "Nutrition project for the elderly," *Journal of the American Dietetic Association* 60(April 1972).

2. D. M. Watkins, "Nutrition for the elderly of today and tomorrow," *Nutrition News*, National Dairy Council (April 1975).

3. A. A. Albanese, "Nutrition and health of the elderly," *Nutrition News*, National Dairy Council (April 1976).

4. H. B. Brotman, "The fastest growing minority: The aging," *American Journal of Public Health* 64(1974):249–52. (See also other articles in this issue.)

5. E. N. Todhunter, *Food Acceptance and Food Attitudes of the Elderly as a Basis for Planning Nutri-*

tion Programs (95 pages). Nashville: Tennessee Commission on Aging, 1974.

6. T. W. Elwood, "Nutrition concerns of the elderly," *Journal of Nutrition Education* 7(1975):50–52.

7. G. M. Keown and R. N. Klippstein, *Concerns of the Aging: Nutrition* (40 pages plus slide set script). Ithaca: Division of Nutritional Sciences, Cornell University, 1975.

8. E. N. Todhunter and the Technical Committee on Nutrition, *Nutrition: Background and Issues, 1971 White House Conference on Aging* (35 pages). Washington, D.C.: Government Printing Office, 1972.

9. D. B. Rao, "Problems of nutrition in the aged," *Journal of the American Geriatrics Society* 21(1973):362–67.

10. J. Pelcovits, "Nutrition education in group meals for the aged," *Journal of Nutrition Education* 5(1973):118–20.

11. S. N. Gershoff et al, "Studies of the elderly in Boston: 1. Effects of iron fortification on moderately anemic people," *American Journal of Clinical Nutrition* 30(1977):226–34.

12. J. Mayer, "The cruel hoax of food fads," *Family Health* 6(1974):36.

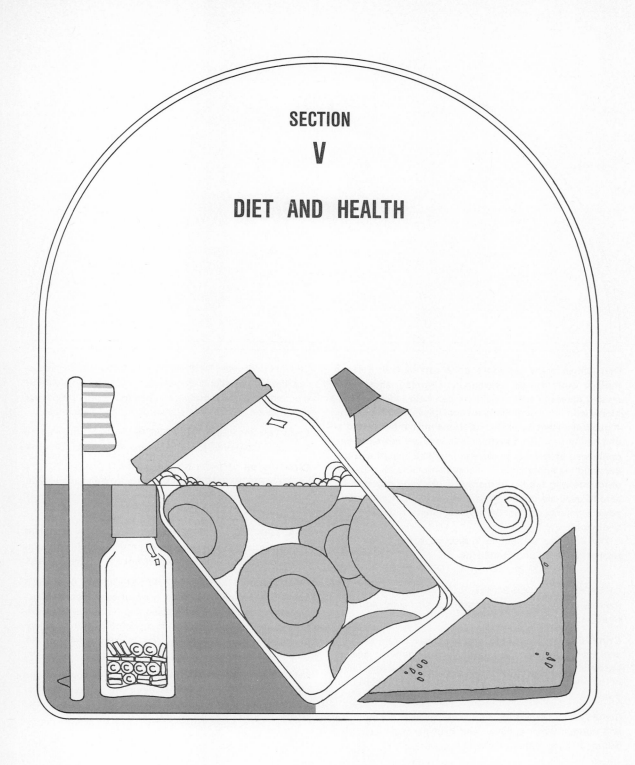

SECTION

V

DIET AND HEALTH

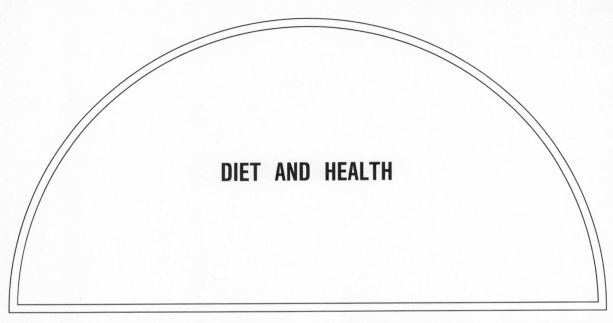

DIET AND HEALTH

Diet can in many instances be a part of both disease therapy and disease prevention. Learning about diet-related diseases and conditions can help individuals afflicted with them participate responsibly in their treatment. A general knowledge of the interrelationship between diet and health can also benefit people who are currently free of disease by helping them maintain their health and understand the importance of diet prescriptions for relatives or friends who are ill. Furthermore, everyone needs to be able to evaluate critically the information that appears in advertisements and in the popular press regarding diet and health.

The chapters in Section V discuss some of the diet-related diseases and conditions.

CHAPTER 20 FOODBORNE ILLNESSES discusses illnesses caused by bacteria, parasites, or toxins, and how to avoid them.

CHAPTER 21 RESISTANCE discusses the role of nutrients in maintaining the body's lines of defense against bacteria and other foreign agents; includes an evaluation of the effects upon "colds" of daily ingestion of more than the RDA for vitamin C.

CHAPTER 22 ANEMIAS discusses the various nutritional and nonnutritional anemias and explains the hazards of self-medication without medical supervision.

CHAPTER 23 GASTROINTESTINAL DISORDERS discusses the interrelationship between nutrition and various gastrointestinal abnormalities—peptic ulcers, dyspepsia, constipation, diarrhea, malabsorption, and flatulence.

CHAPTER 24 FIBER AND HEALTH evaluates the hypothesis that intake of fiber may help prevent several diseases.

CHAPTER 25 CONDITIONS ASSOCIATED WITH CIRCULATORY PROBLEMS discusses the role of diet in diabetes, atherosclerosis, and hypertension—the major causes of death in the United States.

CHAPTER 26 PROTEIN-CALORIE MALNUTRITION (PCM) discusses various forms of protein-calorie malnutrition and efforts to reduce the prevalence of this disease.

CHAPTER 27 MICRONUTRIENT DEFICIENCY DISEASES compares the more common types of such disorders occurring in developed and developing countries; also discusses the history, causes, and physiological abnormalities of beriberi, pellagra, scurvy, rickets, xerophthalmia, and goiter.

CHAPTER 28 ORAL DISEASES discusses how diet and other factors influence the development or prevention of dental caries and periodontal disease.

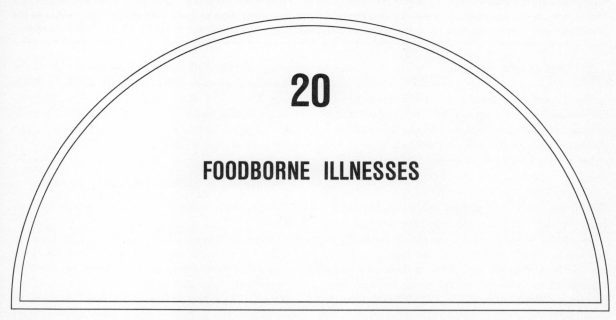

20

FOODBORNE ILLNESSES

The illnesses most commonly associated with food are not related to nutrient content, but rather result from contamination of food. Foodborne illnesses are most often attributable to careless preparation, storage, or serving of foods. Illnesses due to food contamination are extremely common, but fortunately they are usually limited to individuals rather than being epidemic in scope. Cases are generally mild and sometimes go unnoticed; however, each man, woman, and child in this country probably becomes ill at least once every year from eating contaminated food.

It is important to keep in mind that foodborne illness is produced in a person—the *host*—by any one of several different *agents*. The agents may include (1) living matter, such as bacteria, protozoa, molds, and others; or (2) nonliving matter, such as bacterial or fungal toxins and noxious chemicals that occur naturally or are added to food.

CONSEQUENCES OF CONTAMINATION OF FOODS

The general characteristics of most foodborne illnesses are similar. The first or most obvious consequences of food contamination are usually manifest in the gastrointestinal tract, where most contaminants are localized. Some contaminants are absorbed from the intestine and produce ill effects in other body systems.

Symptoms of Foodborne Illnesses

The symptoms of foodborne illnesses vary depending upon the amount or dose consumed and the identity of the offending agent. The most common manifestations include nausea, vomiting, diarrhea, abdominal cramps, and a general feeling of not being well. More serious illnesses may be associated with fever and nervous system abnormalities. Severe vomiting and diarrhea cause excessive loss of body water and ions, which often leads to metabolic and physiological changes. These changes first appear as weakness, fatigue, and depression.

The most damaging effects of food poisoning occur in the very young and the very old. These people, and those who are already weakened by some other disease, may have serious complications or may die of foodborne illnesses that simply cause mild discomfort and gastrointestinal upset in healthy adults.

Food poisoning is produced by living matter (such as bacteria) or nonliving matter (such as toxins or noxious chemicals). The severity of the symptoms and the consequences of food poisoning depend upon the amount and identity of the offending agent consumed, and upon the ability of the body of the individual (the host) to withstand the poisoning.

Incidence of Food Poisoning

The incidence of food poisoning is very difficult to estimate because only a few of the total estimated number of cases are reported to public health authorities. Most of the information available is provided to the Center for Disease Control (CDC) in Atlanta, Georgia, by health departments and other agencies. This chapter relies heavily on data available from the CDC. People who experience the symptoms of food poisoning may take a day off from work or stay home from school, but they usually do not see a doctor. When medical assistance is obtained, these illnesses are rarely studied extensively enough to establish a precise cause because most people are already beginning to recover before the medical investigation begins.

Figure 20-1 shows preliminary numbers for outbreaks of foodborne disease and cases reported to the CDC between 1966 and 1975. Of the 497 outbreaks in 1975, a cause was confirmed in only 191, or 38 percent.

Nutritional Implications

Food contaminants may cause nutrition problems for individuals and for entire populations under some circumstances. Agents of foodborne illness rarely alter the nutritional value of food, but they often cause vomiting and diarrhea, and this leads to poor nutritional status. Wastage of food due to contamination influences the nutritional status of populations; for example, in many countries, a large portion of the food supply (up to half in some tropical countries) never reaches hungry people because crops are ruined between the fields and the marketplace by contamination with bacteria, molds, or rodent excreta.

BEHAVIOR OF BACTERIA

The most frequent causes of foodborne illness that can be diagnosed in this country are related to bacteria. Table 20-1 lists the agents identified as the causes of outbreaks reported to the CDC in 1975. Over 90 percent of the cases in which a diagnosis was confirmed were due to bacterial agents. Knowledge of some basic characteristics of bacteria can help prevent many foodborne illnesses.

Mechanisms of Bacterial Foodborne Illnesses

Two types of food poisoning are caused by bacteria.

An *infection* results from eating food that is contaminated with certain species of *living* bacteria. *Intoxication* is caused by eating food that contains a *preformed toxin* produced by bacteria.

In infections, the bacteria consumed continue to multiply in the intestine, where they produce their toxins and/or invade the intestinal wall. Illness usually does not occur until 36 to 48 hours or longer after eating contaminated food. The time of onset of symptoms (incubation period) after eating depends upon the number of bacteria present in the food and their generation or reproduction time in the intestine. Even after the symptoms are no longer present, the infected person may continue to eliminate living, disease-producing organisms in the feces. These can be transmitted to other people if hands are not washed frequently and proper sanitation is not practiced.

Illness from intoxication usually occurs quickly—between 1 and 12 hours after eating and occasionally up to 24 hours after, depending upon which toxin is consumed. The toxin is present in the food before it is eaten—the bacteria that produced the toxin may or may not be alive in the food at the time it is consumed. Some toxins are destroyed by proper cooking, but others are not.

Distribution of Bacteria

Bacteria are found almost everywhere—in the air we breathe, in the water we drink, on our skin, and throughout our gastrointestinal tracts. The difficulty

Many harmful bacteria are able to grow under the same environmental conditions that support human life. Consumption of harmful living bacteria may cause an infection of the host; consumption of a toxin produced by bacteria causes an intoxication of the host.

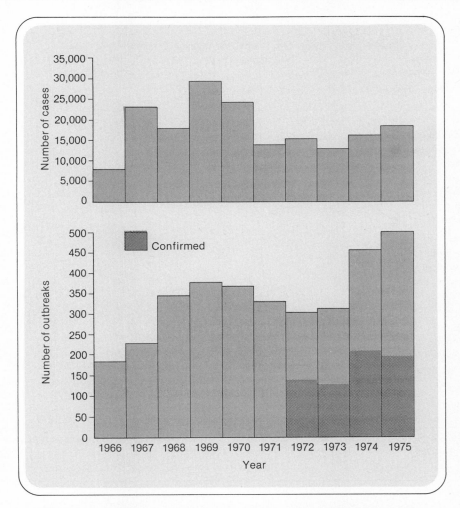

FIGURE 20-1. Foodborne disease outbreaks and cases reported to the Center for Disease Control, 1966–1975. SOURCE: Center for Disease Control, *Foodborne and Waterborne Disease Outbreaks, Annual Summary, 1975,* Department of Health, Education, and Welfare Publication (CDC) 76-8185, 1976, p. 7.

in getting rid of bacteria can be seen by carefully washing your hands and then touching your fingers to a sterile agar dish that contains the nutrients needed by many bacteria (Figure 20-2). If the dish is then kept for several hours at the proper temperature, you can see the colonies of bacteria that have grown from bacteria transferred from your "clean" hand.

Most of the bacteria around or inside us are harmless, but bacteria capable of producing disease are also present. Harmful bacteria normally occur in small numbers and are prevented from multiplying

TABLE 20-1. Confirmed Foodborne Disease Outbreaks and Cases by Causative Agent, 1975

Type of Agent	Outbreaks		Cases	
	Number	Percent	Number	Percent
Bacterial				
Clostridium botulinum	14	7.3	19	0.3
Clostridium perfringens	16	8.4	419	5.7
Salmonella	38	19.9	1,573	21.3
Shigella	3	1.6	413	5.6
Staphylococcus	45	23.6	4,067	55.1
Suspect group D, *Streptococcus*	1	0.5	50	0.7
Other bacteria	6	3.1	282	3.8
Chemical				
Heavy metal	4	2.1	50	0.7
Monosodium glutamate	3	1.6	9	0.1
Mushroom poison	5	2.6	5	0.07
Toxins from fish	25	13.0	86	1.1
Other chemicals	6	3.1	38	0.5
Parasitic				
Dibothriocephalus latum	1	0.5	1	0.01
Trichinella spiralis	20	10.5	193	2.6
Other parasites	1	0.5	1	0.01
Viral				
Hepatitis A	3	1.6	173	2.3
Total Known	191	99.9	7,379	99.9

SOURCE: Center for Disease Control, *Foodborne and Waterborne Disease Outbreaks, Annual Summary, 1975,* Department of Health, Education, and Welfare Publication (CDC) 76-8185, 1976, p. 7.

by the harmless bacteria, which greatly outnumber them.

Conditions for Growth

The conditions necessary to support microorganisms are similar to those needed by humans. Bacteria need moisture, a source of nutrients, and the proper alkalinity of the solution surrounding them. Some bacteria need oxygen, others grow only in the absence of oxygen, and still others survive best in the presence of only a small amount of oxygen.

Most bacteria related to illness grow best at temperatures close to the normal human temperature, 37°C (98.6°F). However, slow growth may occur even at 5°C (40°F) or in some cases up to 65°C (140°F) (Figure 20-3). At low temperatures (for example, below freezing), growth is arrested, but bacteria are not killed. When they are rewarmed, they can again multiply. Some bacteria and most

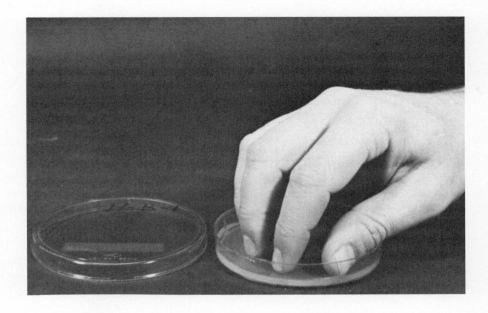

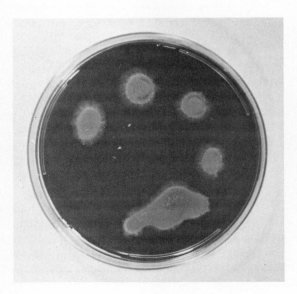
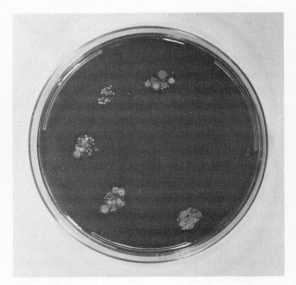

FIGURE 20-2. The hand (previously contaminated with spoiled food) was washed, and then the fingertips were touched to the agar plate. Several bacteria colonies developed after the hand was simply rinsed in water and even after it was also washed with soap and water. (Photos courtesy of Central Soya Company, Inc., from their publication *Sanitation Simplified,* by Dr. Joseph Rakosky, Jr.)

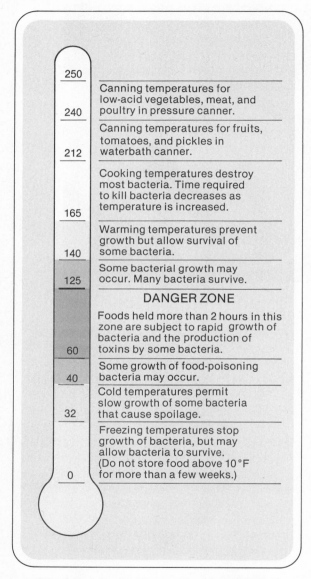

250 — Canning temperatures for low-acid vegetables, meat, and poultry in pressure canner.

240

212 — Canning temperatures for fruits, tomatoes, and pickles in waterbath canner.

Cooking temperatures destroy most bacteria. Time required to kill bacteria decreases as temperature is increased.

165

Warming temperatures prevent growth but allow survival of some bacteria.

140

Some bacterial growth may occur. Many bacteria survive.

125

DANGER ZONE

Foods held more than 2 hours in this zone are subject to rapid growth of bacteria and the production of toxins by some bacteria.

60

Some growth of food-poisoning bacteria may occur.

40

Cold temperatures permit slow growth of some bacteria that cause spoilage.

32

Freezing temperatures stop growth of bacteria, but may allow bacteria to survive. (Do not store food above 10°F for more than a few weeks.)

0

FIGURE 20-3. Temperature guide for food safety—keep hot foods hot and cold foods cold. SOURCE: *Food and Home Notes,* USDA, Office of Communication, June 16, 1976.

SECTION V / DIET AND HEALTH

346

molds can survive extremely high or low temperatures for many years by forming spores, a resting form much like plant seeds. When the proper conditions are restored, the spores germinate and the bacteria reproduce.

Bacterial Infection from Food

The organisms most often involved in bacterial infection from food are *Salmonella, Shigella, Streptococcus,* and *Clostridium perfringens.* Table 20-2 summarizes some basic information about these types of food poisoning.

Salmonella. There are more than 1,700 types of *Salmonella,* but only 200 types were isolated from cases or suspected cases in 1975. There were about 23,000 infected people detected in 1975—and this figure does not include the people who may have been infected and did not seek care or were not cultured to determine the cause of illness. Not all of the 23,000 people known to be infected had gastrointestinal symptoms, and not all cases were due to contaminated food. In fact, only 1,573 cases were proven to be due to contaminated food. This is probably a gross underestimate of the importance of food in transmitting salmonellosis. The most serious bacterial infection, typhoid fever, results from *Salmonella typhosa.* There were 551 proven cases in 1975—again, this probably represents only a fraction of the total. Even with modern therapy, one or two deaths occur out of every 100 cases of typhoid fever. Most people with other types of salmonellosis recover in two to five days.

Salmonella bacteria most frequently are found in poultry, eggs and egg products, raw meats, milk, and fish. They are not detectable by looking at, tasting, or smelling the food. Proper cooking of food prior to serving destroys the *Salmonella* bacteria. Meat and poultry should be heated thoroughly to at least 75°C (165°F) using a thermometer that measures internal temperature. After cooking, poultry should be kept hot or refrigerated immediately. Poultry stuffing should be cooked outside the fowl, thus reducing the risk of contamination, and assuring that a sufficiently high temperature is reached at the center of the bird and at the center of the mound of stuffing.

When fowl is cut on a wooden cutting board, *Salmonella* are easily trapped in the grooves of the wood. The board must be thoroughly scrubbed with soap and rinsed for at least 30 seconds with scalding water to be sure that the bacteria are removed or killed. Failure to clean the board thoroughly may lead to infection of the next food placed on the board. Using an unwashed board for cutting uncooked foods, such as salad, is especially hazardous.

Salmonella bacteria frequently occur in eggs with cracked shells. These eggs should never be used unless they are thoroughly cooked. Cream-filled pastries and custards made with contaminated eggs often cause salmonellosis. Foods made with eggs must be cooked immediately after they are prepared and then kept refrigerated until served. Cake batters containing eggs should not be tasted before they are baked.

Recent isolated cases of salmonellosis have been traced to pet turtles whose containers were cleaned in the kitchen. Careless handling around the sink probably led to splattering turtle feces onto surfaces where food was prepared.

Shigella. *Shigella* bacteria are found in food contaminated with human or animal feces. These bacteria usually cause fever and gastrointestinal symptoms similar to those caused by *Salmonella,* but the illness is usually milder. In 1975, there were only three outbreaks of foodborne illness with 413 cases due to *Shigella,* while there were nearly 11,000 cases of *Shigella* infection. The peak incidence of reported cases is in children aged one to four years. One waterborne outbreak of shigellosis was reported in 1975. It involved 56 people who drank untreated ground water from a semipublic water system.

Most cases of shigellosis subside in less than a week, but some can be so severe that the intestinal mucosa becomes ulcerated, and the stools contain mucus and often blood. An epidemic of this infection occurred in Guatemala in 1969. This dysentery affected over 100,000 people, and there were over 8,000 deaths.

Personal cleanliness is the key to preventing spread of this infection throughout the illness and particularly during the recovery phase. The disease can be spread up to a month or more after a person's symptoms have disappeared. During this time, the infected person is a convalescent carrier of live bacteria in the feces, which may be transmitted to food served to others in the household. People who have recovered from shigellosis should not handle food unless they use extreme care to maintain cleanliness. Public health authorities carefully monitor people with shigellosis (and salmonellosis) and their immediate contacts. Generally, an infected person must have at least three consecutive stool cultures test negative for these bacteria before they are permitted to resume food-handling jobs.

Streptococcus. Foodborne outbreaks of streptococcal infection ("strep") are now rare in the United States, but they continue to occur sporadically. Table 20-1 shows only one known foodborne outbreak in 1975, and that resulted from beef contaminated by a food handler. The bacteria are also transmitted through unpasteurized milk from infected cows, and egg, tuna, or chicken salads, and other high-protein foods prepared by an infected food handler.

Complications of streptococcal infection include scarlet fever, rheumatic fever, and kidney disease. A person who has this infection should be given antibiotics. People in contact with the infected person should be examined to detect those who may be symptom-free but are still carriers. This infection is often spread by a carrier who sneezes on food or has a small infected cut on the hand that harbors *Streptococci.*

TABLE 20-2. Foodborne Illnesses Due to Bacterial Infection

Illness	Causative Agent	Symptoms of Illness	Foods Usually Involved	How Introduced into Food	Preventive or Corrective Procedures
Salmonellosis	Over 1,700 types of *Salmonella* bacteria	Gastrointestinal illness, nausea, diarrhea, abdominal discomfort, occasional vomiting	Meat and poultry, comminuted foods, egg products, custards, shellfish, soups, gravies, sauces, warmed-over foods	Fecal contamination by food handlers; raw contaminated meat, poultry, and eggs; unpasteurized milk	Good personal habits of food handlers, sufficient cooking and refrigeration of perishable foods, elimination of rodents and flies, thorough cooking, food served hot or cold as appropriate
Typhoid fever	Salmonella typhosa	Fever, intestinal upset, headache, constipation or diarrhea, rose spots on trunk of body, stupor or delirium	Moist foods, dairy products, shellfish, raw vegetables, water	By food handlers and other carriers	Prohibition of carriers from handling food, strict personal cleanliness during food preparation, elimination of flies, thorough cooking, food served hot or cold as appropriate
Bacillary dysentery (shigellosis)	*Shigella* bacteria	Fever and gastrointestinal symptoms; may produce mucus and bloody diarrhea	Foods contaminated with excreta on unclean hands	By unsanitary food handling, flies	Strict personal cleanliness in food preparation, refrigeration of moist foods, exclusion of carriers from handling food, thorough cooking, food served hot or cold as appropriate

Perfringens food poisoning	Clostridium perfringens	Diarrhea and abdominal pain in from 4 to 22 hours, usually lasting about 12 hours	Meat that has been boiled, steamed, braised, or partially roasted, allowed to cool several hours, and subsequently served either cooled or reheated	Contaminant of meat	Refrigeration of meat between cooking and use
Streptococcal food infection Beta type: scarlet fever and strep throat	Beta hemolytic Streptococci	Usually upper respiratory symptoms (sore throat, fever)	Foods contaminated with nasal or oral discharges from case or carrier; infected cuts; bruises	Coughing, sneezing, handling	Exclusion of food handlers with known strep infections, proper cooking and refrigeration of foods
Alpha type: intestinal	Enterococcus group; pyogenic group	Nausea, vomiting, diarrhea	Foods contaminated with excreta on unclean hands	By unsanitary food handling	Exclusion of food handlers with known strep infections, thorough cooking of food, refrigeration of moist food during storage periods

Clostridium Perfringens. This type of food poisoning is almost always associated with meat, especially when it is served in restaurants or other large feeding establishments where food is held for a long time on steam tables. There were 419 people who contracted this poisoning in 1975; beef was the vehicle of transmission in 10 of the 16 outbreaks, and single outbreaks were due to chicken, turkey, pork, fish, multiple vehicles, and an unspecified vehicle. The infection often occurs because people do not realize that although *Clostridia* bacteria are destroyed by heat, their spores withstand boiling for several hours. The spores that survive cooking can germinate into bacteria if cooked meat is left standing at room temperature.

Refrigeration immediately after heating prevents rapid reproduction of these bacteria, but larger pieces of meat (such as a roast) cool slowly, especially at the center. Leftover meat dishes should be thoroughly reheated, and leftover gravy should be brought to a rolling boil before serving. Cold sliced meat should be served directly from the refrigerator—not left at room temperature before eating.

Bacterial Intoxication from Food

The two most important types of bacterial intoxication are caused by *Staphylococcus* and *Clostridium botulinum*. Table 20-3 compares the foodborne illnesses caused by these organisms.

Staphylococcus. The *Staphylococcus* ("staph") bacterium is especially troublesome because its toxin is not destroyed by boiling or baking. Therefore, the only protection against this type of food poisoning is to prevent the food from being contaminated; food must be kept refrigerated so that the organisms do not grow and produce their toxin.

Staphylococcus organisms are present in the nose and throat and on the skin of normal, healthy people. They are also present in dust and air. These bacteria can easily be transmitted to food by people who have cuts or infections on their hands, who sneeze in the vicinity of food, or touch their noses while handling food.

Staphylococci grow in a wide variety of moist foods, especially those that contain protein (such as meat, poultry, eggs, and fish). This type of food poisoning is often associated with picnics or buffet banquets, where food is kept standing at room temperature for two hours or more. This is enough time for the bacteria to grow and produce their toxin.

Clostridium Botulinum. These bacteria produce the most deadly poison in the world. It has been estimated that only 16 ounces of this toxin would kill the population of the entire world.

The dormant spores of these organisms are abundant in soil and dust. However, the potent toxin is only formed by the organism in its nonspore, growing form. The bacteria usually grow only in the absence of oxygen (anaerobic conditions). Therefore, we should be aware of the possible presence of these bacteria in food kept at room temperature in a relatively air-free environment, such as cans or jars.

Most of the illness caused by the toxin of *Clostridium botulinum* (botulism) occurs from improper home canning. Since 1899, 72 percent of botulism outbreaks have been traced to home-processed foods and only 9 percent to commercially processed foods. (The source of the other 19 percent is unknown to the CDC.) Toxin-forming bacteria grow best in canned foods that contain little or no acid (such as meat, beans, asparagus, peas, or corn). Fruits, fish, and condiments are other important vehicles. These foods are not adequately sterilized even after boiling for 6 hours. The *Clostridium* spores can be killed by steaming in a pressure cooker under 15 pounds of pressure for 10 minutes. The growth of *Clostridium botulinum* in meat products sold in cans or oxygen-free packages is inhibited by the addition of the preservative nitrite.

Botulism is relatively rare, with only 2,000 cases known to the CDC since 1899. Of the 19 cases reported in 1975, 14 were traced to home food processing, 2 to commercially prepared food, and 3

TABLE 20-3 Foodborne Illnesses Due to Bacterial Intoxication

Illness	Causative Agent	Symptoms of Illness	Foods Usually Involved	How Introduced into Food	Preventive or Corrective Procedures
Botulism	Toxins of *Clostridium botulinum*	Double vision, difficulty in swallowing and speaking, dizziness, progressive paralysis, especially of respiratory system	Improperly processed or unrefrigerated foods of low acidity	Soil, dirt, spores not killed in inadequately heated foods	Foods with pH over 4.0 should be pressure cooked before canning, home-canned foods should be boiled 20 minutes after removal from can or jar: discard all foods in swollen, unopened cans; do not taste suspicious foods
Staphylococcus food poisoning	Toxin of *Staphylococcus*	Gastrointestinal symptoms; occur within 2 to 4 hours after eating	Cooked meats, chopped or comminuted foods, cream-filled or custard pastries, other dairy products, hollandaise sauce, bread pudding, potato salad, salads of chicken, fish, and other meats, warmed-over foods	Usually by food handlers through nasal discharges or purulent local skin infections (acne, pimples, boils, scratches, cuts)	Refrigeration of moist foods during storage periods, minimal use of hands in food preparation, exclusion of unhealthy food handlers

were not determined. Prior to 1949, the death rate was about 60 percent, but with modern treatment it is now less than 20 percent. Death occurs from respiratory paralysis.

The toxin formed by *Clostridium botulinum* is destroyed by adequate cooking. Home-canned foods should be boiled for at least 20 minutes after removal from the can to destroy any toxin that might be present. However, food that might contain the toxin should never be eaten. Even a small taste of food contaminated with the organism may contain enough poison to make a person very ill.

Food Safety Guidelines

Measures to prevent illness caused by bacteria are based on knowing (1) methods of food contamination, (2) conditions that permit bacterial growth, and (3) conditions that inhibit growth or kill bacteria. A few general guidelines will help you protect yourself and your friends and family. We have mentioned some of these in the above discussion of bacteria, but now we will focus on general preventive procedures. Some of the guidelines also apply to other types of food contamination that will be discussed later.

Avoiding Transmission. Disease-causing bacteria may be present in dust, soil, and on the skin of food handlers. Therefore, washing is the first step in the preparation of all food—washing hands before handling the food and washing fresh foods (such as fruits and vegetables) that may be contaminated with microorganisms from soil, dust, or previous dirty hands. Fresh foods should be washed even if they will be peeled. Organisms on the surface of an unwashed carrot, for example, may be transferred by a peeler or knife to the part of the food you will eat. Cooking utensils, kitchen counters, and cutting boards should also be carefully cleaned because they can transmit bacteria from a contaminated food that will later be cooked (therefore, usually making it

safe) to a food that will be eaten raw (therefore, not safe).

The feces of humans and other animals provide an ideal diet for many bacteria. Consequently, fecal contamination of food is a frequent source of food poisoning (as well as being responsible for many viral diseases, such as polio and hepatitis). It is important to be aware that a few sheets of toilet tissue do not obstruct the transmission of bacteria (or viruses). While flies and rodents do act as transmitters of fecal bacteria, human fingers are far more commonly the culprits!

Many bacteria are carried by pets (dogs, cats, turtles, birds, and fish). Even the cleanest, most-loved dog that is allowed to play under the dinner table can be the source of bacteria or other organisms that end up in food on top of the table.

Health of Food Handlers. Many disease-producing organisms are transmitted by food handlers. Obvious sources are pimples, infected cuts or boils, the nose, and the mouth. Public health records are filled with epidemics that can be traced back to one well-meaning cook in a restraurant whose minor infection contributed to the illness, and sometimes death, of many people. Coughs and sneezes in home kitchens can have similar repercussions on the health of the entire family.

Maintaining Proper Temperature of Food. Figure 20-3 shows the temperature preferences of bacteria for reproduction. Food-handling guidelines are based on this information.

1. Foods should be kept below 5°C (40°F) or over 60°C (140°F).
2. Warm food placed in the refrigerator should be spread out in a shallow container to hasten cooling.
3. Frozen foods should not be allowed to thaw or stand at room temperature prior to cooking or serving.
4. Foods should never be left at room temperature for

more than an hour if they have been improperly cooked or handled.

5. Refrigerators should be defrosted when necessary and gaskets around the door should fit tightly in order to maintain temperatures below 5°C (40°F).

PARASITIC INFESTATION

Parasites enter the human body by several routes. Some, such as flukes and hookworm, enter through the skin; others are usually found in foods. Parasites cause blood loss and diarrhea, which rob the body of nutrients. They also use up some of the dietary energy, vitamins, and minerals needed by their host. Some of the most significant and common foodborne parasites are the protozoa *Entamoeba histolytica*, the tiny roundworm *Trichinella spiralis*, and the beef, pork, and fish tapeworms. The characteristics of human encounters with these microorganisms are summarized in Table 20-4.

Entamoeba histolytica

This protozoan parasite causes amoebic dysentery, which is similar in symptoms to the dysentery produced by the *Shigella* bacteria. It also occasionally invades the liver, lung, and brain, and may form abscesses in these tissues.

Entamoeba histolytica may be found in water supplies polluted with sewage or may be transmitted by contaminated food. They also are found in the hair of household pets, such as dogs and cats. Flies and unwashed hands may carry these protozoa to the dinner table.

Many more people are infested with this parasite than show symptoms of dysentery. The number of cases per year is not known, since this is not a reportable disease and rarely are stool samples in this country examined for protozoan parasites. The development of symptoms or illness appears to be more common in poorly nourished people. Fletcher and Jepps, who worked in Malaya over fifty years ago, noted that "Amebiasis is a disease of poverty and want" and "dysentery vanishes before comfort and prosperity."[*]

Trichinella spiralis

Larvae of this tiny nematode parasite are found in cysts in the muscles of garbage-fed hogs. During digestion of improperly cooked pork, the larvae are liberated within the gastrointestinal tract of humans. Nausea, vomiting, diarrhea, and abdominal pain occur as early as 24 hours after ingestion of infested pork, but the more serious consequences do not occur until 4 to 16 weeks later. These parasites mate and spread larvae throughout the body via the lymph and circulatory systems. Muscular pains, swelling of the eyelids, chills, and weakness may occur as the larvae form cysts in the host's muscle tissue. The possibility of this disease may seem remote to you, but 193 cases of trichinosis were diagnosed in twenty foodborne outbreaks in the United States in 1975. It is likely that thousands of cases exist that have not caused symptoms serious enough to warrant extensive muscle biopsies necessary for confirmation. The United States has a longer way to go in controlling trichinosis in pork than most other developed countries of the world.

Tapeworms

The larvae of tapeworms gain access to human beings when cow, pig, or fish muscle meats containing these parasites are insufficiently cooked or eaten raw. Many infestations cause only mild intestinal irritation, but the pork tapeworm (*Taenia solium*) may form cysts in the brain, spinal cord, eye, heart, or other organs. Drugs can eliminate the tapeworms from the intestine, but there is no treatment for the cysts except surgical removal. Fortunately, cysts do

[*] P. E. Sartwell, ed., Maxcy-Rosenau *Preventive Medicine and Public Health*, 10th ed. (New York: Appleton-Century-Crofts, 1973), p. 209.

TABLE 20-4. Foodborne Illnesses Due to Parasites

Illness	Causative Agent	Symptoms of Illness	Foods Usually Involved	How Introduced into Food	Preventive or Corrective Procedures
Amoebic dysentery	*Entamoeba histolytica* (protozoa)	Abdominal pain, diarrhea or constipation, mucus and occasional blood flecks in stool, headache, fatigue	Foods contaminated with excreta on unclean hands; fouled drinking water or milk	By flies, human feces used to fertilize garden vegetables, water, food handlers; mechanism of transmission is poorly understood.	Protection and purification of water supplies, strict personal cleanliness, exclusion of flies, roaches, and other insects; proper nutrition of host results in decreased susceptibility to and seriousness of infection
Tapeworms	Parasitic larvae: in pork, *Taenia solium;* in beef, *Taenia saginata;* in fish, *Dibothriocephalus latus*	None or mild intestinal irritation in most cases; pork tapeworm may result in fatal cysticercosis; fish tapeworm may cause vitamin B$_{12}$ deficiency, anemia, and spinal cord degeneration	Raw or insufficiently cooked beef, pork, or fish that contain living larvae	Muscle containing cysts with living larvae	Cook fish thoroughly, avoid serving raw fish; deep freezing for several days before eating meat
Trichinosis	Larvae of *Trichinella spiralis* (worm)	Nausea, vomiting, diarrhea, abdominal pain; swelling of eyelids, muscle pains, weakness, chills after 4 to 6 weeks	Raw or insufficiently cooked pork or pork products	Raw pork from hogs fed uncooked, infected garbage	Thoroughly cook pork and pork products at temperatures over 150°F, preferably to 160°F

not develop very often, but if they do, they are rarely located in vital areas and therefore cause little difficulty. If the cysts are located in tissues such as the brain, where surgery is difficult or impossible, body function may be seriously compromised or life may be lost.

The fish tapeworm may reach 30 feet in length and one person may harbor as many as 100 worms. Only one case was reported to the CDC in 1975; however, fish tapeworm is far more common than this in certain population groups. In western Alaska and the Baltic countries nearly 100 percent of the population is infected. In the Great Lakes area of the United States, smaller percentages are infected. Eskimos, Japanese, Jews, Russians, and Scandinavians have high infection rates, probably because of their preference for raw or undercooked fish.

In addition to the burden of sharing food intake with the fish tapeworms and the general intestinal discomfort, infected people have a more serious problem. The fish tapeworm prodigiously concentrates vitamin B_{12} in its own tissues, thus soaking up nearly all the dietary intake of this vitamin (a true parasitism) and causing severe anemia.

Tapeworm infestations can be avoided by simply using the proper precautions in food storage and preparation. The cysts of both beef and pork tapeworms are killed by thorough cooking, quick freezing, or curing or salting of meats. Fish tapeworms are killed by thorough cooking or by deep freezing for at least 48 hours.

OTHER TOXINS

Most illness caused by ingestion of food results from the bacteria and parasites we have just discussed. We have not discussed the role of food in the transmission of viral illnesses, except for hepatitis and polio, which were mentioned in passing. Some viral illnesses certainly are transmitted by contaminated food, but a discussion of the epidemiology of viral illnesses goes beyond the scope of this book. A large number of other substances that occur naturally in food, are added to food, or are produced by molds can also make people sick. These illnesses are much less frequent, but a few are mentioned below to alert you to potential problems.

Shellfish Poisoning

This type of food poisoning has been increasingly more common in recent years. It is often associated with the "red tides" along coastal waters. The ocean is colored red by poisonous plankton at certain times of the year and shellfish feed on these plankton. Eating poisoned mussels and clams may cause allergic skin reactions, intestinal upset, or the more serious toxemia—poisoning of the body through the blood. Symptoms may begin in 10 to 15 minutes. There is no specific antidote or cure, but artificial respiration for 12 or more hours may save a person's life.

Prevention rests upon supporting vigorous public health law enforcement and proscriptions on harvesting shellfish from contaminated waters. Individuals should consume shellfish obtained only from reputable sources.

Mycotoxins

The poisons produced by molds or fungi are called *mycotoxins*. One of these, *aflatoxin*, is produced by a mold that grows on peanuts. This mold grows best under moist conditions and is usually associated with harvesting or storage of nuts when the weather is rainy or the ground is damp. If peanut kernels are discolored, shriveled, or broken, or if the nuts appear to be rancid, the risk of this toxin is great enough that they should be discarded. Aflatoxin is a known cancer-causing agent when fed to laboratory animals.

Another mycotoxin, *patulin*, is formed by certain molds that cause storage rot of apples. Such apples usually would not be eaten, but this toxin has been found in cider made from rotted apples. The same toxin given in sufficient amounts intravenously (not by mouth) to rats may be lethal.

These observations might make you hesitant to drink cider, but let's ask some questions and perform some rather simple calculations to help make an informed decision whether you should drink it. You may be able to avoid unfounded fears (overreaction) or irresponsible nonchalance (underreaction). The questions we must ask are:

1. How much patulin is harmful to experimental animals?

2. How much patulin is harmful to humans?

3. How much patulin is in food?

4. How much food provides a harmful amount of patulin?

The answers are:

1. The index used by toxicologists to measure fatal doses of poisons is called the LD_{50}. This index is the amount of a poison that causes death (*lethal dose*) in 50 percent of the experimental animals studied. The LD_{50} for patulin in rats is 15 to 35 milligrams per kilogram of body weight.

2. If we assume that the LD_{50} for patulin in humans is the same as that for rats (15 to 35 mg/kg body weight), we can use a typical human body weight (such as 60 kg) to calculate the toxic range for humans.

15 mg/kg × 60 kg = 900 mg

35 mg/kg × 60 kg = 2,100 mg

Therefore, 900 to 2,100 milligrams of patulin would be lethal to half the people who weigh 60 kilograms.

3. The original research paper reported that the concentration of patulin ranged from 6 to 150 milligrams per litre in the contaminated cider analyzed.

4. To be most careful, let's consider the greatest possible risk of harm. We use the lowest harmful dose (LD_{50} = 900 milligrams of patulin) and the highest reported contamination levels (150 milligrams of patulin in a litre of cider) to calculate the amount of food that would be harmful. In order to consume 900 milligrams of patulin, you would have to drink 900/150 litres, or 6 litres, of cider—much more than you are likely to drink!

This evaluation gives no clear-cut answer to the practical question "Should you, or should you not, drink cider?" This decision must be made by each individual on the basis of a realistic appraisal of the degree of risk involved, the possibility of cumulative effects from other dietary chemicals handled similarly by the body, and how well you like cider. One way to reduce the degree of risk is to select cider that has the least probability of contamination by the toxin-producing mold. Juice derived from apples grown on farms that do not use fungicides to kill molds is more likely to contain the toxin than juice from apples that have been protected from these organisms by judicious spraying.

Factors Influencing Toxicity Studies

The calculations above include many assumptions, but an effective thought pattern is illustrated. This line of reasoning helps put into perspective the potential health hazards of any toxin in food. Other factors that should be considered when a more thorough analysis is made of the safety implications of research regarding toxic substances (chemical or biological) in food include:

1. *Criteria for toxicity.* The LD_{50} is based upon death as an index of toxicity. It is also important to know nonlethal but harmful effects of smaller doses.

2. *Dosage and time.* In most instances, a single dose of a toxin is more hazardous than the same amount given over a more prolonged time. On the other hand, it is important to know the effects of consuming a small amount of a toxin-containing food every day.

3. *Route of administration.* If a toxin is given intravenously, the entire dose reaches the blood and circulates through the body. The toxicity of some poisons taken orally is reduced because they are altered during digestion or they are not completely absorbed.

4. *Metabolism.* Many chemicals are metabolized in the body to a less toxic or nontoxic form. In a few cases, the chemical is changed to an even more toxic form.

TABLE 20-5. Some Toxins and Nutrient Inhibitors
Naturally Present in Foods

Food	Toxin or Inhibitor	Action	Counteraction
Beans, lima and soy	Antitrypsin	Prevents protein digestion	Heat to inactivate
	Lipoxidase	Destroys vitamin A	Heat to inactivate
Cabbage, kale, rutabaga	Goitrogens	Prevent synthesis of thyroxine (can lead to goiter if dietary intake of iodine is low)	Consume only as part of a varied diet
Egg white	Avidin	Binds biotin	Heat to inactivate
Fish, clams	Thiaminase	Destroys thiamin	Heat to inactivate
Mushrooms, certain species and toadstools	Five cyclopeptides, such as muscarine	Cause nausea, vomiting, abdominal pain in early phases; salivation, sweating, constricted pupils, slow heart rate; then severe kidney, liver, and nervous degeneration (50% fatal)	Do not eat wild mushrooms or those sold in places that might not be careful about their products
Potato (immature or sprouting)	Solanine	Vomiting and diarrhea (loss of nutrients)	Avoid such potato products

5. *Excretion and/or storage.* The retention of toxins is governed by the same solubility principles that apply to water-soluble and fat-soluble vitamins. Water-soluble toxins are excreted most readily. Fat-soluble toxins are more likely to be stored and to cause cumulative effects.

Naturally Occurring Toxins

Toxic chemicals occur naturally in many foods. However, for two reasons, they rarely create a practical hazard to health (see Chapter 12). First, they usually are present in very small concentrations. Second, if a varied diet is eaten, toxin-containing foods are not consumed in large amounts.

Table 20-5 summarizes some of these chemicals. Solanine, for instance, causes vomiting, diarrhea, abdominal pain, and/or jaundice. To avoid this toxin, the green part of sprouting potatoes should not be eaten. Also, as most people know, mushrooms should not be eaten unless there is certainty that they are not one of the types that contain toxins such as muscarine.

Other chemicals, such as oxalic acid (which occurs in certain green vegetables), can interfere with (*inhibit*) the absorption of certain nutrients. Foods that contain such chemicals should not be totally avoided—they are all good sources of specific nutrients—but they should be consumed only as part of a varied, nutritionally appropriate diet.

STUDY QUESTIONS

1. What determines the severity of the symptoms and the consequences of food poisoning?

2. What is the difference between an infection and an intoxication?

3. What conditions determine whether bacteria grow in food?

4. Where do the bacteria *Salmonella, Shigella, Streptococcus,* and *Clostridium perfringens* grow and how can you avoid infection from them?

5. How can the toxins of *Staphylococcus* and *Clostridium botulinum* be avoided?

6. What general measures can be taken to avoid transmission of most disease-causing bacteria and toxins?

7. How are most foodborne parasites transmitted?

8. What factors should be considered when evaluating the hazard of consuming a noxious substance?

SUGGESTED READING

1. Expert Panel on Food Safety and Nutrition, Institute of Food Technologists, "Botulism: A scientific status summary." Reprinted in *Nutrition Reviews* 31(1973):265–71.
2. I. D. Morton, "Toxic substances in foods," *Journal of Human Nutrition* 31(1977):53–60.
3. H. G. Day, "Food safety—Then and now," *Journal of the American Dietetic Association* 69(1976):229–34.
4. M. E. Potter et al, "A sausage-associated outbreak of trichinosis in Illinois," *American Journal of Public Health* 66(1976):1194–96.
5. E. V. Morse et al, "Canine Salmonellosis: A review and report of dog to child transmission of Salmonella enteritis," *American Journal of Public Health* 66(1976):82–84.
6. "Patulin: A carginogenic mycotoxin found in cider," *Nutrition Reviews* 32(1974):55–56.
7. J. L. Goodard, "Incident at Selby Junior High," *Nutrition Today* 2(1967):2–16.
8. A. P. Farah, "Can your kitchen pass a health inspection?" *Family Health* 7(1975):32.
9. "Chemical preservation for prevention of mycotoxin production," *Nutrition Reviews* 34(1976):31–32.
10. M. C. Gupta, A. K. Basu, and B. N. Tandon, "Gastrointestinal protein loss in hookworm and roundworm infection," *American Journal of Clinical Nutrition* 27(1974):1386.

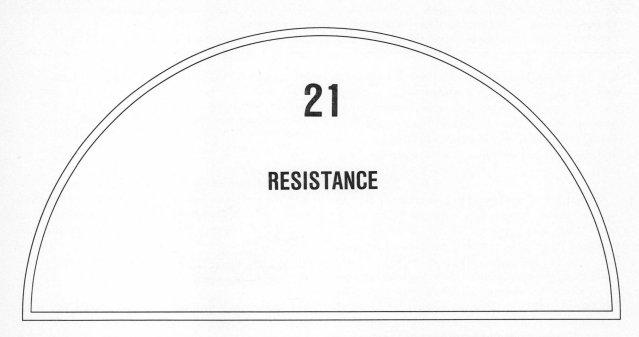

21

RESISTANCE

In this chapter we discuss the roles nutrients play in our defenses against a broad spectrum of infections and foreign agents and in our recovery from such illnesses. An individual's general nutritional status influences the many processes involved in defending the body against invasion, controlling agents that gain entry to the body, and assisting in repair and recovery. For purposes of this discussion, these processes are called *resistance*.

The general nutrition student must have some familiarity with the concept of resistance to appreciate the contribution of an appropriate diet in maintaining health. This information will also help you evaluate advertising claims about products that purport to build up or improve resistance.

LINES OF DEFENSE

The general concept that nutrition is important for the maintenance of health has stimulated a great deal of research designed to explain how nutrients contribute to prevention of illness and to resistance. The body has several lines of defense, and nutrients have specific roles in each.

Protection from Invasion: The Physical Barrier

The first line of defense against bacteria, parasites, viruses, molds, and other agents is simply a physical barrier that prevents their gaining entrance to the body. This barrier includes the skin and the membranes lining nasal passages, lungs, and gastrointestinal tract. Vitamin A is necessary for maintaining the integrity of the cells of these membranes, and vitamin C is necessary for formation of the cement and fibers that hold the cells and membranes together. People who are deficient in these nutrients and in thiamin, riboflavin, niacin, and protein, have a reduced resistance to infections.

Cuts, blisters, and other wounds increase susceptibility to infections because the physical barrier is broken. An adequate intake of nutrients that help heal wounds (zinc and vitamin C) is necessary so that these points of entry for disease-causing organisms can close properly.

Antibody Formation—Blood Defense System

Antibodies, the large, complex proteins found in the gamma globulin portion of the blood plasma,

Resistance to offending agents depends upon a person's nutritional status, general health, and socioeconomic variables.
Vitamin A, vitamin C, and zinc help prevent bacterial invasion of the body.
Results of animal experiments do not always mean that the same results would occur in human experiments.

are the second line of defense. They are produced by the body soon after first contact with an offending agent. Antibodies neutralize, kill, or precipitate such agents and then the white blood cells digest them. The relationships between antibody formation and the roles of individual nutrients are very complex.

Complexities of Research and Isolated Results. Various animal species can form antibodies to the same toxins and bacteria that attack humans. Researchers often study antibody formation in animals as a basis for developing theories regarding resistance to infection in people. However, the response of experimental animals under tightly controlled laboratory conditions does not always correlate with human resistance. Outlining a few of the complexities of this type of research can help you understand why much still remains to be learned about the specific roles of nutrients in this line of resistance.

1. Species variability: Ethics—and life itself—forbid many studies of humans; therefore, most nutrition and biochemical studies are conducted with experimental animals. Often, however, the response of a mouse differs from that of a rather similar rodent, the rat. There may be even less correlation with the effects observed in a dog or monkey. Findings from these species therefore cannot always be generalized to humans.

2. Agent variability: Antibody response is very specific. It depends upon idiosyncracies of the host and the bacteria being tested. Bacteria that cause typhoid fever do not stimulate the production of the same antibody as cholera bacteria. A vaccination against smallpox virus does not result in antibodies that protect against polio virus. Horse serum antibodies against tetanus (lockjaw) toxin are slightly, but significantly, different from the human antibodies against tetanus toxin. Therefore, it is likely that nutrients function somewhat differently in each situation.

3. Nutritional status: Overall nutritional status influences resistance. However, in research studies, a deficiency of a single nutrient is created in order to evaluate any linkage between that nutrient and an abnormality in antibody response. The researcher must be certain that

the animals are well nourished in all other respects, or a true cause-and-effect relationship cannot be proved. Such experiments are important to understanding nutrient functions, but they must be interpreted cautiously, since rarely do humans exhibit a severe deficiency of a single nutrient (Chapter 27).

Much has been learned from extensive work with animals and more limited human studies. Nevertheless, you must keep these problems in mind in order to evaluate research results. This approach is especially important because often simplistic interpretations of nutrition research are presented in the popular press.

Experimental Animals. Research has shown that antibody formation is impaired by a deficiency in experimental animals of pyridoxine, pantothenic acid, and several of the amino acids. Calcium has little effect, but there appears to be a negative correlation between iron nutriture and the ability to form antibodies. The roles of vitamins A, C, D, and E are not well defined.

Human Studies. The correlation between nutrient status and antibody production in humans is less conclusive than for experimental animals. Impairment of antibody response to yellow fever vaccine occurs in protein-deficient children. Pantothenic acid and pyridoxine deficiencies produced in human volunteers caused decreased ability to form certain (but not all) antibodies. However, other studies report that malnourished children exhibit a normal ability to produce antibodies to polio vaccine.

Lymphoid Tissues—Cellular Defense System

The *lymphoid system* consists of a number of specialized tissues throughout the body that produce cells called *lymphocytes*. Some lymphocytes circulate in the blood as one type of white corpuscle, but most are fixed in tissues such as the tonsils, lymph glands, spleen, appendix, and areas of the

Impairment of antibody formation occurs in experimental animals deficient in pyridoxine, pantothenic acid, several amino acids, and possibly other nutrients. In humans the role of nutrients in antibody formation is less precisely defined. The effectiveness of the lymphoid tissues in resistance is impaired in malnourished children.

intestine. The thymus gland (which is large in infants, but becomes smaller with age) appears to be the director of the lymphoid system.

Lymphocytes produce toxic substances and several special chemicals that destroy harmful organisms (and probably mutant or counterfeit cells) that arise in the host. The red, firm skin reaction produced in people who have a positive skin test for tuberculosis, mumps, Valley Fever, and some other infections is brought about by the cellular defense system.

The correlation between nutrition and resistance as related to the lymphoid system is not as well understood as antibody formation. The effects of deficiencies of a single nutrient have not been extensively studied, but indirect evidence indicates that the lymphoid system of children who are deficient in protein and/or calories does not operate normally. For example, autopsies of children who have died of malnutrition show that their thymus glands and other lymphoid tissues are smaller than those of children who died of other causes. Malnourished children are often unable to develop positive skin tests when infected with tuberculosis and certain fungus organisms. This indicates poor resistance to these types of infections and impaired growth and reproduction of their tissue lymphocytes. Similar but less dramatic results are seen in adults who have marginal protein deficiency.

EPIDEMIOLOGICAL STUDIES

Epidemiological studies linking nutrition and resistance are difficult to interpret because the most severely malnourished children are often also those who are most exposed to unhealthful conditions. It is difficult to sort out the relationships between resistance and the specific effects of diet, physical environment, economic circumstances, social habits, genetic factors, and exposure to disease-causing organisms.

Statistics do show two correlations.

1. Malnutrition worsens infectious disease and increases the likelihood of fatality. For instance, measles is a major cause of death among malnourished children in developing countries, but in the United States a child with this infection usually only misses a few days of school.

2. Infection worsens nutritional diseases. A marginally nourished person will often be free of obvious signs of nutritional deficiency, but the stress of an infection worsens nutritional status and may precipitate a frank deficiency disease.

RECOVERY FROM ILLNESS

Many diseases impose an increased need for energy and nutrients upon the body. Fever may cause the loss of up to 4 grams of nitrogen (the breakdown products of body protein) per day in sweat. Most of this may be the same nitrogen that would have been excreted in urine, but far more energy is required to produce sweat than urine. Even mild infections increase metabolic losses of vitamins and minerals. Since the macro- and micronutrients of diseased or injured tissues are broken down and to a great extent excreted, nutrient needs during recuperation from illness are comparable to those during periods of growth or pregnancy.

When a person is recovering from surgery nutrient needs are especially great. Much new tissue and, perhaps, blood must be synthesized. The maintenance of nutritional status in order to preserve resistance is paramount. It is fairly common for poorly nourished people who have had surgery or a serious illness to succumb to infection because of impaired resistance during their recovery period.

Energy needs for activity are reduced when a person is bedridden, but the physiological stress of most illnesses causes an overall increase in energy needs. Fever is evidence of a loss of energy (as heat), and therefore energy sources must be provided in the diet or by intravenous feedings. If energy is not supplied, body tissues will be broken down to meet this need.

Nutritional status during illness is often worsened

Epidemiological studies show that infectious diseases are more deadly in malnourished people, and nutritional deficiencies are worsened by infections.

TABLE 21-1. Drug–Nutrient Interactions

Type of Drug	Effect on Nutrient
Antacids	Decreased absorption of iron and phosphate
Antibiotics	Varied effects due to alteration of bacterial population of intestine (changes in bacterial synthesis and utilization of vitamins; nutrient losses due to diarrhea)
Anticancer drugs, such as methotrexate	Interfere with folate metabolism
Anticonvulsants	Cause low serum folate levels
Antidepressants and antihistamine agents	Stimulate appetite and nutrient intake
Aspirin and barbiturates	Increased excretion of vitamin C
Diuretics	Increased urinary excretion of water, sodium, and potassium
Ethanol (grain alcohol)	Increased zinc loss in urine
Isoniazid (antituberculosis)	Interferes with pyridoxine metabolism
Metformin (a hypo-glycemic agent)	Decreased absorption of vitamin B_{12}
Mineral oil	Reduced absorption of fat-soluble vitamins
Penicillamine	Increased excretion of pyridoxine
Tetracycline	Reduced availability of calcium because the drug binds the mineral in bone

by loss of appetite or by nausea and vomiting after eating. One difficulty in meeting nutrient requirements in patients with certain types of cancer is that the disease distorts taste perception and many foods are no longer appealing. Stores of fat and fat-soluble vitamins may be adequate during a brief illness, but reserves of water-soluble vitamins are quickly depleted. Since protein storage is minimal, the only possible way to meet daily protein needs is for muscles and other tissues to be broken down into amino acids, which are then rebuilt into the proteins necessary for maintaining minimal body functions.

Sometimes the therapy for a disease worsens nutrition problems. Radiation therapy and many drugs may cause nausea and vomiting. The patient may understandably refuse to eat as a result. Some drugs

that affect nutritional status are listed in Table 21-1.

When a person is ill a specific diet should be recommended by a doctor or therapeutic dietitian. Attention must be given to selecting foods that are acceptable to the patient and also provide protein, energy, and other specific nutrients needed in excess of normal requirements. Illness should not be interpreted as a time to let the body rest from digesting food. On the contrary, the increased need for nutrients (and fluids) should be considered a vital part of caring for a sick person.

HOW HIGH CAN YOU BUILD RESISTANCE?

There is no evidence (with the possible exception of vitamin C, which we discuss later) that the use of

Nutrient needs increase during illness and convalescence because damaged tissues must be replaced, energy is lost as body heat (fever), and some drugs impair the utilization of nutrients. These problems are further complicated if the patient does not eat.

nutrient supplements in amounts greater than the RDA reduces the chances of infections or builds up resistance. Such beliefs are popular, but generally rest on fallacies and misunderstandings.

Common Misunderstandings

The idea that healthy people need extra nutrients can be traced to three misconceptions.

1. Some people fail to realize that the scientists who establish the RDA take into account the needs for maintaining health. The RDA is a recommendation well in excess of the minimal requirement of the average person. It is set at a level high enough to meet the needs of most (not just the average) people.

2. People do not understand that when the body's needs for most micronutrients are met, additional intakes are not absorbed, are dumped out in the urine or bile, or produce ill effects.

3. Many people have the idea that if a little of something is good, a lot is better. This is false in terms of nutrients; a lot may actually cause serious health problems. For example, vitamin A deficiency causes ulcers of the cornea of the eye, but a dose only slightly higher than the RDA over a long period of time causes skin changes, generalized itching, blurring of vision, loss of hearing, and headaches.

Nutrients As Drugs

There is no evidence that the use of any nutrient supplement in amounts greater than the RDA has any effect whatsoever on sex drive, the aging process, or symptoms of nutrient-deficiency diseases that are avoidable by consuming nutrients in amounts equal to the RDA. However, for certain diseases large doses of vitamins or minerals may be prescribed by a physician. In these situations, the nutrients act in the body as drugs. The effect of large doses (called *pharmacological amounts*) is quite different from the metabolic role of vitamins consumed in amounts provided by the diet (Table 21-2).

Next time you are tempted by an advertisement for nutrient supplements, remember two facts:

1. A drug is used by a physician to treat a specific disorder that is proven to respond to that drug.

2. Since drugs are not normal constituents of the body, they alter existing processes. Physicians do this purposefully and they are alert to possible harmful effects. Self-prescription of drugs is dangerous.

Vitamin C and Resistance

Vitamin C is the micronutrient most often used by the general public in pharmacological doses. The following questions relate to vitamin C, but the same questions should be asked when you evaluate any hypothesis that claims a specific nutrient cures a disease.

What Is the Dosage versus the RDA? The adult RDA for vitamin C is 45 milligrams. Some proponents of vitamin C recommend a daily intake of 200 to 400 milligrams, but many people consume as much as 1,000 to 5,000 milligrams every day—20 to 100 times the RDA.

Might a High Dosage Be Harmful? The medical literature contains several case reports (though as yet no large, conclusive studies) that indicate vitamin C may be dangerous to some people. Large amounts may cause blood clotting problems for people who have sickle cell anemia (most of whom are blacks), inhibit the effectiveness of certain drugs, and make it difficult for a doctor to diagnose diabetes and liver disease.

Vitamin C is metabolized in the body to oxalic acid, which is normally excreted. High concentrations of this acid can cause the formation of crystals or *stones* of oxalic acid salts in the kidneys. Vitamin C may also contribute to the formation of *uric acid* stones. People with gout may have high uric acid levels, so large doses of vitamin C may worsen the disease.

Another possible, though not proven, hazard is that when a person consistently takes supplemental vitamins in excess of the RDA, the body becomes

Vitamins and minerals consumed in pharmacological amounts by healthy, well-nourished people are not absorbed, are excreted in the urine, or function in the body as drugs.

TABLE 21-2. Effects of Varying Doses of Some Essential Nutrients

Substance	Physiological Dose	Pharmacological Dose and Use	Toxic Dose and Manifestations of Toxicity
Vitamin A	5,000 IU	50,000–100,000 IU Acne, Darier's disease	100,000–500,000 IU Headache, nausea, vomiting, pseudotumor cerebri
Vitamin B$_6$	2 mg	50 mg Toxic symptoms of oral contraceptives	10,000 mg Abnormal hepatic enzymes
Niacin	20 mg	2,000–6,000 mg Hypercholesterolemia	100 mg Cutaneous itching 1,000 mg Carbohydrate intolerance 2,000–6,000 mg Gastritis, emotional unrest
β-Tocopherol	15 mg	300–1,200 mg Cardiovascular disorders	1,000 mg/kg (experimental animals) ↑Deposition of cholesterol in aorta ↓Hepatic tolerance to ethanol
Vitamin D	400 IU	50,000–100,000 IU Hypophosphatemic rickets	1,000–3,000 IU (children) Hypercalcemia 150,000 IU (adults) Renal failure
Vitamin C	45 mg	100–2,000 mg Colds, bladder infections	2,000–4,000 mg Reproductive failure, interferes with tests for glycosuria, reverses effects of anticoagulants, may induce nephrolithiasis, inactivates vitamin B$_{12}$, induction of vitamin C-dependent syndrome

NOTE: Pharmacological doses of essential nutrients may equal or exceed the minimal toxic levels. They may or may not be accepted as proper treatment.
SOURCE: Adapted from R. E. Hodges, ''Ascorbic Acid,'' in *Present Knowledge in Nutrition,* 4th ed. ⓒ 1976, The Nutrition Foundation, Inc. Also used by permission of the author.

accustomed to these doses. When supplements are stopped, signs of vitamin C deficiency may appear. Several case reports are on record of pregnant women taking large doses of vitamin C and their babies developing scurvy-like symptoms on a normal diet. However, no controlled studies have been done—nor are they likely to be done in humans because of medical ethics—to test whether there is a causal relationship between these two observations.

Does the Nutrient Produce the Effect Claimed? In the case of vitamin C, does it affect resistance to colds? Research to evaluate the effect of a vitamin upon a disease must be carefully designed according to the following criteria:

1. There must be two groups of people studied. One group receives the vitamin; the other takes a pill called a *placebo*, which looks and tastes exactly the same but contains no vitamin. Everything else affecting the health and diets of these two groups must be comparable. The larger the groups, the greater is the confidence that can be placed in the results of the experiment if differences are slight.

2. Neither the subjects nor the researchers know which pill is the vitamin and which is the placebo until after the study is completed and the results are analyzed; someone else holds this information. Such studies are called *double-blind* experiments.

3. There must be some way of measuring the *incidence* (number of new cases in a population) or severity of the disease so the results in the two groups can be compared. This is especially important when studying a disease such as a cold, which is difficult to measure by laboratory tests.° The diagnosis of a cold depends more on how an individual feels than on measurable changes.

° This problem is even more serious in current investigations of the effects of additives on hyperkinetic children, where laboratory tests for hyperkinesis do not yet exist.

Four studies of vitamin C are summarized in Table 21-3. Three of these studies met the above criteria; one was not double-blind. The results of these studies are not directly comparable because different indexes were used to measure the effectiveness of the nutrient supplement. However, each study showed that vitamin C reduced one or more of the measures related to colds. The greatest effect seemed to be on the severity of the cold (days of illness or confinement) rather than on the number of colds. The subjects who took vitamin C were sick, on the average, about half a day less than those who took the placebo.

How Much Is Effective? This question is best answered by comparing the results of several studies. Table 21-3 shows that there was little difference in the reduced incidence or severity of colds in subjects taking 200 milligrams of vitamin C compared to those taking 1,000, 2,000, 3,000, or 4,000 milligrams. The effectiveness of the lower dosage is especially important in light of the possible hazards of high doses. Note also that a basic piece of information was omitted in all these studies—the amount of dietary vitamin C consumed was not determined by the researchers. If the diets of the people studied were inadequate in this nutrient, the same results (improved resistance) may have been obtained simply by consuming the RDA or 45 milligrams of vitamin C.

Does the Possible Benefit Outweigh the Possible Risk? The final choice regarding supplemental vitamin C depends upon your interpretation of existing research reports. The primary considerations include evidence supporting the benefits, evidence supporting the risks, and how the dosages of the nutrient (45, 200, 1,000, or 5,000 milligrams) correlate with both benefits and risks.

TABLE 21-3. Effects of Vitamin C on the Cold

Measure	Navajo Study[a] Age (years)		Canada Study[b]	Minnesota Study[c]	NIH Study[d]	Literature Review of Nine Studies
	6–10	10–15				
Dosage (mg)						
Routinely	1,000	2,000	1,000	200	1,000	
For colds	Same	Same	4,000	Same	3,000	
Duration of study	14 weeks	14 weeks	2 months			
Number of subjects	641 (both age groups)		418	—	311	
Measure of effectiveness						
Percentage of subjects free of illness	—	—	26 (vitamin C) 18 (placebo)	—		
Number of colds	—	—	—	15% fewer colds in vitamin C group	1.27 (vitamin C) 1.36 (placebo)	0.09 fewer colds for those taking vitamin C
Days of illness						
Vitamin C group	26% fewer	33% fewer in girls	1.3	1.1	6.59	0.11 day less for those taking vitamin C
Control group		No difference in boys	1.87	1.6	7.14	
Comment	Strongest correlation for nasal discharge and cough		Primary effect on severity of illness based on days confined to house		Placebo was visibly different from vitamin C pill; data indicate that double-blind was broken	

[a] J. Coulehan et al., "Vitamin C prophylaxis in a boarding school," *New England Journal of Medicine* 290(1974):6–10.
[b] T. W. Anderson, B. W. Reid, and G. H. Beaton, "Vitamin C and the common cold: A double-blind trial," *Journal of the Canadian Medical Association* 107(1971):503–508.
[c] D. W. Cowan et al., *Journal of the American Medical Association* 120(1942):1267.
[d] T. R. Karlowski et al., "Ascorbic acid for the common cold: A prophylactic and therapeutic trial," *Journal of the American Medical Association* 231(1975):1038.

SOURCE: Adapted from M. Morrison, "What About Vitamin C?" *FDA Consumer* (October 1974), p. 29.

STUDY QUESTIONS

1. What factors influence resistance to offending agents?

2. Which nutrients help prevent bacterial invasion of the body?

3. How do results of animal experiments contribute to our knowledge about human nutrition?

4. What deficiencies cause impairment of antibody formation in experimental animals? In humans?

5. How is the role of the lymphoid tissues in resistance affected by malnutrition?

6. What two correlations regarding nutritional status and infectious diseases have been shown by epidemiological studies?

7. How do nutrient needs change during illness and convalescence?

8. What happens to vitamins and minerals consumed in pharmacological amounts?

9. How do you evaluate a claim that a micronutrient cures a disease?

SUGGESTED READING

1. R. K. Chandra, "Iron and immunocompetence," *Nutrition Reviews* 34(1976):129–32.

2. L. Schlesingel and A. Stekel, "Impaired cellular immunity in marasmic infants," *American Journal of Clinical Nutrition* 27(1974):615–21.

3. B. S. Worthington, "Effect of nutritional status on immune phenomena," *Journal of the American Dietetic Association* 65(1974):123.

4. J. J. Vitale and R. A. Good, eds., "Nutrition and immunology: Symposium," *American Journal of Clinical Nutrition* 27(1974):623–63.

5. H. McFarlane, "Nutrition and immunity," Chapter 45 in *Present Knowledge in Nutrition*. 4th ed. New York and Washington, D.C.: The Nutrition Foundation, 1976.

6. R. E. Hodges, "Ascorbic acid," Chapter 13 in *Present Knowledge in Nutrition*. 4th ed. New York and Washington, D.C.: The Nutrition Foundation, 1976.

7. M. C. Latham, "Nutrition and infection in national development," in *Food: Politics, Economics, Nutrition and Research*, P. H. Abelson, ed. American Association for the Advancement of Science, 1976.

8. T. R. Karlowaki et al, "Ascorbic acid for the common cold: A prophylactic and therapeutic trial," *Journal of the American Medical Association* 231(1975):1038–42.

9. V. Herbert, "Megavitamin therapy: Facts and fictions," *Food and Nutrition News* 47(March-April 1976).

10. "Hazards of overuse of vitamin D," *Nutrition Reviews* 33(1975):61–62.

11. M. I. Irwin and B. K. Hutchins, "A Conspectus of research on vitamin C requirements of man," *Journal of Nutrition* 106(1975):821.

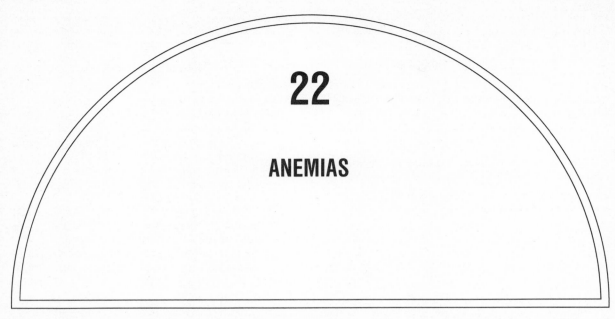

22

ANEMIAS

Anemia is the most common disorder that results from nutrient deficiency. Although anemia is generally not life-threatening, it is a significant health problem in the United States because it affects so many people and impairs their abilities to perform optimally. The abnormalities associated with anemia occur at the cellular level, but they result in restricted functional capacity of the entire body.

PREVALENCE

The *prevalence rate* of anemia (the number of cases that exist in a defined population at a given point in time, for example, at the time a survey is done) in the United States is difficult to determine. This is true partly because health authorities have not agreed upon a definition of anemia (see the section "Indexes of Anemia"). The overall prevalence rates of 10 to 20 percent or more of the United States population reported in the HANES (Figure 18-5) are alarming. In other local studies of children, whether from low-, middle-, or high-income families, up to 40 percent have been found to be anemic! Not all people with anemias have dietary deficiencies, but the majority of them do. Why does

such a large segment of our population suffer from anemia? What is wrong with our approach to correcting this problem? Why are so many of us apparently not able to make proper food selections and avoid deficiencies that cause anemia?

Lack of money to buy food can account for only a small percentage of the anemia in this country. The best sources of iron and the other needed nutrients (beans, liver, enriched cereal products, many vegetables) are less expensive than most poorer sources. Food Stamps have made these foods accessible to many people who might otherwise not be able to afford them. Also, the School Lunch program offers these foods to millions of children, but much of the food goes from cafeteria line, to tray, to the garbage.

Possible explanations for the majority of anemia cases are that people lack information, that not enough effort has been made by nutritionists to motivate people, or that people simply do not care or think enough about their own health or about what it takes to raise healthy children. The recent emphasis on personal responsibility for health in this country may help decrease the prevalence of this condition. Most anemia can be avoided, but pre-

The majority of the American population falls within age or sex groups considered to be vulnerable to nutritional anemia. Anemia is a group of conditions characterized by decreased amounts of hemoglobin within the red blood cells and/or a deficiency of red blood cells, resulting in reduced capacity to transport oxygen to the tissue cells throughout the body.

vention depends upon the ability and desire to make thoughtful food choices based upon an understanding of its causes and knowledge of diet patterns that protect against it.

MEANING OF ANEMIA

The word *anemia* is frequently used, along with the terms *tired blood* and *low blood*, but few people really understand what goes wrong—and why— when they have this problem. *Anemia* is a combination of the prefix *an-* (lack of, or without), the root *-em-* (blood, h*em*e), and the suffix *-ia* (condition of). The literal meaning, "a condition of lack of blood," refers to a relative not an absolute—deficiency. To understand this terminology, we must know a bit more about blood.

Composition of Blood

Blood is actually a mixture of many things; there is no chemical formula or structure for it. Doctors speak of blood as a tissue, just as they refer to liver tissue or heart tissue. The major difference between blood and other tissues is that some of the blood cells are suspended in flowing liquid instead of being stationary. Thus, blood has both a fluid component and a cellular component.

The cellular component of blood consists of many types and subtypes of cells. Some are red, others are white, still others are small pieces of cells called *platelets* (which are necessary for blood clotting). During various stages of their life cycles, blood cells reside in different parts of the body—bone marrow, spleen, storage vessels, and the circulatory trees.

The fluid component of blood is called *plasma*. When the red and white blood cells are separated from whole blood, the remaining translucent, yellowish fluid is plasma. This fluid is largely water, but it is more viscous (sticky) than water because it contains 6 to 8 percent protein. Some of the plasma proteins were listed earlier in Table 2-2.

Indexes of Anemia

Many different tests provide evidence of anemia. Most of these are indirect and provide information about the functional capacity of the blood (Figure 22-1).

Hematocrit. The *hematocrit* is the volume of red blood cells as a percentage of the total volume of blood in a sample. This direct measurement indicates whether adequate blood cells are present at a given moment in the circulatory system—usually in the venous side of the system.

Hemoglobin Concentration. The concentration of hemoglobin provides an indication of the potential capacity of the blood to bind and transport oxygen throughout the body.

Serum Iron Content. The serum iron content indicates how much iron is either in a free state or bound to the protein, transferrin. This provides an estimate of the body's stores or reserves of iron for manufacturing hemoglobin if there is an increase in demand—as in hemorrhage or pregnancy.

The normal values for these indexes (given in Figure 22-1) have been established by studies on limited groups of people. In spite of several decades of use, these normal values have not been validated in all racial and ethnic groups of all ages and body sizes. Therefore, there is some disagreement among experts on the significance of values that lie just outside these normal ranges. Because of this, the results of large surveys of populations may show different prevalence rates for anemia, depending upon the cutoff point used in the definition of anemia for the survey. Such problems plague many epidemiological studies, but usually results of large surveys are quite close to each other.

Anemia decreases the availability of energy within body cells and leads to compensatory overwork of the heart and circulatory system.

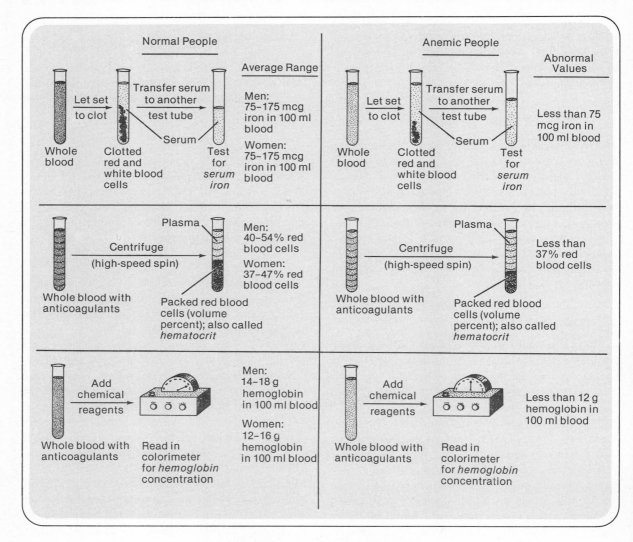

FIGURE 22-1. Tests for anemia.

Effects of Anemia

Anemia may be manifest by a decreased number of red blood cells, decreased hemoglobin, ineffective hemoglobin, or all of these. Any of these conditions will mean that less oxygen is delivered to the cells.

Lack of oxygen at the cellular level causes a metabolic slowdown comparable to a dietary lack of energy-providing macronutrients. When body cells are inadequately oxygenated, the heart and circulatory system speed up in an effort to circulate the blood faster through the lungs (where oxygen enters the system) and then out to the tissues. The more severe the anemia is, the greater the burden on the heart (which itself is operating less effectively due to lack of oxygen reaching cells in the heart).

When a mildly anemic person exercises or has fever, signs of anemia may be noticed. The increased cellular need for oxygen will cause pounding of the heart and skipped beats (palpitations).

The paleness associated with anemia is not easily detected until the condition is moderately advanced. It can be detected most readily by examining the areas of the body where capillaries are closest to the surface of the skin—eyelids, membranes of the mouth, and skin under the fingernails. Signs of anemia such as pallor must be investigated by laboratory tests to determine the cause, severity, and appropriate therapy.

TYPES OF ANEMIAS

Anemia is often caused by nutrient deficiencies, but it may be due to scores of other disorders.

Nutritional Anemias

Many nutrients are involved either directly or indirectly in the production of red blood cells and hemoglobin and in other blood functions such as clotting. These nutrient roles were discussed in Chapter 6.

Blood Cell Abnormalities. Almost all deficiencies eventually cause reduced numbers of red blood cells and reduced transport of oxygen through the body. The type of blood cell abnormality that results from lack of a nutrient depends upon the function(s) of the missing nutrient.

Red blood cells are formed by the division of existing immature blood cells in the interior of bones, called the *bone marrow* (Figure 22-2).° Folic

° In the fetus and during some diseases, blood cells are also produced in the liver and spleen.

acid and vitamin B_{12} are necessary for this division and maturation. During maturation, hemoglobin is synthesized from iron, amino acids, and other small molecules; pyridoxine and copper also play important roles in hemoglobin synthesis. The blood cell abnormalities differ, depending upon whether cell division or hemoglobin synthesis are obstructed.

In mild iron deficiency, the number of red blood cells may be normal, but they are small (*microcytic*, meaning "small cells") and contain less hemoglobin (Figure 22-3). This lower concentration of hemoglobin prevents the cells from carrying normal amounts of oxygen, and the cells lose some of their red color (*hypochromic*, meaning "low color"). Lack of copper or pyridoxine also results in decreased hemoglobin and less intense red color of the cells.

Lack of folic acid or vitamin B_{12} hinders the capacity of parent red cells in the bone marrow to divide on schedule or mature properly. The resulting cells are abnormally large, inadequate in numbers, quite fragile, and susceptible to breakdown earlier than the normal 120 day lifespan. Deficiencies of these vitamins also impair white blood cell production and function.

Under the microscope, the appearance of red blood cells will be similar in folic acid and vitamin B_{12} deficiencies. This makes it difficult to decide which nutrient is causing the anemia. To make matters even more confusing, large doses of folic acid will cure anemia due to vitamin B_{12} deficiency, but folic acid does not cure the nerve damage caused by lack of vitamin B_{12}. If a person takes extra folic acid for a "tired, run-down condition," but actually is deficient in vitamin B_{12}, the anemia will go away but the nerve destruction will continue to worsen. This predicament is especially dangerous because it is very difficult for a physician to recognize the nerve damage until it becomes quite severe and possibly has progressed beyond the point where it could be cured; the lost nerve functions may never be restored.

Other types of nutritional anemias also exist. A deficiency of vitamin E causes the red cells to be

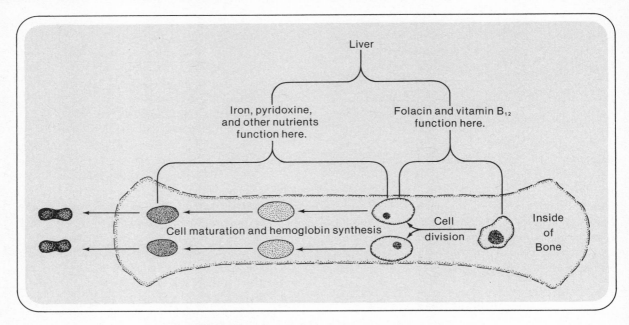

FIGURE 22-2. Normal production of red blood cells.

abnormally large, this nutritional anemia is rare except in premature infants and people with malabsorption diseases.

The anemias associated with pellagra and scurvy (Chapter 27) may resemble either iron or folic acid–vitamin B_{12} deficiency—or a mixture of these abnormalities. The diets of people with pellagra and scurvy are usually inadequate in several nutrients.

Causes. Nutritional anemias are caused by inadequate dietary intakes of one or more nutrients. Different circumstances that are common in certain groups of people often lead to such imbalances. Many of these were mentioned in Section IV, but they are summarized here.

1. A newborn infant may have a nutritional anemia if its mother's diet was deficient. Premature infants are vulnerable to anemia due to iron or vitamin E deficiency because these nutrients are primarily transferred to the fetus during the last few weeks in utero of a normal length pregnancy. The need to supplement a baby's diet with iron-rich food (such as cereal) depends upon its stores of this mineral accumulated before birth.

2. The toddler, still carrying a bottle everywhere it goes, is a prime candidate for anemia. Such a child often gets most of its energy from milk (a poor source of iron) and therefore has little appetite for other iron-rich foods. This nutritional anemia can occur even when body weight is normal or excessive—the problem is often not recognized by the parents.

3. School-age children who have not learned to like vegetables (especially the green, leafy types) miss excellent sources of iron and folacin. Enriched cereal and baked goods can help supply iron and three of the B vitamins, but if most of these foods contain large amounts of sugar, the overall nutrient density of the child's diet is diluted. Also, grain products are not a good source of folacin.

4. Teen-agers have heightened needs for must nutrients because they are growing rapidly and are usually more active than older people. Their daily diets are often repetitive. If the foods eaten most frequently are

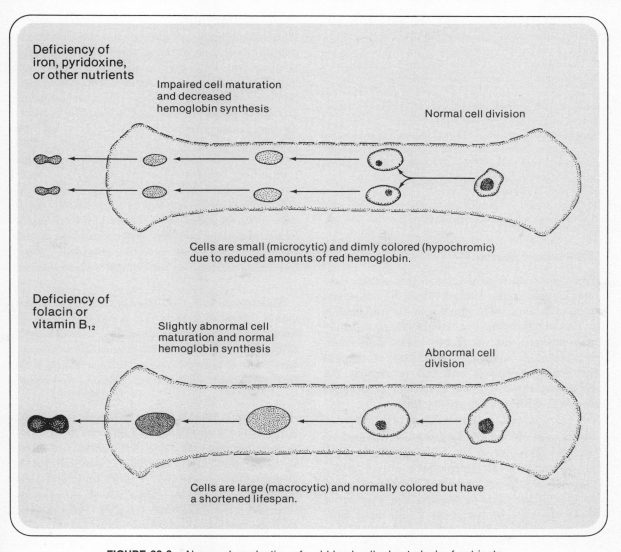

Deficiency of iron, pyridoxine, or other nutrients

Impaired cell maturation and decreased hemoglobin synthesis

Normal cell division

Cells are small (microcytic) and dimly colored (hypochromic) due to reduced amounts of red hemoglobin.

Deficiency of folacin or vitamin B₁₂

Slightly abnormal cell maturation and normal hemoglobin synthesis

Abnormal cell division

Cells are large (macrocytic) and normally colored but have a shortened lifespan.

FIGURE 22-3. Abnormal production of red blood cells due to lack of nutrients.

soft drinks, candy, and milk shakes (poor sources of the raw materials needed for red blood cell formation), nutritional anemias are almost inevitable.

5. In men, a nutritional anemia is very frequently associated with excessive reliance upon alcohol as a dietary source of energy. Nonalcoholic adult males usu-ally consume sufficient amounts of foods that supply the nutrients needed for red cell formation. In fact, about one-fourth of the iron in their bodies is present in the storage form.

6. Women rarely have significant iron reserves unless they pay particular attention to their needs for this

nutrient. The pregnant woman who fails to acquire prenatal supervision or delays it until the last few months of pregnancy will probably be deficient in iron and possibly in folacin. Both she and her infant may suffer complications at or soon after delivery because of her negligence. Disregard for dietary advice from a doctor, nurse, or nutritionist causes the same consequences.

7. Elderly people often suffer from anemia because of their overall reduced food intake and failure to consume foods rich in iron and/or folacin. Production of stomach acid is diminished in some older people, and therefore dietary iron is not absorbed well.

8. Vegetarians of all ages must plan their diets carefully (Chapter 12) to avoid the risk of anemia.

Nonnutritional Anemias

Deficiencies of iron or folacin account for most of the anemia in the United States, but these are not the only causes. The conditions discussed below may produce the same run-down feelings and paleness as anemias due to dietary deficiencies. Self-prescription of nutrient supplements to correct other disease processes will fail to remedy the anemia and allow the real condition to progress unchecked, with possible risk of life.

Blood Loss. Blood may be lost in many ways that are less obvious than a cut. Stomach ulcers allow blood to leak into the gastrointestinal tract. If this continues, a significant amount of blood may be lost even though the ulcer is painless and may occur without any signs or symptoms. If the total daily blood loss exceeds 50 to 60 millilitres, the stools may then give warning by their black color and stickiness. If bleeding is slight-to-moderate and intermittent, significant iron losses will occur and yet stools will usually appear normal. For example, 50 millilitres of blood (10 teaspoonfuls) lost in the stools each day is equal to a loss of 25 milligrams of iron. To replace this amount, a person would have to consume as much as 200 to 250 milligrams of iron above the RDA of 10 to 18 milligrams per day.

(Remember only 10 to 15 percent of iron in the diet is absorbed. Higher percentages may be absorbed by people whose iron stores are depleted.) In order to keep up with this rate of iron loss, a person would have to eat enormous amounts of iron-rich foods— 30 ounces of hog liver, 14 cups of enriched farina, 23 cups of prune juice per day. Clearly, it would be far easier (and probably less expensive) to have the ulcer treated than to eat such quantities of foods. And the risk of massive hemorrhage or intestinal perforation from ulcer disease would be reduced once treatment was effective.

Blood loss may also occur in the intestines due to other diseases and parasite infestation. Iron supplements alone do not cure these disorders, and if proper medical attention is not obtained, massive bleeding may occur in later stages of these diseases.

Malabsorption. Malabsorption of nutrients causes a form of anemia that is not correctable by taking vitamins or minerals orally. The underlying disease must be treated. Malabsorption syndromes have several different causes, such as allergies, infections, tumors, blood vessel diseases, and others.

Pernicious Anemia. Though pernicious anemia is associated with vitamin B_{12}, it is not caused by a dietary deficiency. It is due to the absence of intrinsic factor (see Chapter 4), which is necessary for the absorption of vitamin B_{12}. Failure to diagnose and treat this anemia by injections of vitamin B_{12} throughout the affected person's life results in spinal cord degeneration and death.

Sickle Cell Anemia. One of several anemias caused by a genetic disorder is sickle cell anemia. As many as 7 to 8 percent of American blacks have a mild form of sickle cell anemia, called *sickle cell trait.* Two or three percent of blacks also may have *hemoglobin C trait.* These and hundreds of other disorders of hemoglobin may show up as mild cases of anemia; they do not respond to dietary treatment.

Nutrition-conscious adults may safely donate blood three, or perhaps four, times a year without developing nutrient deficiencies. At the same time, they receive a medical checkup for anemia.

BLOOD DONATIONS

This discussion of anemia might make you skeptical about the wisdom of donating blood. But several facts may alleviate this fear. When you offer to give blood, a fingertip blood sample is taken first. This blood sample is tested to be sure you are not anemic. A check of your height, weight, pulse, and blood pressure lend additional margins of safety because nutritional status and reserves may be inferred from these measurements. Indeed, a visit to a bloodmobile is an inexpensive and convenient way to find out whether you are even marginally anemic or have certain other measurable disorders (such as high blood pressure or some types of heart disease).

Another reason not to fear blood donation is that healthy people have a reserve of red blood cells in the spleen and other parts of the circulatory system that can be mobilized quickly. They also have a phenomenal capacity to increase red cell production to compensate for blood loss, whether it is voluntary or accidental.

Some people feel faint after a blood donation. This is not primarily due to oxygen insufficiency, but is caused by the decreased volume of fluid in the circulatory system. Within a few hours the body normally compensates for this by shifting body water from the tissue cells into the circulatory system.

The juice or soft drink offered to blood donors is more than a courteous thanks; it helps compensate for the fluid loss. It is also a subtle way to keep the donor at rest while drinking the beverage and within the area supervised by the physician or nurse, should any problem arise. Within four to six hours for most donors and 24 hours for nearly all donors, the blood volume will be normal.

Iron is obviously donated along with the blood. In a pint of blood there will be 200 to 250 milligrams of iron. Spread over a year, this is 0.6 to 0.7 milligram per day. Dietary intake must be 3 to 7 milligrams every day above normal needs to rebuild iron stores. For adult males, this margin is easily achieved without much effort. For women, especially those who are menstruating, careful selection of iron-dense foods is necessary. Blood donations are accepted from an individual no more frequently than every three months—the minimum time for a nutrition-conscious person to restore the iron reserves.

STUDY QUESTIONS

1. How common is anemia in the United States?

2. What is the result of anemia at the cellular level?

3. How does anemia affect the heart and circulatory system?

4. How does the appearance of red blood cells help a doctor diagnose the cause of a nutritional anemia?

5. What are some nonnutritional anemias?

6. What are the benefits and risks of donating blood?

SUGGESTED READING

1. Committee on Nutrition of the Mother and Preschool Child, Food and Nutrition Board, *Iron Nutriture in Adolescence*. Washington, D.C.: National Academy of Sciences, 1976.
2. J. D. Cook et al, "Serum ferritin as a measure of iron stores in normal subjects," *American Journal of Clinical Nutrition* 27(1974):681–87.
3. E. N. Todhunter, "Iron, blood and nutrition," *Journal of the American Dietetic Association* 61(1972):121.
4. J. W. Suttie, "Vitamin K and prothrombin synthesis," *Nutrition Reviews* 31(1973):105–109.
5. C. C. Johnson and M. F. Futrell, "Anemia in black preschool children in Mississippi: Dietary and hematologic findings," *Journal of the American Dietetic Association* 65(1974):536.
6. C. A. Finch, "Iron metabolism," *Nutrition Today* 4(1969):2–7.

23

GASTROINTESTINAL DISORDERS

Any disease or abnormal function of the gastrointestinal tract may lead to impaired digestion and absorption, and, therefore, affect the nutritional status of a person. Food-related gastrointestinal disorders range in severity from mild discomfort due to certain types of food poisoning (Chapter 20) to a proposed relationship between diet and intestinal cancer (Chapter 24). Between these extremes are many common conditions—peptic ulcers, dyspepsia, constipation, and others—that trouble large numbers of people. Not all these disorders are caused by diet, but understanding the relationship of nutrition to their management may permit some relief of distress or forestall development of nutritional complications.

PEPTIC ULCERS

Peptic ulcers are erosions or circumscribed loss of tissue of the gastrointestinal lining or mucosa. They occur most often in the first portion of the small intestine (the *duodenum*) but may also occur in the stomach and esophagus. These ulcers are more common among people with type O blood than those with types A, B, or AB. Peptic ulcers are two to four times more frequent in men than in women.

Peptic ulcers probably result from an interplay between environmental factors (diet is only one of these) and genetic factors that leads to a general failure of the mucosa to withstand the destructive action of gastric juice. Factors suspected of contributing to this failure are:

1. reduction in cellular resistance,
2. loss of intracellular substances normally protecting the mucosa,
3. excessive secretion of hydrochloric acid,
4. diminished secretion of mucus,
5. or a combination of any of these.

The nervous system may also contribute to the production of peptic ulcers by altering the muscular contractions that control the emptying of the stomach, increasing the stomach secretions, and decreasing the blood flow through the stomach cells.

The abdominal discomfort of peptic ulcers varies in severity, frequency, type of pain (dull, burning, gnawing, sharp), and location of pain. Nausea and vomiting or an unpleasant sensation of hunger may

Dietary modifications recommended for a person with a peptic ulcer include distributing food intake among five or six small meals, maintaining appropriate body weight, selecting dietary sources of the nutrients needed for healing wounds, and avoiding certain foods that are poorly tolerated by the individual.
Dyspepsia is most often caused by emotional problems or nondietary disorders.

---

be present. Some people who develop massively bleeding ulcers have no discomfort at all to warn them of the disease.

Dietary restrictions of all sorts have been prescribed for people with peptic ulcers, but most of these have not been effective and some have proven harmful. The recommendation that patients drink milk or cream at hourly intervals is highly controversial because of the high fat and cholesterol content of these foods. (Studies have indicated that "heart attacks" are more common in ulcer patients on high-fat, high-cholesterol diets than among other people.) Various antacids and prescription drugs, along with other modifications in habits, are probably safer treatment for ulcer disease—but drugs also have complications.

It is generally agreed that dividing the day's total food intake into five or six small meals rather than the usual two or three meals reduces the symptoms of ulcers and hastens healing. It is important that people with ulcer disease include in their diets the nutrients required for tissue repair—adequate protein, vitamin C, and zinc. Adequate amounts of these nutrients are available from foods (supplements should not be necessary) if care is taken in diet planning. If overweight is present, professional guidance is required to achieve normal or ideal body weight while also permitting healing of the ulcer. There is no evidence that coarse or spicy foods delay healing, or that a soft or bland diet hasten healing. Tobacco, alcohol, caffeine-containing beverages (coffee and colas),° and certain drugs (especially aspirin and antiarthritis drugs) often complicate the treatment of ulcer disease. Some people find that certain foods cause worsening of symptoms; these should then be avoided.

A rigid dietary regimen does not necessarily prevent the recurrence of ulcer disease and may be self-defeating. If the prescribed diet is tastelessly bland and preferred foods are not allowed, patients will "cheat" on the diet and probably will not follow other recommendations either.

The information provided here is not intended to replace the need for careful medical evaluation and supervision of people who have ulcer disease or symptoms of peptic ulcers. This discussion merely gives a framework for understanding some of the processes of ulcer disease and a rationale for carrying out whatever dietary modifications are advised. Prevention of complications requires early diagnosis, intensive education, support and encouragement, and an integrated approach to the development of sound health practices.

DYSPEPSIA

Dyspepsia (difficult digestion) describes a general condition in which the coordinated muscular functions of the stomach or intestines are disturbed. The person with dyspepsia experiences one or several complaints: nausea, heartburn, bitter taste, bad breath, foul and/or acidic burping, lack of appetite, a pain or fullness beneath the breastbone, and a feeling of fullness or bloating (especially after meals).

Dyspepsia may be caused by a disease of the stomach, liver, gall bladder, kidney, pancreas, or intestine. It is also observed in diabetes, hypertension, atherosclerosis, and cancer. Emotional tension, however, is associated with over half of the cases of dyspepsia.

The main line of therapy is not dietary, but correction of the underlying problem. When emotional behavior contributes to a digestive disturbance, the patient and the doctor together must seek to uncover and correct the psychological problem. In such cases, use of dietary measures alone may lessen the symptoms but not alter the cause of the condition.

° Recent reports indicate that substances other than caffeine in coffee, tea, and cola beverages worsen ulcer symptoms and delay the healing process.

The incidence of true constipation is not as high as many people might assume.
Prolonged, mild diarrhea or severe, short-term diarrhea can rob the body of dietary nutrients and nutrient stores, thus retarding the recovery and repair processes.

CONSTIPATION

Many myths linger among the general public about constipation. The most prevalent myth is that everyone should have a normal bowel movement every day. Despite what you might surmise from advertisements for laxatives, the important consideration is simply that the feces should be eliminated frequently enough to maintain personal comfort— whether this occurs twice a day, daily, or every third day. Failure to appreciate this concept has created unnecessary concern for many people and forced countless children to spend hours in the bathroom instead of being outside playing. If the child were out getting some exercise, this would probably be a better stimulus to defecation than parental harangues.

Constipation is indeed a problem for many people, especially pregnant women (Chapter 14) and elderly people (Chapter 19). Other people simply do not take the time or they resist the urge to defecate. They may maintain a routine that is so irregular they are not aware of this physiologically important action. Other causes of constipation include use of some nonabsorbable antacids, other drugs, thyroid disorders, lead poisoning, and mental depression.

The consequences of habitual constipation may be not only rectal and anal discomfort, but associated sensations of bloating, excessive flatulence, headache, dizziness, weakness, and poor appetite. These associated symptoms may cause a person to alter eating habits, thus, perhaps, resulting in poor dietary selections and nutrient imbalances.

Very little well-designed research has been carried out on the treatment of constipation. But it is known that most people, after a bit of effort, can cure their constipation without recourse to laxatives. Exercise and an additional four to six glasses of fluids are generally recommended. A large breakfast with a regular toilet stop for a relaxed ten minutes each morning often works wonders after three or

four weeks. Occasionally it may be necessary to use a water-retaining colloid (such as agar) with 12 ounces of water at bedtime in order to relieve the dryness of stools. Nondigestible carbohydrate within the intestine (Chapter 24) presumably acts as a mechanical stimulant in aiding defecation. The gases produced by bacterial metabolism of intestinal contents also produce a laxative effect.

Many commercial laxatives increase the ionic concentration within the intestine by an irritant effect. This causes additional fluid to seep or ooze into the intestines, and also increases motility by stimulating muscular contractions and softening the intestinal contents. Excessive reliance upon laxatives may impair the absorption of iron and calcium, and ultimately lead to the need for more potent cathartics or enemas.

DIARRHEA

Diarrhea may be caused by anxiety, a minor infection, parasites, toxins, and many other disorders. Protein or folacin deficiency and pellagra may also cause diarrhea.

Even minor diarrhea, if prolonged, can significantly affect nutritional status. This is especially true for infants, young children, the aged, and the debilitated. If nutrients move rapidly past the mucosal cells, there is less opportunity for them to be absorbed by the villi. Even more significant are the protein and mineral losses when tissue fluids pass from the blood and body cells into the intestine and are excreted with the diarrheal stools. Strong irritants or toxins and infections destroy the cells lining the intestine. The protein content of these cells as well as other nutrients pass out of the body with the frequent, fluid stools.

The major objective of treatment for diarrhea is to correct its cause. Drugs sometimes reduce the severity of diarrhea by partially paralyzing the muscles and decreasing the activity of glandular cells of the intestinal wall. Bananas, boiled skim

Malabsorption may be caused by nutritional deficiencies, several diseases of the gastrointestinal organs, congenital abnormalities, sensitivity to components of food, and many other disorders.
Flatulence may be caused by swallowing air or by production of gas during the metabolism of nondigestible raffinose sugars by intestinal bacteria.

milk, and apple skins (which contain pectin) may diminish diarrhea. The most important role of the diet, however, is replacement of the lost fluids and nutrients. Mineral and fluid replacement may begin with salty broths; warm, weak tea; and diluted fruit juices. Orange juice and bananas help to replace the potassium losses. Thin cooked cereals provide energy, fluids, and micronutrients, but concentrated sweets and starches are not tolerated well early in the treatment period.

MALABSORPTION

A discussion of all malabsorption syndromes goes far beyond the scope of this book. Just a few are mentioned here.

Dietary deficiency of folacin or deficiency of vitamin B_{12} (either dietary or due to lack of intrinsic factor) results in failure of the normal reparative processes of the intestinal cells. The surface of the lining becomes smooth and flat, rather than bristling with villi, thus decreasing the absorptive surface and reducing the absorption of many nutrients.

A cycle of nutrient deficiency, which begets malabsorption, which in turn begets more nutrient deficiency, is epitomized by iron deficiency in the face of failure of stomach acid production. As many as 16 percent of patients with iron deficiency anemia lack stomach hydrochloric acid, and an even larger percentage show superficial wasting of the stomach lining. In younger people these changes may be reversed upon iron replenishment, but in older individuals the changes persist and are not explainable.

Malfunctioning of any gastrointestinal organ may lead to impaired nutritional status. *Hepatitis* and *mononucleosis* impair the synthesis by the liver of bile salts important for fat absorption. *Cystic fibrosis* and *pancreatitis* diminish the secretions of digestive enzymes by the pancreas. *Gall bladder disease,* or *gall stones,* impairs fat digestion.

Some children have congenital abnormalities of the intestinal cells that cause malabsorption. For example, people with disaccharid*ase* deficiency lack the enzymes necessary for cleaving sucrose, lactose, or maltose into simple sugar, thus rendering it unavailable for absorption. Lactose intolerance, a reduced capacity to absorb the sugar of milk, is more common among blacks and Orientals than among Caucasians. The severity of symptoms caused by this disorder varies greatly among individuals.

A few people are born with a sensitivity to certain components of food, such as the protein *gluten* (found in wheat and other cereal products). The cause of gluten sensitivity is unknown, but the disease can cause serious weight loss, weakness, and diarrhea. In severe cases, the patient resembles a person who is starved. Elimination of wheat, oats, barley, and rye from the diet and reliance on special gluten-free foods combined with thoughtful diet planning, enables most people with this condition to maintain fairly normal routines.

FLATULENCE

Excessive intestinal gas production, or *flatulence,* is a problem for many people. Flatulence can be more serious than just a "social problem." It can be accompanied by headache, dizziness, slight mental confusion, and reduced ability to concentrate.

In the majority of cases, the excessive gas simply represents air swallowed because of anxiety. Large volumes of air also enter the stomach when chewing gum or talking while chewing food. Intestinal gas is sometimes produced by the metabolism of intestinal bacteria. It is currently thought that in some instances flatulence is primarily due to bacterial metabolism of small polysaccharides known as the *raffinose* group of sugars. These carbohydrates are chains made of galactose, glucose, and fructose. Four- and five-sugar polysaccharides that contain additional galactose also belong to this group. Raffinose sugars are found in highest concentration in leguminous seeds such as beans and peas.

Humans have little of the enzyme necessary for

digesting raffinoses, but the bacteria *Clostridium perfringens* do have this enzyme. This organism grows under the conditions that exist in the *terminal* portion of the intestine—beyond the portion where simple sugars are optimally absorbed. Therefore, the simple sugars released from raffinoses are primarily utilized by bacteria rather than humans. Bacterial metabolism produces carbon dioxide, and some hydrogen, nitrogen, oxygen, and methane. The latter gas causes the odor associated with flatulence.

STUDY QUESTIONS

1. How should a person with a peptic ulcer modify his/her diet?

2. What causes dyspepsia?

3. What are the causes of constipation?

4. Why is diarrhea a threat to health?

5. What nonnutritional disorders cause malabsorption?

6. Why does the consumption of large amounts of beans or peas cause flatulence in some people?

SUGGESTED READING

1. "Laxatives: What does regular mean?" *FDA Consumer* 9(1975):16–21.
2. "Severe diarrhea in children," *Nutrition Reviews* 33(1975):286–87.
3. C. T. L. Huang et al, "Fecal steroids in diarrhea: I. Acute shigellosis," *American Journal of Clinical Nutrition* 29(1976):949–55.
4. "Coffee drinking and peptic ulcer disease," *Nutrition Reviews* 34(1976):167–68.
5. "Beliefs about the ulcer diet," *Journal of the American Dietetic Association* 60(1972).
6. "Diet, bacteria and the colon: Symposium," *American Journal of Clinical Nutrition* 29(1976):1409–84.
7. C. Garza and N. S. Scrimshaw, "Relationship of lactose intolerance to milk intolerance in young children," *American Journal of Clinical Nutrition* 29(1976):192–96.
8. Several articles on diet and gastrointestinal diseases, *Journal of the American Dietetic Association* 60(1972).

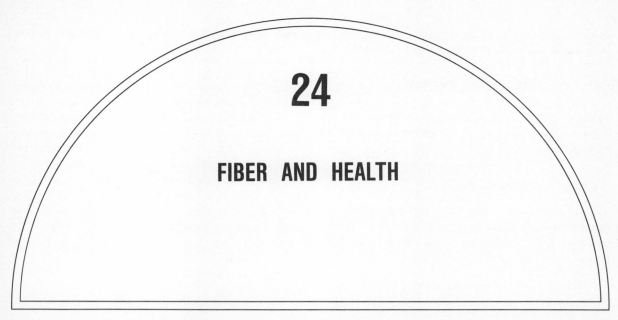

24

FIBER AND HEALTH

The relationships between fiber and several diseases are among the newest and most active areas in nutrition research. So many studies are in progress that the discussion to follow may be outdated shortly after it is written. Although the final answers regarding these relationships remain beyond the horizon of nutrition knowledge, there are several practical purposes for including this discussion on fiber and health.

1. Some basic information about fiber is given.

2. The discussion can help you understand why many answers to nutrition questions are elusive.

3. It illustrates how researchers apply the scientific method of reasoning and investigation to try to answer these questions.

4. It exposes the exploits of overenthusiastic journalists and authors (who have not mastered point 3), and shows how misinterpretation of data may lead to nutrition problems.

THE SCIENTIFIC METHOD

Training in the scientific method of thinking encompasses more than rote memorization. A major educational objective is to sharpen the students' powers of observation, especially of events that do not conform to the expected (such as the observa-tion of families with repeated sets of twins, bleeding disorders that only occur in males, or diseases found only in certain populations or geographic areas). If two or more relatively unexpected conditions are observed under the same circumstances, the scientist develops an hypothesis (or several hypotheses) to explain the observations. Then experiments are carefully designed to test the strength of the hypothesis and find out whether the relationship is cause-and-effect, accidental, or due to an additional cause or condition independently related to each observation.

The discussion to follow requires an understanding of two terms. *Epidemiological investigations* are studies of the distribution and dynamics of diseases or conditions affecting population groups. Observations during such studies raise questions that may be tested in controlled experiments. However, it is difficult, if not impossible, to prove on the basis of epidemiological observations alone that two observations are causally related.

An *hypothesis* is an idea that is not proven but is assumed to be true for purposes of argument or further investigation. Hypotheses may lead to new knowledge, but they should not be mistaken for facts.

FIBER-HEALTH CORRELATION

The correlation between fiber and health developed first from an epidemiological observation that led to an hypothesis.

Epidemiological Observations

Researchers observing the black population in east Africa south of the Sahara Desert noted a lower incidence of the following conditions than existed among Americans and Western Europeans:

1. Ischemic heart disease (the primary cause of heart attacks)
2. Cancer of the colon and rectum
3. Appendicitis
4. Hemorrhoids and varicose veins
5. Diverticular disease of the colon
6. Phlebitis and resulting blood clots to the lungs
7. Obesity

Development of the Hypotheses

Researchers sought possible explanations for these observations. Diets vary in different regions of Africa, but in the areas studied, the people eat relatively large amounts of cornmeal, beans, bananas, and potatoes—a diet quite different from that of most Americans and also different in some ways from diets in other areas of Africa. Therefore, the scientists proposed their first hypothesis.

Hypothesis I. Differences in diet may contribute to the difference in incidence of coronary heart disease, cancer of the colon, appendicitis, hemorrhoids, diverticulosis, phlebitis, and obesity.

This hypothesis does not take into account possible correlations with other differences, such as availability of medical care, life expectancy (and coincidentally the incidence of these diseases in older versus younger people), obesity, exercise, prevalence of intestinal parasites, intestinal bacteria, quality of drinking water, and many other genetic and cultural factors.

Note that the statement of the hypothesis uses the conditional form of the verb, "may contribute." In scientific publications, a researcher should be careful to maintain this grammatical tense. In the popular press, this reservation is often lost after the first paragraph or is buried at the end of the article. Journalists may also make other word changes that make hypotheses sound like definitive results:

Scientist says:	Popular press says:
Theory	Discovery
Implications	Findings
Suggests	Shows
Contributes to	Causes

Since seven disorders were cited in the original hypothesis, researchers had at least seven possible correlations to study. Several of these disorders are gastrointestinal, so the investigators sought some common factor related to digestion or absorption. Fiber is a poorly defined term, even among nutritionists, but it is generally accepted that food high in fiber helps to alleviate constipation. The African diet is higher in fiber than the American diet, so the researchers postulated a second hypothesis.

Hypothesis II. Differences in the fiber content of the diet may contribute to differences in the incidence of the diseases cited.

Note that this hypothesis disregards any other dietary differences between the two populations, such as energy intake in relation to energy needs, fat and other nutrient composition of the diet, specific foods that provide fiber in the diet, animal versus vegetable protein intake, and other variables.

TESTING HYPOTHESIS II

Investigation of Hypothesis II requires several lines of inquiry in order to examine how dietary differences in populations and the physiological effects of fiber might be related to the diseases cited.

The hypotheses regarding the effects of fiber upon health do not take into consideration other differences in the nutrient composition of the diet or epidemiological differences in health status, lifestyle, physiological factors, and cultural factors. Africans eat more fiber than Americans; in the African diet, fiber is supplied primarily by corn and beans rather than wheat.

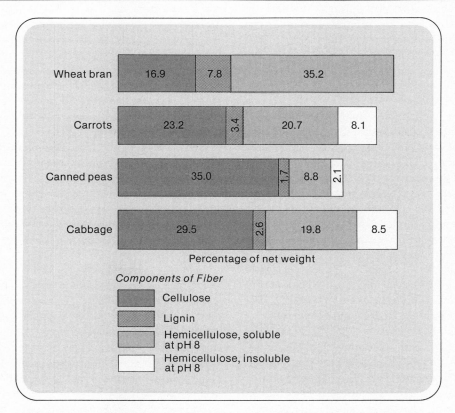

FIGURE 24-1. Variation in amount of components of fiber in several foods. SOURCE: R. D. Williams and W. H. Olmsted, *Journal of Nutrition* 11 (1936):433.

Dietary Considerations

Several dietary factors must be considered. First, we need to define the word *fiber* and then to compare the amount of fiber and the types of fiber-containing foods consumed by the different population groups.

Definition of Fiber. Dietary fiber is loosely defined as the nondigestible components of food. This broad group may be broken down into several family members. The main subgroups are nondigestible carbohydrates (such as cellulose, hemicellulose,

pectic substances, gums) and noncarbohydrates (such as lignin). Very little information is currently available regarding which fiber family members are present in various foods. Results of some analyses done many years ago are shown in Figure 24-1 as examples of the wide differences in the fiber composition of foods.

This information is important since each member of the fiber family may have different physiological effects on the body. Current knowledge of fiber has been compared to what scientists knew about B vitamins fifty years ago. The dietary factor originally called *vitamin B* was later shown to be several separate nutrients, each with different functions in the body, and these vitamins are not all found in the same foods. The family members that make up fiber will most likely be shown to exhibit a comparable individuality.

Crude fiber, another important term, is determined in a laboratory—not in the body. It is a measure of the components (mainly cellulose and lignin) that remain after chemical digestion of food by strong, hot acid and alkali. (This is the only currently available laboratory technique for simulating physiological digestion.) Food composition tables list crude fiber, which is usually less than dietary fiber, but the relative amounts of these two forms vary from food to food. In some foods, dietary fiber is seven times greater than crude fiber; in other foods, these two values are almost the same.

Amount of Fiber. It is important to consider in at least semiquantitative terms the amount of fiber we might want to add to the average American diet to improve health.

The 1965 USDA Household Survey (Chapter 13) found that the average American diet provides approximately 4 grams of crude fiber, whereas studies in Africa have reported average crude fiber intakes of about 25 grams—a difference of approximately 21 grams. In Chapter 21, however, we mentioned that it is sometimes informative to evaluate the results of more than one study. Let's see whether doing this sheds any light on the fiber hypothesis.

A relationship between fiber and its possible effects on health has been deduced by some investigators from observed changes in the American diet during this century and coincidental increases in the incidence of some (but not all) of the diseases cited in the hypothesis. The average American diet in 1909 to 1913 provided approximately 6 grams of fiber. Therefore, the decrease during this century is about 2 grams of crude fiber.

A similar relationship between disease experience and diet history may also be inferred from another study. Differences were observed between pairs of brothers, where one lived in Boston and the other in Ireland. The men who lived in Ireland had lower incidence of cardiovascular diseases than their brothers; their average daily intake of crude fiber was 6.4 grams. The men who immigrated to Boston had higher incidence of cardiovascular diseases; their diet contained only about 3.6 grams of crude fiber. There was a difference in fiber consumption of about 3 grams each day.

These two sets of comparisons raise the question of whether a 2- or 3-gram increase in the amount of fiber consumed by most Americans would have the same effect (if any) as the 21-gram increase suggested by the original observation of Africans. The importance of this question will become clear when we consider the possible problems due to high intake of fiber.

Dietary Source of Fiber. A comparison of the dietary sources of fiber for the two populations studied may help evaluate the fiber hypothesis and its possible dietary implications. Americans derive most of their dietary fiber from wheat, potatoes, fruits, and vegetables; Africans south of the Sahara Desert derive most of their dietary fiber from corn and beans. (Wheat is eaten to a significant degree in Africa only by people who live north of the Sahara, not by the population studied.) This difference in diet patterns calls into question the value of increasing fiber intake by additional amounts of wheat bran and whole-grain cereals. It is possible (though certainly not proved) that the effect upon disease incidence may be attributable to components of fiber found in higher concentrations in corn or beans, but in lower concentrations in wheat products.

Now, let's compare the dietary sources of fiber in the other epidemiological investigation—changes in the United States during this century. Chapter 13 (Figure 13-1) pointed out that since 1910, there has been approximately a 50 percent reduction in consumption of flour and cereal products; this is also true of potatoes. On the other hand, there has been an increase in the consumption of nonfibrous foods

Increased fiber intake speeds the passage of food through the intestine, increases water content and bulk of the feces, and perhaps changes the types of bacteria that reside in the intestine.

---

such as meats and milk. The student who is learning critical nutrition thought patterns should at this moment be considering *another* question about how changes in diet patterns (other than fiber) might correlate with changes in disease patterns.

Physiological Effects

Another line of investigation regarding Hypothesis II involves clarification of the physiological effects of fiber. Experiments have shown several physiological differences between populations that consume small versus relatively large amounts of crude fiber.

Transit Time. Researchers can measure how long it takes a bolus of food to travel through the gastrointestinal tract by giving the subject a colored pill to swallow and then examining the color of each stool passed thereafter. Such studies have shown that transit time for most of the Africans on high-fiber diets is about 40 hours; for Americans this time is about 80 hours.

Fecal Weight and Volume. The feces of subjects who consume high-fiber diets usually weigh more than the feces of people who consume low-fiber diets. The increase in weight is about 10 to 20 times the actual weight of the fiber consumed. This is largely attributed to water absorbed by the nondigestible fiber. For example, 25 grams of fiber would increase fecal weight by about 250 to 500 grams—this approximates the weight of from 1 cup to 1 pint of water.

Consumption of fiber increases the elimination of some energy-containing substances, but this does not alter total energy retained within the body, because humans lack the enzymes to digest such substances. There is currently no evidence that the amount of fiber in the diet has any effect upon the energy derived from other macronutrients in the diet. However, the effect of fiber on absorption of nutrients is a subject of investigation.

Other Changes. Certain intestinal bacteria metabolize fiber for their own nutrient needs. Thus, a high-fiber diet influences the numbers and species of organisms in the intestine—some bacteria increase and others decrease. Changes in the intestinal bacteria population may alter production of intestinal gas, which in turn may explain the changes in transit time. Gaseous distention of the rectum may stimulate more frequent defecation but with reduced fecal volume. (Fecal volume is influenced by the bulk of bacteria excreted with the feces. Up to a quarter of the volume of a stool may be bacteria.)

Another factor to consider is that fiber binds bile salts and fatty acids, which are carried on to the terminal portion of the intestine where they may be metabolized to gases—again, stimulating defecation. Thus, many complex processes are probably affected by the amounts and types of fiber in the diet.

Correlation with Disease

Several theories that may explain the role of fiber in reducing the incidence of disease(s) are being investigated.

Constipation. The relief of constipation is thought to be related to the water-absorptive properties of nondigestible fiber. Some studies indicate that the fiber in bran is a better laxative than the fiber in fruits and vegetables. One form of fiber (lignin) may, however, counteract the laxative effect of cellulose and hemicellulose (two other forms of fiber). Therefore, the types of fiber present in a food may cause opposite results, and the effects on transit time may depend on the proportions of the various forms of fiber in a food.

Cancer of the Colon. Several theories have been proposed to explain why fiber intake may reduce the risk of this disease. All the theories are based on the possibility that a diet high in fiber-containing foods has some type of effect on *carcino-*

gens (cancer-causing agents) in the diet or on substances that are converted into carcinogens by bacterial metabolism. A high-fiber diet may have the following effects:

1. Stimulate the growth of certain intestinal bacteria that metabolize carcinogens to nonharmful substances.
2. Speed up the passage of carcinogens through the intestine, thus reducing the time that the mucosa is exposed to the carcinogen.
3. Increase the water content of the intestine, thus reducing the concentration of carcinogens as they pass the intestinal cells.

Some scientists believe that one or more of these theories will be proved to be true, but others think the statistical correlation between diet and this type of cancer is stronger for the amount of dietary fat and protein intake rather than for the fiber intake.

Another matter of concern to some investigators is that cancer of the stomach is usually high in populations where cancer of the colon is low, and the opposite pattern is also true. Stomach cancer has a higher mortality rate than colon cancer. So, if diet affects both types of cancer, changing to a diet that reduces colon cancer may at the same time introduce the factor that causes stomach cancer. Thus, the solution to one problem may create the other problem—a worse situation.

Coronary Heart Disease and Atherosclerosis.
The research that is designed to investigate the correlation between fiber and cardiovascular disease is mainly based upon the ability of fiber to bind with bile salts in the intestine.

Cholesterol has an undetermined relationship to coronary heart disease and atherosclerosis (Chapter 25). It is metabolized in the liver to bile salts, which travel to the gallbladder and then to the intestine. Some bile salts are normally reabsorbed from the intestine and recirculated to the liver (Figure 24-2). Fiber may hold bile salts in the intestine long enough for them to be metabolized by bacteria, thus

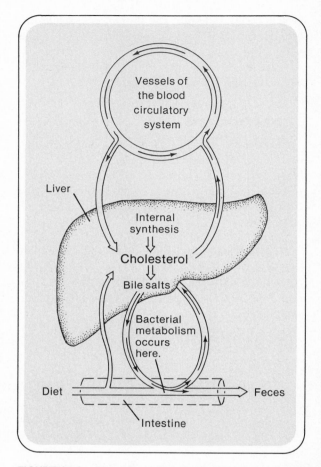

FIGURE 24-2. Circulation of cholesterol into, out of, and within the body.

siphoning them off into the feces. One hypothesis currently under investigation is that this process indirectly reduces serum cholesterol because more cholesterol must be converted into bile salts to replace those that are metabolized by intestinal bacteria. Research into these relationships is complicated by many factors (dietary, genetic, physiological, and others) that alter bile salt metabolism and serum cholesterol. Yet, this line of research may uncover useful information about coronary heart disease and atherosclerosis, which

The nutritional implications of increasing fiber intake largely depend upon the differences between the amounts of fat, cholesterol, phytate, and micronutrients in the high-fiber foods added to the diet and the amounts of these substances in the low-fiber foods omitted from the diet.

together have accounted for more than one-third of the total death rate in the United States each year since 1950.

Another consideration in comparing data from the surveys of Africans and Americans is that heart disease and atherosclerosis usually affect older people. There are fewer elderly people in the African population because death often comes in early adult or middle life. Therefore, fiber may be only coincidentally related to a lower cardiovascular death rate.

NUTRITIONAL IMPLICATIONS

Before you alter your diet in any way, you should ask, "What are all the nutritional implications of this dietary change?" In some cases, unexpected benefits may accrue, while other alterations may be detrimental either physically or financially.

Fat and Cholesterol

In some instances, increasing fiber intake may improve other aspects of a diet, depending upon which foods are added as sources of fiber and which foods are omitted in order to keep energy intake from becoming excessive. Increasing fiber intake may reduce fat and cholesterol consumption and therefore be beneficial (see Chapter 25). For instance, substitution of beans, fruits, and vegetables (high in fiber) for meat and dairy products (low in fiber) reduces fat and cholesterol intake. On the other hand, substituting whole-grain products with high fiber content for milled cereal products has little effect upon fat intake and no effect upon cholesterol intake.

Minerals

Another hypothesis (again, not proved) may make you somewhat hesitant to alter your diet radically. Many foods (such as whole-grain cereals) that are good sources of fiber are also high in phytate (Table 24-1). Phytate has been shown to bind calcium, iron zinc, and other trace elements, and thereby reduce their absorption from the intestine into the blood.° The significance of this effect upon mineral absorption must be considered in light of the facts that anemia due to iron deficiency is a major health problem in the United States and calcium intakes are below the RDA for many teen-agers, children, and elderly people. The amount of phytate in foods should be kept in mind if the amount of fiber in a diet is changed.

The amount of dietary phytate that causes a change in trace element absorption is not yet defined. Recent studies have shown that male subjects who consumed 30 grams of wheat bran a day for three weeks had reduced serum cholesterol levels, but they also had lower levels of iron in their serum (see Chapter 22). This finding suggests that the benefit (lower serum cholesterol) should be weighed against the hazard (lower iron stores) for each individual. Overall health and nutritional status must be considered.

PATTERN OF REASONING

It may be frustrating that this discussion provides no clear answers for planning an advisable intake of fiber. But the purpose of this chapter would be defeated if a conclusion were drawn for the reader. The objectives of this chapter have been to illustrate the steps in evaluating any hypothesis and to point out the need to ask relevant questions. A few questions that might be applied to other possible cause-and-effect relationships are:

1. What is the hypothesis? Does the writer clarify the difference between coincidental observations and causal relationships?
2. What other factors are disregarded in the development of the hypothesis?

° It has been hypothesized that certain types of fiber also bind minerals and reduce their absorption.

TABLE 24-1. Approximate Crude Fiber and Phytate Content per Serving of Food

Food	Crude Fiber (g/serving)	Phytate (g/serving)
Cereal, ½–⅔ cup		
All-bran	3.0	1.5
40% bran	0.9	0.4
Wheat bran	0.8	2.0
Most other cooked or ready-to-eat cereals	Trace–0.3	Trace–0.1
Bread, 1 slice		
Whole wheat, pumpernickel	0.4	Less than 0.2
Raisin, rye, French, italian, enriched white	0.05–0.2	Less than 0.05
Fruits, medium size or ½ cup		
Apple (with skin)	2.0	0
Watermelon	1.5	0
Prunes, dried peaches	1.5	0
Honeydew, bananas	1.0	0
Berries	1.0	0.02
Peaches, apricots, citrus fruits, fruit cocktail	0.5	0
Fruit juice	0.2	0
Vegetables, ½–⅔ cup		
Parsnips, peas, brussels sprouts	2.0	Less than 0.2
Pork'n beans	2.0	2.0
Beans, lima	1.5	3.0
Beans, kidney	1.0	0.7
Broccoli, carrots	1.0	Less than 0.2
Green beans, corn, celery, turnip, tomato, greens	0.5–1.0	Less than 0.1
Potato (with skin)	0.8	0.5
Potato chips, spinach	Less than 0.5	Less than 0.1
Nuts, ½ cup	1.0–2.0	1.2
Sunflower seeds, 1 cup	2.0	1.0

SOURCE: K. W. McNutt, "Perspective—Fiber," *Journal of Nutrition Education* 8, no. 4 (Oct.–Dec. 1976): 150–52. Table adapted from data compiled by Harland and Oberleas from unpublished data; B. K. Watt and A. L. Merrill, *Composition of Foods: Raw, Processed, Prepared,* Agriculture Handbook No. 8 (Washington, D.C.: U.S. Department of Agriculture, Agricultural Research Service, 1975); and D. Oberleas, "Phytates," in *Toxicants Occurring Naturally in Foods,* F. M. Strong, ed. (National Academy of Sciences, 1973), pp. 363–71.

3. What are the meanings of the words used? Is accuracy compromised in order to put the hypothesis into terminology that is quickly grasped by the nonscientist?

4. Are epidemiological observations tested by controlled experiments?

5. Is evidence provided that links the diet pattern being considered to all health claims or conditions cited, or are there merely loose associations?

6. How is the amount of nutrient consumed related to the potential benefits and hazards of the dietary change?

7. How do the answers to the above questions differ for people under varying conditions of energy needs, nutrient needs, age, sex, food preferences, and socioeconomic factors?

8. What are the total nutritional implications of the dietary change?

Few people are willing to go through this detailed analysis. This, indeed, is one reason that the general reader is often misled about nutrition by popular writers.

STUDY QUESTIONS

1. What hypotheses have been postulated regarding the effects of fiber upon health?

2. How does average fiber intake compare between Africans and Americans? Between Americans today and Americans in 1910?

3. What are the proven physiological effects of fiber?

4. What physiological effects of fiber are currently under investigation?

5. What mechanisms are being researched that may explain the role of fiber in preventing cardiovascular disease? In preventing colon cancer?

6. What factors must be considered when we try to determine the nutritional implications of increasing fiber intake?

7. What questions may be asked when evaluating popular articles regarding nutrient–health hypotheses that originated from epidemiological observations?

SUGGESTED READING

1. A. I. Mendeloff, "Dietary fiber," Chapter 38 in *Present Knowledge in Nutrition*. 4th ed. New York and Washington, D.C.: The Nutrition Foundation, 1976.

2. J. Trowell, "Definition of dietary fiber and hypotheses that it is a protective factor in certain diseases," *American Journal of Clinical Nutrition* 29(1976): 417–27.

3. "Food and fibre: Fifth Annual Marabou Symposium," *Nutrition Reviews* 35(March 1977):1–72.

4. F. C. Bing, "Dietary fiber in historical perspective," *Journal of the American Dietetic Association* 69(1976):498–505.

5. G. A. Leveille, "Dietary fiber," *Food and Nutrition News* 47(February 1976).

6. "Zinc availability in leavened and unleavened bread," *Nutrition Reviews* 33(1975):18–19.

7. J. G. Reinhold, K. Nasr, A. Lahimgarzadeh, and H. Hedayat, "The effects of purified phytate and of phytate-rich bread upon metabolism of zinc, calcium, phosphorus and nitrogen in man," *Lancet* 1(1973):283–349.

25

CONDITIONS ASSOCIATED

WITH CIRCULATORY PROBLEMS

Several diseases have an impact upon the circulatory system and are of nutritional importance because diet is a factor in their prevention, treatment, and/or course. These diseases include atherosclerosis, the condition associated with heart attacks and strokes; hypertension, or high blood pressure; and diabetes.

Of all the illnesses that are related to diet, these have the greatest impact upon health and are the most significant causes of death in the United States; they account for 49 percent of all deaths of all age groups in 1974.

COMMON CHARACTERISTICS

Atherosclerosis, hypertension, and diabetes appear to be quite different one from another in underlying cause and disturbance of physiology, but there are several common elements related to their prevention, therapy, and outcomes.

Obesity

The most significant common factor is obesity. Since overweight is generally most prevalent in affluent countries, these disorders are sometimes grouped together and called the "diseases of advanced societies" or "diseases of the overdeveloped nations." The correlation between obesity and circulatory diseases may be described in several ways, but the following statistics should point out the hazards of obesity:

1. Eighty percent of people who have diabetes are overweight.
2. The risk of a heart attack is 50 percent greater in overweight people than in matched control groups who are not overweight.
3. One-fifth to one-third of all people with hypertension are markedly overweight.

These facts suggest that weight control on a life-long basis is of great importance in preventing these life-threatening diseases, or at least aiding in their management.

Interdependence

Each of the three diseases may be accompanied by one or both of the others. For example, people

Atherosclerosis, hypertension, and diabetes are associated with circulatory problems. The specific causes of these problems are unclear, but several risk factors—including diet patterns—appear to contribute to their frequency and severity in certain population groups.

with hypertension or diabetes quite often develop heart disease in which *arteriosclerosis* plays a role. The degree of overlap of these conditions and the order of their appearance varies among individuals. Because there are common abnormalities accompanying these disorders, treatment or control of one condition will generally ameliorate another or retard its progression.

Vulnerable Groups

Each of the conditions associated with circulatory problems is more common among certain groups in the population. These groups are considered to be *vulnerable* for one reason or another, such as race, sex, lifestyle, diet, or occupation. Epidemiological studies (Chapter 24) have provided some information about the populations most likely to develop certain diseases and the preventive measures that should be directed to these populations. For instance, a statistician may show that dietary factor A (such as sodium intake or fat content of the diet) correlates most closely with the incidence of a certain disease in people who are between 45 and 65 years old; males rather than females; people who also have disease Y; people who have certain lifestyles; or other population characteristics. Such epidemiological observations suggest that the major efforts of health educators should be directed toward reducing or eliminating the offending dietary factor from the diets of vulnerable groups. This is a more efficient use of disease-prevention resources than trying to change the diet patterns of the entire population. (The groups most vulnerable to each circulatory disease are discussed on the following pages in the context of the disease.)

The application of statistical information has appropriate uses, but it also has certain limitations. It can be used to predict the probability of the disease in a population; however, it cannot predict whether a given individual within a population group will develop the disease.

Multiple Risk Factors

Several factors appear to be linked to the causes of atherosclerosis, hypertension, and diabetes. Some (such as obesity) influence all three diseases; others are unique to one disorder.

The multiple risk factor concept is important when we try to evaluate statements such as "factor X is the cause of disease A." In diseases with more than one probable cause, the situation is best explained by saying "factor X contributes (or may contribute) to disease A." This takes into account the role that factor Y (any other risk factor) may have in the development of the disease. For instance, smoking contributes to the development of heart attacks, but obesity and hypertension also contribute. So we cannot state that smoking is *the* cause of heart attacks, which would erroneously imply that it is the only cause.

Prevention

Another factor common to these conditions is that preventive measures may reduce their incidence, progression, severity, and/or complications. The most effective prevention programs often involve the efforts of several groups and individuals:

Patients must be educated and motivated to accept their share of responsibility for preventing the onset or minimizing the consequences of these diseases.

Responsible organizations must implement such education programs and give screening tests to identify people with early stages of these conditions—when the diseases are easier to control. Screening programs are probably worthwhile for hypertension and arteriosclerosis detection, since intervention will likely reduce complications and progression. Mass screening programs for diabetes may not be cost-effective, because there is only meager evidence that early detection and treatment alter the outcome of the disease. If obesity and/or

Obesity worsens atherosclerosis, hypertension, and diabetes.

Measures to prevent any one of these circulatory problems—atherosclerosis, hypertension, or diabetes—often lessen the consequences of another that may also be present.

hypertension and/or arteriosclerosis are also present, then diabetes screening programs may have a favorable impact on morbidity and mortality.

Professionals must provide accessible services, treatment plans must be followed, and disease-specific care must be integrated with general care (called *primary care*) of the patient, so that both the disease and the social and environmental circumstances in which it develops are dealt with.

Despite the efforts of interested groups to reduce the incidence and toll of circulatory problems, these conditions will continue to be the major causes of death in the United States until the individuals who are currently free of disease acquaint themselves with—and practice—measures that can reduce the risk of developing the diseases later in life.

DIABETES

Several very different diseases are known as diabetes (which means "syphon" or "to go through"). The most common is *diabetes mellitus*, associated with abnormal handling of glucose and insulin; this is the condition referred to in this book simply as *diabetes*. Other forms include *diabetes insipidus* (an inability to retain water due to a pituitary gland or hypothalamic malfunction in the release of antidiuretic hormone), *bronzed diabetes* (due to an improper handling of iron, *hemochromatosis*), *renal diabetes*, and many others.

Diabetes may be divided into two general categories with respect to cause:

- Cases where a cause can be determined (such as infection, destruction of the pancreas, or certain hormonal disorders)
- Cases where a known cause cannot be found

The latter category accounts for over 90 percent of all cases. In these cases, the diabetes is probably an hereditary disease of metabolism in which there is an inadequate supply of *effective insulin* and most often an accompanying blood vessel disease. The condition is usually diagnosed on the basis of the amount of glucose in the blood, and confirmed by tests that measure insulin levels in blood. The most damaging aspect of the disease is the long-range development of abnormalities of the small blood vessels (*microvasculature*) and, to a lesser extent, the large blood vessels.

Incidence

The National Commission on Diabetes found that between 1965 and 1973, the number of people affected with diabetes increased by more than 50 percent, and in 1975, as many as 10 million Americans (nearly 5 percent of the population) were affected. The commission estimated that every 15 years the number of people with diabetes will double. Only about half of the people who have diabetes are aware that they have it. Diabetes is 50 percent more common among women than among men. People with incomes below $5,000 per year are three times as likely to have diabetes as other income groups.

Symptoms

Symptoms of diabetes may develop slowly over several months or years, or they may develop in only a few days. The abnormalities that may alert the physician or patient to the possibility of diabetes include excessive thirst, excessive urination, and excessive appetite despite weight loss. In more advanced cases, the person may tire easily, feel drowsy, experience a generalized itching, or have recurrent infections and poor wound healing.

Forms of Diabetes

There are two major clincial forms of diabetes; their characteristics are given in Table 25-1. *Maturity-onset diabetes* is usually manageable, but long-term complications may develop, and occasionally acute complications occur. *Growth-onset (juvenile) diabetes* accounts for only about 5 percent

Control of the most common type of diabetes is easier if a person learns about the disease and follows a doctor's advice about diet, medication, exercise, and lifestyle.

Characteristic	Maturity-Onset	Juvenile-Onset
Age of onset	Over 35 years old	Children
Onset	Gradual	Often abrupt
Control	Manageable	More difficult
Weight	Overweight	Underweight
Blood sugar	Narrow range	Broad fluctuation
Ketosis	Rare	Common

TABLE 25-1. Characteristics of the Two Major Clinical Forms of Diabetes

of the people who have diabetes. If untreated, it may progress to mental depression, nausea, vomiting, coma, shock, and ultimately death.

It is important for patients to understand how to handle their diseases. Nondiabetics who realize that these two forms exist can relate appropriately to diabetics. Too often people think that all diabetics are very fragile and must lead sheltered lives, but most diabetics can be taught to manage their diseases and pursue normal activities.

Metabolic Abnormalities

Several metabolic problems are associated with diabetes.

Lack of Effective Insulin. The best-understood abnormality is an inadequate supply of effective insulin. Some diabetics actually have decreased supplies of insulin, but the adjective "effective" takes into account the possibilities that insulin may be synthesized but not released from the pancreas, it may function ineffectively when it is released, or the organs of the body may not respond normally to the insulin. A recent discovery is that some diabetic patients apparently lack insulin binding sites, have an inadequate number of sites, or have weak binding sites on their cells, so that insulin is unable to promote the entry of glucose into such cells. These studies, which must be confirmed and extended before being put into practice, may offer new tools to diagnose diabetes by a relatively simple method and to study in a test tube the genetics or inheritance patterns of this common disease.

Since insulin is necessary for the movement of glucose from the blood into many of the cells that metabolize it, the blood glucose concentration of diabetics builds up after a meal, while the cells remain "hungry." As the blood flows through the kidneys, much of the excess glucose passes into the urine and is excreted, often accompanied by large volumes of water and loss of essential minerals. The loss of minerals, which are part of the body's pool of alkali (bases), leaves the body in an acidic condition—hence, the term *diabetic acidosis*.

In severe, poorly controlled diabetics, blood glucose levels fluctuate from high to low. The low points are accompanied by sweating, dizziness, and possibly coma. These fluctuations often may be reduced by weight loss; planning the timing, quantities, and nutrient composition of meals; and balancing exercise and eating. Sometimes, diabetics also must take insulin as an injection or as an oral drug to stimulate insulin action in the body.

Effective patient education about the management of diabetes together with the use of drugs have changed diabetes from a disease that was often fatal in young adulthood to an abnormal metabolic condition compatible with a fairly normal routine and considerably increased—if not normal—life expectancy.

Blood Vessel Disease. The damage from diabetes results from changes in the small blood vessels (microvasculature). It is not yet known whether these blood vessel changes are a part of the same genetic abnormality that causes the problem of ineffective insulin. An interrelationship between the two abnormalities is supported by the observation in diabetics that the eye and the kidney—the organs most often affected by blood vessel changes—are bathed in high concentrations of glucose because their cells (in contrast to most other body cells) do not require insulin for the entrance of glucose. Recent studies tend to show that when high blood sugar levels are brought under control with insulin, the blood vessel changes observed in eye examinations improve.

Complications

Some complications of diabetes are short-term and others are long-range. The short-term complications of uncontrolled diabetes are loss of glucose (hence, energy), water, and minerals in the urine; a condition of *ketosis;* and possibly coma and shock.

Loss of Glucose. The loss of glucose in the urine causes gradual weight loss, excessive hunger, and listlessness. Water is needed to keep the sugar dissolved in the urine; therefore, sugar and water loss in the urine lead to dehydration and thirst.

Sugar in the urine is associated with urinary tract infections, possibly because bacterial growth is supported by the presence of glucose. The interaction between infection and diabetes is a double-edged sword. First, infections create a metabolic stress that is more difficult to control for a diabetic than for a nondiabetic. Second, diabetics are more susceptible to infections, and they recover from infections more slowly. (Defective resistance due to poorly functioning white blood cells may also underlie this observed tendency to more frequent infections among diabetics (Chapter 21).

Ketosis. Ketosis results from unusual metabolism of macronutrients for the release of energy—not from the fluctuations in circulating glucose. In the absence of effective insulin, glucose cannot be fully used for energy release. Storage fat is therefore broken down into fatty acids and then into acetyl CoA. Ketosis develops due to the same metabolic

changes that occur during low-carbohydrate weight-reduction diets (Chapter 9). In diabetics, the acidity of body fluids (acidosis) may increase enough to cause coma and death in only a day. If insulin (along with other corrective steps) is given at an early stage, acidosis and ketosis may be reversed in only a few hours.

Long-Range Complications. Long-range complications that involve the blood vessels are of two types. One type is atherosclerosis, the same process that occurs in nondiabetics. Another process is unique to diabetics—it occurs in the supporting tissues of small blood vessels, particularly those that supply blood to the kidney, retina of the eye, skin, and nervous system. Gradual blood vessel narrowing diminishes nourishment of various tissues, with ultimate consequences such as kidney failure, blindness, ulcers of the feet, and gangrene.

Role of Diet

The main objectives of diet planning related to diabetes are maintenance of normal body weight and spacing of energy intake to coincide with periods of greatest energy expenditure. Beyond these generalizations, the role of the diet depends upon the existing health of an individual, just as for nondiabetics.

Prevention. Diabetes is at least in part a genetic disorder. Therefore, it cannot be either caused or cured by any specific diet pattern, though the manifestations may be worsened by poor diet patterns. However, since there is an overlap between diabetes and atherosclerosis (diabetics are twice as prone to heart disease as nondiabetics), the diet patterns that may reduce other circulatory diseases may also lessen the severity of diabetes. Diet modification is most important for people with family histories of diabetes. These people are more likely than others to develop the disease at some future time. The National Commission on Diabetes (in its 1975 report to the United States Congress) stated that for every 20 percent of excess weight, the chance of being diabetic more than doubles. Prevention of diabetes therefore has as a cornerstone the prevention of obesity.

Control. Diabetics who are taking insulin injections or pills must balance their food intake in relation to the type of insulin used, its peak action, and their exercise patterns. Low-carbohydrate diets for diabetics have been abandoned in recent years, because such diets led to high intake of fat. This appears to complicate the blood vessel disorder and may well reduce the survival rate of diabetics. However, sucrose restriction appears to be wise, since sucrose causes wide swings in blood insulin levels (making control difficult) and sometimes increases plasma triglycerides (which may complicate a concomitant atherosclerosis process). As we mentioned before, control of the blood glucose level is now considered to be important in retarding the development or progression of microvascular disease in the eyes of diabetics, and may also retard the progression of microvascular disease in other organs.

ATHEROSCLEROSIS

*Arterio*sclerosis is a general term for the degeneration of arteries that results in a thickening and hardening of the arterial walls. *Athero*sclerosis is one type of arteriosclerosis, a condition characterized by accumulation of lipids in the arteries. This disorder is the underlying cause of most heart disease and plays a major role in strokes (caused by abnormalities of the circulatory system within the brain).

Incidence

In 1974, there were approximately 900,000 deaths from cardiovascular diseases out of 1,900,000

total deaths. Atherosclerosis accounts for 80 to 85 percent of the cardiovascular deaths.°

These percentages and large numbers may seem impersonal and irrelevant, but these same statistics tell us that among your college classmates, three males out of fifteen will have a heart attack before age 60. One of these three will die within a week; for the other two, the chances of dying within the next five years will be five times greater than for those who have not had a heart attack.

Risk Factors

Predicting who will have a heart attack is not as simple as having fifteen classmates throw dice. The dice can be loaded—to win or to lose in terms of heart disease—depending upon several *risk factors* (Figure 25-1).

Hereditary Risk Factors. Hereditary risk factors (such as sex or ethnic makeup) are beyond an individual's control. Atherosclerosis in older people affects both sexes with similar frequency, but it is less common among premenopausal women than among men of the same age. This disease is more common in some families than others, but this may be due to both genetic and environmental conditions.

Body build and psychological makeup also influence the incidence of atherosclerosis. These risk factors are genetically determined to a certain degree, but they can be partially controlled by an individual.

Environmental Risk Factors. Environmental factors are at least in part controllable by the indi-

°Conditions such as rheumatic heart disease, myocarditis, congenital heart abnormalities, and many others, are also considered cardiovascular diseases. But these are not diet-related syndromes and therefore will not be discussed in this book. One should realize the broader meaning of the term *cardiovascular disease* when trying to evaluate comments and statistics regarding this group of disorders.

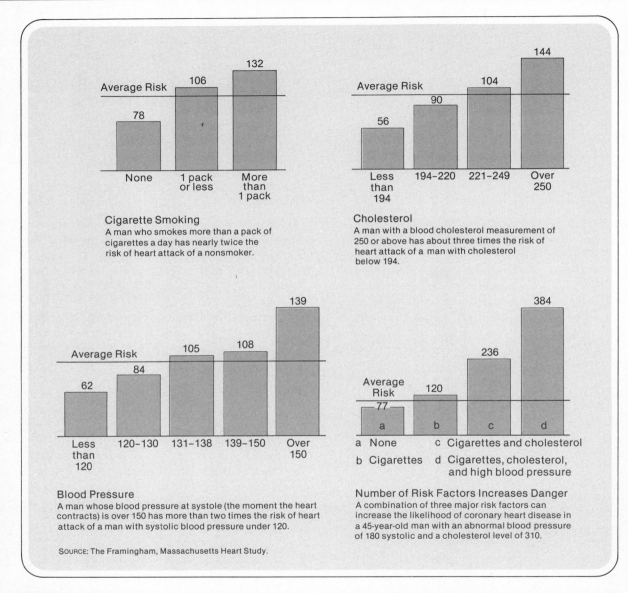

FIGURE 25-1. Risk factors in heart attack. These graphs demonstrate the extent to which particular risk factors increased the danger of coronary heart disease for 30- to 62-year-old men in Framingham, Massachusetts. Portions of columns below the horizontal line indicate lower-than-average risk. Portions of columns above the line indicate higher-than-average risk. (From *Coronary Heart Disease: Risk Factors and the Diet Debate* by L. M. Hursh. © 1975, National Dairy Council. Courtesy of National Dairy Council.)

Elevated serum lipids can indirectly lead to reduction of blood flow to tissues by involvement of the clotting mechanism or by lipid accumulation within the lining of blood vessels, thus narrowing their diameter.

vidual—especially cigarette smoking. Exercise reduces the risk of cardiovascular disease; it helps to combat obesity and provides other benefits for the circulatory system that are not fully understood.

Abnormalities

To understand how the accumulation of blood lipids in the arteries harms the body, we must answer these questions:

1. What are blood lipids?
2. How does their accumulation affect circulation?
3. How are these changes related to heart attack and stroke?

Total Blood Lipids. Cholesterol, triglycerides, phospholipids, and lipoproteins are included in the total blood lipids. Disagreement persists among scientists regarding many aspects of diet and circulatory diseases, but most of them agree that the risk of atherosclerosis increases with elevation of cholesterol. Triglyceride level usually, but not always, fluctuates parallel to cholesterol level, and similar variations occur in lipoproteins.

Circulation. If the blood is rich in lipids, some of these molecules may become stuck between the inner and middle linings of blood vessels (for unknown reasons). These sticky deposits may occur in isolated places of the blood vessels or be distributed throughout the length of several vessels.

Isolated deposits are called *plaques*. These tend to form elevations of the lining of the blood vessels. The elevations disturb the flow of blood in the same way that a stone sticking up in a fast-moving stream causes water to swirl around it. The swirling currents of blood damage blood cells and *platelets*. Platelets are fragments or pieces of cellular cytoplasm in the blood that originate from giant cells in the bone marrow. They are easily damaged. When injured, they are able to trigger a very complex process of blood clotting that begins when injured platelets interact with a blood protein called *fibrin-*

ogen. The damaged cells, platelets, and fibrinogen may form a clot (or *thrombus*) in an artery. If the clot attaches to the vessel wall, it grows larger as other cells stick to it. Eventually, the thrombus can close off the vessel completely (as in *coronary thrombosis*). Sometimes, a piece of the thrombus breaks loose, travels into the narrowing part of a branching arteriole, and occludes one of the branches. Either of these processes blocks the passage of blood into the occluded vessel. If other vessels remain open, the results may not be catastrophic, but if no other vessels supply the tissues downstream, then those tissues will quickly die.

Damage of a lesser, but significant degree, can also occur when fat deposits reduce the diameter of the blood vessels and simply lessen the amount of blood trickling through (Figure 25-2). This narrowing does not cause death, but it impairs cellular function. In the brain, this causes confusion, disorientation, speech problems, drowsiness, and other warning signs that a stroke may be imminent. Narrowing of the blood vessels also increases the resistance to blood flow within the vessels, thus placing an additional burden on the heart. Chest pain and shortness of breath are signs of vascular insufficiency in the heart.

Role of Diet

Several atherosclerosis risk factors are influenced by diet, but not all potential problems can be solved by diet modifications. Scientists uniformly agree that overweight (obesity) is a risk factor and that weight reduction—reduction of energy intake—is the first dietary step in the retardation and prevention of atherosclerosis. The second step is to lower blood cholesterol and other lipids.

Otherwise healthy people who show only slightly abnormal blood lipids generally do not get the same benefits from certain dietary changes as do people with more advanced lipid disorders. Diet therapy must be tailored to fit the type and severity of the individual's lipid disturbance.

Several dietary patterns are considered by scientists to increase the risk of atherosclerosis. Therefore, a diet should be selected that allows a person to maintain an appropriate body weight and also takes into account all other diet risk factors.

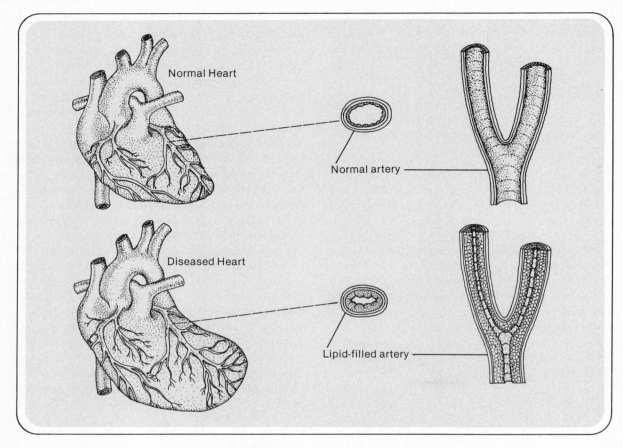

FIGURE 25-2. Normal and diseased hearts.

Prescribed Dietary Changes. For people with elevated blood lipids, a chart has been developed that recommends using a dietary guideline or a combination of different dietary guidelines, depending upon which blood lipid(s) is (are) high. The diet instructions are designed to reduce the risk of atherosclerosis; they can be suited to the disease as it occurs in each person. This type of prescribed diet should not be confused with the general preventive measures.

Preventive Dietary Changes. There is strong disagreement among nutrition scientists regarding what dietary patterns should be recommended to the general (healthy) public to reduce the risk of cardiovascular disease. Different groups of researchers insist that the major dietary risk factor is an excessively high intake of one or a combination of the following: all carbohydrates, sucrose, all fat, saturated fat, or cholesterol. Other dietary changes that have been proposed to reduce the risk of atherosclerosis include substituting "hard" for "soft" drinking water, and reversing the quantities of copper and zinc in the diet. These theories are only speculations at this time but may prove to be of significance.

In the absence of definite research findings to guide our food habits, the best policy is to try to honor a moderate approach to diet and lifestyle. This involves moderation in our intake of all the above nutrients, including the use of eggs, dairy products, and animal fats. Of course, tobacco and nonprescription drug use should be curtailed at the same time as dietary practices are improved.

Fat. The American Heart Association recommends that fat intake be limited to about 35 percent of the total energy consumed, but for diet planning, this percentage needs to be converted into grams of fat. On a 3,000 Cal diet, this would be

$$3,000 \times 0.35 = 1,050 \text{ Cal}$$
$$1,050 \text{ Cal} \div 9 \text{ Cal/g} = \text{about } 117 \text{ grams of fat}$$

If energy needs are only 2,000 Cal, it would equal 78 grams of fat.

Another rough guideline for reducing fat intake is based on the fact that most Americans now derive about 45 percent of their energy from fat. Therefore, they have to shift approximately 10 percent of the energy of the diet from fat to another macronutrient. On a 3,000 Cal diet, this would mean reducing fat intake by roughly 2 tablespoons of fat.

$$3,000 \times 0.10 = 300 \text{ Cal}$$
$$300 \text{ Cal} \div 9 \text{ Cal/g} = 33 \text{ grams of fat}$$

From a 2,000 Cal diet, about 22 grams of fat should be replaced by other energy sources. Table 25-2 shows the amount of fat that may be eliminated from the diet by making certain substitutions.

TABLE 25-2. Quantities of Dietary Fat Reduced by Various Means

Food	Fat (g)	Comment	Savings (g)
Candy bar, chocolate, 2 oz.	20	Substitute hard candy	20
Ice cream, ⅙ qt.	5	Substitute sherbet (1 g fat)	4
Margarine, 1 T.	12	Use only ½ T.	6
Milk, whole, 1 cup	9	Substitute 1 cup of skim milk	9
Pie, 1 slice		Substitute fruit (no fat) or gelatin (no fat)	
Apple	18		18
Custard	15		15
Pecan	37		37
Potatoes, french fries or hash browns, 1 cup	10	Substitute baked potato	10
		If ½ T. margarine is added	4
Poultry, fish, or meat (fried), each tablespoon of fat taken up during frying	14	Broil	Varies—check amount of fat poured into skillet and amount left after cooking
Salad, mixed green, with 1 T. salad dressing	14	Substitute fruit or tomatoes with ½ cup creamed cottage cheese (5 g fat)	9

Polyunsaturated/Saturated Fat. Many scientists recommend a greater intake of polyunsaturated fat relative to saturated fat. This does not mean that total fat intake should be increased. Adding vegetable fat (margarine and other imitation dairy products) to the diet—without concurrently reducing animal fat—increases the risk factor related to total fat intake.

Substituting vegetable oil for animal fat improves the polyunsaturated/saturated fat (P/S) ratio of the diet (review Figure 2-5), thus minimizing one dietary risk factor. On the other hand, simply cutting down saturated fat both reduces total fat intake and increases the P/S ratio, thus minimizing two dietary risk factors.

Cholesterol. Cholesterol content is high in many foods, such as meat, eggs, and dairy products (Table 25-3), that also supply saturated fat. Therapeutic diets prescribed by physicians sometimes contain as little as 300 milligrams of cholesterol, but there is no generally agreed upon dietary cholesterol intake that is recommended for preventive diets. There is a limit to the value of completely omitting cholesterol from the diet, because when the dietary intake of cholesterol drops below a certain level, the body starts to synthesize cholesterol. The range of cholesterol intake below which the body begins this synthesis is not the same for everyone; it depends in part upon the individual's level of serum cholesterol.

Some people do not respond to low-cholesterol diets even when they have markedly elevated blood cholesterol. This indicates an abnormal rate of synthesis of cholesterol (perhaps on a genetic basis, and not simply overeating) or very efficient intestinal absorption of cholesterol and bile salts.

Total Carbohydrates and Sucrose. An optimal intake of total carbohydrates has not been determined, but a diet that obtains 35 percent of energy from fat and 15 percent from protein, leaves 50 percent for carbohydrates and alcohol. Sucrose and perhaps some other simple sugars are also considered to be risk factors, but again there is little information about the amounts of sucrose associated with increased risk of atherosclerosis. Sucrose intake may be reduced by omitting it from beverages such as tea and coffee, cutting down (or out) soft drinks, and not adding it to cereals or other foods. Pastries, other desserts, and dried fruits contain much more sucrose than fresh or unsweetened canned fruits (review Table 2-1). A large proportion of sucrose enters the American diet as candy and other snacks.

HYPERTENSION

Hypertension is technically not a disease; it is a physiological abnormality that can result from a variety of diseases. It is reflected by blood pressure measurements that exceed established norms.° Lowering the blood pressure usually reduces the complications of a disease for the patient. It may or may not alter the progression of the disease (such as kidney failure) that causes the hypertension. Lowering the blood pressure reduces the burden on the heart and lessens the chances of stroke and heart attacks.

In some cases, hypertension can only be corrected by curing the underlying disease or condition, while in others, it can be controlled by diet, drugs, and other types of intervention.

Prevalence

Hypertension afflicts about 33 million people 18 to 74 years old. Seven percent of people 18 to 24 years old and 22 percent of those 35 to 44 years old have definite or borderline hypertension. One-third of the white population over 45 have hypertension as compared to over half of the black population in this age group. Many people are unaware that they

° For normal, working adults the norm is up to 140/90, as measured in the upper arm (if the arm is not "too obese" or "too muscular").

TABLE 25-3. Cholesterol Content of Various Foods

Poultry, Meats (3 oz.)	Cholesterol (mg)	Fish and Seafood (3 oz.)	Cholesterol (mg)	Dairy Products and Eggs	Cholesterol (mg)	Foods Made with Animal Products	Cholesterol (mg)
Chicken		Bass, whiting, carp, sole, pollack, pike, perch	50–70	Butter, 1 T.	35	Cake, 1 piece	
White	67			Chicken fat, 1 T.	9	Angel food	0
Dark	77			Cheese, 3 oz.		Sponge, 66 g	162
Gizzards	166	Clams	43	American	77	Yellow, 75 g	33
Turkey		Cod	70	Cheddar	84	Cream puff, 130 g	188
White	65	Crab	85	Cottage	8	Custard, ½ cup	139
Dark	86	Flounder	43	Swiss	85	Ice cream, 10% fat, ½ cup	27
Brains	1,700	Haddock	51	Cream, 1 T.		Ice milk, ½ cup	13
Heart	233	Halibut	51	Cheese	16	Mayonnaise, 1 T.	10
Kidneys	683	Herring	82	Half and half	6	Muffin, 40 g	21
Liver	372	Lobster	72	Sour	8	Corn	28
Sweetbreads	396	Oysters	43	Whipping	20	Noodles, ½ cup	25
Beef	80	Salmon	40	Egg, whole, 50 g	252	Pie, ⅛	
Lamb	83	Sardines	119	White, 33 g	0	Lemon	117
Pork	76	Scallops	45	Yolk, 17 g	252	Pumpkin	70
Sausage	53	Shrimp	128	Lard, 1 T.	13	Popover	59
Veal	86	Trout	47	Milk, 1 cup		Potato salad, ½ cup	81
		Tuna	55	Buttermilk	5	Pudding (mix), ½ cup	15
				Nonfat	5	Waffle	119
				Whole	34	White sauce, ½ cup	17
				Yogurt, low fat, 1 cup	17		

NOTE: All foods of plant origin contain no cholesterol, including fruits, vegetables, cereals, grains, nuts, vegetable oils, and some imitation egg, dairy, and meat products.
SOURCE: R. M. Feeley, P. E. Criner, and B. K. Watt, "Cholesterol Content of Foods," *Journal of the American Dietetic Association* 61 (1972): 134–49.

have this problem. Screening programs conducted periodically in many communities could minimize the consequences of hypertension, but only a small percentage of people who have abnormal screening results bother to follow through and acquire medical supervision. Also, many people who know they are hypertensive fail to take the medicine prescribed or to follow the diet recommended by their doctor. Of the nearly 13 million people in 1972 who, based on the Health Interview Survey, knew they had hypertension, only 60 percent were under medical treatment.

Abnormality

Blood pressure is normally regulated by an interplay of several hormones and certain nervous reflexes. These work together to balance the amount of blood (blood volume) within the circulatory system, and the space available for that blood within the circulatory system. If the amount of blood increases or if the space within the circulatory system decreases, blood pressure goes up. Normally, the body can readily adjust to these changes, but people with hypertension do so poorly or not at all. Sodium and, to a lesser extent, potassium, magnesium, and calcium play key roles in controlling both of the above factors.

Blood Volume Increase.   When the kidneys are unable to transfer salt and water efficiently from the blood to the urine, the blood volume increases. This may result from many causes. Some of these are (1) abnormalities of the hormones that control the excretion of water and sodium by the kidneys, (2) high concentrations of body sodium that hold water within the blood or tissues (as in edema), and (3) complex interrelationships between these two.

Space within the Circulatory System.   The space within the circulatory system, or the volume capacity of the system, normally increases when the muscles surrounding blood vessels relax and become flabby, thus permitting greater stretching of the

vessels. The diameter of these vessels enlarges, and so their capacity to hold blood increases. As the circulatory tree relaxes, the pressure within decreases. In response to this lower pressure, the kidneys return more salt and water until the circulatory tree fills up with fluid. As it fills up, the blood pressure rises. The kidneys sense this rising pressure, and begin to excrete more water and minerals, chiefly sodium, until the blood pressure returns to a lower, normal level. Thus, the kidneys play a pivotal role in maintaining the proper volume of fluid within the circulatory tree, and also help to keep the blood pressure in the system within a normal range. It is important to remember, though, that the state of contraction or relaxation of the muscles in the walls of the blood vessels that make up the circulatory system also affect blood pressure, and the tone of these muscles can change in fractions of a second in response to hormonal or nervous stimulation.

Cause

The diseases that are known to cause hypertension explain only about 20 percent of all existing cases. These diseases include blood vessel abnormalities, certain tumors, and the abnormal release of hormones from the kidneys, adrenals, thyroid, or pituitary glands. Many of these are curable by surgery. Other cases are related to changes in the elasticity of the blood vessels (such as in diabetes or arteriosclerosis). The other 80 percent of cases cannot be cured, since the causes are unknown; however, most of them can be controlled.

Sodium intake has a variable influence upon blood pressure. Its inconsistent effect may be explained by genetic and environmental factors that alter the sensitivity of individuals to this nutrient. The muscle cells of arteries and arterioles contain sodium, potassium, magnesium, and calcium. In people with hypertension, there is a disturbance in the balance of these minerals in the muscle cells. Such people are thought to be hypertensive because of these cationic changes that cause the actomyosin in the arterioles to be hypersensitive to normal hormone and nervous stimulation. What causes these cationic imbalances in unknown.

The state of current knowledge is summarized here.

1. Some people are very sensitive to sodium; the degree of their hypertension closely parallels their sodium intake.

2. Some people do not develop hypertension even on very high sodium diets.

3. Some people continue to show hypertension even on very low sodium diets.

Scientists are seeking clues to this disease by studying rats. For several generations, the researchers select and mate only the rats that are most sensitive to salt; thus, these experimental animals have a *genetic sensitivity* to salt. The longer these rats eat salt, the greater is the hypertensive effect. Offspring of these rats, fed large amounts of salt from birth, develop high blood pressure that is not reduced if salt is withheld from the diet later in life.

The implications of these rat studies for humans are yet undetermined. One of the current limitations to controlling hypertension by restricting sodium intake is that we lack a way of detecting which people are sensitive to sodium (as are the genetically selected rats) and which are not. The possibility of a high incidence of sensitivity, however, suggests that salt consumption should be seriously considered as *one* factor in the development of hypertension for the general public.

The following information may help you decide how much salt you want to consume. In the United States, current salt intake varies between 6 and 18 grams per day per person. A hazardous intake level has not been defined, but in northern Japan, where sodium intake (primarily monosodium glutamate) is about 26 grams per day, approximately 40 percent of the population is hypertensive.

Minimal salt requirements for normal healthy people depend to a large extent upon the amount of sweating that occurs. If a person sweats heavily, intakes of salt in excess of 15 grams per day may be required. On the other hand, diets of 1 to 2 grams per day are often prescribed for (though probably not often followed by) patients with high blood pressure.

Low sodium intakes present little hazard. Since many foods naturally contain sodium, a diet containing a variety of foods, but with no added sodium, should supply adequate amounts to meet minimal needs. Table 25-4 shows the sodium content of several foods.

TABLE 25-4. Sodium Content per Serving of Foods

Food	Sodium[a] (mg/serving)	Food	Sodium[a] (mg/serving)
Fruits		Fats	
Most fruits or fruit juices	5–25	Butter or margarine, 1 T.	46
		Vegetables[b]	
Dairy Products[b]		Most fresh vegetables (asparagus,	
Egg, whole, 1	50–60	brussels sprouts, cabbage, let-	
Ice cream		tuce, etc.)	5–25
Regular	84	Turnip, ½ cup	26
Soft	109	Beet, diced, ½ cup	37
Yogurt	120	Celery, diced, ½ cup	75
Milk (whole, skim, 2%)	122	Vegetable soups, reconstituted	200–250
Cheese, 1-inch cube		Tomato juice, 6 oz.	364
Cheddar	120	Potato salad	450
Swiss	107	Potato chips, 100 g	1,000[c]
American	199	Pork and beans with tomato sauce	900
Buttermilk	319	Sauerkraut	1,755
Cottage cheese	400–600	Corn	
		Fresh	Trace
Meats, Poultry, Fish[b]		Frozen	2–5
Lamb, ¼ lb.	60	Canned	604
Beef chuck, boneless for stew	64	Green peas	
Ham, fresh, ¼ lb.	65	Fresh	2
Chicken, diced	90–120	Frozen	184
Pork sausage, cooked, 4-inch link	125	Canned	548
Beef sirloin without bone, ½ lb.	134	Beans, lima	
Calf liver, ¼ lb.	135	Fresh	5
Clams, raw, 1 pt.	163	Frozen	175–200
Oysters	175	Canned	585
Haddock, ¼ lb.	200	Green beans	
Flounder, ¼ lb.	270	Fresh	8
Bacon, 2 medium strips	306	Frozen	3–9
Bologna, 1 oz.	369	Canned	564
Frankfurter, 1 medium	500–600	Carrots	
Tuna, 3¾ oz.		Fresh	52
Packed in oil	750	Frozen	—
Packed in water	40	Canned	581
Canned beef and vegetable stew	1,007	Spinach	
Corn beef hash	1,188	Fresh	90
Dried beef, uncooked, 1 oz.	1,219	Frozen	93–107
Canned chili con carne with beans	1,354	Canned	548

SOURCE: C. F. Adams, *Nutritive Value of American Foods in Common Units,* Agriculture Handbook No. 456 (Washington, D.C.: U.S. Department of Agriculture, Agricultural Research Service, 1975).

TABLE 25-4. Sodium Content per Serving of Foods (*continued*)

Food	Sodium[a] (mg/serving)	Food	Sodium[a] (mg/serving)
Cereals, Baked Goods, Desserts		Condiments	
Shredded wheat, oatmeal, macaroni, rice, and similar products	Low in sodium[d]	Lemon juice, vinegar, wine, sugar, molasses, jams, jellies, preserves, maple extract, vanilla, walnut extract	Low in sodium
Graham cracker, 1	53		
Bread, 1 slice	100–200		
Cake, pie, or doughnuts, 1 piece	100–200	Mayonnaise, 1 T.	84
Gelatin dessert, 1 cup	122	Peanut butter, 1 T.	97
Fig bars or chocolate chip cookies,		Salad dressing	
4	140	Most types, 1 T.	100–200
Muffin, 1 medium	176	Italian, 1 T.	300
Popcorn, 1 cup		Pickle relish, 1 T.	107
Salted	175	Tomato catsup, 1 T.	156
Unsalted	Trace	Chili sauce, 1 T.	201
40% bran flakes, wheat flakes, or		Cocoa, 1 oz.	
sugar-coated cereals	250–300	Processed with alkali	203
Roll or biscuit, 1 medium	240–270	Not processed with alkali	Trace
Macaroni and cheese, 1 cup	270	White sauce; $\frac{1}{4}$ cup	250
Pudding made with milk, 1 cup	322	Baking powder, 1 tsp.	330
Pancake, 6 inch, 1	412	Salt, $\frac{1}{4}$ tsp.	530
Pizza with cheese and sausage, 14		Peanuts, 1 cup	
inch, $\frac{1}{8}$	488	Salted	602
Oyster crackers, 1 cup	495	Unsalted	7
Bouillon, 1 cube	960	Olives, green, 10 small	686
Cheese crackers, 4 oz.	1,250	Pickle, 1 medium	
		Dill	928
		Sour	879

[a] Sodium values do not apply to vegetables cooked in salted water or seasoned with salt. Moderately salted vegetables have approximately the same amount as commercially canned vegetables.

[b] 1 cup unless otherwise noted.

[c] This is a high value. Sodium content varies.

[d] Sodium content is increased when these cereals are cooked in salted water; for example, $\frac{1}{4}$ teaspoon of salt in cooking water increases sodium content by 530 milligrams.

STUDY QUESTIONS

1. Which three important disorders are associated with the circulatory system and may be affected by diet patterns?

2. Why does obesity affect these disorders?

3. How do measures to prevent one of these problems affect the consequences of another?

4. How may the most common type of diabetes be controlled?

5. If one of your parents is diabetic but you have never had symptoms of the disease, how can you minimize the risk of the disease becoming manifest?

6. What are three hereditary risk factors of atherosclerosis? What are three risk factors that you can control?

7. How may elevated serum lipids lead to reduction of blood flow to tissues (a heart attack or stroke)?

8. What dietary guidelines may help reduce the risk of atherosclerosis?

9. How may the consequences of hypertension be reduced?

10. What causes hypertension?

11. How does sodium in the body influence blood pressure for people? Why may this mechanism not maintain a normal blood pressure in hypertensive people?

SUGGESTED READING

1. R. E. Shank, J. F. Mueller, A. M. Gotto, L. Scott, M. J. Albrink, H. M. Perry, and R. E. Hodges, "Nutrition in Cardiovascular Diseases Series," *Journal of the American Dietetic Association* 62(1973):613–42.

2. I. S. Wright and D. T. Fredrickson, eds., *Cardiovascular Diseases: Guidelines for Prevention and Care.* Inter-Society Commission for Heart Disease Resources for the Department of Health, Education and Welfare. Washington, D.C.: Government Printing Office, 1973.

3. F. A. Kummerow et al, "Additive risk factors in atherosclerosis," *American Journal of Clinical Nutrition* 29(1976):579–84.

4. H. C. McGill and G. E. Mott, "Diet and coronary heart disease," Chapter 37 in *Present Knowledge in Nutrition.* 4th ed. New York and Washington, D.C.: The Nutrition Foundation, 1976.

5. L. M. Klevay, "Coronary heart disease: The zinc/copper hypothesis," *American Journal of Clinical Nutrition* 28(1975):764–74.

6. K. M. West, "Prevention and therapy of diabetes mellitus," Chapter 35 in *Present Knowledge in Nutrition.* 4th ed. New York and Washington, D.C.: The Nutrition Foundation, 1976.

7. L. Lamberg, "Diabetes: Researchers discover some new links in the puzzle," *Today's Health* 53(1975):32–35, 53–55.

8. J. W. Anderson, "Metabolic abnormalities contributing to diabetic complications: II. Peripheral nerves," *American Journal of Clinical Nutrition* 29(1976):402–408.

9. W. B. Kannel, "Some lessons in cardiovascular epidemiology from Framingham," *The American Journal of Cardiology* 37(1976):269–82.

10. W. B. Kannel, "Prevention of heart disease in the young coronary candidate," *Primary Care* 4(1977):229–43.

26

PROTEIN–CALORIE MALNUTRITION (PCM)

The form of malnutrition that causes the greatest loss of life and the most significant impairment to health around the world is *protein–calorie malnutrition (PCM)*.° Severe PCM rarely occurs in the United States, but we have all seen pictures in newspapers of children in other countries with this devastating condition. Many Americans wish to help these children and seek avenues to direct their concern. Some people alter their own diets, others contribute money to international organizations, and many spend time raising funds for philanthropic groups. These personal efforts help a few children, but long-term solutions must be built upon a deeper understanding of the nutritional problems involved, their causes, and the effectiveness of preventive and curative measures.

VARIATIONS OF PCM

Protein–calorie malnutrition describes several deficiency states that have certain similarities and some important differences.

° Many international nutritionists prefer the term *protein–energy malnutrition (PEM)*.

Marasmus and Kwashiorkor

Protein–calorie malnutrition primarily due to an inadequate intake of energy is called *marasmus*. The form of PCM that occurs when energy intake is adequate, but dietary protein is deficient is called *kwashiorkor*. Most often the condition is at some point between these two extremes. Vitamin and mineral deficiencies almost always accompany PCM as well.

Age and Appearance. Marasmus occurs throughout the preschool years. Marasmic children, who are literally starved, seem to be reduced almost to just skin and bones, but they have enlarged abdomens. Their eyes are deep-set and their cheeks are shallow. They often look like miniature old people who are grossly underweight.

Kwashiorkor usually occurs during the second or third year of life. Its onset often coincides with cessation of breast feeding by the child. Protein deficiency causes water to be abnormally retained in the tissues. This water retention, called *edema*, may be so severe that body weight is normal—the pounds of water mask the fact that little muscle tissue remains. The child's face appears full—almost moon-shaped—and the feet and hands are puffy. Edema may not be noticed on casual observation, but if an examiner or mother presses firmly on the skin for a few seconds and then the finger is pulled away, a depression will remain until water gradually seeps back into the compressed tissue spaces.

Skin. The appearance of the skin differs in these two conditions. If a marasmic child has been adequately fed in the past, the skin that used to cover normal muscles hangs loosely around the skeleton. In kwashiorkor, the skin is coarsened in spots. In black children, it has light or depigmented spots; in Caucasians and Orientals, there are dark or heavily pigmented areas. Ulcers and sores develop, and the area around the nose and mouth appears chapped, cracked, flaky, or sometimes oily. A rash is often seen on various parts of the body, especially the groin. These changes may be due to both lack of protein and coexisting vitamin deficiencies.

Behavioral Changes. The behavioral changes that occur are similar in both forms of PCM. A child with either form is initially irritable, but later becomes too weak and listless even to cry. Figure 26-1 shows an African child and her father during the time she had kwashiorkor and after her recovery. The psychological changes associated with this disease affect the family, as well as the patient—an important point when one attempts to treat a victim of PCM.

Body Weight. The onset of PCM is easier to diagnose when a chronological growth chart is kept regularly for the child. Affected children show a plateau in the rate of weight gain before more debilitating changes occur. Some nutritionists in developing countries think that the growth chart—a very simple, inexpensive diagnostic tool—offers one of the most effective keys for reducing the death rate of preschool children. Its usefulness is dependent, however, on mothers learning to understand and respect the importance of regularly bringing

their family to be weighed at a health clinic. A reduction in the rate of height gain and muscle wasting can often be avoided if weight gain plateaus are noted soon enough for the health worker to initiate nutrition intervention.

Other Disorders. Protein–calorie malnutrition routinely causes the liver and spleen to enlarge in their futile attempts to maintain normal functions. Anemia and decreased resistance to many types of infection and parasitic infestation also occur. Death often results from a disease (such as measles or dysentery) that imposes an overwhelming stress on the poorly nourished child.

Mild to Moderate Forms

The number of children in the world with extreme PCM is relatively small compared to the tens of millions with mild to moderate forms of the disease. Statistics are misleading because children cannot live very long with severe kwashiorkor or marasmus. Either they are rehabilitated or they die—usually the latter. In countries where these conditions are most prevalent, accurate statistics are not kept on death rates. Indeed, in many areas children are not even counted among the living in census figures until they survive their first or second birthday.

Children who are afflicted with mild forms of PCM that persist over many months, fall far below the weight and height standards for their ages. They are anemic and have skin lesions, frequent respiratory diseases, and other infections. Most are not bedridden, but they tire easily, are apathetic, and perform poorly in school.

Adult Forms

Although PCM is less life-threatening once growth has been achieved, this same deficiency state also takes its toll among adults. Depending upon the degree of deficiency, repercussions range from gen-

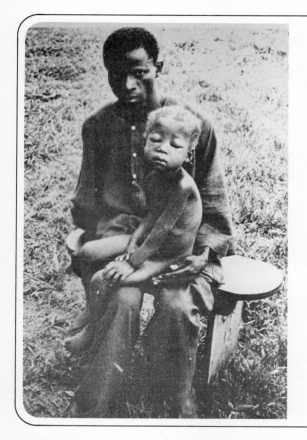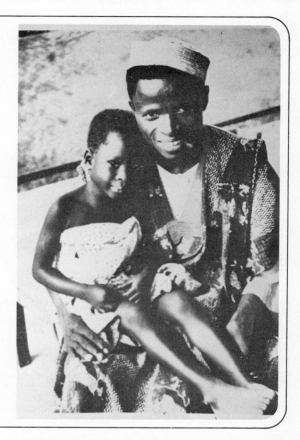

FIGURE 26-1. Child and father—during kwashiorkor and after recovery. The expressions on their faces (even the way the father is holding his daughter) show the emotional toll of this condition. (Reproduced by permission of Dr. David Morley, Tropical Child Health Unit, Institute of Child Health, University of London.)

eralized lack of energy with concomitant decreased work and earning capacity to frank starvation and death. Malnutrition of wage-earning parent(s) may indirectly affect the health of the entire family, which suffers from lack of food-purchasing power.

CAUSES OF PCM

The interrelationships among some of the causes of PCM are shown in Figure 26-2. The middle and lower parts of this chart include many physiological abnormalities discussed elsewhere in this book. The top of the chart summarizes factors that interrupt access to food. The complexity of the problem is apparent. Obviously, not all the factors can be neatly compartmentalized and the same effects may result from multiple causes.

Economic Factors

Protein–calorie malnutrition may result from poverty of an individual or an entire country. It may

The causes of PCM are linked to many social problems of developing countries—such as poverty; lack of sanitation, education, and health care systems; and cultural factors.

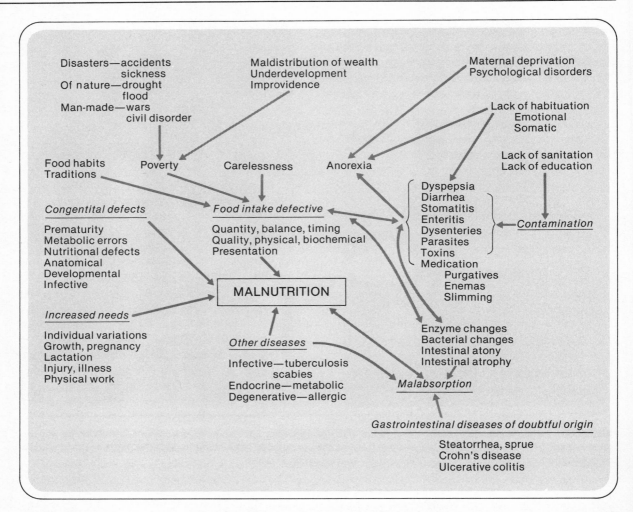

FIGURE 26-2. Some causes of malnutrition. This chart was developed by Dr. Cicely D. Williams, who first described kwashiorkor in the medical literature and postulated that this disease might be linked to a deficiency of protein. (Adapted from "Malnutrition" by C. D. Williams, in *The Lancet* 2 (August 18, 1962):342. © 1962, The Lancet. Also used by permission of the author.)

be worsened by maldistribution of wealth. Economic underdevelopment is often accompanied by extremely limited food delivery and preservation systems. Without good transportation networks, foods cannot reach hungry people even short distances away. If farms and markets are linked by small, dirt roads, the rainy season may bring to a halt the delivery of food. Natural disasters, such as droughts, floods, or earthquakes, can worsen or initiate PCM. During wars and civil disorders, adult males die in battles, while women and children die at home from lack of food, curtailment of health services, and lack of other life-sustaining necessities.

The less developed countries do not have the resources to provide concurrently adequate sanitation, education, and health care—all of which play interdependent roles in preventing PCM. Lack of sanitation systems predisposes children to infectious and parasitic diseases spread by sewage and its contamination of food and water. Lack of an educational system hinders efforts to teach people about efficient agricultural methods, food needs, and health practices that relate to nutritional status.

Lack of health care facilities and trained personnel often mean that many developing societies must rely upon the services of midwives, witch doctors, and herbal medicine. These resources, if properly utilized, may provide adequate care for some health needs, but tribal medicines often fail to correct relatively simple nutritional disorders. In such cases, ignorance (despite the availability of food) leads to unnecessary death.

Behavioral Factors

Psychological problems of varying complexity may contribute to malnutrition. Kwashiorkor may be due in part to emotional problems generated by disruption of the maternal–child relationship when breastfeeding stops. In some cultures, the child is taken away from the mother at the time of weaning and lives temporarily with the grandmother or another relative. This separation, or maternal deprivation, may be so traumatic that the child refuses to eat, regardless of what is offered.

Kwashiorkor is a word from the Ga language used in West Africa. It means "the disease that the older child gets when the next child is born." Long before scientists understood this disease, a clue to one of its causes was recognized by the people who saw their children die from it. The Africans believed that evil spirits caused jealousy between siblings; scientists today cite the psychological problems involved. Either terminology points to a change in the personal interactions, or psychodynamics, within the family as a factor in the development of kwashiorkor.

Infant Feeding Practices

Marasmus is caused by an overall deprivation of food; children simply do not get enough energy to survive. On the other hand, kwashiorkor is related to the type of food given when the child is weaned. The diets associated with kwashiorkor around the world all have similar nutrient characteristics—adequate energy, but insufficient protein.

In Southeast Asia, infants who develop marasmus are fed little more than the water in which rice was cooked. If sugar is added to the rice water, the disease appears more like kwashiorkor. Other infant foods associated with kwashiorkor resemble dried milk in appearance (white, powdery products), but mothers do not know that these foods contain little or no protein. For example, in South America, cornstarch is often given; in Africa, children are fed a coarse, white flour made from cassava (a tuber resembling our potato), which contains only about 1 percent protein. Ignorance combined with poverty guides the mothers to use these cheaper products instead of milk when they stop breastfeeding.

The consequences of feeding such foods to a child are even more serious if the powder is reconstituted with polluted water. Lack of sanitation imposes further risks once a child begins to crawl, then toddle, beyond adult supervision. The child may wander into unsanitary areas where anything may be picked up and eaten.

Infant feeding often suffers when family planning is not practiced. If the family is large and poor, psychological factors may lead to rejection of the newborn simply because its food requirements compete with those of other children who have already established emotional bonds with their parents.

Protein–calorie malnutrition in developing countries can be eradicated only by integration of nutrition programs with other aspects of national development.
Every method of nutrition intervention has some advantages and some limitations.

PREVENTION OF PCM

Although lack of food is the underlying cause of PCM, countless international efforts have proven that food distribution programs are little more than short-lived stopgap measures in preventing this condition. An American tourist visiting a developing country may bemoan the lack of hospitals to care for malnourished children, but local doctors and government planners know that pouring funds into expensive facilities and sophisticated therapy is financially prohibitive—and a futile effort. Children who had been hospitalized for months and supposedly cured of their PCM frequently return a short time later to a health care facility in the same condition that required their initial admission. Without other approaches to correcting the cause of the PCM, the relapse–rehabilitation cycle is repeated until death occurs.

Development Planning

Children will continue to die of PCM until developing countries can progress economically to the point of generating enough productivity or capital to support solutions for all the problems shown in Figure 26-2. Feeding programs and nutrition education must be recognized in program planning, but only at a level consistent with other aspects of development. If a single component of the development plan is funded to the detriment of any other, the effectiveness of the overall solution will be diminished.

When national resources are limited, a country must set priorities regarding use of funds for education, health care, and other needs. The importance of nutrition is interwoven in all aspects of development. A few basic examples of these developmental interrelationships are:

1. Economic growth is necessary to generate funds for agricultural and social development, but malnutrition reduces work capacity and therefore hampers economic growth.

2. Hungry children cannot glean maximal benefits from funds allocated to education, but lack of schools stymies efforts to teach people about food and health.

3. Population expansion dilutes food resources, but parents who know that many of their children will die at a young age of malnutrition or other diseases have good reason for rejecting family planning.

Nutrition Intervention Programs

Planners and international organizations (such as the World Health Organization, Pan American Health Organization, World Bank) recognize the value of allocating some of their resources to nutrition programs. These efforts are often integrated into broader health plans. Experience has proven that effective multilateral aid programs require the endorsement of the entire political structure of the host country, as well as the cooperation of health personnel. Commitment to the project by both the political and medical leaders helps to ensure its continuation. Selection of the most appropriate nutrition intervention program depends on the degree of development of other services in the country. For instance, a school feeding program is of little value if the children most in need do not attend school. Other examples of the merits and limitations of various nutrition intervention programs are summarized in Table 26-1. Under certain circumstances, more than one intervention program—each directed toward a different population group—is the best approach to improving nutritional status and stimulating overall development of the country.

EFFECTS ON MENTAL DEVELOPMENT

Impairment of mental development in children who have PCM is a worldwide concern. It is difficult, however, to establish a direct cause-and-effect relationship between malnutrition and mental development. Disease, use of health services, heredity, poverty, and psychological and cultural influences all impact on nutritional status; these same variables affect mental development. Evaluation of mental development in children (well-nourished versus malnourished) is complicated by the fact that quality of education, environmental stimuli, and parent–child relationships also affect learning patterns, which in turn are used to measure mental development. It is difficult to break into this cycle in order to measure causes and effects among these many variables.

Hunger and Behavior

There is little question that a hungry child has a shortened attention span. Hunger may also cause behavioral problems that inhibit learning for a child, who in turn disrupts the education of other students in a class. These effects of hunger can usually be corrected before permanent brain damage occurs. Yet, a child who has consistently performed poorly in school because of being hungry may become so discouraged and so accustomed to failure that it is almost impossible for that child to catch up with peers even after nutritional status is improved.

Cellular Alterations

A lasting, irreversible effect of malnutrition on the development of the nervous system seems to depend upon the age at which the nutritional deprivation occurs and the severity of the deficiency. The consequences of malnutrition are most serious among young children. This appears to be linked to the fact that the brain attains about 80 percent of its growth during the first four years of life. Severe caloric and nutrient impoverishment during this critical period seem to cause the most damaging alterations in the development of brain cells.

Studies of the intellectual performance of children who have recovered from severe malnutrition yield conflicting results. Some people show no residual effects, while others are seriously retarded for life. Social or family factors may contribute to the

different degree of rehabilitation achieved by individuals.

Animal Experiments

Animal experiments help researchers separate the role of nutrition from other factors affecting mental development. It is possible to study changes that arise from extreme protein and energy deprivation—deficiencies more severe than those experienced by the majority of children with PCM.

Severe undernutrition of young pigs, rats, and mice alters the lipid, protein, and mineral composition of the brain. It decreases the growth and division of brain cells, and causes changes in brain wave patterns.

Studies of monkeys with PCM have revealed behavioral changes. The animals were listless and apathetic, and avoided new objects placed in their cages. This avoidance behavior pattern, if it is indeed comparable to what occurs in humans, may partly explain the retarded learning patterns of malnourished children.

PROTEIN–CALORIE MALNUTRITION IN THE UNITED STATES

The severe forms of PCM are almost always thought of as problems of developing countries, but these deficiencies also occur in the United States.

Children

The few cases of severe PCM found among North American children are usually due to extreme poverty. This condition has been recognized in Public Health Service hospitals that care for Indians living on reservations in the Southwest. Milder conditions have also been seen in urban hospitals. Although financial deprivation is part of the cause, PCM in the United States is also associated with parental ignorance or frank child neglect. Protein–calorie

413

TABLE 26-1. Nutrition Intervention Programs

Program	Advantages	Limitations
Food Distribution		
Supplemental feeding programs through health care facilities	Motivate people to return to clinic for more comprehensive supervision of interrelated health problems and for family planning	Food may be used by nondeficient members of the family or sold to meet what the family considers more pressing needs
School feeding programs	Decrease absenteeism and increase effectiveness of funds allocated for education; may be combined with other aspects of health and nutrition education	The most deprived and malnourished children do not attend school
Rehabilitation Centers		
Requiring family participation in therapy	Mothers are taught how to prevent recurrence of PCM while their children are being treated in the rehabilitation center.	The diet of many families is dependent upon income earned by a working mother; participation of the mother in such programs therefore reduces income for purchasing food
Without family participation in therapy	PCM is temporarily reversed	High rate of remission
Either of the above	Child may survive past most vulnerable age	Family may lack money to practice preventive measures learned
Education		
School system	Lessons may include nutrition, food preparation and sanitation, agriculture, interrelated health practices	Slow process; teachers must first be educated; many children do not attend school in less developed countries
Public education via radio and television in village centers	Inexpensive way to reach many people	Causes of malnutrition (therefore the appropriate message) may vary within broadcasting area; no way to personalize or reinforce message and thus assure behavior modification

Food Production and Processing

Home gardens	Increase food availability; crops can be planned to meet specific nutrient needs; indirectly increase funds available for related health services	Impossible in cities where causes of PCM are most complex; require time and training; subject to droughts and floods or insect and rodent destruction
Fortification and/or enrichment	Inexpensive method if food processing technology is already available; reaches many people if proper food is selected for fortification; not dependent upon education	No effect on home-grown food unless local mills are used as enrichment centers; certain micronutrients cannot be added
Formulated food mixtures	If properly designed, can be relatively inexpensive and formulated to correct specific nutrient deficiencies; not dependent upon education	May require agricultural change to supply all foods needed; will be rejected by those most in need if marketed and promoted as "food for poor people"; processing facilities for preparation are often distant from population most in need

malnutrition of varying degrees occurs occasionally among children fed vegetarian diets.

Adults

Nutrition surveys (Chapter 13) show little evidence of average protein intakes below the RDA among the general population—except in pregnant and lactating women. Energy intakes fall below recommended standards more frequently than protein intakes.

General malnutrition does occur in low-income groups, especially among the elderly. Severe malnutrition is also seen in alcoholics. Deficiencies similar to PCM sometimes result from drug therapy, intestinal malabsorption, and certain diseases, including psychiatric problems that cause people to refuse to eat.

Hospital Patients

It has recently been recognized that some hospitalized patients show evidence of PCM, as detected by reduced skin fold thickness and low serum protein levels. The relationship of PCM to the disease type that caused the hospital admission, length of stay in the hospital, and predisposing factors is not clear, although some cases are apparently due to inadequate attention to patients' nutritional requirements by the hospital staff. In the recent past, and occasionally now, conditions such as pellagra, beriberi, scurvy, and PCM were found in some hospitals for the retarded and mentally ill. Protein–calorie malnutrition appears to be quite common among people suffering from chronic diseases, such as malignancies, psychiatric disorders, liver failure, intestinal malfunction, and other "wasting" conditions.

STUDY QUESTIONS

1. How do the two severe forms of PCM differ?

2. What social problems are linked to the cause of PCM?

3. Why does adding sugar to rice water cause a child to develop kwashiorkor instead of marasmus?

4. Name three nutrition intervention programs; for each of these, explain what other components of national development are necessary in order for the program to be effective.

5. How does hunger affect learning capacity?

6. Under what circumstances does PCM have the most detrimental effect on brain development?

7. What are the primary causes of PCM in the United States?

SUGGESTED READING

1. M. Gebre-Medhin and B. Vahlquist, "Famine in Ethiopia—a brief review," *American Journal of Clinical Nutrition* 29(1976):1016–1020.

2. "A starved child of the new vegetarians: A case history," *Nutrition Today* 8(1973):10–12.

3. R. E. Olson, ed., *Protein-Calorie Malnutrition.* New York: Academic Press, 1975.

4. "Cicely Williams: Marking her eightieth year," *Nutrition Reviews* 31(1973):329–84.

5. Subcommittee of the Committee on International Nutrition Programs, Food and Nutrition Board, "Present knowledge of the relationship of nutrition to brain development and behavior," National Academy of Sciences. Reprinted in *Nutrition Reviews* 3(1973):242–46.

6. J. Dobbing, "Nutrition and brain development," Chapter 44 in *Present Knowledge in Nutrition.* 4th ed. New York and Washington, D.C.: The Nutrition Foundation, 1976.

7. M. F. Elias and K. W. Samonds, "Exploratory behavior and activity of infant monkeys during nutritional and rearing restriction," *American Journal of Clinical Nutrition* 27(1974):458–63.

8. J. Van Duzen, J. P. Carter, and R. Vander Zwagg, "Protein and calorie malnutrition among preschool Navajo Indian children: A follow-up," *American Journal of Clinical Nutrition* 29(1976):657–62.

9. R. H. Barnes, "Dual role of environmental deprivation and malnutrition in retarding intellectual development," *American Journal of Clinical Nutrition* 29(1976):912–17.

10. J. G. Chopra, "Enrichment and fortification of foods in Latin America," *American Journal of Public Health* 64(1974):19–26.

11. Advisory Committee on Technology Innovation, Board of Science and Technology for International Development, Commission on International Relations. *Food Science in Developing Countries: A Selection of Unsolved Problems.* Washington, D.C.: National Academy of Sciences, 1976.

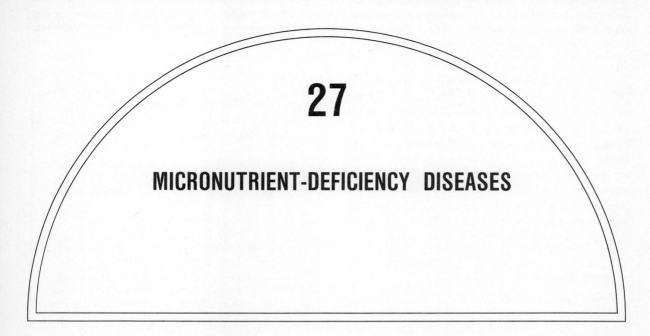

27

MICRONUTRIENT-DEFICIENCY DISEASES

Deficiency diseases due to severe inadequacy of only a single vitamin or mineral are extremely rare in the United States. However, diseases such as scurvy, beriberi, rickets, and blindness due to vitamin A deficiency continue to be major health problems throughout the world. Occasionally, one of these conditions occurs in a person whose diet lacks only the one crucial micronutrient, but most often, people show signs of several deficiencies at the same time. Multiple deficiency conditions of varying degrees of severity also occur in the United States.

The manifestations of these conditions and their consequences upon health—indeed, upon life itself—are influenced by factors that nutritionists and physicians have only recently begun to put into perspective:

1. Severity of the deficiency (mild to severe)
2. Capacity of the body to store certain nutrients (for instance, fat-soluble or water-soluble vitamins) to different degrees
3. The combination of coexisting nutritional deficiencies (PCM as well as micronutrient deficiencies)
4. Coexisting disorders (such as cancer, infections, or diarrhea) that may alter nutrient needs or nutrient utilization

5. Normal physiological conditions (such as pregnancy) that increase nutrient needs
6. Socioeconomic and psychological barriers to selection of an appropriate diet

This chapter discusses the major micronutrient-deficiency diseases, their causes and manifestations, and how such conditions may be prevented under various circumstances.

RECOGNITION OF MICRONUTRIENT DEFICIENCIES

Medical and public health education programs have only recently reintroduced the subject of micronutrient deficiences into the curricula. The long neglect or oversight of this aspect of nutrition in training programs for health personnel came about largely because early work in nutrition focused on single micronutrient-deficiency diseases. Such conditions were, indeed, seen in many people in the United States until about forty years ago. However, as researchers correlated certain vitamins or essential minerals with the disease characteristics resulting from each micronutrient deficiency, it became a simple matter to diagnose and treat such clear-cut cases of malnutrition. Appropriate programs were also introduced to prevent deficiencies. As scourges such as scurvy, rickets, and pellagra disappeared, the successes on the nutrition front contributed to a false sense of security among the general public and in the community of health professionals. It was assumed that nutrient deficiencies were no longer a serious threat to the health of the majority of our population. As a result, for the past quarter century, nutrition has received little attention in the education of health professionals in the United States.

Recent Advances

As medical advances have led to the conquering of more and more diseases (such as scurvy and infections), and as chronic diseases have become more prominent, researchers have begun to direct their attention to the microenvironment of cells and cellular chemistry. What they are finding is that many diseases and conditions do not have a single cause, such as a specific vitamin deficiency or bacterium, but often have multiple causes. This new appreciation for the multicausality concept has, in several ways, enhanced the ability of doctors to recognize nutrient deficiencies.

1. It has led to the realization that deficiency diseases usually represent a combination of several overlapping disorders, or multiple causes. The condition may closely resemble one disease, but the patient may also have a few characteristics of several others.

2. Researchers have also begun to examine the relationships between nutrient deficiencies and the severity of manifestations of nonnutritional diseases (such as measles).

3. Other new lines of investigation are the influences of nutritional status upon the recovery rates and lengths of recovery periods following surgical procedures and many medical or nonsurgical diseases.

Another hindrance to the recognition of the broad implications of micronutrient deficiencies was the lack of instruments that were sensitive enough

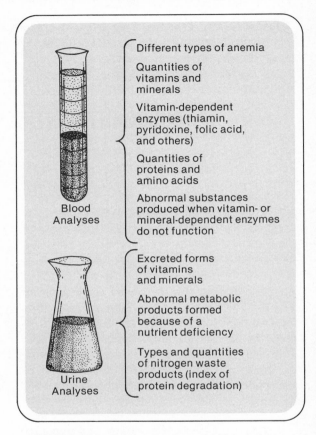

FIGURE 27-1. Tests to evaluate nutritional status.

to detect mild or moderate dietary deficiencies. Newer laboratory tests and equipment using small urine and blood samples (Figure 27-1) can now be used to diagnose deficiency states in their early phases. These more sensitive procedures have shown that even mild deficiencies produce measurable impairment to the body's ability to maintain optimal performance.

The growing emphasis upon nutrition in health education, the increasing awareness of the multicausality of disease, and the availability of diagnostic tools have all enhanced the capability of physicians to recognize and treat the types of deficiency diseases that are most common today. However,

Micronutrient-deficiency diseases develop slowly, produce signs and symptoms similar to other disorders, are often indistinguishable in their early stages, and impair many processes throughout the body.

deficiency diseases have not been eliminated from the United States. They continue partly because people do not recognize the manifestations of micronutrient-deficiency diseases or they put off seeking medical therapy until their disease becomes complicated and difficult to cure. The subtle, progressive, and cumulative effects of nutrient deficiencies are discussed below.

Progression of Deficiency

Deficiency diseases worsen in a rather insidious pattern; they do not occur overnight. Metabolic functions are restricted long before symptoms appear.

Some body functions are more sensitive to a micronutrient deficiency than others. For instance, in the case of pyridoxine, as dietary intake or absorption decreases, the concentration of the vitamin in the blood falls. Then, the pyridoxine-dependent enzymatic reactions become less active and select cells behave sluggishly. Later, anemia and more serious neurological complications occur. The warning clues are there early in the deficiency, but generally they are not detectable without clinical laboratory tests.

Another factor that determines the progression of deficiency diseases is the capacity of the body to store micronutrients. In general, there are larger reserves of the fat-soluble vitamins (A, D, E, and K). The other vitamins and minerals, which are soluble in the aqueous fluid of the interior of cells, blood, and urine, are more readily lost from the body.

Nonspecificity of Early Signs

The initial manifestations of micronutrient deficiencies are not clearly recognizable as evidence of a nutritional disorder. For instance, the early signs of deficiency of any B vitamin (marginal anemia, low body weight, and changes in the skin) may also be caused by nonnutritional disorders (such as parasites, respiratory and gastrointestinal infection,

or skin diseases caused by fungus infection). Since these conditions are often prevalent in marginally or poorly nourished people, it is difficult to identify the specific underlying disorder or the degree to which these symptoms are caused by dietary deficiencies or other factors.

The sequence, severity, and type of cellular abnormalities caused by nutritional deficiencies depend upon the specific function of each vitamin or mineral that is deficient. In many instances, however, the same general symptoms occur. For instance, a deficiency of any one of several micronutrients may impair the production or survival of red blood cells and therefore cause an anemia (Chapter 22). Or, abnormalities of the nervous system may be caused by a deficiency of calcium, vitamins B_6 or B_{12}, folic acid, magnesium, or other micronutrients. Laboratory tests are helpful in diagnosing the specific cause (nutritional or otherwise) of such symptoms, but this may be difficult in the early stages of a deficiency.

Recognition of marginal deficiencies may also be delayed if people attribute lethargy and loss of appetite to tensions at work or other emotional problems. The early symptoms of micronutrient deficiencies are quite similar to the symptoms of some of the depressive aspects of stress. However, the causes of such symptoms are usually discovered only after careful medical examination and testing. Once the cause is determined, the appropriate treatment may be prescribed.

Broad Effects

Because of the numerous nutrient-dependent functions that occur in cells throughout the body, most deficiencies exhibit widespread manifestations. The parts of the body that usually show the first signs of deficiency are those that are wearing out and being rebuilt with the greatest frequency: membranes of the gastrointestinal tract, skin (especially on the face and around the mouth), hair, fingernails, and blood cells.

Isolated deficiency diseases are usually associated with monotonous diets; multiple deficiency diseases are usually associated with inadequate food intake; and secondary deficiencies are usually due to conditions that impair the intake, absorption, or utilization of nutrients.

A severe deficiency of each vitamin or mineral has certain unique manifestations, but these occur rarely. It is more important to be aware that deficiency of any of several nutrients may at some time during the dietary deprivation state be associated with depressed growth rate, impaired reproductive capacity, skin or hair changes, lethargy or mental depression, anemia or weakness, wasting of muscles, and, if severe and prolonged, death.

CAUSES OF MICRONUTRIENT DEFICIENCIES

Since micronutrient-deficiency diseases encompass a broad spectrum of disorders, the causes cannot be neatly classified. The specific condition in any one individual may reflect dietary inadequacies and a multitude of other factors. However, there are similar patterns, which result in isolated deficiencies (lack of one nutrient), multiple deficiencies (lack of several nutrients), or secondary nutrient deficiencies (not due to dietary lack).

Isolated Deficiencies

Diseases due to the lack of a single micronutrient frequently result from a diet that includes a limited selection, rather than limited amounts, of foods. Such monotonous diets may lead to scurvy (caused by lack of vitamin C) or vitamin A blindness in otherwise well-nourished people who do not consume sufficient amounts of certain fruits and vegetables. Beriberi (caused by lack of thiamin) and pellagra (caused primarily by lack of niacin) are also associated with monotonous but calorically adequate diets. Beriberi is linked to a diet that contains mainly unenriched, *polished* rice (the thiamin-rich husk has been removed) and lacks other sources of this vitamin (such as meat, vegetables, or whole-grain or enriched cereals). Pellagra often occurs in people who derive most of their energy from corn or cornmeal. These foods are low in both niacin and

the amino acid tryptophan, which can be converted to niacin.

Rickets, another isolated deficiency disease, is not due to a monotonous diet; it can develop in people who select a rather broad and varied diet. This disease is caused by a lack of biologically available vitamin D and is most often due to a combination of two factors—an inadequate dietary supply of vitamin D and a lifestyle that does not include sufficient exposure to sunlight.

Multiple Deficiencies

A person who simply does not eat enough food will exhibit a combination of symptoms of micronutrient deficiencies and of PCM (Chapter 26). Multiple deficiencies can also occur, however, in people who consume adequate (or even excessive) amounts of energy. The person who skips breakfast and has cocktails followed by meat, potatoes, and coffee for both lunch and dinner is probably deficient in vitamin A, folacin, riboflavin, and calcium. It is likely that a person who completely omits cereal products from the diet will be deficient to some degree in niacin, thiamin, and riboflavin—unless the diet is planned with care.

Secondary Deficiencies

Secondary nutrient deficiencies are deficiencies primarily caused by nonnutritional disorders. For instance, many diseases cause a loss of appetite or nausea and vomiting, which impair nutritional status. The emaciation of cancer is caused both by a loss of appetite and the rapid growth of cancer cells, which use up the available dietary nutrients. Intestinal parasites cause secondary nutritional deficiencies because they use large amounts of dietary nutrients for their own metabolism. Disease of any part of the gastrointestinal tract may cause a malabsorption syndrome and therefore precipitate a nutrient deficiency even when dietary intake is adequate.

Socioeconomic and Cultural Factors

Micronutrient deficiencies occur both in the United States and around the world. However, the causes of these diseases are generally different in developing versus developed countries.

Multiple micronutrient-deficiency diseases are often found in *developing countries* among people who have PCM. The causes are often similar to the factors, such as food habits and lack of sanitation, discussed in Chapter 26. Improper planning of agriculture, crop failures, or seasonal fluctuations in food availability also distort the nutrient balance of the diet. Inadequate intake of a single vitamin or mineral in the absence of PCM may be attributable to lack of that micronutrient in the food supply or cultural patterns that lead to omission from the diet of foods that are major sources of that nutrient.

In *developed countries,* isolated micronutrient deficiencies are more often due to improper selection of foods than to unavailability of foods. Multiple dietary deficiencies usually are caused by social isolation (as among the elderly), ignorance, drug interactions, extreme poverty, or reliance upon a monotonous diet. People who consume large volumes of alcohol and those who frequently use psychomimetic drugs often decrease their food intake to such a degree that they become deficient in several nutrients.

PREVENTION

Great strides have been made in alleviating the suffering and reducing the loss of life caused by micronutrient deficiencies. An awareness of the preventive measures used in both developed and developing countries can help us appreciate the progress that has been made and perhaps minimize

the possibility of the reappearance of such disorders in the future.

Developed Countries

Many nutrient-deficiency diseases were fairly common in the United States as recently as the 1930s. The discovery of micronutrients and information regarding dietary sources of each led to the virtual disappearance of these conditions. The development of economical laboratory procedures for the synthesis of vitamins enabled doctors to prescribe these nutrients for poorly nourished patients. Such syntheses also made possible the enrichment of cereal products, as well as the fortification of dairy products.

In the United States, the threat of many vitamin and mineral deficiencies also has been lessened by socioeconomic changes. Increased availability of fruits and vegetables throughout the year has been made possible by improved transportation and food preservation methods. Eradication of deficiency diseases is closely linked to an improved standard of living, which has made possible a general upgrading of the quality of diets in the United States. Public assistance, including first the Commodity Distribution Program and more recently the Food Stamp Program; Women, Infants, and Children (WIC) Program; School Breakfast and Lunch Programs; and Elderly Feeding Programs, have increased the accessibility of food. However, surveys continue to report nutrient and energy intakes below the RDA in many groups. Elimination of existing marginal deficiencies requires correction of problems such as social isolation and lack of information about appropriate food selection.

Developing Countries

Countries that lack the technology for fortification or enrichment, the facilities for preserving and transporting fruits and vegetables out of season, and a national budget to fund broad public assistance programs, rely upon other methods for preventing these deficiency diseases.

In tropical and subtropical climates, a wide variety of fresh foods are grown throughout the year. Papayas, mangos, cashews and a variety of melons and squashes are especially good sources of vitamins A and/or C. Often, however, people must be educated to select sources of each nutrient, depending upon what foods are currently being harvested.

Vitamin D deficiency is less of a threat in many developing countries because children wear little or no clothing and they spend much of their time in the sunshine. Organ meats and fish oils, which are not frequently eaten in developed countries, help to protect against deficiency diseases in developing countries. Also, soups or stews made with beans, vegetables, and bony cuts of meat are often eaten; their nutrient-rich juices are consumed by people rather than by garbage disposals.

Breastfeeding, which avoids many dangers of food contamination and helps to ensure an adequate diet early in life, is continued in many countries well into the second year of childhood. It is not uncommon in some African cultures for the diet of a three- or four-year-old child to be supplemented with breast milk.

Currently, several large-scale international efforts are underway to eradicate vitamin A deficiency. Education is considered important in parts of the world where the disease coexists with excellent, but unused, sources of this nutrient. Elsewhere, people are being taught to grow and prepare foods that are rich in carotene. Training of local health auxiliaries and physicians to recognize the early signs of this disease and to prescribe appropriate diet changes are beginning to reduce the number of children that are blinded by this deficiency.

CLASSICAL DEFICIENCY DISEASES

During their lifetimes, few North Americans will see or hear about any person who is afflicted with a severe micronutrient deficiency. The purpose of the discussion to follow is not to frighten you into selecting an appropriate diet, but rather to point out that such deficiencies do indeed exist—and they have serious consequences.

This discussion also puts into perspective the gradual accumulation of information regarding the role of micronutrients in maintaining health. An understanding of deficiency diseases did not occur instantaneously. This knowledge has evolved over centuries, and researchers have yet to explain the mechanisms that link many nutrients and the abnormalities characteristic of their deficiency states. The annals of nutrition are filled with stories of long pursuits of vitamins and essential minerals, and of explanations of their functions. Only a few of these can be mentioned here.

Beriberi

Beriberi is the disease caused by a deficiency of thiamin. It occurs most frequently in Asian countries where polished rice is the staple food, but it also occurs occasionally among alcoholics in developed countries. This disease contributed to the deaths of many prisoners-of-war in Asia during World War II, and to a lesser extent during the Korean and Vietnam conflicts.

History. The first clue to the correlation between diet and beriberi was uncovered during the latter part of the nineteenth century, when this disease was a major cause of death in Japan, especially among sailors. The Director General of the Japanese Navy found that addition of barley, milk, and meat to the rice diet of his sailors resulted in an almost complete disappearance of beriberi.

About the same time, another critical piece of information resulted from an experiment in Java. A Dutch physician named Eijkman found that if he fed chickens polished rice, they developed a nerve disease similar to human beriberi unless they were also fed the rice husk. Eijkman hypothesized that a

A deficiency of thiamin initially affects the nervous and muscular systems, ultimately resulting in heart failure. This condition is called *beriberi*.

toxin or organism in the polished rice was overcome by something in the rice husk.

Years later, the pieces of this puzzle began to fit together when chemists treated rice husks with different solutions (water, alcohol, alkali, or acid) that selectively dissolved out various components of the husks. Feeding each of these solutions to different groups of animals with beriberi and watching the responses of these animals identified which fluid contained the antiberiberi factor. Then the scientists concentrated their efforts on this rice husk extract.

Further laboratory tests and separations gave researchers a progressively purer substance—less and less of the extract was needed to cure beriberi. Chemical analysis of the purified substance told them the amount of carbon, hydrogen, oxygen, nitrogen, and sulfur in the unknown factor. This information helped chemists devise other tests to reveal how these atoms were grouped within the vitamin molecule. The next step in the discovery was the synthesis of this molecule from simple laboratory chemicals. The identity of thiamin was finally proved when the synthetic vitamin (of known chemical structure) was given to thiamin-deficient animals and then to humans, and shown to cure beriberi.

This same general pattern of investigation has led to the discovery of all the presently known vitamins. The solvent separation procedure and subsequent feeding experiments allowed scientists to distinguish fat-soluble vitamin A from water-soluble vitamin B as early as 1912. The tedious process of separating the many vitamins within these groups and identifying their structures continued for the next four and a half decades. The structure of vitamin B_{12}, the last vitamin to be discovered, was determined in 1947.

Abnormality. The manifestations of thiamin deficiency depend upon the severity of the deficiency and coexisting conditions such as protein deficiency or alcoholism that may worsen the disease. Moderate deficiency results from a diet that contains only about 0.2 or 0.3 milligram per 1,000 Cal. It causes gradual development of nervous system symptoms such as weakness; a tingling sensation or numbness of the fingers, toes, and area around the mouth; and later, tingling or numbness of the arms and legs. A decreased attention span, combined with nervous and muscular problems, reduces work capacity.

Severe deficiency (resulting from diets that contain less than 0.2 milligram thiamin per 1,000 Cal) affects the cardiovascular system. The heart enlarges, edema develops, and even mild exertion makes the heart beat rapidly. As the disease progresses, appetite is lost, digestive problems and constipation occur, and the nerve damage worsens. The patient dies of heart failure.

The most acute type of thiamin deficiency (called *Wernicke's encephalopathy*) usually occurs in developed countries among alcoholics. Abnormalities include weakness or paralysis of eye muscles and an unusual way of walking. Memory and thought processes are often seriously impaired. Mental confusion, coma, and death may ensue within a few hours.

The course of beriberi is usually more dramatic in infants than in adults. The symptoms may worsen rapidly and a thiamin-deficient child who has appeared healthy may die quickly of heart failure.

Pellagra

Pellagra is usually associated with niacin deficiency, but it is almost always accompanied to a lesser degree by a lack of several B vitamins, protein, and other nutrients as well.

History. The pursuit of an understanding of pellagra is an excellent example of how epidemiological observations ultimately led to the solution of a nutrition problem (Chapter 24). For centuries, this disease was known to exist in populations where corn was the staple in the diet; it occurred more frequently and with greater severity in the spring than during other seasons. At the turn of the century, pellagra affected thousands of Americans, but,

A deficiency of niacin (and other nutrients) results in abnormalities in the skin, nervous system, and gastrointestinal tract. This condition is called *pellagra*.

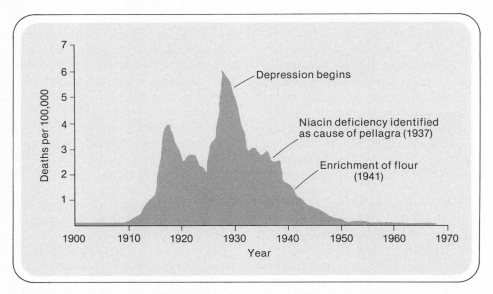

FIGURE 27-2. Incidence of pellagra during this century. (Adapted from "Nutrition in the United States—1900 to 1974" by W. A. Gortner, in *Cancer Research* 35(1975):3246. © 1975, Cancer Research, Inc. Also used by permission of the author.)

for some unknown reason, it was most common in the southeastern portion of the United States. In 1914, the Public Health Service sent Dr. Joseph Goldberger to this area to find out why it occurred.

To appreciate Goldberger's perceptiveness you must realize that at this time Pasteur's discoveries of the role of bacteria in disease permeated the thought patterns of scientists. A few investigators were developing concepts about "vital amines" in foods, but this idea had limited impact within the scientific community. Goldberger's first approach to pellagra followed the more conventional ideas. He, his wife, and fourteen colleagues became a "filth squad"—they ate and were injected with various biological materials (including excreta) from pellagra patients. When none of these materials transmitted the disease, the germ theory waned, and the investigator sought new avenues of inquiry.

The critical clue that redirected Goldberger's thinking was the observation that the disease occurred in poorly fed people but not in well-fed doctors and nurses who lived in close contact with pellagra patients. He hypothesized that that disease could be prevented by altering the diet. He tested the hypothesis by feeding some of the patients a diet including meat and milk. These patients recovered, whereas other patients (his control subjects) failed to improve while on their regular diets, which were predominantly cornmeal, molasses, and fatty meat called fatback.

Despite Goldberger's report of the curative effects of an improved diet in 1914, reduction in the incidence of pellagra was slow (Figure 27-2). In 1928 (the year before Goldberger's death), there remained an estimated 120,000 Americans who suffered from pellagra. The prospects for eradication of this disease improved in 1937 with the isolation of a form of niacin (nicotinamide). In 1941, niacin, along with other nutrients, was added to enriched cereal products. During the following decade, pellagra was almost completely eradicated.

Abnormality. The symptoms of pellagra can be described by the three D's—dermatitis, dementia, and diarrhea.

Dermatitis. The skin rash of pellagra is most severe in parts of the body exposed to sunlight—the hands and neck, the arms below shirt sleeves, and the legs below pants cuffs. The sensitivity of the skin to sunlight explains the old idea that pellagra mainly occurred in the springtime. Actually, the deficiency was there long before spring. It worsened as winter progressed and food stores became depleted; then warm weather brought the niacin-deficient people outside into the sunshine, and the signs of the disease became manifest.

The skin of pellagrins does not usually appear inflamed (like a pimple or infection), but rather is toughened in spots, coarse and bumpy to the touch, and red. In severe cases, it looks like a sunburn, and the exposed underlayers of skin are vulnerable to infection.

Dementia. The word *dementia* means mental deterioration, but the nervous system damage in pellagra ranges in severity from dizziness and loss of balance to tremors, depression, and delirium. It is no coincidence that Goldberger found many pellagrins in mental institutions. The cause (inadequate diets in mental hospitals) and effect (mental deterioration) of this disease locked these patients into a vicious cycle.

Diarrhea. Pellagra causes several abnormalities of the gastrointestinal tract; one of these is diarrhea. Other signs are cracked and painful skin around the mouth, and an inflamed and sensitive tongue. The stomach fails to produce acid, so that iron absorption is decreased. The intestinal mucosa loses its bristly structures (villi) that are necessary for maximal absorption. It is no wonder, therefore, that pellagrins exhibit broad, general symptoms of malnutrition (anemia, muscle wasting, and reduced height and weight).

Some of the abnormalities of pellagra may be attributed to a coexisting lack of protein and micronutrients. The absence of fruits, vegetables, and dairy products in the diets of pellagrins studied by Goldberger no doubt caused a deficiency of a variety of nutrients other than niacin.

Scurvy

Scurvy, the disease caused by lack of vitamin C, is perhaps the deficiency disease best known to nonnutritionists. The pictures in elementary school health books of people with swollen, bleeding gums leave a more lasting impression than do the less demonstrable signs of scurvy such as skin bruises, anemia, or bone changes.

History. The abnormalities of scurvy were described in the Ebers Papyrus about 1550 B.C. and in the later writings of Greeks and Romans. In more modern history, there is reason to believe that scurvy hindered the success of early attempts to explore the Western Hemisphere, because the richest sources of vitamin C (fresh fruits and vegetables) were not among the easily stowable rations that accompanied seafaring adventurers. Many of the men who died at sea succumbed, not in battle or shipwrecks, but simply for lack of a tiny six-carbon molecule—vitamin C. A teaspoonful of this vitamin would have been more than enough to prevent the disease in a sailor for a six month voyage.

It was, in fact, an experiment among sailors in 1747 that is usually credited with proving that scurvy was curable by altering the diet. The experiment was similar to that done 140 years later in Japan to cure beriberi, but in this case the sailors were British, the investigator was James Lind, and the dietary modification included six different test substances.

Lind found that the sailors who were given vinegar, sea water, elixir vitriol, or a mixture of herbs and garlic, contracted scurvy as often as those with no dietary changes (his controls). Cider seemed to help a bit, but addition of two oranges and a lemon each day provided the best protection. "Limeys," the nickname for British sailors, originated from a

A deficiency of vitamin D, calcium, or phosphorus causes decreased incorporation of calcium and phosphorus into growing regions of bones and teeth in children (a condition called *rickets*) and impaired maintenance of support tissues in the bones of adults (a condition called *osteomalacia*).

---

regulation instituted in 1795 that lime (the name then used for lemon) juice be given daily to sailors on all British ships. This policy was later endorsed by other countries, but its earlier use by Britain, and therefore the protection of these sailors against scurvy, might have been one factor explaining why Britannia ruled the seas for so many years.

Although the scurvy preventive property of citrus fruits was realized by Lind in 1747, almost two centuries passed before the important factor within these fruits—ascorbic acid—was isolated and synthesized in 1932. In the intervening years, many people died of scurvy. As recently as 1912, this disease took its toll among Captain Scott and his crew during their explorations of the South Pole.

Abnormality. The gross manifestations of scurvy appear to be explained by the fact that lack of vitamin C impairs the function of cells that form connective tissue, bones, and the inner portion of teeth (called *dentine*). Increased capillary fragility, impaired blood flow through tiny vessels, and defects in the formation of connective tissue are thought to contribute to the slow healing of cuts, bruises, and other wounds, and the aching in joints and muscles of patients with this deficiency disease.

The first visible abnormalities of scurvy occur after about five months on a deficient diet and they might be easily overlooked. The hair follicles, especially those on the thighs and buttocks, become more prominent. This happens because the follicles are plugged with the protein, keratin. The hairs within the follicles grow in coils (like springs) until they finally force their way through the skin surface. The tiny capillaries that normally nourish the hair-producing cells hemorrhage, and the skin becomes flecked with minute bumps that look bruised. As the disease progresses, these lesions spread all over the body. Hemorrhages also occur within the heart and other muscles, in and around the joints, and in the kidneys, thus impairing multiple body functions. Severe scurvy is usually associated with anemia and bone changes that are recognizable on X rays.

Scurvy causes dramatic changes in the tissues of the mouth; they become red and swollen. The slips of gum tissue (*gingiva*) that separate the bases of the teeth are often the most seriously affected. Hemorrhages within the mouth are not considered to be life-threatening, but because they make eating painful, food intake diminishes and overall nutritional status plummets. The severity of the oral changes is in part influenced by the state of oral hygiene.

Rickets and Osteomalacia

The terms *rickets* and *osteomalacia* describe the same bone disease. Different names are used because the manifestations of vitamin D, calcium, or phosphorus deficiency depend upon whether the bones are growing, as in children (rickets), or the nutrient deficiency impairs the maintenance of the bones, as in adults (osteomalacia).

History. The soft bones, bowed legs, and chest deformities characteristic of rickets were first described in the English medical literature 300 years ago. Calcium and phosphorus were implicated in the development of this disease around 1900, when it was observed that these minerals were not normally absorbed by rachitic children. As the role of vitamins began to be appreciated, early nutritionists realized that "fat-soluble A" contained two essential dietary substances. Oxidation destroyed the dietary factor (later shown to be vitamin A) that prevented eye lesions, but oxidation did not affect the other factor (vitamin D) that cured rickets. The latter component was isolated in 1930 and its chemical structure was demonstrated years later.

Although rickets has not caused as many deaths over the years as other deficiency diseases, there is evidence that this abnormality used to be widespread. It occurred to the greatest degree in northern countries that had limited sunshine and most seriously in smoggy industrial cities. The autopsy records of Baltimore children under two years old

A deficiency of vitamin A causes progressive damage to the eye, ultimately resulting in blindness. This condition is called *xerophthalmia.*

who died between 1926 and 1942 showed that signs of rickets occurred in over 50 percent of those examined, although these children died from some other cause. Severe rickets was noted in more than 12 percent of these death records.

The story of vitamin D is continuing to unfold. Scientists have recently discovered that enzymes located in the liver and kidneys alter this nutrient to produce several forms of vitamin D that behave much like hormones. Although rickets is usually preventable with small amounts of dietary vitamin D or small amounts produced in the skin on exposure to sunlight, some children have a genetically caused type of rickets that can only be cured by continuous administration of several hundred times the average requirement of this vitamin. It has been shown that many of these children are born without the enzyme(s) necessary for the transformation of vitamin D to DHCC, the hormonal form (Chapter 7). In some cases, synthetic DHCC can be given therapeutically. However, the dosage must be minute because DHCC is many times more potent than vitamin D. An excessive amount of DHCC would be lethal in a very short time.

Abnormality. The basic defect in rickets and osteomalacia is the decreased incorporation of calcium and phosphorus into the growing regions of bones and teeth in children, and impaired maintenance of support tissues in the bones of adults. Lack of deposition of calcium causes the bones to become soft, but the site of deformity depends upon the pressures exerted on the growing bones at the time the deficiency occurs. In an infant, the back of the skull may be flattened due to the pressure exerted by the weight of its head while lying in the crib. If the disease occurs in a crawling child, the knees and wrists are most disfigured, and the rachitic toddler or preschool child develops bowed legs.

Potentially the most dangerous deformities are those of the chest. The breastbone (sternum), which is linked by cartilage to the ribs, may be forced inward or outward. If the softened ribs move in-

ward, chest expansion and breathing may be impaired. This causes reduced lung volume and may or may not lead to lung and heart complications, depending upon severity.

Rickets also causes delayed tooth eruption and thinning of the protective enamel layer of teeth. Also, a reduction of muscle tone, combined with skeletal deformities, forces affected children to waddle rather than walk. Another common sign of this disease in infants is the delayed closure of the "soft spots" (fontanelles) on the top of the head.

Osteomalacia causes bone softening, deformity, and increasing vulnerability to fracture. This condition most often affects the pelvis, but collapse of vertebrae may also occur. Osteomalacia usually results from a combination of dietary inadequacy, lack of exposure to sunlight, and frequent pregnancies (which deplete nutrient stores).

Other conditions, such as malabsorption syndromes, parathyroid gland disease, kidney diseases, and inborn errors of metabolism, may lead to rickets or osteomalacia. These other conditions are currently responsible for more cases of deranged calcium and phosphorus handling than dietary deficiency of vitamin D.

Xerophthalmia

Of all the vitamin deficiency diseases, xerophthalmia is probably least known among Americans. But its effects are much more devastating to children around the world than the conditions described by more easily pronounceable names. *Xerophthalmia* means a condition of (*-ia*) dryness (*xeros*) of the eye (*ophthalmos*). This name describes the early signs of a deficiency, but the disease may culminate in total blindness. Vitamin A deficiency is the *major cause of blindness* in most developing countries.

History. Although the term *fat-soluble* A was coined in 1912, many years passed before the unique structure and properties of vitamin A were distinguished from those of other fat-soluble vitamins. In the course of investigations, it was discovered that plant pigments called *carotenes* could be converted by the body into a substance that had the same disease-preventive properties as vitamin A.

Abnormality. The first indication of vitamin A deficiency is *night blindness*—a change that is not detectable by a doctor when examining a child. This condition is not so severe that the child cannot see at all, but vision is impaired after dusk. Early diagnosis is further complicated because the child is often too young to realize that his or her inability to see is abnormal. The examiner may only learn of night blindness by asking the mother whether the child stumbles or moves hesitantly when light is dim.

The next stage of this disease is associated with a dryness of the membranes around the eyelids. Secretion of tears diminishes, and then frothy, foamy white deposits (*Bitot spots*) appear, usually at the junction of the white and colored portions of the eye. More severe deficiency results in a dryness, and therefore dullness, of the cornea accompanied by a reddening of the membranes and the white of the eye.

These changes may be corrected if vitamin A is given in time, but if the deficiency becomes more severe, ulcerations of the cornea develop, followed by infection. The next stage is perforation of the cornea, which begins to bulge. Finally, the lens of the eye becomes detached and drops (*prolapses*) out of its normal position. The lesion heals with scar tissue and blindness results. Life continues, but in a senseless darkness that might have been prevented if the parents had known what to feed the child or if someone had recognized the presence of the disease before it was too late to save the child's eyesight.

Goiter

Goiter usually results from a deficiency of iodine, which triggers a series of hormonal reactions that culminate in enlargement of the thyroid gland. Goiter may also be caused by other diseases, hormonal abnormalities, hereditary factors, or excessive intakes of iodine.

A few foods (primarily in the cabbage family) contain substances called *goitrogens*. These inhibit the incorporation of iodine into the hormone thyroxin. The body senses a decrease in the production of thyroxin, and hormonal signals are sent from the pituitary to the thyroid. These signals cause the thyroid to enlarge in an effort to produce more thyroxin. Goitrogen-containing foods rarely are consumed in sufficient amounts to create a problem in people whose diets supply adequate iodine, but they may contribute to the development of goiter in areas of the world where the soil and water are abnormally low in iodine.

In parts of the Midwest and Great Lakes areas of the United States, the soil contains low levels of iodine and the freshwater fish available are not good sources of this nutrient. Populations living in coastal areas are more likely to have adequate intakes of this mineral because foods grown in these areas are richer in iodine (because the soil contains more iodine) and ocean fish are good sources of iodine. Iodine also inadvertently enters the food supply through certain manufacturing processes; milk and baked goods may be high in iodine.

Iodized salt (which contains potassium iodate) is a major source of this nutrient for most Americans, but not all salt is iodized. Check the box in the kitchen where most of your food is prepared to see what kind of salt you use. Those who, for medical reasons, must follow a low-salt diet must assure that other sources of iodine are included in their diets.

Other Diseases

Clinical nutritionists can recite the causes and abnormalities of many more diseases caused by a deficiency of a single nutrient. The people who take care of patients must be aware of the nutritional deficiencies that frequently accompany diseases of

An understanding of how nutrients help prevent disease has evolved over centuries; their role in preventing disease continues to be investigated.

TABLE 27-1. Clinical Signs of Various Deficiencies Found in the HANES Population, Aged 1 to 74

Nutrient Deficiency	High Risk	Moderate Risk	Low Risk
Protein		Hepatomegaly (1.4)	
Riboflavin		Cheilosis (1.0) Nasolabial seborrhea (1.0)	Conjunctival injection, eyes (1.0)
Niacin	Filiform papillary atrophy of tongue (1.8)	Fungiform papillary hypertrophy of tongue (4.2) Fissures of tongue (4.5)	Serrations or swelling of tongue (5.6)
Thiamin		Absent knee jerks (1.0) Absent ankle jerks (1.7)	
Vitamin D		Bowed legs[a] (3.3) Knock knees[a] (1.3)	
Vitamin A and/or essential fatty acids		Follicular hyperkeratosis, arm (4.0)	Dry, scaling skin (xerosis) (2.5)
Vitamin C		Bleeding and swollen gums (2.5)	Diffuse marginal inflammation (17.5) Swollen red papillae of gingivae (6.5)
Iodine	Thyroid enlargement, Groups II (1.0)	Thyroid enlargement, Group I (3.7)	
Calcium		Positive Chvostek's sign (6.8)	

NOTE: Numbers in parentheses indicate the percentage of the population examined showing positive signs of deficiency.
[a] The clinical signs listed here indicate a moderate risk of having had the deficiency.
SOURCE: *Preliminary Findings of the First Health and Nutrition Examination Survey, United States, 1971–72: Antrhopometric and Clinical Findings*, U.S. Department of Health, Education and Welfare Pub. No. (HRA) 75-1229 (Washington, D.C.: Government Printing Office, 1975).

other origin or result from physician-initiated therapy of certain diseases. The complexity of these interrelationships goes far beyond the concerns of nonmedical personnel and this book.

HANES RESULTS

The HANES (Chapter 13) examined a subgroup of the entire survey population for clinical signs of deficiencies of various nutrients. Each sign was categorized as being a low, moderate, or high risk for a particular nutrient deficiency. Table 27-1 summarizes the results of the clinical examination of people 1 to 74 years old. The numbers in parentheses indicate the percentage of people with positive clinical signs suggestive of nutrient deficiency.

The micronutrient for which the smallest percentage of the population demonstrated clinical deficiency signs was riboflavin. Low risk signs were most prevalent for vitamin C and niacin deficiency. One of the moderate risk signs was positive for calcium in 6.8 percent of the population; for vitamin A and/or essential fatty acids in 4.0 percent of the population; and for thiamin in 1.7 percent of the population. The only vitamin for which a high risk factor was found to be positive in more than 1 percent of the population was niacin. The thyroid enlargement noted may have been caused by either inadequate or excessive intakes of iodine or by other nonnutritional disorders.

STUDY QUESTIONS

1. What factors affect the manifestations of micronutrient-deficiency diseases?

2. What has caused the increased awareness of the importance of micronutrient deficiencies?

3. What are some characteristics common to several micronutrient-deficiency diseases?

4. What generally causes isolated deficiency diseases, multiple deficiency diseases, and secondary deficiency diseases?

5. How has the incidence of micronutrient-deficiency diseases been reduced in developed countries? In developing countries?

6. What are the basic steps in the process of discovering an essential nutrient?

7. What causes beriberi? How is it characterized?

8. What causes pellagra? How is it characterized?

9. What causes scurvy? How is it characterized?

10. What is rickets? What is osteomalacia?

11. What causes xerophthalmia? How is it characterized?

12. What causes goiter? How is it characterized?

SUGGESTED READING

1. Y. Itokawa, "Kanehiro Takaki: A biographical sketch," *Journal of Nutrition* 106(1976):581.
2. C. E. Butterworth, "The skeleton in the hospital closet," *Nutrition Today* 9(1974):4–8.
3. D. A. Roe, *A Plague of Corn: The Social History of Pellagra.* Ithaca: Cornell University Press, 1973.
4. K. M. Hambidge et al, "Zinc nutrition in preschool children in the Denver Headstart program," *American Journal of Clinical Nutrition* 29(1976):734–38.
5. W. K. Simmons, "Xerophthalmia and blindness in northeast Brazil," *American Journal of Clinical Nutrition* 29(1976):116–22.
6. F. R. Ellis, S. Holesh, and T. A. B. Sanders, "Osteoporosis in British vegetarians and omnivores," *American Journal of Clinical Nutrition* 27(1974): 769–70.
7. H. A. P. C. Oomen, "Vitamin A deficiency, xerophthalmia, and blindness," Chapter 9 in *Present Knowledge in Nutrition.* 4th ed. New York and Washington, D.C.: The Nutrition Foundation, 1976.
8. E. N. Todhunter, W. J. Darby, and K. W. McNutt, "A bedside library for nutrition scholars," Chapter 53 in *Present Knowledge in Nutrition.* 4th ed. New York and Washington, D.C.: The Nutrition Foundation, 1976.
9. M. W. Moncrieff, "Rickets," *Nutrition* (London) 29(1975):221–25.
10. J. L. Spivak and D. L. Jackson, "Pellagra: An analysis of 18 Patients and a review of the literature," *The Johns Hopkins Medical Journal* 140(1977): 295–309.

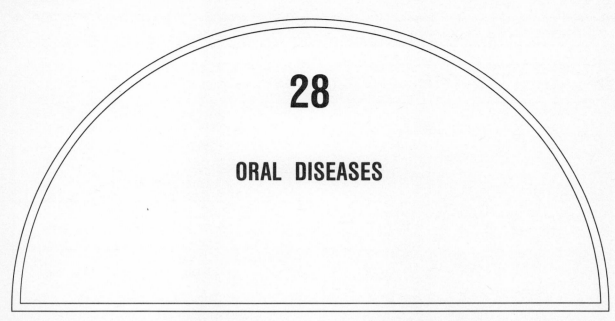

28

ORAL DISEASES

Oral diseases are the most prevalent health problems in the United States. These conditions primarily include *dental caries* and *periodontal disease*.

Bacteria have a pivotal role in the production of these diseases, but dental caries and periodontal disease are not truly infectious diseases. Tissue invasion by microorganisms is only one step in a complex sequence of events that result in oral disease. Other contributing factors include diet composition, eating patterns, oral hygiene practices, and genetics. All these influences may contribute to the growth of microorganisms that eventually can rob us of our teeth—and often the health of our entire bodies.

THE ROLE OF NUTRIENTS

Nutrients play a role in oral health at the time of tooth formation and also during the maintenance and preservation phases. Thus, diet is an important factor in oral health throughout life.

The composition of teeth is quite similar in many ways to that of bones. Both are made of a protein matrix, or honeycomb type of structure, interspersed with calcium, phosphorus, magnesium, and carbon. Teeth also contain lesser amounts of fluorine, zinc, manganese, iron, and a dozen other ele-

ments. Mineralization within the protein matrix causes the hardness of the outer portion (*enamel*) of the teeth (Figure 28-1). The inner, nonmineralized part of a tooth is soft tissue, comparable in many ways to the marrow of bone. The cells here are normally well supplied with blood, which provides oxygen and nutrients.

The tooth–bone analogy fails, however, in terms of cellular growth and repair. Once the adult (*deciduous*) teeth have attained maximal size, there is no further growth or mineralization. Teeth cannot repair themselves as can bone.

Nutrients such as calcium, phosphorus, and vitamin D, which participate in tooth formation, are especially important while growth continues. Optimal calcification of *dentine*, the inner tooth structure, is dependent upon adequate vitamin C. Vitamin A is important for the calcification and development of the outer surface, or enamel.

A proper balance of nutrients is also necessary to nourish all the cells in other tissues of the oral cavity. Tooth eruption out of the gum tissue is delayed in severe rickets and PCM. Chapter 27 described the damage of tissues in the mouth that accompanies scurvy and pellagra.

The nutrients available to a child during its de-

Nutrients are used in the structure of teeth, to nourish the nonmineralized tooth tissue, for the calcification process, and to maintain other tissues in the oral cavity.

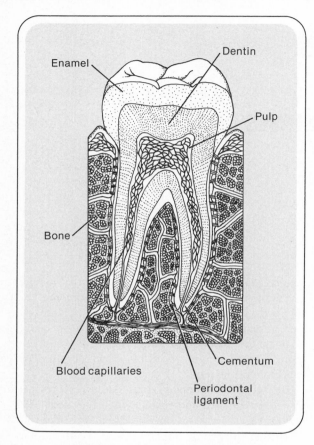

FIGURE 28-1. The anatomy of the tooth.

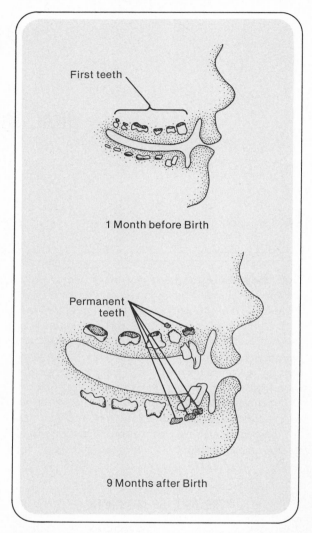

FIGURE 28-2. A baby's jaws and teeth. (Redrawn from an illustration courtesy of National Dairy Council.)

velopment within the uterus and the first years of life affect tooth formation. Protein and other nutrients are necessary for the early phases of tooth formation, which precede the appearance of the tooth above the gum surface (Figure 28-2). The young of experimental animals that have been fed diets extremely low in trace elements are born with congenital malformations of the mouth.

Nutritional status and oral health are interdependent. Malnutrition may cause damage to teeth and oral tissues; on the other hand, diseases of the teeth and mouth may cause malnutrition. A sore tongue, bleeding gums, or fungus infection within the mouth can be a strong deterrent to eating. Lack of teeth or poorly fitted dentures are also significant barriers to maintaining a nutritionally adequate diet.

PREVALENCE

The prevalence of the two diet-related oral diseases varies in different age groups.

Dental Caries

Dental caries is commonly referred to as *tooth decay* or *cavities*. The word *caries* is derived from a Greek term meaning "rotten."

The prevalence of caries is greatest in children aged six to nine, but 75 to 90 percent of children entering the first grade have already experienced this condition. This disease continues to be a major health problem through the teen years. The Ten-State Nutrition Survey and the HANES reported a high prevalence of caries and evidence of widespread oral illness, even among the adult population.

Periodontal Disease

Gum inflammation, or *gingivitis,* is the first stage of periodontal disease. The severe form, commonly known as *pyorrhea,* involves the separation of teeth from the tissues that support them in the jaws.

Periodontal disease is the major cause of tooth loss after age thirty-five, but this disease is not limited to adults. The early stages of inflammation are often recognized by dentists in children. For example, the National Health Survey, 1963–1965, found that in 39 percent of the children aged six to eleven periodontal disease had begun. This was not considered to be a serious threat to the children at the time, but such findings emphasize the need for early dental checkups and parental supervision of health practices that can prevent worsening of periodontal disease during adolescence.

Many young people have swollen gums that bleed easily. This is a definite sign of periodontal disease, which will eventually lead to more severe problems. The end stage of this condition—loss of teeth—affects 18 percent of the United States population, or over 40 million Americans. It has been estimated that half of the people over age 65 have lost all their teeth.

The most prevalent form of periodontal disease results from poor oral hygiene. Advancing age, poor alignment of the teeth, certain diseases (such as diabetes), and other factors contribute to the development of oral disease, but in most cases these are not the primary causes. Periodontal disease is highly correlated with lower socioeconomic status, which in turn correlates with less frequent opportunities for dental care and preventive measures.

Why is periodontal disease so common? Part of the explanation may come as a surprise to students if their parents have insisted upon regular checkups and professional care of their teeth. It may be difficult to believe, but half the American children under age fifteen have never been to a dentist! Another contributing factor is that one person in three in the United States receives no dental care, except for emergency treatment.

MECHANISM OF CARIES PRODUCTION

An understanding of how caries are produced is fundamental to any program aimed at caries prevention.

Plaque Formation

Plaque is a gelatinous mass composed of oral microorganisms and a matrix of cell debris, saliva glycoproteins, and polysaccharides produced by the microorganisms.

The first step in plaque formation requires the presence of bacteria in the mouth; cavities cannot be produced in germ-free experimental animals, regardless of the nutrient composition of their diets. The bacteria most strongly incriminated in current studies of plaque formation include several strains of *Streptococcus,* but primarily *Streptococcus mutans.* These bacteria initially adhere loosely to the tooth

433

Bacteria present in the mouth link together the glucose units from sucrose molecules to form dextrans, which are sticky filaments that adhere to the tooth surface.

Plaque is a combination of dextrans and living bacteria that can convert any simple sugar to enamel-destroying acid.

surface. When conditions are right for their growth, they multiply rapidly, forming colonies.

The next step is the synthesis of specialized polysaccharides called *dextrans*. These chains, or filaments, contain glucose units, but they can only be made from the glucose half of a sucrose molecule. Dextrans are not made from simple glucose. Dextran filaments are produced and excreted by bacteria, forming a gummy mass that allows all the components of plaque to adhere to the tooth surface.

Acid Production

Bacteria within plaque are very much alive and metabolically active. They can utilize almost any sugar (sucrose, glucose, fructose, lactose, maltose) as a source of energy. Streptococcal bacteria cannot completely break down sugars to release carbon dioxide and water as human cells do (Chapter 5). Instead, their metabolic systems stop at the point where lactate is formed. This acid is capable of dissolving tooth enamel—gradually etching and then eroding the tooth surface. Once this process has begun, it can only be stopped—never reversed. To prevent further damage, tooth and bacterial debris must be cleaned out, and the decayed areas filled with plastic or metal(s). Some metals (such as gold and silver) used in fillings act as poisons to bacterial enzyme systems, thus minimizing recurrent caries in the same spot.

Nonplaque Caries

Plaque is an integral part of caries formation on the smooth surfaces of teeth, but caries can develop in the back teeth (molars and bicuspids) without plaque formation. The jagged structures of these teeth make it possible to grind food more efficiently, but food can collect in these pits and fissures, safe from the reach of toothbrush bristles. Bacteria residing in these same crevices can adhere to the tooth surface without the need for sticky dextrans. The threat of decay in molars and bicuspids is even greater because the types of bacteria that thrive under these environmental conditions are metabolically capable of converting complex carbohydrates such as starch, as well as simple sugars, into corrosive lactic acid.

EVOLUTION OF PERIODONTAL DISEASE

Bacterial plaque also plays a role in periodontal disease. In this condition, the accumulation of plaque occurs along the line where gum and teeth meet. In periodontal disease, the oral structure initially affected is not the tooth, but the gum. Irritating substances that are excreted by the bacteria in plaque seep into the crevices between tooth and gum. Consequently, the tissues become inflamed and tender, often swollen, and bleed easily.

As plaque accumulation progresses, the bacteria closest to the tooth surface die and their remains gradually mineralize, forming a hard deposit called *calculus* or *tartar*. Calculus may further irritate the gum, but it probably would cause little damage if it were not covered by plaque, which still contains living metabolically active organisms. These bacteria excrete into the area between the gums and the teeth enzymes that aid in the breakdown of oral tissues.

In the more advanced stage of periodontal disease, the fibers that secure the gums to the teeth are destroyed and the teeth become loosened. The gap between teeth and gums widens and allows further penetration of bacteria and food residues. Eventually, the damage extends deeper, finally reaching the bone that supports the teeth. Thus, the teeth are completely separated from supporting structures.

PREVENTION

All the factors that contribute to the cause of oral diseases must be considered in preventive programs.

Bacteria within plaque that occur along the line where gum and teeth meet, excrete substances that irritate gum tissue and eventually cause the destruction of the fibers that hold teeth in place in the mouth.

The risk of oral diseases is reduced by exercising good oral hygiene during the adult years as well as during childhood.

Oral Hygiene

The primary goal of oral hygiene is to maintain the teeth free of plaque. Most people can accomplish this by regular oral self-care. Plaque should be carefully removed at least once a day. It is preferable to clean the teeth in the evening before retiring, because saliva contains ions that reduce the acidity within the mouth, but salivation decreases during sleep. Therefore, the acid produced by any bacteria remaining on the teeth during sleep is less efficiently neutralized.

Thorough Brushing. Brushing is part of the process of removing plaque from surfaces that can be reached by a toothbrush. The contour, tufting, texture, or power of the brush is less important than the thoroughness of the procedure.

Dental Floss or Tape. Dental floss or tape should be as handy in the bathroom as the toothbrush. Even the most probing toothbrush cannot reach spaces between the teeth—an excellent hideaway for destructive bacteria.

Since individual mouths vary in structure, alignment of teeth, and condition of the gums, no generalized pattern of brushing and flossing is effective for everyone. A dentist or dental hygienist can recommend the best method for scouring hidden pockets and crevices unique to your mouth.

Disclosing Wafers. Disclosing wafers contain a dye similar to that used for years by dentists to locate plaque. They are a relatively new tool for fighting plaque, and are now widely available in drugstores. The wafers are chewed and then the saliva–stain mixture is swished between the teeth for about 30 seconds. The dye primarily adheres to plaque, allowing a person to see where the decay-causing organisms remain.

Use of disclosing wafers adds about a minute to the oral hygiene routine, but it may save hours in a dentist's chair. The first use of these wafers can impress upon a hasty or inefficient tooth brusher the extent of residual plaque. It can also point out the tooth areas most often overlooked during brushing and flossing. If the cumulative cost (about a nickel each) prohibits regular use, this check can be made periodically to monitor thoroughness of cleansing.

Professional Care. Thorough periodic cleaning of the teeth by a dentist or dental hygienist removes all plaque and calculus. The dentist can also recognize early stages of decay, and thus more serious complications can be avoided.

The importance of professional care continues beyond the cavity-prone years. Detection by the dentist of the first signs of periodontal disease may make it possible to slow down or arrest the progressive damage. Early diagnosis and treatment can make a crucial difference in whether you eventually lose your teeth. The foods you can eat, your mouth comfort, lifestyle, and general health status will someday all be affected by the condition of your teeth and gums.

Diet and Eating Habits

The risk of oral disease can be minimized if you keep in mind how bacteria use various nutrients and you use this knowledge when selecting foods for meals and snacks.

Carbohydrates play various roles in caries production. Sucrose is especially damaging, because it supports both bacterial growth and dextran formation. The lactose in milk, and the fructose, glucose, and sucrose found in fruits, vegetables, and other foods can all support bacterial growth. Once plaque has formed in the mouth, all these simple sugars can be metabolized by bacteria to form acid.

Starch, such as that found in bread, cereal, potatoes, and other foods, can also be converted into caries-causing acid, but this can be accomplished

Frequent exposure of the teeth to foods containing carbohydrates (especially sticky foods and those high in sucrose) increases the risk of oral diseases.

only by bacteria that reside in the crevices of back teeth.

The amount of time resident bacteria are in contact with energy sources is a crucial determinant in plaque formation and acid production. Exposure can be minimized by avoiding snacks and minimeals, cleaning the teeth thoroughly, and avoiding sticky forms of food (especially those containing, or eaten in conjunction with, sucrose).

The most damaging types of food are those that appear in the mouth frequently. Repeated use of hard candy, breath-sweetening mints, or chewing gum is like continuously feeding nutrients to the acid-forming bacteria. The simple sugars in fruit juice can be damaging to the teeth if a toddler sucks on a bottle of fruit juice all day or goes to bed with one. Parents who pay dentist bills justifiably complain when children constantly sip soft drinks, but the same parents should be aware that sipping coffee with milk (lactose) and sugar (sucrose) throughout the day presents the same hazard to their own oral health.

Sticky foods are more of a dental threat than beverages that are quickly consumed. For example, sugar-coated cereals, granolas, dried fruit, and caramels are more cariogenic than fruit juice or soft drinks because the sticky foods are forced into crevices during chewing and adhere to tooth surfaces. Since their sugars remain in the mouth for a longer time, there is a greater probability that they will be converted into acid.

Formulated Foods

Another approach to prevention of oral diseases involves the alteration of the composition of foods. For example, sweet-tasting substances are being evaluated as possible substitutes for the sugars currently used in prepared foods. They are being tested for caries-prevention capacity as well as safety and other properties. The most promising sugar substitute appears to be a five-carbon substance called *xylitol* (Figure 28-3). Studies in Sweden show that people who chew gum containing xylitol twice a day have a reduction in tooth decay comparable to that achieved by substituting xylitol for most of the sucrose in their diets.

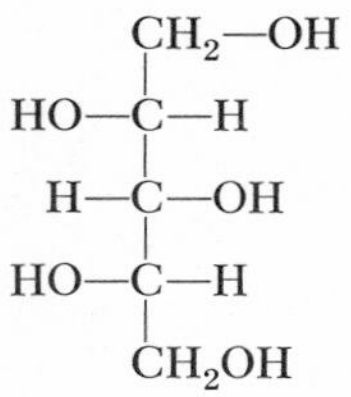

CH2—OH
HO—C—H
H—C—OH
HO—C—H
CH2OH

FIGURE 28-3. Structure of xylitol.

Another possibility being explored is the addition of phosphate to foods. Under some circumstances, caries may be reduced by adding phosphate, but certain forms of phosphates may be toxic in large doses. The use of phytates (which are polyphosphate molecules) must be weighed against the possible disadvantages caused by formation of nonabsorbable complexes with calcium, iron, magnesium, and other minerals.

Fluoridation

Most measures to improve oral health hinge upon personal values—individual choice and family proprieties—but fluoridation of the water supply is a community decision. The effectiveness of fluoridation is well documented: 20 to 60 percent reduction in dental caries has been achieved by adding fluoride to the water supply. Many communities have yet to elect this procedure despite the fact that it only costs between 5 and 15 cents per person annually within the area served by most public water supplies. On the other hand, the cost for dental care for children in areas with fluoridated water supplies is less than half the cost of care in nonfluoridated areas.

Fluoridation is not always hindered solely by political, philosophical, or financial deterrents. Many parts of the United States still lack water systems that are adaptable to fluoridation. In such areas, fluoride capsules taken regularly by individuals can help to lower the risk of oral disease. The limitation of this approach is that studies have shown that less than half of families to whom these capsules were made available continued to use them for any significant length of time.

Cultural Patterns

Dollars, research, and education will continue to be poured into oral health, but it is difficult to change people. Americans are not as aware of the importance of cleaning the teeth as are people in other countries, or, perhaps, we just fail to put our awareness into practice. For example, in many countries, toothpicks are placed on the table and used—even in the nicest restaurants. But Americans rarely use toothpicks, especially not in public. Another aid to caries prevention is brushing after lunch in the restrooms at school or in the office. Again, this is simply not the thing to do in the United States, but it is in other countries.

People in some of the developing countries of the world use more common sense about oral health than Americans. African children, for instance, may never have seen a toothbrush (much less be able to afford one), but traditions have taught them to protect their teeth. They break a twig from a tree, chew on it enough to soften the fibers slightly, and thus have a cleaning tool that can function as well as any toothbrush. This procedure often is more efficient, because these people move the twig around their mouths while doing other things at the same time, rather than dashing through a haphazard tooth-cleaning routine that is confined to the bathroom.

Genetics

Despite maximal efforts to prevent dental diseases, some people appear to be more prone to these conditions than others. The influence of genetics on oral health is poorly understood but strongly indicated. People who are more susceptible to these diseases can only hope to reduce the severity of their disease by strict observance of all possible preventive measures.

STUDY QUESTIONS

1. How are nutrients used in the oral cavity?

2. What are the two most prevalent oral diseases?

3. How is plaque formed?

4. What are the steps that lead to caries?

5. How can plaque formation lead to the need for false teeth?

6. How can the risk of oral disease be reduced by the individual? By the community?

7. What types of foods pose the greatest danger to oral health?

SUGGESTED READING

1. "Frequency of eating and dental caries prevalence," *Nutrition Reviews* 32(1974):139–41.
2. "Dental caries prevalence and trace elements other than fluoride," *Nutrition Reviews* 32(1974):120–22.
3. "Malnutrition and oral health in children," *Nutrition Reviews* 32(1974):44–47.
4. "Protein deficiency and tooth and salivary gland development," *Nutrition Reviews* 32(1974):24–26.
5. R. J. Andlaw, "Diet and dental caries: A review," *Journal of Human Nutrition* 31(1977):45–52.
6. J. P. Frazier et al, "Provider expectations and consumer perceptions of the importance and value of

dental care," *American Journal of Public Health* 67(1977):37–43.

7. J. H. Freeland, R. J. Cousins, and R. Schwartz, "Relationship of mineral status and intake to periodontal disease," *American Journal of Clinical Nutrition* 29(1976):745–49.

8. L. Kramer et al, "Dietary fluoride in different areas in the United States," *American Journal of Nutrition* 27(1974):590–94.

9. A. T. Brown, "The role of dietary carbohydrates in plaque formation and oral disease," Chapter 48 in *Present Knowledge in Nutrition.* 4th ed. New York and Washington, D.C.: The Nutrition Foundation, 1976.

10. I. Jenny, "Preventing dental disease in children: An ecological approach," *American Journal of Public Health* 64(1974):1147–55.

SECTION
VI

THE FUTURE OF NUTRITION

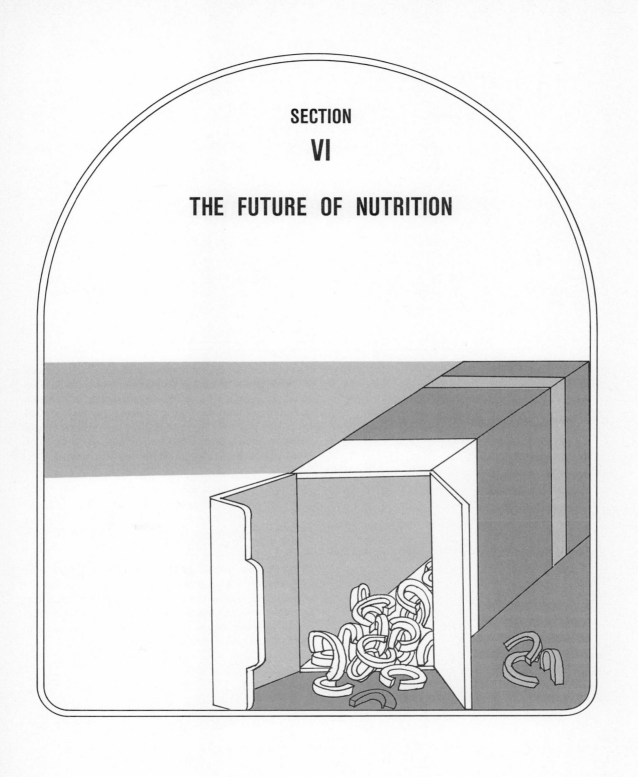

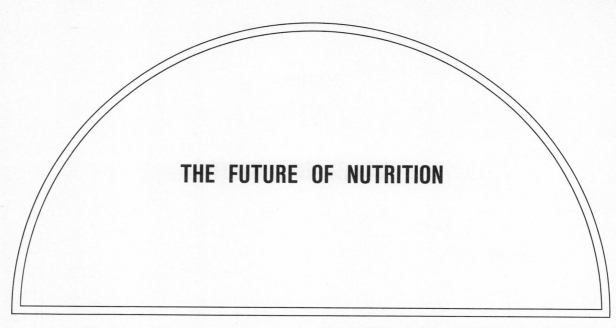

THE FUTURE OF NUTRITION

The science of nutrition, like every science, encompasses an ever-increasing body of knowledge. Your need to learn about nutrition and to apply newly available information will continue throughout your lifetime. This final section discusses how nutrition knowledge can be increased and its application expanded by researchers, by individuals who are not scientists, and by society as a whole.

CHAPTER 29 EXPANDING NUTRITION KNOWLEDGE discusses how to find reliable sources of nutrition information, how to evaluate information you hear or read about nutrition, and how to use nutrition information on food labels.

CHAPTER 30 HORIZONS OF NUTRITION deals with basic research leading to the growth of nutrition knowledge, efforts to solve the world food problem, current and projected research that will affect your life in the future, and the roles of several segments of society in improving the nutritional status of individuals.

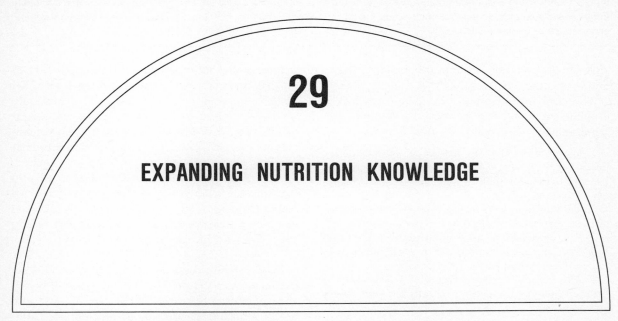

29

EXPANDING NUTRITION KNOWLEDGE

College courses are selected by students for a variety of reasons. Some are required for graduation, some are prerequisite for more advanced studies, and others offer knowledge basic to a chosen career. Elective courses are generally taken to provide background knowledge that can be expanded at leisure after graduation. For many students, nutrition courses fall into this latter category of learning experiences.

This book has presented concepts based on present scientific information and its application to questions of current interest, but the science of nutrition encompasses an ever-expanding body of knowledge. Future discoveries will affect the lives of all people. The goal of this chapter is to facilitate your ability to continue expanding your nutrition knowledge in the years to come.

NUTRITION RESOURCES

Many researchers who have spent a lifetime pursuing evasive vitamins and feeding various diets to rats are no doubt surprised that society has recently become very interested in the subject of food.

This public discovery of nutrition has had a variety of repercussions. Advertising agencies have capitalized on this interest in food commercials, the sales of diet-related paperback books have soared, and most astute political candidates include an anti-hunger plank in their campaign platforms. This atmosphere has created an excellent "environment for learning" (in educational terminology), but the climate is also ripe for the public to be misled.

Whom Can You Believe?

Almost every person who conveys nutrition information to the public (including your authors) has certain biases and perspectives. In most instances, these do not work against the best interests of the public, but sometimes, because of its presentation or its interpretation, the message is detrimental.

Expanding nutrition knowledge outside the classroom is made more difficult because of the communication gap between scientists and the press (who are primary sources of information for the general public). To make matters worse, the credibility of certain scientists is sometimes questioned because of their professional affiliations with government, industry, or, at times, academia. This condemnation-by-association leads some people to disregard the statements of certain nutritionists before listening to and evaluating what is said.

The resultant dilemma is the natural product of our current social and political atmosphere. Depending upon your point of view:

1. Government may be viewed as conscientiously protecting the quality of the food supply or strangled by red tape to the detriment of both consumers and suppliers.

2. The food industry is seen as capitalistic exploitation or competitive free enterprise.

3. Consumerism is a long-overdue expression of society's rights or an opportunity for a vocal minority to impose its desires upon the broader society.

4. The free press is the strength of a democracy or license to purvey whatever news sells the most papers and advertising.

Researchers, teachers, and the general public all become entangled in these broad controversies.

Nonscientists are no doubt dismayed by conflicting information about nutrition that is reported from supposedly authoritative sources. Their confusion might be less if they realized that disagreements among scientists are the fodder for growth of nutrition knowledge. Differences of opinion regarding the methodology and design of an experiment or the interpretation of the significance and meaning of data from an experiment provide a check-and-balance that can be the best possible way of directing the application of science. This intellectually stimulating scientific environment, however, often leaves the consumer confused because most people lack the background or interest to probe far below the surface of nutrition controversies. Under these circumstances, it is helpful to know where you can go for a reliable, balanced answer to questions of concern.

Organizations

"Nutrition" is rarely listed in the yellow pages of the telephone book, but the following suggestions may help locate a source of nutrition information.

Professional Societies. Several disciplines related to food and nutrition have professional societies. Their membership is broad enough to take into account different points of view. Standards for membership vary among societies, but most members are currently working in the field and presumably must keep abreast of the latest information. Several of these societies joined together in 1974 to form the National Nutrition Consortium. These societies (Appendix A29-1) each maintain a staff and facilities for answering questions that fall within their own area of expertise.

Public Health Agencies. Every state health department has a person who is the director or supervisor of nutrition services. Many county and city health departments also employ nutritionists. Community clinics, especially those for children, infants, and pregnant women, usually have nutritionists on their staffs. Programs for the elderly sponsored by the Administration on Aging also utilize nutritionists.

Colleges and Universities. Nutritionists in colleges and universities may be located in several departments. Teachers may not be able to allot academic time to consumer inquiries, but most can suggest an appropriate source of information. Land grant institutions are staffed to answer questions from the general public related to food and nutrition.

Other Health-Related Groups. Other groups, such as the American Heart Association, the National Foundation for the March of Dimes, the American Diabetes Association, and the Red Cross, often provide consumer services related to nutrition. Local chapters of such organizations may exist in your community.

Hospitals and Health Maintenance Organizations (HMO). Hospitals and HMOs often have staff nutritionists. Consultations are usually given on a fee-for-service basis or as part of a prepaid medical plan.

Dental and Medical Associations. State and local dental and medical associations (or societies) sometimes keep a roster of professionals qualified in nutrition. Occasionally these organizations can refer a physician to a dietitian who does fee-for-service patient consultations. However, such services should only be provided by dietitians who communicate with the physician regarding the total medical status of the patient.

Individuals

Because of their training and the nature of their work, nutritionists develop expertise of different types and differ in their ability to answer consumer questions.

The Meaning of Degrees. A critical reader always checks the qualifications of a source of information. The string of letters behind an author's name is usually (but not always) an indication of the person's expertise in nutrition. However, a Ph.D., M.D., D.Sc., M.S., M.A., or M.P.H. is hardly a guarantee that the person is well informed on a specific topic.

Nutritionists are found in a variety of disciplines. The strength as well as the complexity, of this science is that it overlaps biochemistry, physiology, medicine, home economics, food technology, bacteriology, toxicology, and many other disciplines (see Figure 29-1). No one person can possibly maintain an expertise in all these areas. For example, it is unrealistic to expect a food technologist to know the effect of sugar intake on diabetes, or to ask a physician how much vitamin C is destroyed by cooking asparagus. The inquirer, therefore, should ask a scientist what his or her major interest is before addressing specific questions. When an "expert" in the appropriate field is located, he or she should be asked whether there are other scientists who do not

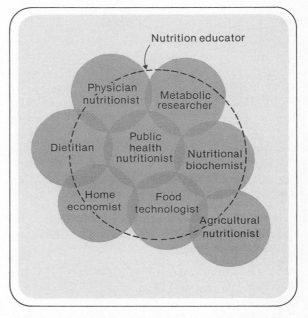

FIGURE 29-1. Overlapping expertise and training within nutrition. (Adapted from "Nutrition teaching in preventive medicine" by W. H. Sebrell, Jr., and T. B. VanItallie, in the *Archives of Environmental Health* 4 (June 1962):68. © 1962, Heldref Publications. Also used by permission of the authors.)

share the viewpoint expressed by this person. The response to this question may indicate how much confidence to place in that individual's opinion.

Specialist and Generalist. Certain tradeoffs must be kept in mind when advice is sought from nutritionists. Some of the most brilliant nutritionists of necessity become so engrossed in their narrowly defined area of research that they are not aware of what consumers consider problems at the moment. Others who are more involved in applied nutrition, have a breadth of information in all areas but lack the depth. Society ultimately benefits from the contribution made by each group, but when seeking information, you should not expect from one what is the strength of the other.

Communication Tips. Conversations with professional nutritionists can be frustrating if you are seeking brief, simple answers. Scientists are very precise in their thinking, and their conversations usually involve a lengthy clarification of the conditions under which any given statement is, and is not, valid. This is why most authoritative nutritionists are not popular on television talk shows, and why they communicate poorly, if at all, with the press. Their critical thinking pattern makes them less than sympathetic if you have not given serious thought and study, commensurate with what is easily available, before asking a question.

EVALUATION OF NUTRITION INFORMATION

Misinterpretation of nutrition information often occurs because people fail to read carefully or they overlook the real significance of numbers as they actually appear or are spoken.

Grammatical Rules

The following suggestions may uncover possible pitfalls in interpretation of nutrition information. These grammatical patterns may unintentionally slip into conversations or print, but they can be a warning that information should be examined critically. If a writer is careless about *how* something is said, the reader should be careful about *what* is said.

Multiple Subject–Multiple Object. Sentences with multiple subjects and objects can mislead the reader. For instance:

> "Sugar, fat, cholesterol, and salt cause diabetes, cancer, hypertension, and heart attacks."

You might assume that each dietary factor is required to cause all the diseases, that all the dietary factors must interact before causing any of the diseases, or many other permutations of these combinations of causes and effects.

Incomplete or Unquantified Comparatives. Incomplete or unquantified comparatives leave the reader in the dark or open to make any implied—but not stated—assumptions:

> "Fiber content is lower in the American diet."

Lower than what? It is important to know how much lower and also how much each diet contains before proceeding to evaluate other correlations.

Opinion. Personal opinion is often subtly woven into nutrition articles, even those without by-lines. "In other words" is a phrase that should send up a red flag for a critical reader. "It is thought," "It is believed," "It appears," should make you immediately question "By whom?" "On what basis?"

Generalizations. Generalizations are easily misinterpreted. "Many nutritionists recommend" may mean a majority of the professional nutritionists in this country or it may mean a much smaller group.

Qualifiers. It may be helpful to mark qualifiers in an article to avoid being misled. "May," "seems to," "perhaps," "probably," and "assuming" should alert the reader that everything in that statement is a supposition and not a fact. Qualifiers can easily be forgotten if several pages of text go on to elaborate on a supposition.

Juxtaposition of Sentences. The juxtaposition of two sentences can lead a reader to draw a correlation even though it was never stated by the author. For instance:

> "The American diet in 1942 provided half as much meat as the diet in 1976. Many recruits in World War II were found to be in poor health."

The author never says that the recruits were in poor health because their diets contained half as much meat as the 1976 diet, but the reader has been led to make this correlation.

Undefined Terms. Undefined terms plague the nutrition literature. The phrase "A nutritious food" is used too loosely by many people. It conveys no information about the nutrient content of the food or its relative contribution to meeting nutrient needs. "Harmful to health," "beneficial to your body," and "good for you" can be meaningful terms, but only if they are explained further.

Connotations. Connotations of words can broaden the communication gap—intentionally or unintentionally. "Full of energy" has a different implication from "full of calories," but both mean about the same thing. "Gassing tomatoes" leaves a different impression from "tomatoes stored in a gaseous atmosphere." The following are pairs of words that have quite different connotations although their meanings are synonymous in many contexts.

full of calories ⟷ full of energy
coarse ⟷ textured
slippery ⟷ smooth
manipulate ⟷ alter
filler ⟷ carrier
dissect ⟷ separate
stiffen ⟷ stabilize
synthetic ⟷ formulated
cheap ⟷ inexpensive

Mathematical Rules

Mathematics is considered such a precise science that numbers should not be misleading. They need not be—if you read carefully.

Reading Labels on Graphs. Understanding labels on graphs is important for correct interpretation of numbers. Often, a graph does not use zero as the lowest value. This saves space and allows the reader to visualize small, but significant, changes. However, it places a responsibility on the reader to know what degree of change corresponds with a significant deviation from normal.

Graphs that present changes compared to 100 percent of a certain index clearly indicate trends, but unless you understand the meaning of the 100 percent standard, it is difficult to interpret the significance of fluctuations from this initial value. In graphs of nutrient consumption trends, check whether the values refer to the weights of nutrients eaten, the amount eaten as a percentage of the amount eaten earlier (for instance, in 1978 compared to 1913), or the energy provided by that nutrient as a percentage of total energy intake. All three of these types of graphs are useful, but each conveys different information.

Dosages of Nutrients. Dosages of nutrients are often cited in nutrition literature, and it is helpful to compare these values to the RDA. Few people keep a table of RDA values at their fingertips and most of the exact numbers memorized for this course will probably be beyond your recall six months from now. It is rarely necessary to know the RDA to the last decimal point, but it would help to recall whether a nutrient is needed in milligram or gram quantities, maybe even a bit closer than that.

Students are better than teachers at devising easy ways to memorize lists of names and numbers. The best method we know is a senseless string of syllables and rounded-off numbers that approximate the RDA in milligrams—perhaps Table 29-1 will help you in the future. Vitamin B_{12}, the micronutrient with the lowest RDA (3 micrograms), and protein, the nutrient with the highest RDA (46 to 56 grams), are not included in Table 29-1.

Toxicity Calculations. Toxicity calculations are difficult unless you are familiar with certain mathematical conversions, but occasionally such efforts may be worthwhile. Chapter 20 gives an example of such calculations in the context of a naturally oc-

TABLE 29-1. Guide to Remembering Approximate RDA Values

Approximate Adult RDA	Nutrients	Initials of Nutrients Needed in Approximately the Same Amount
Less than 1 mg	Iodine Folacin	IF
1–2 mg	Thiamin Riboflavin Pyridoxine	TRiP
10–20 mg	Zinc Iron Niacin	ZIN
50 mg	Ascorbic acid (vitamin C)	A
1,000 mg	CAlcium Phosphorus	CAP

curring toxin. The questions that should be posed are the same when trying to put into perspective the hazard of any noxious substance—whether it occurs naturally, is produced by a bacterium or fungus, or is added during food processing.

Many writers do not try to help their readers through these calculations. They may state ill effects without also stating toxic doses and the amount of toxin in food. The reader is often left without an answer to the question that applies to everyday life. People who understand the fundamentals of toxicology outlined in Chapter 20 are able to ask appropriate questions to put hazards in perspective.

Anecdotes

Anecdotes fill the pages of many books that bear nutrition-related titles. These stories tell of people with a broad array of disorders—warts, infertility, dandruff, recurrent crying spells, upset stomach, irritability, terminal cancer—who have been miraculously cured by taking nutrient supplements or making a dietary change. These stories provide a glimmer of hope for people who feel they have no other recourse; they also sell thousands of books and trillions of vitamin and mineral capsules.

Such books must be read very carefully. Earlier chapters of this book have pointed out the need to consider all variables that may affect a physiological change and the importance of carrying out well-controlled studies that compare the effects of a placebo and a nutrient. The interpretation of anecdotes is further limited because the abnormal condition is frequently self-diagnosed by people who have no way of knowing what other diseases (psychological or physiological) can cause the same disorder.

It is incorrect to say that ingestion of nutrient supplements never coincides with remission of symptoms or disease. However, we can say that, with few exceptions, there is no evidence that vitamins or minerals in excess of recommended nutrient needs cause reversal of these conditions. In some conditions, the progress of some patients coincides

Information on food labels can help expand nutrition knowledge, but consumers must understand the importance of the designated serving size, the meaning of the U.S. RDA, and several points that, if disregarded, may cause misinterpretation of this information.

with changes in their psychological state. Some people call it faith or the will of God; others claim it is mere coincidence; some call it positive thinking; still others, more scientifically oriented, try to monitor fluctuations in brain waves and coincidental changes in physiologically measurable indexes.

The study of these phenomena borders on another frontier of medical knowledge. The untapped potential of the human brain has not been thoroughly explored. The influences of the mind on physiological function (psychosomatic effects) have been recognized, but these effects have not yet been explained through carefully controlled research. Until these correlations are understood and harnessed for the benefit of humanity, you can only keep in mind that a possible explanation of "vitamin cures" may be linked to the fact that people believe the cure will work.

Usually, it is a waste of time to try to convince a person who has been cured that his or her micronutrient supplement was not the cause of the cure. It may be worthwhile, however, to know how to discuss such stories with other people—those who are curious and might be easily persuaded to believe in the cure, yet not so emotionally involved that they lose sight of reason. The following questions will not apply to every situation or story, but they may lead a discussion toward patterns of thought that will be helpful for people who have not studied nutrition.

1. Was the person's diet adequate or inadequate before the cure?
2. Was the cure measurable or was it just a change in the way the person feels? Who measured the effect?
3. Was the cure part of a controlled test of the effect of the micronutrient?
4. What else might have caused the cure?

USING FOOD LABELS

Compared to full-color advertisements for miracle diet books, fascinating true-life stories of nutrient cures, and entertaining television celebrities who are self-proclaimed nutrition experts, it seems terribly boring to turn to the label on a can of beans to expand your nutrition knowledge. This is not the only way to learn, but it offers certain advantages:

- It is easily accessible information.
- Its validity is carefully controlled.

Much of the print on food packages is not there by chance or fancy, but because of government regulations. These regulations are always being expanded and revised, depending upon consumer needs and use and upon the growth of knowledge in the field. Nutrition-related information that currently appears on many food packages includes the categories described below.

Ingredient Labeling

The part of the label that lists the ingredients of the product in order of their predominance can be helpful in estimating nutrient content. Order of predominance can be misleading, however, unless you read carefully. For example, enriched flour may be listed as the predominant ingredient of a pastry; since enriched flour has a relatively high nutrient density for several micronutrients, you might assume this to be true for the pastry also. However, if the ingredients listed after the enriched flour include sugar, molasses, and corn syrup, it is quite possible that the sum of these foods that supply only energy is greater than the amount of enriched flour in the pastry. Similar confusion regarding the significance of the listing sequence arises when a food contains several types of flour or several sources of fat. Knowledge of the nutrient similarities of various types of foods helps to put ingredient labeling information into perspective. Another way to guess how much of an ingredient is present is to find a spice or condiment in the list (such as salt); any ingredient listed after the condiment is present in relatively small amounts—probably less than a gram per serving.

Nutrition Quality Guidelines

The FDA has developed standards of nutrient and ingredient composition for certain groups of foods. Products are not required to meet these criteria, but only the foods that measure up to these standards can bear the following statement:

> "This product provides nutrients in amounts appropriate for this class of foods as determined by the U.S. Government."

The minimum levels of nutrients for frozen heat-and-serve dinners are shown in Table 29-2. Few consumers will ever even wonder about how much thiamin is in a TV dinner, but if they look for—and find—the quality guideline statement, they have some assurance that the dinner has a relatively high nutrient density, as shown in Table 29-2.

Standardized Foods

The labels of certain foods do not list all ingredients. Instead, laws require that the product meet carefully defined standards if it bears a specific commonly used name (such as mayonnaise). The details of these regulations are quite complex, but in many ways they guard against the consumer's being misled while shopping. The standards for standardized foods can be obtained by writing to the FDA.

Nutrition Information Panel

The nutrition information panel, which became a mandatory part of the food labeling regulation in 1975, is required only if (1) a nutrient is added to a food, or (2) a claim is made in advertising or on the package that in any way conveys a message related to nutrition.

This panel may be used voluntarily by the manufacturer on any other product, but if it is used, it must comply in every way to the regulation. For instance, a label cannot state protein content with-

TABLE 29-2. Minimum levels of Nutrients for Frozen Heat-and-Serve Dinners

Nutrient	Minimum Levels	
	For each 100 Cal of the Total Components	For the Total Components
Protein, g	4.60	16.0
Vitamin A, IU	150.00	520.0
Thiamin, mg	0.05	0.2
Riboflavin, mg	0.06	0.2
Niacin, mg	0.99	3.4
Pantothenic acid, mg	0.32	1.1
Vitamin B_6, mg	0.15	0.5
Vitamin B_{12}, mcg	0.33	1.1
Iron, mg	0.62	2.2

out also providing information about energy value and the other nutrients that must be listed on the label. Consumer awareness of the nutrition information panel is gradually increasing, but the information given is not always understood.

Standard Information. The first point that must be understood is that the values on the label (Figure 29-2) refer to the amount of nutrients in one serving of the food. People who eat more or less than the serving size amount must adjust all other values accordingly. The amounts of energy (in Calories) and macronutrients (in grams) per serving are listed below the serving size description.

The bottom part of the label tells the percentage of the U.S. RDA of protein and seven other nutrients (calcium, iron, vitamin A, vitamin C, thiamin, riboflavin, and niacin) provided by one serving of the food. The protein value at the bottom of the label takes into account the quality of the protein,

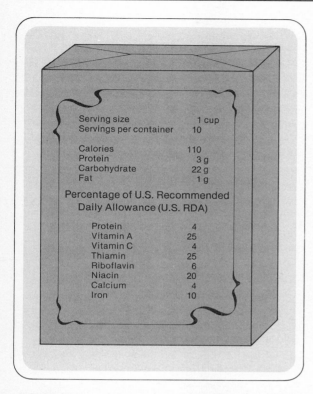

Serving size	1 cup
Servings per container	10
Calories	110
Protein	3 g
Carbohydrate	22 g
Fat	1 g

Percentage of U.S. Recommended Daily Allowance (U.S. RDA)

Protein	4
Vitamin A	25
Vitamin C	4
Thiamin	25
Riboflavin	6
Niacin	20
Calcium	4
Iron	10

FIGURE 29-2. Nutrition information panel on a food label.

as well as its weight. For foods with a PER (Chapter 2) equal to casein, 45 grams of protein is equal to 100 percent of the U.S. RDA. Foods with a PER less than casein must contain more protein—65 grams—in order to be labeled as containing 100 percent of the U.S. RDA for protein.

Optional Information. U.S. RDA values have been established for twelve other vitamins and minerals (see Table 8-2). The manufacturer may list any of these with no requirement of listing the other optional nutrients.

Manufacturers may also elect to provide on the label the content of cholesterol, saturated and polyunsaturated fat, and/or sodium. This type of label-

ing must include a statement that the information is provided for persons whose physician has recommended dietary modifications.

Potential Problems. Appropriate use of nutrition labeling information requires an understanding of several points.

1. The values given are a measure of nutrients present after processing, but they do not make any allowances for nutrient losses caused by the consumer who overcooks or repeatedly reheats food.

2. The percentage U.S. RDA values are rounded off at various intervals. (Values less than 10 percent are rounded to the nearest 2 percent, 10 to 50 percent are rounded to the nearest 5 percent, and over 50 percent are rounded to the nearest 10 percent.) This treatment of numbers is important when a comparison of the nutrient content of two products is being made. Nutrition labels do not convey useful information about small differences in nutrient content.

3. The greatest potential hazard of nutrition labeling is that the consumer may assume that only the nutrients listed on the label are needed.

The third problem seems to be unavoidable because information is not currently available to establish U.S. RDA values for many nutrients. Also, if too many nutrients were listed, the consumer would be so overwhelmed that the information would rarely be used.

The problem is partially alleviated by the fact that in a particular food, the amounts of some of the nutrients required to be on all information panels often parallels the amounts of some other nutrients not required on the label. The presence of one nutrient therefore often indicates the presence of another. This principle is not applicable, however, when foods are fortified with an "indicator nutrient." For instance, foods that are good sources of iron usually also provide other trace elements that travel into the food supply along with the iron. However, if a food is fortified with iron, the value for iron on the label does not indicate a comparable increase in trace element content.

Advantages of the Label

Nutrition labeling information cannot currently be used to assess total daily intake because many fresh and processed products are not labeled. The usefulness of the label, therefore, is mainly for:

- Learning which foods are better sources of each nutrient
- Learning the energy value of food
- Approximating nutrient density
- Determining relative macronutrient composition of a food

Although the label does not provide sufficient information to answer all consumer questions, teaching people to use the values that are available remains an enormous challenge to nutrition educators.

STUDY QUESTIONS

1. Where in your community (besides at your college or university) might you be able to find a person to answer questions about nutrition?

2. How can you determine whether a person is qualified to provide the type of nutrition information you seek?

3. What grammatical patterns might be misleading in the context of nutrition discussions?

4. How much bread must you eat daily to consume a toxic dose of potassium bromate if this additive is present in bread at a level of 75 milligrams of potassium bromate per kilogram of bread and if a toxic dose is 75 milligrams of potassium bromate per kilogram of body weight?

5. How can anecdotes about vitamin cures be misleading?

6. What information is availabe on food labels?

SUGGESTED READING

1. K. W. McNutt, "Public understanding of nutrition: Implications for education programs," *Contemporary Nutrition* (March 1977).

2. P. L. White, "The perfect environment for nonsense," *Nutrition News* National Dairy Council (October 1973).

3. "Nutrition misinformation and food faddism," *Nutrition Reviews Supplement* 32(1974):1–74.

4. "Standards of identity," *Nutrition Reviews* 32(1974):29–31.

5. J. Mayer, "How to find the facts about good nutrition," *Family Health* 9(1977):32, 66.

6. O. C. Johnson, "The Food and Drug Administration and labeling," *Journal of the American Dietetic Association* 64(1974):471.

7. M. L. Ross, "What's happening to food labeling?" *Journal of the American Dietetic Association* 64(1974):262.

8. *Nutrition Labeling: How It Can Work for You.* Bethesda: The National Nutrition Consortium, Inc., 1975.

9. L. M. Henderson, "Programs to combat nutritional quackery," *Journal of the American Dietetic Association* 64(1974):372.

10. R. N. Podell et al, "The public seminar as a nutrition education approach," *Journal of the American Dietetic Association* 67(1975):460–63.

11. "Nutrition beliefs: More fashion than fact," *FDA Consumer* 10(1976):24–27.

12. E. Newman, *Strictly Speaking* New York: Bobbs-Merrill Publishing Co., 1974.

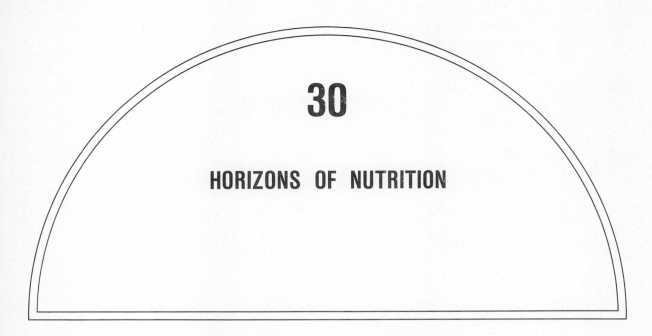

30

HORIZONS OF NUTRITION

Chapter 29 provided guidelines for how an individual might continue to learn about nutrition after completion of this course. This final chapter deals with how nutrition knowledge is expanded at the research level, and current and projected programs that apply research to the needs of society. By the time you reach this chapter, the amount of material already covered may seem monumental, and you may ask, "Why bother with what nutritionists do not know?"

The first reason is that future advances may very closely affect your life.

The second reason is that your peers will be among the people who solve these problems. Some of your classmates may be part of the team that clarifies the role of nutrition in many diseases and devises ways to balance world population and the food supply.

The third reason is that public participation in determining the direction of science and health care has soared in recent years and will increase even more in the future. The interdependence between science and society mandates that nonscientists become involved in such decisions and express their wishes, concerns, and priorities.

PATTERNS OF PROGRESS

Nutrition research is conducted in conjunction with other scientific research and it is linked to social transitions.

Other Sciences

Nutritionists build upon and contribute to a knowledge base shared by many disciplines. The foundation of nutrition knowledge dates back to Hippocrates, but the modern science of nutrition began to grow only two centuries ago when Lavoisier began his study of respiration. Table 30-1 lists highlights in the historical development of knowledge that is today considered basic to nutrition. These advances are listed chronologically and categorized under several subheads showing how progress was made concurrently in various areas of nutrition research. The contributions of several basic sciences to nutrition are summarized below.

Biochemistry and Physiology. Most publications of nutrition discoveries prior to the 1930s appeared in journals of biochemistry or physiology. Many of

Scientists from many disciplines have contributed to the growth of nutrition knowledge, and nutrition researchers have contributed knowledge to these disciplines.

TABLE 30-1. Historical Highlights in Nutrition

Year	Defining Nutrient Needs	Digestion	Respiration and Energy Production
1700			
1750		The stomach (mid-1700s) was believed to digest food by mechanical grinding and putrefaction. Reaumur (1752) demonstrated that chemical changes occur during digestion; he studied birds that regurgitated their food. Spallanzani (1780), using metal grid tubes and sponges that were swallowed and then retrieved, studied digestion in birds, animals, and himself.	Lavoisier and Laplace (1783) showed that respiration is a form of combustion; they measured the temperature change in an ice bath calorimeter using a guinea pig. Lavoisier and Seguin (1789) measured oxygen inhaled and carbon dioxide exhaled by men at rest, at work, and after eating.
1800		Prout (1824) identified hydrochloric acid in gastric juice. Schwann (1833) identified pepsin in gastric juice. Beaumont (1833) studied digestion in a man who had a bullet wound that left an opening (fistula) to his stomach.	Liebig with Pettenkofer, Voit, and Rubner (1824) expanded studies on respiration.

Essential Macronutrients			Micronutrients	
Protein	Fats	Carbohydrates	Minerals	Vitamins
			Iron (1713) was identified in blood.	
				Lind (1753) showed that intake of lemons and oranges can cure scurvy.
Magendie (1816) showed in dogs that nitrogen-containing foods are necessary for life.			Iodine (1812) was isolated.	
Prout (1824) summarized the elements of organized bodies as albuminous (protein), oleaginous (fat), and saccharine (carbohydrate).				
	Chevreul (1828) showed that fats are a combination of glycerol and fatty acids.			
Mulder (1838) introduced the word *protein*.				
Boussingault (1839) showed that animals cannot use atmospheric nitrogen as plants do.				

TABLE 30-1. Historical Highlights in Nutrition (*continued*)

Year	Defining Nutrient Needs	Digestion	Respiration and Energy Production
1850	Early attempts (mid-1800s) to find the cheapest and most nutritious diet for the poor and unemployed.		
1900	Voit (Germany) and Atwater (United States) (late 1800s) proposed nutritional standards based on the kinds and amounts of food eaten by healthy people. Chittendon, Sherman, and others (1904) attempted to measure protein and mineral needs.		Atwater (late 1800s) introduced the bomb calorimeter for measuring energy value of food. Atwater and Benedict (1904) developed a respiration calorimeter for humans. Lusk (early 1900s) studied intermediary metabolism using calorimeters.

Essential Macronutrients			Micronutrients	
Protein	Fats	Carbohydrates	Minerals	Vitamins
	Boussingault (1845) proved that carbohydrates could be converted metabolically to fat.	Schmidt (1844) identified sugar in blood. Fehling (1849) introduced a chemical method for measuring glucose. Bernard (1856) discovered glycogen in the liver.		
Lawes and Gilbert (1850s) showed, by feeding farm animals, that all proteins are not of equal nutritive value. Fick and Wislicenus (1866) showed that nitrogen excretion does not increase in men when mountain climbing and therefore proved that muscular activity does not occur at the expense of tissue protein.				
			Studies (late 1800s) began on the need for minerals in the diet of farm animals.	Eijkman (1896) showed the effects of brown rice in preventing and curing beriberi.
Osborne and Mendel (1900s) expanded the concept of variation in the nutritive value of protein.				Hopkins (1906–12) proposed that accessory growth factors are necessary for growth and health of experimental animals. Funk (1912) introduced the word *vitamine*.

TABLE 30-1. Historical Highlights in Nutrition (*continued*)

Year	Defining Nutrient Needs	Digestion	Respiration and Energy Production
	Vitamin requirements (1930s) were studied on the basis of growth, body tissue content, and cure and prevention of deficiency symptoms. The first *RDA* (1943) was published.		
1950	FAO/WHO (1950s) began to coordinate dietary requirements of different countries.		

Essential Macronutrients			Micronutrients	
Protein	Fats	Carbohydrates	Minerals	Vitamins
	Many studies (1913–15) on fat-soluble vitamins were in progress.			McCollum and Davis, and Osborne and Mendel (1913–15) discovered two unknown but essential dietary factors named vitamins A and B. Vitamin C (1917) was discovered. Vitamins D and E (1922) were discovered. Studies (1926) showed that vitamin B is more than one factor. The coenzyme role of vitamins (1932) began to be studied.
	Burr and Burr (1929) demonstrated that linoleic acid is an essential nutrient.			
Rose and co-workers (1938) identified eight essential amino acids for adults. Block and Mitchell (1946) introduced the chemical score method of evaluating protein value based on amino acid composition.				Vitamin B_{12} (1947) was discovered.
	Investigations (1950s) indicated a possible relation between lipids and coronary-vascular disease.		Trace element investigations (1950s) began to increase.	

the leading nutritionists today never took a course entitled "Nutrition," though they have taught the subject and, more importantly, their investigations have generated the facts that fill this book.

Bacteriology.   Many metabolic pathways were studied in microorganisms long before researchers worked out the details of how animals utilize nutrients.

Animal Husbandry and Agriculture.   Research designed to help farmers grow larger livestock, produce more eggs and milk, and harvest greater yields of plant products provided information that led to basic concepts related to human nutrition. These studies have also increased the availability of food and nutrients to humans, thus reducing the prevalence of malnutrition.

Physics, Engineering, and Mathematics.   Physics, engineering, and mathematics have provided many of the analytical tools essential for nutrition research. Instruments that measure ultraviolet light and fluorescence, and isotopes were not discovered by nutritionists, but these tools opened the door to nutrition investigations that previously had been impossible. New methods, such as gas–liquid chromatography, nuclear magnetic resonance, mass spectrophotometry, and electron-spin resonance, allow nutritionists to probe the intricacies of trace element functions, subtle shifts in vitamin structure and binding during metabolic reactions, and numerous other questions.

Space Technology.   Computers have revolutionized nutrition research. And NASA engineers call upon nutritionists to help feed their astronauts.

Social Stimulus

Much of nutrition research reflects changes in society. The soaring world population has stimulated studies designed to develop new food resources and to increase the nutritional value of traditional foods. The diminishing availability of oil has challenged nutritionists around the world to produce food with the least possible use of energy resources. Environmental concerns have led nutritionists to query how conditions outside the body may alter nutrient needs.

Consumerism influences the direction of research in basic science, food safety, and product development. The increasing role of government in delivery of health services and in provision of other needs, including food, has had an impact upon both the generation and the application of nutrition knowledge. During 1975, the International Year of the Woman, several nutrition symposia began to focus attention upon a relatively unexplored topic—the nutrient needs of females.

WORLD FOOD PRODUCTION

The most pressing demand upon nutritionists today is to alleviate the imbalance between food supplies and food demands of the world's population. Failure to solve this problem will lead to social upheaval combined with unprecedented mass starvation. When the World Food Conference convened in Rome in 1974, representatives of many underfed countries described their plight with clenched fists—not outstretched hands. Their hostility due to the inequitable distribution of the world food supply was evident, and, had there been any doubt before, the conferees left Rome convinced that this is a world problem and not solely the burden of developing countries.

Defining the Essentials

The complexity of the world food problem cannot be conveyed in the short space available here. However, the Protein Advisory Group of the United Nations, in an analysis of the problem, defined the

The solution of the world food problem requires research, technological assistance, and the efforts of people in many fields not directly related to nutrition.

most essential needs quite succinctly as water, improved seeds, and more fertilizer. The major pressure on the world food supply is the population increase. Solution of the problem is made more complex because unforeseen climatic disruptions such as floods and droughts complicate projections of food production needs and hamper food distribution efforts.

Research Needs

Part of the solution to the world food problem must come from research laboratories. The development of cereals and legumes of higher protein content and better protein quality offer some hope, but many of the higher-quality strains of corn and wheat are even more dependent upon adequate fertilizer, water, and optimal growing conditions than the standard strains. In many areas, the primary need is for energy—simple sources of Calories—rather than for protein.

Nutritionists and food technologists are also seeking ways of expanding or converting other protein sources into available foods. Conservation and increased utilization of fish resources and *marine farming* are growing areas of research. In many parts of the world, animals such as large rodents or aquatic mammals that are not now used as foods may be eaten in the future. Another possibility is to domesticate animals such as antelopes that can graze in marginal lands not suited for agriculture.

Vegetable protein mixtures will undoubtedly be used much more during your lifetime, but problems remain due to the flatulence caused by bean products, naturally occurring toxins or nutrient inhibitors in many plant foods, and the amount of energy needed to extract and concentrate vegetable protein.

Microorganisms that can convert oil by-products into their own cellular protein may someday appear on dinner plates in the United States, but this is not feasible at present. (Bacterial and yeast protein fed in large amounts cause diarrhea and other compli-

cations, perhaps due to their high content of DNA and RNA.) Another line of microbiological research is based on bacterial conversion of human waste into essential nutrients. This recycling of chemicals, if perfected, could allow astronauts to survive for extended periods of time without needing a large external source of energy and nutrients.

Technological Assistance

Another approach to alleviating the imbalance between people and food is to help developing countries improve their capability for protecting their foods from rodents, insects, and microorganisms, and for improving their food preservation and distribution systems. These changes will come slowly, but such programs also provide employment and reduce the necessity of purchasing imports. They make food available in a form that can be transported to the more isolated segments of the country where poverty and malnutrition are often most severe.

Material and technical assistance is currently influenced by the oil shortage. The cost of fertilizers (by-products of oil) has soared in recent years beyond the means of many farmers in developing countries. Fuel is also necessary for operating agricultural machinery, powering irrigation systems, transporting seeds and other goods to farmers, and distributing foods from farms to markets. Therefore, and two major recommendations related to assistance programs are:

1. Aid should be as fuel, rather than food.
2. Emphasis should be given to small-scale, labor-intensive agriculture.

This approach reduces the dependence upon equipment that requires fuel, while at the same time it increases employment. Small-scale farms can diversify their planting to include both cash crops and food consumed at home.

The results of research related to food and nutrition will affect your diet and your health in years to come.

Careers for the Concerned

The broad solution to correcting the existing food deficit requires input from many disciplines. Students who are considering a career that may allow them the opportunity to help solve the world food problem need not restrict their options solely to nutrition.

More land must come under cultivation, but climate, terrain, quality of soil, and other obstacles restrict these efforts. Engineers are needed to build dams, irrigation systems, wells, and water desalination plants. The monetary system must make credit available to carry farmers from seed and fertilizer purchasing season through the harvest and sale of crops; economists must address themselves to this problem. Expanded extension programs are needed to educate farmers, especially when new crops or methods are introduced. Research on products that can be cultivated under local growing conditions must be conducted by agriculture scientists and soil chemists. A general improvement of public health services, education, and family planning are all integral parts of the community and national development that must coincide with efforts to augment food production and distribution. These advances are dependent upon a dedicated cadre of workers in many different fields.

CURRENT AND PROJECTED STUDIES

Scientists sometimes say—half jokingly, half seriously—that "truth changes with the morning mail." Each experiment published in monthly journals adds a new piece of information to current puzzles and investigations. As studies begin to fit the pieces together, the final picture may be quite different from what was initially anticipated. The direction of nutrition research may change in the future, but an awareness of several areas of current and projected studies can sharpen predictions regarding

solutions to nutrition enigmas within the crystal ball today.

Animal Feeding

Nutritionists are currently investigating livestock feeding methods that use the existing food resources most efficiently. When grain is fed to cattle, the energy captured as beef is only about 30 percent of what was fed. On the other hand, cattle can convert carbohydrates that are not utilizable at all by humans into digestible nutrients. These two concepts have led to increased production of grass-fed beef, which will probably be used more in the future.

Other research on livestock feeding is beginning to show that the amount of saturated fat in meat can be reduced by altering the composition of livestock feed. This research may be applied to other animal products such as poultry and dairy products.

Home Preparation of Food

New methods of home preparation of food often create a need for additional research. The growing popularity of microwave ovens, for instance, is beginning to influence the interest of scientists in the effects of this method of cooking on the nutritive value of food. Use of crock pots raises questions about the amount of vitamins remaining in food cooked slowly at a low temperature and the possibility of bacterial contamination under these conditions when foods are not handled carefully.

The rising popularity of home gardens and home preservation has coincided with many cases of food poisoning that were traced to ignorance of the meaning of pressure conditions during heating or to substitutions for the proper seals, jars, or cooking vessels. This change in consumer handling of food may stimulate the development of equipment that is easier and safer to use on a small scale in the kitchen. In the meantime, people must be taught the importance of safe techniques for home canning and freezing.

Safety of Additives

The GRAS review (Chapter 12) and the projected increase in use of food additives have contributed to the establishment in 1974 of the National Center for Toxicological Research (NCTR) for evaluating the safety of chemicals added to food. This facility is equipped to maintain experimental animals in a germ-free environment and to store computerized information regarding diet composition, food consumption, growth, and laboratory analyses on body fluids and microscopic examination of tissues. Thus, the investigators have access to critical data spanning several generations on any animal in which adverse effects appear when fed a specific compound. The NCTR will not provide answers overnight, but it will generate a data base needed to evaluate the long-term effects of specific amounts of additives upon health.

Trace Elements

In the early 1970s, the USDA established a special research facility in North Dakota that focuses on the investigation of trace elements. The physiological function and human requirements of essential minerals, their distribution in food, the factors that alter absorption and utilization, their role in disease, and their toxic effects are several of the avenues of research being conducted at these laboratories.

Nutritive Value of Food

The USDA is currently compiling and computerizing volumes of previously unavailable information on the nutritive value of food. The data bank provides information on various brands of food and on many nutrients not listed in the USDA *Handbook*

Number 8. Several sections of the new nutrient composition handbook were published in 1977.

Future analyses of nutritive value must take into consideration factors that were understood poorly, if at all, a few years ago. These include the interaction of nutrients with other components of a food (such as phytate, oxalate, and fiber) and protein-bound forms of micronutrients. Many questions remain about the absorbability or utilization of various forms of micronutrients (such as folacin and iron) that occur in foods.

Biochemistry and Physiology

Scientists who specialize in the biochemical and physiological role of nutrients will someday provide more thorough answers to important questions about nutrition, such as:

1. What factors predispose an individual to obesity?
2. What role does nutrition play in brain development?
3. How do nutrients and hormones interact?
4. Can dietary modifications alter the progress of certain diseases?
5. What effects do large intakes of nutrients have?
6. What is the role of diet in the cause of cancer and in the therapy of patients with cancer?

NUTRITION EDUCATION

The improvement of the nutritional status of people is dependent not only upon research but also upon transmitting information to people and helping them use this knowledge. Formal nutrition education began in the United States early in this century. It grew rapidly during the 1940s and was stimulated by several national conferences in 1941, 1952, 1957, and 1962 under the auspices of the federal Interagency Committee on Nutrition Education (ICNE). The White House Conference on Nutrition in 1969 and the follow-up conference in 1971 continued to emphasize the importance of education in alleviating the consequences of improper food selection patterns in this country.

Curriculum Development

In recent years, nutritionists have made more of an effort to combine their expertise with that of educators. Basic concepts regarding nutrition were developed during the late 1960s by the ICNE and some state departments of education formulated curriculum guides for nutrition education. Some of these have been the basis of excellent programs, but others have collected dust or been tossed into trash cans. The more recent interest in nutrition education has resurrected some of these guides and stimulated the development of others, but many roadblocks remain before large-scale programs can be implemented.

Dilemma of Teachers

Teachers are currently overloaded with material to be taught, and time allotted to nutrition must be sequestered from other topics such as drug education, mental health, venereal disease, and other growing social concerns. Teachers therefore need ways to integrate nutrition concepts with other mandatory curricular material. They also need the support of administrators, food service personnel, school health workers, and—of prime importance—parents and the broader community. Nutritionists must also be organized to assist in education programs and to serve as resources for information beyond the training of most teachers.

Program Development

For many years, the major sources of information for classroom use in nutrition were generated by the Department of Agriculture, especially by the home economics experts in the agricultural extension program. The Agricultural Research Service of the USDA prepared many related materials for students and consumers. Their efforts were complemented by programs developed by the educational branches of several food-related trade associations.

In 1968, the USDA began a new project called the Expanded Food and Nutrition Education Program (EFNEP), which provides in-service training in nutrition to several thousand people. The EFNEP aides in this program teach food and nutrition to neighbors in their own communities.

The current interest of the United States Congress in nutrition indicates that in the future even more federal monies may flow for both classroom and community education programs. Some of the funds designated for the School Lunch Program, administered by the USDA, may now be used to develop an education component in coordination with school food service.

As these and other programs expand, there will be an even greater demand for designing education messages and methods that are appropriate for specific audiences. Core concepts may be woven through all programs, but different emphases must be given, depending upon individual nutrient needs, existing dietary patterns, and the multitude of factors that influence food selection.

Training of Personnel

Although education of students and the broader public is the ultimate goal of nutritionists, many other people must be trained to communicate nutrition information.

A few schools of education are developing courses in nutrition for future teachers. Others are offering summer workshops and in-service training for educators already in the classroom. The impact of these programs is not as immediate as public education, but knowledge invested in teachers will spread outward like ripples in a pond.

Schools of public health train many nutritionists who later work in various health programs. There is a growing need to include more nutrition in the training of health professionals such as nurses, physician's assistants, dental hygienists, and other health care extenders and educators.

Nutrition education for physicians is another area where progress is being made, but much more remains to be accomplished. Most doctors who graduated from medical school a decade ago received only a smattering of training in the diagnosis and treatment of nutritional disorders. Now, many medical schools are beginning to give greater emphasis to this topic. In some instances, a separate nutrition course is offered; in others, nutrition lectures are incorporated into other curricula such as biochemistry, physiology, or specialities of clinical medicine. Several nutrition professorships and nutrition centers have been established in cooperation with medical schools, but more physicians who specialize in teaching nutrition to medical students are needed.

Looking Ahead

Efforts to improve nutritional status must be integrated into the changing system of health care delivery in this country. It is realistic to say that almost any program initiated today will only begin to have a significant impact ten years from now. Nutrition educators must coordinate their efforts with other health planners so that current training programs will mesh with other aspects of health education. This approach is necessary in order to provide personnel with the qualifications to complement projected systems of health care and consumer health education.

COLLABORATIVE EFFORTS

The ultimate question that ties together the significance of whatever lies beyond the current nutrition horizon can be stated simply: "Will the body of knowledge encompassed by the discipline of nutrition develop and be used in a way that contributes to the improvement of the health of individuals?"

An affirmative answer might be justified on the grounds of current and projected research, the growing momentum of nutrition education programs, the unprecedented public interest in diet and health, and many other favorable trends. However, if the present interest in nutrition is to have a lasting impact upon health, contributions must be made by several segments of the population. All of these should be part of a collaborative, integrated effort that will not happen simply by chance.

Federal Government

Several groups within the federal government have acknowledged the need for a national nutrition policy that addresses not only domestic, but international, issues. Recommended guidelines for such a policy were submitted by the National Nutrition Consortium (see Chapter 29), in 1974, to the Senate Select Committee on Nutrition and Human Needs. The suggested goals and measures to attain these goals are summarized in Appendix A30-1.

The expansion of the role of the federal government in planning and supporting nutrition programs will largely depend upon decisions made by the President and members of Congress. Implementation of programs is executed by various agencies, most of which currently fall within the DHEW and USDA. Enforcement of many regulations related to food and nutrition is largely the responsibility of the FDA (a part of DHEW), but other groups such as the Federal Trade Commission (FTC), which regulates the advertising of food, and the Environmental Protection Agency (EPA), which makes many decisions related to food safety, are also involved. These organizations interpret and carry out the mandates of legislators, but they are dependent upon Congress for their powers and budget.

Food Industry

The producers and suppliers of food also have a role in improving nutritional status. The primary responsibility is to ensure the safety of products by developing and abiding by the highest possible standards for good manufacturing procedures. The food industry also has the responsibility of offering to the consumer foods from which an appropriate diet can be selected. The array of foods in the market should be broad enough to meet the variable nutrient needs of the entire population. Since some people have special dietary needs due to diseases, the industry must define its corporate responsibility in terms of the risk of expending capital for research, development, and marketing of foods for this relatively small market. The responsibility of the food industry for nutrition education is a controversial topic. Such a precedent exists in some other industries; for example, some automobile dealers support high school driver education, alcoholic beverage producers sponsor alcohol abuse education programs, and life insurance companies have spearheaded many programs in health and safety education.

For about twenty-five years, a few food companies and trade associations have indeed been providing nutrition materials for classroom and consumer education. In the last decade, support for these and many other programs in both education and research has expanded. Public nutrition education may be accomplished through the existing mechanisms for marketing foods, but such efforts must be carefully designed and evaluated.

Health Care Deliverers

The health care delivery system also has a responsibility in improving the nutritional status of people. Professionals and paraprofessionals must be able to diagnose and treat nutritional disorders. On a cost/benefit basis, however, it is much more efficient to prevent nutrition problems than to cure them. In the long run, well-planned and implemented preventive programs (such as early disease detection and health education) prove to be much less costly in dollars and time, and much more beneficial in quality of life than efforts to treat severely ill patients.

The importance of including nutritionists on the preventive medicine team is beginning to be recognized by prepaid medical plans, which lose money when their members become sick. Similar roles are evolving for nutrition counselors in private practice, who work with patients in cooperation with the physician caring for coexisting medical problems. Public health programs involving nutritionists are yet another way of approaching a solution to current nutrition problems.

Each Individual

Consumers can interact with each of the above segments of society that have a role in improving nutrition status. They can convey their ideas to legislators, and support or oppose these people at the voting machine on the basis of their responsiveness to nutrition concerns. They can influence products on the market by the power of the dollar, and express their agreement or dissatisfaction with products by direct contact with consumer affairs officers. They can seek preventive health and nutrition education programs, and make diet selections consistent with what they have learned.

In the future, you will no doubt eat many meals without considering the nutritional value of food. There will be times when nutrition is not very important compared to other interests and concerns. Hopefully, however, your nutrition knowledge will be flexible enough to guide you in developing sound, practical dietary patterns that help maintain health. It is the hope of your authors that mastering and using nutrition knowledge will not stop when you close this book.

STUDY QUESTIONS

1. What basic sciences have contributed to our present knowledge of nutrition?

2. Cite the contributions to solving the world food problem that might be made by people in five different fields of work.

3. Why should the nonscientist be interested in research in the health fields?

4. Was nutrition taught in your high school? Why or why not?

5. What can you do to increase the application of nutrition knowledge to the improvement of health?

SUGGESTED READING

1. E. N. Todhunter, "Chronology of some events in the development and application of the science of nutrition," *Nutrition Reviews* 34(1976):353–67.

2. C. R. Stadler, D. D. Sanford, J. M. Reid, and N. D. Heidelbaugh, "Skylab menu development," *Journal of the American Dietetic Association* 62(1973):390.

3. A. Berg, N. S. Scrimshaw, and D. L. Call, eds., *Nutrition, National Development and Planning.* Cambridge, Mass.: MIT Press, 1975.

4. W. J. Darby, "Nutrition, food needs and technologic priorities: The World Food Conference," *Nutrition Reviews* 33(1975):225–34.

5. P. Handler, "Does it matter how many of us there will be?" *Food Technology* 29(1975):46–52.

6. J. Mayer, ed., *U.S. Nutrition Policies in the Seventies.* San Francisco: W. H. Freeman, 1973.

7. *White House Conference on Food, Nutrition and Health, 1969. Final Report.* Washington, D.C.: Government Printing Office, 1970.

8. R. P. Shafer, "Government control of individual behavior—Its right and proper role," First annual Rosenhaus lecture, *American Journal of Public Health* 64(1974):390–93.

9. C. D. Williams, "Grassroots nutrition—Or, consumer participation," Martha Trulson Memorial Lecture, 1972, *Journal of the American Dietetic Association* 63(1973):125.

10. E. T. Mertz, "Genetic improvement of cereals," *Nutrition Reviews* 32(1974):129–31.

11. J. Mayer, "Nutrition's future: Food for thought," *Family Health* 7(1975):42.

APPENDIX

TABLE A3-1. Metric Conversions for Selected Household Measures

Common Measures	Metric Measures
Liquid	Millilitres (ml)
1 teaspoon	5
1 tablespoon	15
1 jigger (1.5 oz.)	45
1 cup	240
1 pint	480
1 quart	960
1 gallon	3,840
Solid	Grams (g)
1 ounce	28
1 pound	454

NOTE: One millilitre of water weighs one gram. For most foods, their volume in millilitres approximately equals their weight in grams. When you are making rough estimates, the metric equivalents of one ounce and one pound may be rounded to 30 grams and 450 grams, respectively.

TABLE A3-2. Foods Grouped According to Energy Value

Food	Energy Value (Cal)	(kJ)	Food	Energy Value (Cal)	(kJ)
1–25 Calories			**26–50 Calories**		
Bouillon, 1 cube	5	21	Broccoli, ⅔ cup	26	109
Celery, 1 stalk	7	29	Tomato, 1 medium	27	113
Vinegar, ¼ cup	7	29	Strawberries, ½ cup	28	118
Onion, chopped, 2 T.	8	34	Turnip greens, 1 cup	29	122
Low-calorie salad dressing, 1 T.	10–20	42–84	Carrot, 1 medium	30	126
Lettuce, ½ head	12	50	Ripe olives, 5 large	31	130
Radishes, 10 large	14	59	Vegetable juice cocktail, 6 oz.	31	130
Dill pickle, 1 large	15	63	Bean sprouts, 1 cup	37	155
Chili sauce, 1 T.	16	67	Grapefruit, ½ medium	40	168
Half and half cream, 1 T.	20	84	Mixed vegetables, ½ cup	41	172
Green beans, canned, ½ cup	22	92	Sweet pickle relish, 2 T.	42	176
Marshmallow, 1	23	97	White sugar, 1 T.	46	193
Cucumber, 1 small	25	105	Molasses, 1 T.	50	210
Mushrooms, 1 cup	25	105			

TABLE A3-2. Foods Grouped According to Energy Value (*continued*)

Food	Energy Value (Cal)	(kJ)	Food	Energy Value (Cal)	(kJ)
51–75 Calories			**151–200 Calories**		
Jam and jelly, 1 T.	50–60	210–252	Beer, 12 oz.	151	634
Chicken noodle soup, $\frac{1}{3}$			Chop suey with meat, $\frac{1}{2}$ cup	151	634
can reconstituted	51	214	Tuna fish, $\frac{1}{2}$ cup	158	664
Jelly beans, 5	52	218	Fried chicken, $\frac{1}{2}$ breast	160	672
Grits, $\frac{1}{2}$ cup	62	260	Whole milk, 1 cup	160	672
Orange, 1 medium	64	268	Doughnut, 1 medium	164	689
Vegetarian vegetable soup, $\frac{1}{3}$			Chili with beans, $\frac{1}{2}$ cup	170	714
can reconstituted	65	273	Bacon, 4 slices	172	722
Bread, 1 slice	65–75	273–315	Hash brown potatoes, $\frac{1}{2}$ cup	175	735
French dressing, 1 T.	66	277	Pancakes (4-inch diameter), 3	186	781
Cheddar cheese, 1-inch cube	68	286	Spaghetti (no sauce), 1 cup	192	806
Corn kernels, $\frac{1}{2}$ cup	68	286	**201–300 Calories**		
Tartar sauce, 1 T.	74	311	Hamburger (no bun), 4 oz. raw	202	848
			Cheese souffle, 1 cup	207	869
76–100 Calories			Welsh rarebit, $\frac{1}{2}$ cup	210	882
Coleslaw, $\frac{2}{3}$ cup	80	336	Macaroni and cheese, $\frac{1}{2}$ cup	215	903
Cantaloupe or honeydew, $\frac{1}{2}$ melon	82	344	Meat loaf, 4 oz.	226	949
Egg, 1 large	82	344	Chocolate cake with white icing,		
Orange juice, 6 oz.	84	353	1 piece	232	974
Lima beans, canned, $\frac{1}{2}$ cup	86	361	Chocolate eclair	239	1,004
Nonfat milk, 1 cup	88	370	Animal crackers, 1 pkg.	245	1,029
Chocolate syrup, 2 T.	92	386	Soft-serve ice cream, 1 cup	266	1,117
Mashed potatoes (with milk and			Peanut butter and jelly sandwich	285	1,197
margarine), $\frac{1}{2}$ cup	94	394	Breakfast drink, made with	290	1,218
Peanut butter, 1 T.	94	394	1 cup milk		
Apple, 1 medium	96	403	**301–400 Calories**		
Cornflakes, 1 cup	96	403	TV dinner, complete	300–500	1,260–2,100
			Cream puff	303	1,273
101–150 Calories			Pork chop, 1 medium	308	1,294
Banana, 1 medium	101	424	Boston cream pie, $\frac{1}{6}$ pie	311	1,306
Butter or margarine, 1 T.	102	428	Tuna salad, 1 cup	349	1,466
White sauce, $\frac{1}{4}$ cup	102	428	Bean soup, 1 cup	355	1,491
Soft drink, 12 oz.	110–170	462–714	Lemon meringue pie, $\frac{1}{6}$ pie	357	1,499
Potato chips (2-inch diameter), 10	114	479	Malted milk, 12 oz.	366	1,537
Soybeans (cooked), $\frac{1}{2}$ cup	117	491	Porterhouse steak, lean, 6 oz.	385	1,617
Yogurt, 1 cup	120–150	504–630	**Over 401 Calories**		
Potato salad, $\frac{1}{2}$ cup	124	521	Sunflower seeds, hulled, $\frac{1}{2}$ cup	406	1,705
Chicken chow mein, $\frac{1}{2}$ cup	130	546	Cherry pie, $\frac{1}{6}$ pie	412	1,730
Hot dog (no bun), 1 medium	130–170	546–714	Peanuts, $\frac{1}{2}$ cup	419	1,760
French fries, 10 medium pieces	137	575	Turkey potpie (9-inch), $\frac{1}{3}$ pie	550	2,310
Baked potato, 1 medium	145	609	Pecan pie, $\frac{1}{6}$ pie	577	2,423
Chocolate candy bar, 1 oz.	147	617	T-bone steak, fat untrimmed,	1,395	5,859
Sweet potato, 1 medium	148	622	10 oz.		

SOURCE: C. F. Adams, *Nutritive Value of American Foods in Common Units,* Agriculture Handbook No. 456 (Washington, D.C.: U.S. Department of Agriculture, Agricultural Research Service, 1975).

TABLE A3-3. Energy Values of Some Common Alcoholic Beverages

Beverage	Energy Value (Cal)	(kJ)
Liqueurs or brandies, 1 cordial glass	55–75	231–315
Table wine (12% alcohol), 1 wine glass	87	365
Gin, rum, vodka, whiskey, 1 jigger		
80 proof	97	407
90 proof	110	462
100 proof	124	521
Dessert wine (18% alcohol), 1 wine glass	141	592
Beer, 12 oz.	151	634
Martini, Manhattan, or old fashioned	140–180	588–756

TABLE A3-4. Approximate Basal Metabolic Rates (BMR) of Adults

Men Appropriate Weight lb.	kg	BMR[a] Cal/day	Women Appropriate Weight lb.	kg	BMR[a] Cal/day
133	60	1,630	109	50	1,399
142	64	1,690	115	52	1,429
151	69	1,775	122	56	1,487
159	72	1,815	129	59	1,530
167	76	1,870	136	62	1,572
175	80	1,933	144	66	1,626
182	83	1,983	152	69	1,666

[a]These values are approximately 75 to 125 Cal higher than values published elsewhere.

SOURCE: Adapted from Food and Nutrition Board, National Academy of Sciences–National Research Council, *Recommended Dietary Allowances,* 8th ed. (Washington, D.C.: National Academy of Sciences, 1974).

TABLE A3-5. Minerals Required for Enzyme Function

Mineral	Metabolic sequence	Enzyme
Ascorbate and vitamin E	Oxidation and reduction reactions	
Copper	Phase III of energy release	Cytochrome oxidase
	Amino acid breakdown	Tyrosinase
Iron	Phase III of energy release	Cytochrome oxidase
	Detoxification of hydrogen peroxide	Peroxidase
	DNA/RNA catabolism	Xanthine oxidase
	Phase III of energy release	Ferredoxin
	Oxygen metabolism	Catalase
Magnesium	ATP-ADP-AMP	Phosphotransferases
	Triose-phosphate in glucose central pathway	Pyruvate phosphokinase
Manganese	Urea formation for nitrogen excretion	Arginase
	ATP-ADP-AMP	Phosphotransferase
Magnesium, manganese, and phosphorus	Activation of enzymes in general	
Molybdenum	Hydrogen transfer	Flavo-enzymes
Potassium	Triose phosphate in central glucose path	Pyruvate phosphokinase
Selenium	Oxidation-reduction reactions	Glutathione reductase
Sodium	Energy for membrane transfer	Plasma membrane ATPase
Zinc	Lactate/pyruvate pathway	Lactate dehydrogenase
	Digestion	Carboxypeptidase
	Alcohol metabolism	Alcohol dehydrogenase
	Carbon dioxide metabolism	Carbonic anhydrase

TABLE A4-1. Role of Hormones in Digestion

Hormone	Source	Released in Response to:	Effect
Gastrin	Stomach, duodenum	Food in the stomach	Stimulates production of gastric fluid
Cholecystokinin	Duodenum	Lipids in duodenum	Release of bile from the gallbladder into the duodenum
Enterogastrone	Duodenum	Lipids and acidic chyme	Inhibits secretion of gastric juice: slows peristalsis
Pancreozymin	Duodenum, jejunum	Polypeptides and acidic chyme	Secretion of viscous pancreatic juice and enzymes
Secretin	Duodenum	Peptides and acidic chyme	Secretion of thin, alkaline pancreatic juice

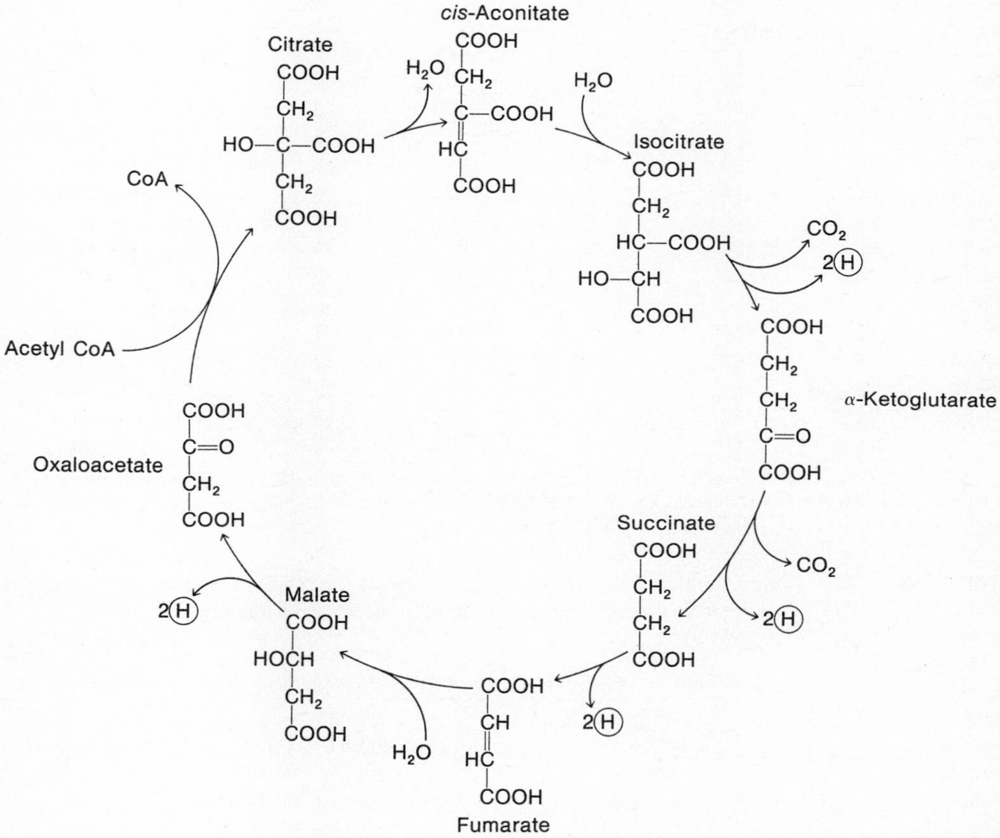

Figure A5–1. Details of Krebs cycle.

Age (years)	Protein	Vitamin A	Vitamin C	Thiamin	Riboflavin	Niacin	Calcium	Iron
Children								
1–3	35	40	67	47	47	45	80	83
4–6	50	50	67	60	65	60	80	56
7–10	55	67	67	80	70	80	80	56
Males								
11–14	70	100	75	93	88	90	120	100
15–18	85	100	75	100	106	100	120	100
19–22	85	100	75	100	106	100	80	56
23–50	90	100	75	93	94	90	80	56
51 +	90	100	75	80	88	80	80	56
Females								
11–14	70	80	75	80	77	80	120	100
15–18	75	80	75	74	82	70	120	100
19–22	75	80	75	74	82	70	80	100
23–50	75	80	75	67	70	65	80	100
51 +	75	80	75	67	65	60	80	56

SOURCE: Reprinted from The National Nutrition Consortium with R. M. Deutsch, *Nutrition Labeling: How It Can Work for You* (Washington, D.C.: The National Nutrition Consortium, 1975). © 1975, The National Nutrition Consortium. Used by permission.

TABLE A8-2. U.S. Recommended Daily Allowances (U.S. RDA) for Children, Infants, and Pregnant or Lactating Women (for use in nutrition labeling of foods)

Nutrient	Children (under 4 years)	Infants (under 13 months)	Pregnant or Lactating Women
Protein	28 g[a]	25 g[a]	65 g[a]
Vitamin A	2,500 IU	1,500 IU	8,000 IU
Vitamin C	40 mg	35 mg	60 mg
Thiamin	0.7 mg	0.5 mg	1.7 mg
Riboflavin	0.8 mg	0.6 mg	2.0 mg
Niacin	9.0 mg	8.0 mg	20 mg
Calcium	0.8 g	0.6 g	1.3 g
Iron	10 mg	15 mg	18 mg
Vitamin D	400 IU	400 IU	400 IU
Vitamin E	10 IU	5 IU	30 IU
Vitamin B_6	0.7 mg	0.4 mg	2.5 mg
Folacin	0.2 mg	0.1 mg	0.8 mg
Vitamin B_{12}	3 mcg	2 mcg	8 mcg
Phosphorus	0.8 g	0.5 g	1.3 g
Iodine	70 mcg	45 mcg	150 mcg
Magnesium	200 mg	70 mg	450 mg
Zinc	8 mg	5 mg	15 mg
Copper	1 mg	0.6 mg	2 mg
Biotin	0.15 mg	0.15 mg	0.3 mg
Panthothenic acid	5 mg	3 mg	10 mg

[a]If the protein efficiency ratio of protein is equal to or better than that of casein, U.S. RDA is 45 grams for pregnant or lactating women, 20 grams for children under 4 years of age, and 18 grams for infants.

TABLE A9-1. Energy and Nutrient-Density Variation
with Food Groups

Food Group[a]	Energy		INQs of Two Nutrients Characteristic of Group[b]	
	(Cal)	(kJ)		
Fruits/vegetables			Vitamin C	Vitamin A
Apple, 1 medium	70	294	1.6	0.3
Applesauce, sweetened	230	986	0.5	0.2
Asparagus	30	126	49.0	20.0
Avocado, 1 medium	370	1,554	3.1	0.8
Beets, 2 medium	30	126	7.0	0.3
Broccoli	40	168	134.0	45.0
Brussels sprouts	55	231	94.0	7.0
Carrot, raw, 1 medium	20	84	8.0	125.0
Corn canned	170	714	3.0	2.0
Corn, fresh, 1 ear	70	294	4.0	2.0
Grapefruit, pink, ½ medium	50	210	34.0	5.0
Green beans	30	126	19.0	10.0
Lemonade	110	462	6.0	0
Lettuce, 1 head	30	126	23.0	32.0
Okra, 8 pods	25	105	26.0	8.0
Orange, 1 medium	65	273	39.0	2.0
Peach, fresh, 1 medium	35	147	8.0	17.0
Peaches, dried	420	1,764	3.0	7.0
Potato, boiled, 1 medium	105	441	8.0	0
Potatoes, mashed with milk and butter	185	770	4.0	0.8
Potatoes, french fried, 10 pieces	155	631	3.0	0
Sauerkraut	45	189	28.0	1.0
Spinach	40	168	48.0	167.0
Strawberries	55	231	61.0	0.8
Summer squash	30	126	27.0	13.0
Sweet potato, baked, 1 medium	155	651	6.0	26.0
Sweet potato, candied, 1 medium	295	1,239	2.0	17.0
Tomato, 1 medium	40	168	40.0	19.0
Tomato catsup, 1 T.	15	63	5.0	6.0
Tomato juice, 8 oz.	35	147	32.0	19.0
Watermelon, 1 wedge	115	483	10.0	10.0
Cereals			Thiamin	Protein
Bagel, 1	165	693	1.3	1.3
Barley, ½ cup	350	1,470	0.5	0.8
Biscuit, 2″ diameter, 1	90	378	1.4	0.8
Bread				
Cracked wheat, 25 g	65	273	0.7	1.1
Raisin, 25 g	65	273	0.2	1.1
Rye, 25 g	60	252	0.5	1.2

TABLE A9-1. Energy and Nutrient-Density Variation (*continued*)

Food Group[a]	Energy		INQs of Two Nutrients Characteristic of Group[b]	
	(Cal)	(kJ)	Thiamin	Protein
Cereals (*continued*)				
Bread (*continued*)				
White, enriched, 25 g	70	294	1.3	1.0
Whole wheat, 28 g	65	273	2.1	1.6
Breakfast cereal				
Corn flakes	155	651	1.6	0.5
Farina, quick	105	441	1.8	1.0
Oatmeal	130	546	2.2	1.4
Puffed oats	100	420	2.2	1.4
Shredded wheat biscuit, 1	90	378	1.0	0.8
Wheat flakes	105	441	2.8	1.0
40% bran flakes	105	441	2.0	1.4
Cake				
Angel food, 53 g	135	567	—	0.8
Brownie, 20 g	95	399	0.7	0.4
Cupcake, iced, 36 g	130	546	0.1	0.5
Fruitcake, 30 g	110	462	0.6	0.6
Gingerbread, 63 g	175	735	0.2	0.4
Pound cake, 30 g	140	588	0.1	0.5
White cake, iced, 71 g	250	1,056	0.1	0.4
Cookies				
Chocolate chip, 2 (20 g)	100	420	0.3	0.7
Chocolate or vanilla sandwiches (packaged), 2 (20 g)	100	420	—	0.7
Fig bars, 2 (28 g)	100	420	—	0.7
Graham crackers, 4 (28 g)	110	462	0.1	0.6
Doughnut (cake type), 32 g	125	525	0.3	0.6
Grits, enriched	125	525	0.6	0.9
Macaroni	190	798	1.9	1.1
And cheese	430	1,806	0.7	1.4
Muffins, corn, 40 g	130	546	0.8	0.8
Noodles	200	840	1.7	1.2
Pancakes, buckwheat, 2	110	462	0.8	1.3
Pastry, Danish (without fruit and nuts), 65 g	275	1,155	0.3	0.6
Pie				
Apple, 135 g	350	1,470	0.1	0.3
Boston cream, 69 g	210	882	0.2	0.7
Butterscotch, 130 g	350	1,470	0.2	0.6
Cherry, 135 g	350	1,470	0.1	0.4
Custard, 130 g	285	1,197	0.4	1.0
Lemon meringue, 135 g	305	1,281	0.2	0.5
Mince, 135 g	365	1,533	0.4	0.3
Pecan, 118 g	490	2,058	0.6	0.4

TABLE A9-1. Energy and Nutrient-Density Variation (*continued*)

Food Group[a]	Energy		INQs of Two Nutrients Characteristic of Group[b]	
	(Cal)	(kJ)		
Cereals (*continued*)			Thiamin	Protein
Pie (*continued*)				
Pumpkin, 130 g	275	1,155	0.2	0.6
Pizza, cheese 75 g	185	777	0.3	1.3
Popcorn, plain	25	105	—	1.4
With oil and salt	40	168	—	0.9
Sugar coated	135	567	—	0.6
Pretzels, twisted, 16 g	60	252	—	1.2
Rice, enriched	225	945	1.6	0.6
Unenriched	225	945	0.3	0.6
Spaghetti	155	651	2.0	1.1
With meat balls	330	1,386	1.2	2.0
With tomato sauce	260	1,092	1.5	1.2
Wafers, rye, 2 (13 g)	45	189	1.4	1.6
Milk			Calcium	Riboflavin
Cheese				
American, 1 oz.	105	441	4.3	1.6
American, processed spread, 1 oz.	80	336	4.6	2.5
Cheddar, 1 oz. (28 g)	115	483	4.2	1.5
Cottage, 6 oz.	180	756	2.0	3.2
Cream, 2 oz.	210	882	0.4	0.9
Parmesan, grated, ¼ cup	160	672	6.7	2.5
Roquefort, 17 g	65	275	1.9	2.3
Swiss, natural, 1 oz.	105	441	5.7	1.4
Cocoa	245	1,029	2.8	2.5
Cream, 1 T.				
Half and half	20	84	1.8	1.4
Light coffee	30	126	1.2	0.9
Sour	25	105	1.1	1.1
Whipped topping (pressurized)	10	42	0	0.7
Whipping, heavy	55	231	0.5	0.5
Custard, baked	305	1,281	2.2	2.2
Ice cream	255	1,071	1.8	1.5
Rice (16% fat)	330	1,386	0.8	0.7
Soft-serve	265	1,113	2.4	2.0
Ice milk	200	840	2.4	2.0
Imitation creamers				
Liquid frozen, 1 T.	20	84	—	0.2
Powdered (with vegetable fat), 1 t.	10	42	—	0.2
Milk				
Buttermilk	90	378	7.6	6.6
Low fat (2%)	145	609	5.6	4.9

TABLE A9-1. Energy and Nutrient-Density Variation (*continued*)

Food Group[a]	Energy (Cal)	(kJ)	INQs of Two Nutrients Characteristic of Group[b]	
Milk (*continued*)			Calcium	Riboflavin
Nonfat (skim)	90	378	7.6	6.6
Whole	160	672	4.1	3.5
Milk, malted	245	1,029	3.0	2.7
Sherbet	260	1,090	0.3	0.3
Yogurt				
Skim milk	125	525	5.4	4.8
Whole milk	150	630	4.2	3.5
Meat			Protein	Iron
Bacon, 2 slices	90	378	2.7	1.8
Beans, 1 cup				
Great northern	210	882	2.7	3.0
Kidney	230	966	2.3	2.6
Lima	260	1,092	2.2	3.0
With franks	210	882	1.8	1.7
Beef, 3 oz.				
Hamburger, lean	185	777	4.4	2.1
Hamburger, regular	245	1,029	3.0	1.4
Rib roast (lean/fat)	375	1,575	1.6	0.8
Round (lean/fat)	165	693	5.4	2.5
Sirloin steak (lean/fat)	330	1,386	2.1	1.0
Sirloin (lean)	170	714	5.5	2.4
Beef potpie, 8 oz.	560	2,352	1.5	0.9
Beef stew, with vegetables	210	882	2.5	1.7
Chicken				
Breast, fried, 3.3 oz.	155	651	5.7	1.1
Broiled, without skin, 3 oz.	115	483	6.2	1.6
Canned, boneless, 3 oz.	170	714	3.8	1.0
Chili				
With beans	335	1,407	2.0	1.6
Without beans	510	2,142	1.8	0.9
Corned beef, canned, 3 oz.	185	777	4.2	2.6
Corned beef hash, 3 oz.	155	651	1.6	1.4
Crabmeat, 3 oz.	85	357	6.2	1.1
Egg, 1 medium	80	336	2.7	1.8
Fish sticks, breaded, 5	200	840	3.4	0.3
Haddock, fried, 3 oz.	140	588	4.3	0.9
Ham				
Boiled, luncheon meat, 2 oz.	135	567	2.9	1.5
Cured, 3 oz.	245	1,029	2.6	1.2

TABLE A9-1. Energy and Nutrient-Density Variation (*continued*)

Food Group[a]	Energy (Cal)	(kJ)	INQs of Two Nutrients Characteristic of Group[b] Protein	Iron
Meat (*continued*)			Protein	Iron
Ham (*continued*)				
Deviled, 2 T. (26 g)	90	378	1.6	0.9
Heart, beef, 3 oz.	160	672	6.0	4.0
Lamb				
Chop, 4.8 oz.	400	1,680	2.2	0.5
Roast, 3 oz.	235	987	3.3	0.8
Liver, beef, 3 oz.	195	819	4.1	4.9
Nuts				
Almonds, ½ cup	425	1,785	1.1	1.0
Cashews, ½ cup	390	1,638	1.1	0.9
Peanut butter, 2 T.	190	798	1.5	0.4
Peanuts, ½ cup	420	1,764	1.6	0.5
Oysters, raw	160	672	4.4	10.5
Peas				
Black-eyed	190	798	2.4	2.2
Split	290	1,218	2.4	1.9
Pork				
Chop, 3.5 oz.	260	1,092	2.2	1.1
Roast (lean/fat), 3 oz.	310	1,302	2.4	1.1
Pork and beans	310	1,302	1.9	1.9
Salmon, canned, 3 oz.	120	504	5.0	0.8
Sardines, in oil, 3 oz.	175	735	4.0	1.8
Sausage				
Bologna, 2 slices (26 g)	80	336	1.3	0.8
Braunschweiger, 2 slices (20 g)	65	273	1.6	2.4
Frankfurter, 1 (56 g)	170	714	1.5	0.6
Pork links, 2 (26 g)	125	525	1.4	0.6
Salami, 1 oz. (28 g)	130	546	1.9	1.0
Vienna, 2 (32 g)	80	336	1.8	1.0
Shrimp, canned, 3 oz.	100	420	7.4	3.3
Tuna, drained, 3 oz.	170	714	5.0	1.2
Veal, roast, 3 oz.	230	966	3.5	1.6

[a]Serving size is 1 cup unless otherwise noted.
[b]Based on an energy requirement of 2,300 Calories.
SOURCE: Excerpted from R. G. Hansen, A. W. Sorenson, and A. J. Wittmer, ''Index of Nutritional Quality Food Profiles'' (Logan, Utah: Utah State University, 1975). © 1975 Utah State University, Used by permission.

TABLE A11-1. A Week's Menus Based on the Thrifty Food Plan

Meal	SUNDAY	MONDAY	TUESDAY	WEDNESDAY	THURSDAY	FRIDAY	SATURDAY
Breakfast	Orange juice French toast Syrup Beverage	Orange juice Ready-to-eat cereal Doughnut Beverage	Peach, sliced Oatmeal Cinnamon toast Beverage	Orange juice Egg Pan-fried potatoes Toast Beverage	Peach, sliced Ready-to-eat cereal Toast Beverage	Apple juice Farina Toast Beverage	Apple, quartered Pancakes Syrup Beverage
Lunch	Beef pot roast Gravy Mashed potato Mixed vegetables Bread Ice milk Beverage	Grilled cheese sandwich Macaroni salad Baked apple Beverage	Frankfurters Sauerkraut Bread Oatmeal cookies Beverage	Beef macaroni soup Saltine crackers Plums Beverage	Noodle soup Peanut butter and jelly sandwich Carrot sticks Graham crackers Beverage	Frankfurter bean soup Saltine crackers Oatmeal cookies Beverage	Cheese sandwich Gelatin (with apple juice and celery) Meringue pie Beverage
Dinner	Beans in tomato sauce Macaroni salad Pear halves Corn bread Gelatin Beverage	Beef stew with vegetables Corn bread Ice milk Beverage	Beef pie with vegetables Refrigerator biscuits Lettuce-wedge with dressing Peanut butter cake Beverage	Fried chicken Rice Gravy Corn Bread Peanut butter cake Beverage	Beef pattie Baked potato Stewed tomatoes Muffin Ice milk Beverage	Cheese rarebit on toast French-fried potatoes Spinach Meringue pie Beverage	Spaghetti with meat sauce Tossed salad (lettuce, carrots, dressing) Bread sticks Ice milk Beverage
Snack	Doughnut	Bread and jelly sandwich	Cheese and saltine crackers	Doughnut	Peanut butter cake	Graham crackers	Ready-to-eat cereal

NOTE: Milk for everyone at least once daily, and for children, teen-agers, and pregnant and nursing women, more often. Spreads for bread and sugar for cereal, coffee, and tea may be added, if desired.

SOURCE: B. Peterkin, "Dietary guidance for food stamp families," *Family Economics Review*, Agricultural Research Service, U.S. Department of Agriculture (Winter 1976):24.

TABLE A17-1. Mean Height and Weight of Children by Age, Sex, and Race, United States, 1971–72

Age (years)	Sex	Mean Height (inches)			Mean Weight (pounds)		
		Total	White	Black	Total	White	Black
1	Male	32.9	33.0	32.4	26.3	26.6	24.8
2		35.7	35.6	36.3	29.6	29.1	31.8
3		38.8	38.8	38.7	34.4	34.5	34.1
4		41.8	41.8	41.9	39.1	39.0	40.0
5		44.4	44.4	44.4	44.2	44.1	45.4
6		46.4	46.3	46.9	48.6	48.2	50.2
7		49.1	49.1	50.0	54.2	54.4	53.2
8		50.8	50.8	50.8	57.7	57.3	60.9
9		53.0	52.9	53.5	70.6	71.0	68.8
10		55.2	55.1	56.2	75.8	75.3	76.2
11		57.5	57.2	58.7	83.0	82.8	84.0
12		60.7	60.8	59.6	98.7	99.6	92.4
13		63.1	63.5	61.2	111.5	114.1	98.5
14		65.5	65.5	66.8	124.0	126.2	120.6
15		67.0	66.9	67.8	133.5	131.0	145.0
16		69.4	69.4	69.2	151.9	153.0	145.2
17		70.0	70.1	69.6	153.7	153.7	155.3
1	Female	31.9	31.8	32.2	23.9	23.7	25.0
2		35.5	35.5	35.3	28.3	28.6	27.0
3		38.7	38.6	39.4	33.9	33.9	33.6
4		41.7	41.7	41.7	37.2	37.0	38.2
5		44.3	44.1	45.4	44.0	43.7	45.8
6		46.6	46.5	47.1	47.7	47.6	48.0
7		49.3	49.3	49.8	53.7	53.4	54.8
8		50.9	50.8	51.4	61.2	60.6	64.7
9		53.5	53.5	53.2	70.5	71.4	62.7
10		55.1	55.0	56.0	75.2	74.7	78.3
11		58.4	58.4	58.5	89.4	88.9	92.4
12		60.5	60.6	60.3	100.4	101.9	95.6
13		63.0	63.1	62.2	117.4	117.7	115.3
14		63.8	63.8	64.2	123.7	124.3	124.6
15		64.8	64.7	65.1	128.7	131.7	116.7
16		63.5	63.4	64.3	121.7	121.0	131.6
17		63.3	63.3	63.3	129.6	129.5	124.8

SOURCE: *Preliminary Findings of the First Health and Nutrition Examination Survey, United States, 1971–72: Anthropometric and Clinical Findings,* U.S. Department of Health, Education and Welfare Pub. No. (HRA) 75-1229 (Washington, D.C.: Government Printing Office, 1975).

Committee on Nutrition
American Academy of Pediatrics
P. O. Box 1034
Evanston, Illinois 60204

American Dietetic Association
620 North Michigan Avenue
Chicago, Illinois 60611

American Institute of Nutrition
9650 Rockville Pike
Bethesda, Maryland 20014

American Society for Clinical Nutrition
9650 Rockville Pike
Bethesda, Maryland 20014

Institute of Food Technologists
221 North La Salle Street, Suite 2120
Chicago, Illinois 60601

Food and Nutrition Board
National Academy of Sciences
2101 Constitution Avenue
Washington, D. C. 20006

Society for Nutrition Education
National Nutrition Education Clearing House
2140 Shattuck Avenue, Suite 1110
Berkeley, California 94704

Goals of a National Nutrition Policy

1. To assure an adequate, wholesome food supply at reasonable cost to meet the needs of all segments of the population, this supply being available at a level consistent with the affordable lifestyle of the era.

2. To maintain food resources sufficient to meet emergency needs and to fulfill a responsible role as a nation in meeting world food needs.

3. To develop a level of sound public knowledge and responsible understanding of nutrition and foods that will promote maximal nutritional health.

4. To maintain a system of quality and safety control that justifies public confidence in its food supply.

5. To support research and education in foods and nutrition with adequate resources and reasoned priorities to solve important current problems and to permit exploratory basic research.

Measures for Attaining the Goals

1. Maintain surveillance of the nutritional status of the population and determine the nature of nutritional problems observed.

2. Develop programs within the health care system that will prevent and rectify nutritional problems.

3. Assist the health professions in coordinated efforts to improve the nutritional status of the population through the life cycle.

4. Develop programs for nutrition education for both health professionals and the general public.

5. Identify areas in which nutrition knowledge is inadequate and foster research to provide this knowledge.

6. Assemble information on the food supply, including food production and distribution, and provide a nutritional input in the regulation of foreign agricultural trade.

7. Determine the nutrient composition of foods and promote and monitor food quality and safety.

8. Cooperate with other nations and international agencies in developing measures for solving the world food and nutrition problems.

SOURCE: *Guidelines for a National Nutrition Policy: A Working Paper,* prepared by The National Nutrition Consortium, Inc. for the Select Committee on Nutrition and Human Needs, U.S. Senate (Washington, D.C.: Government Printing office, 1974). © 1974, The National Nutrition Consortium. Used by permission. This working paper also includes a discussion of programs needed to meet these objectives.

APPENDIX TABLE. Nutritive Values of the Edible Part of Foods

Dairy Products (cheese, cream, imitation cream, milk; related products)

Butter. See Fats, oils, related products.

Food, Approximate Measure, and Weight (in grams)	Measure	Weight (g)	Water (%)	Food Energy (Cal)	Protein (g)	Fat (g)	Carbohydrate (g)	Calcium (mg)	Phosphorus (mg)	Iron (mg)	Potassium (mg)	Vitamin A Value (IU)	Thiamin (mg)	Riboflavin (mg)	Niacin (mg)	Ascorbic Acid (mg)
Cheese																
Natural																
Camembert (3 wedges/4-oz. container)	1 wedge	38	52	115	8	9	Trace	147	132	.1	71	350	.01	.19	.2	0
Cheddar	1 oz.	28	37	115	7	9	Trace	204	145	.2	28	300	.01	.11	Trace	0
Cottage (curd not pressed down)	1 cup															
Creamed (4% fat)																
Large curd		225	79	235	28	10	6	135	297	.3	190	370	.05	.37	.3	Trace
Small curd		210	79	220	26	9	6	126	277	.3	177	340	.04	.34	.3	Trace
Low fat (2%)		226	79	205	31	4	8	155	340	.4	217	160	.05	.42	.3	Trace
Low fat (1%)		226	82	165	28	2	6	138	302	.3	193	80	.05	.37	.3	Trace
Uncreamed (dry curd, less than 1/2% fat)	1 oz.	145	80	125	25	1	3	46	151	.3	47	40	.04	.21	.2	0
Cream	1 oz.	28	54	100	2	10	1	23	30	.3	34	400	Trace	.06	Trace	0
Mozzarella, made with whole milk	1 oz.	28	48	90	6	7	1	163	117	.1	21	260	Trace	.08	Trace	0
Parmesan, grated	1 oz.	28	18	130	12	9	1	390	229	.3	30	200	.01	.11	.1	0
Romano	1 oz.	28	31	110	9	8	1	302	215	—	—	160	—	.11	Trace	0
Swiss	1 oz.	28	37	105	8	8	1	272	171	Trace	31	240	.01	.10	Trace	0
Pasteurized process cheese																
American	1 oz.	28	39	105	6	9	Trace	174	211	.1	46	340	.01	.10	Trace	0
Swiss	1 oz.	28	42	95	7	7	1	219	216	.2	61	230	Trace	.08	Trace	0
Pasteurized process cheese food, American	1 oz.	28	43	95	6	7	2	163	130	.2	79	260	.01	.13	Trace	0
Pasteurized process cheese spread, American	1 oz.	28	48	82	5	6	2	159	202	.1	69	220	.01	.12	Trace	0
Cream, sweet	1 T.															
Half and half (cream and milk)		15	81	20	Trace	2	1	16	14	Trace	19	20	.01	.02	Trace	Trace
Light, coffee, or table		15	74	30	Trace	3	1	14	12	Trace	18	110	Trace	.02	Trace	Trace
Whipping, unwhipped (volume about double when whipped)																
Light		15	64	45	Trace	5	1	10	9	Trace	15	170	Trace	.02	Trace	Trace
Heavy		15	58	80	Trace	6	Trace	10	9	Trace	11	220	Trace	.02	Trace	Trace
Whipped topping (pressurized)	1 T.	3	61	10	Trace	1	Trace	3	3	Trace	4	30	Trace	Trace	Trace	0
Cream, sour		12	71	25	Trace	3	1	14	10	Trace	17	90	Trace	.02	Trace	Trace
Cream products, imitation (made with vegetable fat)																
Sweet																
Creamers																
Liquid (frozen)	1 T.	15	77	20	Trace	1	2	1	10	Trace	29	10[1]	0	0	0	0
Powdered	1 t.	2	2	10	Trace	1	1	Trace	8	Trace	16	Trace[1]	0	Trace	0	0

Table of nutritive values — milk and milk products (continued)

Food	Measure	Grams	Water (%)	Food energy (cal)	Protein (g)	Fat (g)	Carbohydrate (g)	Calcium (mg)	Phosphorus (mg)	Iron (mg)	Potassium (mg)	Vitamin A (IU)	Thiamin (mg)	Riboflavin (mg)	Niacin (mg)	Ascorbic acid (mg)
Whipped topping																
Frozen	1 T.	4	50	15	Trace	1	1	Trace	1	Trace	1	30[1]	0	0	0	0
Powdered, made with whole milk	1 T.	4	67	10	Trace	Trace	1	4	3	Trace	6	10[1]	Trace	.02	Trace	Trace
Pressurized	1 T.	4	60	10	Trace	1	Trace	Trace	1	Trace	1	20[1]	0	0	0	0
Sour dressing (imitation sour cream) made with nonfat dry milk	1 T.	12	75	20	Trace	2	1	14	10	Trace	19	Trace[1]	.01	.02	Trace	Trace
Ice cream. See Milk desserts, frozen.																
Ice milk. See Milk desserts, frozen.																
Milk, fluid																
Whole (3.3% fat)	1 cup	244	88	150	8	8	11	291	228	.1	370	310[2]	.09	.40	.2	2
Lowfat (2%)																
No milk solids added		244	89	120	8	5	12	297	232	.1	377	500	.10	.40	.2	2
Milk solids added																
Label claim less than 10 g of protein per cup		245	89	125	9	5	12	313	245	.1	397	500	.10	.42	.2	2
Label claim 10 or more g of protein per cup (protein fortified)		246	88	135	10	5	14	352	276	.1	447	500	.11	.48	.2	3
Lowfat (1%)																
No milk solids added		244	90	100	8	3	12	300	235	.1	381	500	.10	.41	.2	2
Milk solids added																
Label claim less than 10 g of protein per cup		245	90	105	9	2	12	313	245	.1	397	500	.10	.42	.2	2
Label claim 10 or more g of protein per cup (protein fortified)		246	89	120	10	3	14	349	273	.1	444	500	.11	.47	.2	3
Nonfat (skim)																
No milk solids added		245	91	85	8	Trace	12	302	247	.1	406	500	.09	.37	.2	2
Milk solids added																
Label claim less than 10 g of protein per cup		245	90	90	9	1	12	316	255	.1	418	500	.10	.43	.2	2
Label claim 10 or more g of protein per cup (protein fortified)		246	89	100	10	1	14	352	275	.1	466	500	.11	.48	.2	3
Buttermilk	1 cup	245	90	100	8	2	12	285	219	.1	371	80[3]	.08	.38	.1	2
Milk beverages																
Chocolate milk (commercial)	1 cup															
Regular		250	82	210	8	8	26	280	251	.6	417	300[3]	.09	.41	.3	2
Lowfat (2%)		250	84	180	8	5	26	284	254	.6	422	500	.10	.42	.3	2
Lowfat (1%)		250	85	160	8	3	26	287	257	.6	426	500	.10	.40	.2	2
Eggnog (commercial)		254	74	340	10	19	34	330	278	.5	420	890	.09	.48	.3	4
Malted milk, home-prepared with whole milk	1 cup milk plus 3/4 oz. powder															
Chocolate		265	81	235	9	9	29	304	265	.5	500	330	.14	.43	.7	2
Natural		265	81	235	11	10	27	347	307	.3	529	380	.20	.54	1.3	2
Shakes, thick[4]	1 container															
Chocolate, net wt. 10.6 oz.		300	72	355	9	8	63	396	378	.9	672	260	.14	.67	.4	0
Vanilla, net wt. 11 oz.		313	74	350	12	9	56	457	361	.3	572	360	.09	.61	.5	0

APPENDIX TABLE. Nutritive Values of the Edible Part of Foods (continued)

Food, Approximate Measure, and Weight (in grams)	Water (%)	Food Energy (Cal)	Protein (g)	Fat (g)	Carbohydrate (g)	Calcium (mg)	Phosphorus (mg)	Iron (mg)	Potassium (mg)	Vitamin A Value (IU)	Thiamin (mg)	Riboflavin (mg)	Niacin (mg)	Ascorbic Acid (mg)
Dairy Products (cheese, cream, imitation cream, milk; related products) (continued)														
Milk desserts, frozen														
Ice cream														
Regular (about 11% fat) 1 cup														
Hardened 133	61	270	5	14	32	176	134	.1	257	540	.05	.33	.1	1
Soft serve (frozen custard) 173	60	375	7	23	38	236	199	.4	338	790	.08	.45	.2	1
Rich (about 16% fat), hardened 148	59	350	4	24	32	151	115	.1	221	900	.04	.28	.1	1
Ice milk														
Hardened (about 4.3% fat) 131	69	185	5	6	29	176	129	.1	265	210	.08	.35	.1	1
Soft serve (about 2.6% fat) 175	70	225	8	5	38	274	202	.3	412	180	.12	.54	.2	1
Sherbet (about 2% fat) 193	66	270	2	4	59	103	74	.3	198	190	.01	.09	.1	1
Milk desserts, other 1 cup														
Custard, baked 265	77	305	14	15	29	297	310	1.1	387	930	.11	.50	.3	1
Pudding, from chocolate mix and milk														
Regular (cooked) 260	70	320	9	8	59	265	247	.8	354	340	.05	.39	.3	2
Instant 260	69	325	8	7	63	374	237	1.3	335	340	.08	.39	.3	2
Yogurt 1 container, net wt. 8 oz.														
With added milk solids														
Made with lowfat milk														
Fruit-flavored[5] 227	75	230	10	3	42	343	269	.2	439	120[6]	.08	.40	.2	1
Plain 227	85	145	12	4	16	415	326	.2	531	150[6]	.10	.49	.3	2
Made with nonfat milk 227	85	125	13	Trace	17	452	355	.2	579	20[6]	.11	.53	.3	2
Without added milk solids														
Made with whole milk 227	88	140	8	7	11	274	215	.1	351	280	.07	.32	.2	1
Eggs														
Eggs, large (24 oz./per dozen) 1 egg														
Fried in butter 46	72	100	6	8	1	26	80	.9	58	290	.03	.13	Trace	0
Hard-cooked, shell removed 50	75	85	6	6	1	28	90	1.0	65	260	.04	.14	Trace	0
Poached 50	74	80	6	6	1	28	90	1.0	65	260	.04	.13	Trace	0
Scrambled (milk added) in butter (also omelet) 64	76	95	6	7	1	47	97	.9	85	310	.04	.16	Trace	0
Fats, Oils; Related Products														
Butter														
Regular														
1 T. 14	16	100	Trace	12	Trace	3	3	Trace	7	430[7]	Trace	Trace	Trace	0
1 pat 5	16	35	Trace	4	Trace	1	1	Trace	1	150[7]	Trace	Trace	Trace	0
Whipped														
1 T. 9	16	65	Trace	8	Trace	2	2	Trace	2	290[7]	Trace	Trace	Trace	0
1 pat 4	16	25	Trace	3	Trace	1	1	Trace	1	120[7]	0	Trace	Trace	0
Fats, cooking (vegetable shortenings) 1 T. 13	0	110	0	13	0	0	0	0	0	—	0	0	0	0
Lard 1 T. 13	0	115	0	13	0	0	0	0	0	0	0	0	0	0
Margarine														
Regular														
1 T. 14	16	100	Trace	12	Trace	3	3	Trace	4	470[8]	Trace	Trace	Trace	0
1 pat 5	16	35	Trace	4	Trace	1	1	Trace	1	170[8]	Trace	Trace	Trace	0

Food	Measure	Grams	Water (%)	Food energy (Cal)	Protein (g)	Fat (g)	Saturated (g)	Oleic (g)	Linoleic (g)	Carbohydrate (g)	Calcium (mg)	Phosphorus (mg)	Iron (mg)	Potassium (mg)	Vitamin A (IU)	Thiamin (mg)	Riboflavin (mg)	Niacin (mg)	Ascorbic acid (mg)
Soft (two 8-oz. containers/lb.)	1 T.	14	16	100	Trace	12	2	4	5	Trace	3	2	0	2	470[8]	—	—	—	0
Whipped (6 sticks/lb.)	1 T.	9	16	70	Trace	8	1	3	3	Trace	2	1	0	1	310[8]	—	—	—	0
Oils, salad or cooking	1 T.																		
Corn		14	0	120	0	14	1	4	7	0	0	0	0	—	—	0	0	0	0
Soybean oil, hydrogenated		14	0	120	0	14	2	3	7	0	0	0	0	—	—	0	0	0	0
Soybean-cottonseed oil blend, hydrogenated		14	0	120	0	14	3	4	7	0	0	0	0	—	—	0	0	0	0
Salad dressings, commercial	1 T.																		
Blue cheese — Regular		15	32	75	1	8	2	2	4	1	12	11	Trace	6	30	Trace	.02	Trace	Trace
Blue cheese — Low calorie (5 Cal/t.)		16	84	10	1	1	Trace	Trace	Trace	1	10	8	Trace	5	30	Trace	.01	Trace	Trace
French — Regular		16	39	65	Trace	6	1	1	3	3	2	2	.1	13	—	—	—	—	—
French — Low calorie (5 Cal/t.)		16	77	15	Trace	1	Trace	Trace	Trace	2	2	2	.1	13	—	—	—	—	—
Italian — Regular		15	28	85	Trace	9	2	2	4	1	2	1	Trace	2	Trace	Trace	Trace	Trace	—
Italian — Low calorie (2 Cal/t.)		15	90	10	Trace	1	Trace	Trace	Trace	1	1	1	Trace	2	Trace	Trace	Trace	Trace	—
Mayonnaise		14	15	100	Trace	11	2	3	6	Trace	3	4	.1	5	40	Trace	.01	Trace	—
Mayonnaise type — Regular		15	41	65	Trace	6	1	1	3	2	2	4	Trace	1	30	Trace	Trace	Trace	—
Mayonnaise type — Low calorie (8 Cal/t.)		16	81	20	Trace	2	Trace	Trace	1	2	3	4	Trace	1	40	Trace	Trace	Trace	—
Tartar sauce, regular		14	34	75	Trace	8	1	2	4	1	3	4	.1	11	30	Trace	Trace	Trace	Trace
Fish, Shellfish, Meat, Poultry; Related Products																			
Fish and shellfish																			
Clams, raw, meat only	3 oz.	85	82	65	11	1	—	—	—	2	59	138	5.2	154	90	.08	.15	1.1	8
Crabmeat (white or king), canned, not pressed down	1 cup	135	77	135	24	3	—	—	—	1	61	246	1.1	149	—	.11	.11	2.6	—
Fish stick (4 x 1 x ½"), breaded, frozen, cooked[9]	1 stick or 1 oz.	28	66	50	5	3	—	—	—	2	3	47	.1	—	—	.01	.02	.5	—
Haddock, breaded, fried[9]	3 oz.	85	66	140	17	5	1	2	1	5	34	210	1.0	296	—	.03	.06	2.7	2
Oysters, raw, meat only (13–19 medium Selects)	1 cup	240	85	160	20	4	—	—	—	8	226	343	13.2	290	740	.34	.43	6.0	—
Salmon, pink, canned, solids and liquid	3 oz.	85	71	120	17	5	1	1	Trace	0	167[10]	243	.7	307	60	.03	.16	6.8	—
Sardines, Atlantic, canned in oil, drained solids	3 oz.	85	62	175	20	9	3	2	Trace	0	372	424	2.5	502	190	.02	.17	4.6	—
Scallops, breaded, frozen, fried, reheated	6 scallops	90	60	175	16	8	—	—	—	9	—	—	—	—	—	—	—	—	—
Shad, baked with butter or margarine, bacon	3 oz.	85	64	170	20	10	—	—	—	0	20	266	.5	320	30	.11	.22	7.3	—
Shrimp — Canned meat	3 oz.	85	70	100	21	1	—	—	—	1	98	224	2.6	104	50	.01	.03	1.5	—
Shrimp — French fried[11]	3 oz.	85	57	190	17	9	—	—	—	9	61	162	1.7	195	—	.03	.07	2.3	—
Tuna, canned in oil, drained solids	3 oz.	85	61	170	24	7	—	—	—	0	7	199	1.6	—	70	.04	.10	10.1	—
Tuna salad[12]	1 cup	205	70	350	30	22	—	—	—	7	41	291	2.7	—	590	.08	.23	10.3	2
Meat and meat products																			
Bacon (20 slices/lb., raw), broiled or fried, crisp	2 slices	15	8	85	4	8	3	4	1	Trace	2	34	.5	35	0	.08	.05	.8	—

APPENDIX TABLE. Nutritive Values of the Edible Part of Foods (continued)

Food, Approximate Measure, and Weight (in grams)		Water (%)	Food Energy (Cal)	Protein (g)	Fat (g)	Carbohydrate (g)	Calcium (mg)	Phosphorus (mg)	Iron (mg)	Potassium (mg)	Vitamin A Value (IU)	Thiamin (mg)	Riboflavin (mg)	Niacin (mg)	Ascorbic Acid (mg)
Fish, Shellfish, Meat, Poultry; Related Products (continued)															
Beef,[13] cooked															
Cuts simmered, braised, or pot roasted (piece, 2½ x 2½ x ¾")															
Lean and fat	3 oz.	53	245	23	16	0	10	114	2.9	184	30	.04	.18	3.6	—
Lean only	2.5 oz.	62	140	22	5	0	10	108	2.7	176	10	.04	.17	3.3	—
Ground beef (patty, 3 x ⁵/₈"), broiled															
Lean with 10% fat	3 oz.	60	185	23	10	0	10	196	3.0	261	20	.08	.20	5.1	—
Lean with 21% fat	2.9 oz.	54	235	20	17	0	9	159	2.6	221	30	.07	.17	4.4	—
Roast, oven cooked, no liquid added (2 pieces, 4⅛ x 2¼ x ¼")															
Relatively fat, such as rib															
Lean and fat	3 oz.	40	375	17	33	0	8	158	2.2	189	70	.05	.13	3.1	—
Lean only	1.8 oz.	57	125	14	7	0	6	131	1.8	161	10	.04	.11	2.6	—
Relatively lean, such as heel of round															
Lean and fat	3 oz.	62	165	25	7	0	11	208	3.2	279	10	.06	.19	4.5	—
Lean only	2.8 oz.	65	125	24	3	0	10	199	3.0	268	Trace	.06	.18	4.3	—
Steak															
Relatively fat—sirloin, broiled (piece, 2½ x 2½ x ¾")															
Lean and fat	3 oz.	44	330	20	27	0	9	162	2.5	220	50	.05	.15	4.0	—
Lean only	2.4 oz.	59	115	18	4	0	7	146	2.2	202	10	.05	.14	3.6	—
Relatively lean—round, braised (piece, 4⅛ x 2¼ x ½")															
Lean and fat	3 oz.	55	220	24	13	0	10	213	3.0	272	20	.07	.19	4.8	—
Lean only	2.4 oz.	61	130	21	4	0	9	182	2.5	238	10	.05	.16	4.1	—
Beef, canned															
Corned beef	3 oz.	59	185	22	10	0	17	90	3.7	—	—	.01	.20	2.9	—
Corned beef hash	1 cup	67	400	19	25	24	29	147	4.4	440	—	.02	.20	4.6	—
Beef and vegetable stew	1 cup	82	220	16	11	15	29	184	2.9	613	2,400	.15	.17	4.7	17
Beef potpie (home recipe), baked[14] (piece, ⅓ of 9" diam. pie)	1 piece	55	515	21	30	39	29	149	3.8	334	1,720	.30	.30	5.5	6
Chili con carne with beans, canned	1 cup	72	340	19	16	31	82	321	4.3	594	150	.08	.18	3.3	—
Chop suey with beef and pork (home recipe)	1 cup	75	300	26	17	13	60	248	4.8	425	600	.28	.38	5.0	33
Lamb, cooked															
Chop, rib (cut 3/lb. with bone), broiled															
Lean and fat	3.1 oz.	43	360	18	32	0	8	139	1.0	200	—	.11	.19	4.1	—
Lean only	2 oz.	60	120	16	6	0	6	121	1.1	174	—	.09	.15	3.4	—
Liver, beef, fried (slice)	3 oz.	56	195	22	9	5	9	405	7.5	323	45,390[15]	.22	3.56	14.0	23
Ham, light cure, lean and fat, roasted (2 pieces, 4⅛ x 2¼ x ¼")[16]	3 oz.	54	245	18	19	0	8	146	2.2	199	0	.40	.15	3.1	—

Food	Measure															
Luncheon meat, boiled ham, slice (8/8-oz. pkg.)	1 oz.	28	59	65	5	5	0	3	47	.8	—	0	.12	.04	.7	—
Pork, fresh,[13] cooked																
Chop, loin (cut 3/lb. with bone), broiled	2.7 oz.	78	42	305	19	25	0	9	209	2.7	216	0	.75	.22	4.5	—
Roast, oven cooked, no liquid added, lean and fat (piece, 2½ x 2½ x ¾")	3 oz.	85	46	310	21	24	0	9	218	2.7	233	0	.78	.22	4.8	—
Sausage																
Bologna	1 slice	28	56	85	3	8	Trace	2	36	.5	65	—	.05	.06	.7	—
Braunschweiger	1 slice	28	53	90	4	8	1	3	69	1.7	—	1,850	.05	.41	2.3	—
Brown and serve (10–11 links/8-oz. pkg.), browned	1 link	17	40	70	3	6	Trace	—	—	—	—	—	—	—	—	—
Deviled ham, canned	1 T.	13	51	45	2	4	0	1	12	.3	—	0	.02	.01	.2	—
Frankfurter (8/1-lb. pkg.)	1 frankfurter	56	57	170	7	15	1	3	57	.8	—	—	.08	.11	1.4	—
Salami																
Dry type (12 slices/4-oz. pkg.)	1 slice	10	30	45	2	4	Trace	1	28	.4	—	—	.04	.03	.5	—
Cooked type (8 slices/8-oz. pkg.)	1 slice	28	51	90	5	7	Trace	3	57	.7	—	—	.07	.07	1.2	—
Vienna sausage (7/4-oz. can)	1 sausage	16	63	40	2	3	Trace	1	24	.3	—	—	.01	.02	.4	—
Poultry and poultry products																
Chicken, cooked, bones removed																
Breast, fried,[17] ½ breast (3.3 oz. with bones)	2.8 oz.	79	58	160	26	5	1	9	218	1.3	—	70	.04	.17	11.6	—
Drumstick, fried[17] (2 oz. with bones)	1.3 oz.	38	55	90	12	4	Trace	6	89	.9	—	50	.03	.15	2.7	—
Half broiler, broiled (10.4 oz. with bones)	6.2 oz.	176	71	240	42	7	0	16	355	3.0	483	160	.09	.34	15.5	—
Chicken, canned, boneless	3 oz.	85	65	170	18	10	0	18	210	1.3	117	200	.03	.11	3.7	3
Chicken a la king, cooked (home recipe)	1 cup	245	68	470	27	34	12	127	358	2.5	404	1,130	.10	.42	5.4	12
Chicken and noodles, cooked (home recipe)	1 cup	240	71	365	22	18	26	26	247	2.2	149	430	.05	.17	4.3	Trace
Chicken chow mein, canned	1 cup	250	89	95	7	Trace	18	45	85	1.3	418	150	.05	.10	1.0	13
Turkey, roasted, light and dark meat, chopped or diced	1 cup	140	61	265	44	9	0	11	351	2.5	514	—	.07	.25	10.8	—
Fruits and Fruit Products																
Apples (about 3/lb.)	1 apple	138	84	80	Trace	1	20	10	14	.4	152	120	.04	.03	.1	6
Apple juice, bottled or canned[18]	1 cup	248	88	120	Trace	Trace	30	15	22	1.5	250	—	.02	.05	.2	2[19]
Applesauce, canned																
Sweetened	1 cup	255	76	230	1	Trace	61	10	13	1.3	166	100	.05	.03	.1	3[19]
Unsweetened	1 cup	244	89	100	Trace	Trace	26	10	12	1.2	190	100	.05	.02	.1	2[19]
Apricots																
Raw	3 apricots	107	85	55	1	Trace	14	18	25	.5	301	2,890	.03	.04	.6	11
Canned in heavy syrup	1 cup	258	77	220	2	Trace	57	28	39	.8	604	4,490	.05	.05	1.0	10
Avocados, raw, whole, California, mid- and late-winter	1 avocado	216	74	370	5	37	13	22	91	1.3	1,303	630	.24	.43	3.5	30

APPENDIX TABLE. Nutritive Values of the Edible Part of Foods (*continued*)

Food, Approximate Measure, and Weight (in grams)	Water (%)	Food Energy (Cal)	Pro-tein (g)	Fat (g)	Carbo-hydrate (g)	Cal-cium (mg)	Phos-phorus (mg)	Iron (mg)	Potas-sium (mg)	Vitamin A Value (IU)	Thia-min (mg)	Ribo-flavin (mg)	Niacin (mg)	Ascorbic Acid (mg)
Fruits and Fruit Products (*continued*)														
Banana — 1 banana — 119	76	100	1	Trace	26	10	31	.8	440	230	.06	.07	.8	12
Blackberries, raw — 1 cup — 144	85	85	2	1	19	46	27	1.3	245	290	.04	.06	.6	30
Blueberries, raw — 1 cup — 145	83	90	1	1	22	22	19	1.5	117	150	.04	.09	.7	20
Cantaloupe. See Muskmelon.														
Cherries, sour (tart), red, pitted, canned, water pack — 1 cup — 244	88	105	2	Trace	26	37	32	.7	317	1,660	.07	.05	.5	12
Cranberry juice cocktail, sweetened, bottled — 1 cup — 253	83	165	Trace	Trace	42	13	8	.8	25	Trace	.03	.03	.1	81[20]
Cranberry sauce, sweetened, strained, canned — 1 cup — 277	62	405	Trace	1	104	17	11	.6	83	60	.03	.03	.1	6
Fruit cocktail, canned in heavy syrup — 1 cup — 255	80	195	1	Trace	50	23	31	1.0	411	360	.05	.03	1.0	5
Grapefruit														
Raw, medium, pink or red — 1/2 grapefruit with peel — 241	89	50	1	Trace	13	20	20	.5	166	540	.05	.02	.2	44
Canned, sections with syrup — 1 cup — 254	81	180	2	Trace	45	33	36	.8	343	30	.08	.05	.5	76
Grapefruit juice														
Raw, pink, red, or white — 1 cup — 246	90	95	1	Trace	23	22	37	.5	399	[21]	.10	.05	.5	93
Frozen, unsweetened, diluted with 3 parts water by vol. — 1 cup — 247	89	100	1	Trace	24	25	42	.2	420	20	.10	.04	.5	96
Grapes, Thompson seedless — 10 grapes — 50	81	35	Trace	Trace	9	6	10	.2	87	50	.03	.02	.2	2
Grape juice, canned or bottled — 1 cup — 253	83	165	1	Trace	42	28	30	.8	293	—	.10	.05	.5	Trace[19]
Grape drink, canned — 1 cup — 250	86	135	Trace	Trace	35	8	10	.3	88	—	.03[22]	.03[22]	.3	[22]
Lemonade, frozen, diluted with 4 1/3 parts water by vol. — 1 cup — 248	89	105	Trace	Trace	28	2	3	.1	40	10	.01	.02	.2	17
Muskmelon														
Cantaloupe, orange-fleshed — 1/2 melon with rind — 477	91	80	2	Trace	20	38	44	1.1	682	9,240	.11	.08	1.6	90
Honeydew — 1/10 melon with rind — 226	91	50	1	Trace	11	21	24	.6	374	60	.06	.04	.9	34
Oranges, all commercial varieties, raw — 1 orange — 131	86	65	1	Trace	16	54	26	.5	263	260	.13	.05	.5	66
Orange juice														
Raw, all varieties — 1 cup — 248	88	110	2	Trace	26	27	42	.5	496	500	.22	.07	1.0	124
Canned, unsweetened — 1 cup — 249	87	120	2	Trace	28	25	45	1.0	496	500	.17	.05	.7	100
Frozen concentrate, diluted with 3 parts water by vol. — 1 cup — 249	87	120	2	Trace	29	25	42	.2	503	540	.23	.03	.9	120
Peaches														
Raw — 1 peach — 100	89	40	1	Trace	10	9	19	.5	202	1,330[23]	.02	.05	1.0	7
Canned														
Syrup pack — 1 cup — 256	79	200	1	Trace	51	10	31	.8	333	1,100	.03	.05	1.5	8
Water pack — 1 cup — 244	91	75	1	Trace	20	10	32	.7	334	1,100	.02	.07	1.5	7
Frozen, sliced, sweetened — 1 cup — 250	77	220	1	Trace	57	10	33	1.3	310	1,630	.03	.10	1.8	103[24]

Food	Measure	Grams	Water (%)	Food energy (cal)	Protein (g)	Fat (g)	Carbohydrate (g)	Calcium (mg)	Phosphorus (mg)	Iron (mg)	Potassium (mg)	Vitamin A (IU)	Thiamin (mg)	Riboflavin (mg)	Niacin (mg)	Ascorbic acid (mg)
Pears																
Raw, Bartlett	1 pear	164	83	100	1	1	25	13	18	.5	213	30	.03	.07	.2	7
Canned in heavy syrup	1 cup	255	80	195	1	1	50	13	18	.5	214	10	.03	.05	.3	3
Pineapple																
Raw, diced	1 cup	155	85	80	1	Trace	21	26	12	.8	226	110	.14	.05	.3	26
Canned, crushed, chunks, tidbits, heavy syrup pack		255	80	190	1	Trace	49	28	13	.8	245	130	.20	.05	.5	18
Pineapple juice, unsweetened, canned	1 cup	250	86	140	1	Trace	34	38	23	.8	373	130	.13	.05	.5	80[20]
Plums																
Raw, Japanese and hybrid	1 plum	66	87	30	Trace	Trace	8	8	12	.3	112	160	.02	.02	.3	4
Canned in heavy syrup (Italian prunes)	1 cup[25]	272	77	215	1	Trace	56	23	26	2.3	367	3,130	.05	.05	1.0	5
Prunes, dried, "softenized," with pits																
Uncooked	4 extra large or 5 large prunes[25]	49	28	110	1	Trace	29	22	34	1.7	298	690	.04	.07	.7	1
Cooked, unsweetened	1 cup[25]	250	66	255	2	1	67	51	79	3.8	695	1,590	.07	.15	1.5	2
Prune juice, canned or bottled	1 cup	256	80	195	1	Trace	49	36	51	1.8	602	—	.03	.03	1.0	5
Raisins, seedless, packet (½ oz. or 1½ T.)	1 packet	14	18	40	Trace	Trace	11	9	14	.5	107	Trace	.02	.01	.1	Trace
Rhubarb, cooked, sugar added	1 cup	270	63	380	1	Trace	97	211	41	1.6	548	220	.05	.14	.8	16
Strawberries																
Raw, whole, capped	1 cup	149	90	55	1	1	13	31	31	1.5	244	90	.04	.10	.9	88
Frozen, sweetened, sliced	1 container (10 oz.)	284	71	310	1	1	79	40	48	2.0	318	90	.06	.17	1.4	151
Tangerine	1 tangerine	86	87	40	1	Trace	10	34	15	.3	108	360	.05	.02	.1	27
Watermelon, raw (4 x 8" wedge)	1 wedge with rind and seeds[26]	926	93	110	2	1	27	30	43	2.1	426	2,510	.13	.13	.9	30
Grain Products																
Bagel (3" diam.), made with egg	1 bagel	55	32	165	6	2	28	9	43	1.2	41	30	.14	.10	1.2	0
Barley, pearled, light, uncooked	1 cup	200	11	700	16	2	158	32	378	4.0	320	0	.24	.10	6.2	0
Biscuit, baking powder[27] (2" diam.)	1 biscuit	28	27	105	2	5	13	34	49	.4	33	Trace	.08	.08	.7	Trace
Breadcrumbs (enriched),[28] dry, grated	1 cup	100	7	390	13	5	73	122	141	3.6	152	Trace	.35	.35	4.8	Trace
Bread																
Boston brown bread,[28] canned (slice, 3¼ x ½")	1 slice	45	45	95	2	1	21	41	72	.9	131	0[29]	.06	.04	.7	0
Cracked-wheat bread[28]		25	35	65	2	1	13	22	32	.5	34	Trace	.08	.06	.8	Trace
French bread (enriched)[28] (slice, 5 x 2½ x 1")		35	31	100	3	1	19	15	30	.8	32	Trace	.14	.08	1.2	Trace
Raisin bread (enriched)[28]		25	35	65	2	1	13	18	22	.6	58	Trace	.09	.06	.6	Trace
White bread (enriched),[28] soft-crumb type		25	36	70	2	1	13	21	24	.6	26	Trace	.10	.06	.8	Trace
Whole-wheat bread,[28] soft-crumb type		28	36	65	3	1	14	24	71	.8	72	Trace	.09	.03	.8	Trace

APPENDIX TABLE. Nutritive Values of the Edible Part of Foods (continued)

Food, Approximate Measure, and Weight (in grams)	Water (%)	Food Energy (Cal)	Protein (g)	Fat (g)	Carbohydrate (g)	Calcium (mg)	Phosphorus (mg)	Iron (mg)	Potassium (mg)	Vitamin A Value (IU)	Thiamin (mg)	Riboflavin (mg)	Niacin (mg)	Ascorbic Acid (mg)
Grain Products (continued)														
Breakfast cereal 1 cup														
Hot, cooked														
Corn (hominy) grits, degermed														
Enriched	245	125	3	Trace	27	2	25	.7	27	Trace[30]	.10	.07	1.0	0
Unenriched	245	125	3	Trace	27	2	25	.2	27	Trace[30]	.05	.02	.5	0
Farina, quick-cooking, enriched	245	105	3	Trace	22	147	113[31]	.[32]	25	0	.12	.07	1.0	0
Oatmeal or rolled oats	240	130	5	2	23	22	137	1.4	146	0	.19	.05	.2	0
Wheat, rolled	240	180	5	1	41	19	182	1.7	202	0	.17	.07	2.2	0
Wheat, whole-meal	245	110	4	1	23	17	127	1.2	118	0	.15	.05	1.5	0
Ready-to-eat														
Bran flakes (40% bran), added sugar, salt, iron, vitamins	35	105	4	1	28	19	125	12.4	137	1,650	.41	.49	4.1	12
Bran flakes with raisins, added sugar, salt, iron, vitamins	50	145	4	1	40	28	146	17.7	154	2,350	.58	.71	5.8	18
Corn flakes														
Plain, added sugar, salt, iron, vitamins	25	95	2	Trace	21	32	9	0.6	30	1,180	.29	.35	2.9	9
Sugar-coated, added salt, iron, vitamins	40	155	2	Trace	37	1	10	1.0	27	1,880	.46	.56	4.6	14
Wheat flakes, added sugar, salt, iron, vitamins	30	105	3	Trace	24	12	83	.[32]	81	1,410	.35	.42	3.5	11
Wheat, puffed														
Plain, added iron, thiamin, niacin	15	55	2	Trace	12	4	48	.6	51	0	.08	.03	1.2	0
Presweetened, added salt, iron, vitamins	38	140	3	Trace	33	7	52	1.6[33]	63	1,680	.50	.57	6.7	20[34]
Wheat, shredded, plain	25	90	2	1	20	11	97	.9	87	0	.06	.03	1.1	0
Wheat germ, without salt or sugar, toasted 1 T.	6	25	2	1	3	3	70	.5	57	10	.11	.05	.3	1
Buckwheat flour, light, sifted 1 cup	98	340	6	1	78	11	86	1.0	314	0	.08	.04	.4	0
Bulgur, canned, seasoned 1 cup	135	245	8	4	44	27	263	1.9	151	0	.08	.05	4.1	0
Cake made from cake mix with enriched flour														
Angel food (1/12 of cake) 1 piece	53	135	3	Trace	32	50	63	.2	32	0	.03	.08	.3	0
Coffeecake (1/6 of cake) 1 piece	72	230	5	7	38	44	125	1.2	78	120	.14	.15	1.3	Trace
Cupcake, made with egg, milk (2½''' diam.) 1 cupcake														
Without icing	25	90	1	3	14	40	59	.3	21	40	.05	.05	.4	Trace
With chocolate icing	36	130	2	5	21	47	71	.4	42	60	.05	.06	.4	Trace
Devil's food with chocolate icing (1/16 of cake) 1 piece	69	235	3	8	40	41	72	1.0	90	100	.07	.10	.6	Trace
Gingerbread (1/9 of cake) 1 piece	63	175	2	4	32	57	63	.9	173	Trace	.09	.11	.8	Trace

Food	Measure															
White, 2-layer with chocolate icing (1/16 of cake)	1 piece	71	21	250	3	8	45	70	127	.7	82	40	.09	.11	.8	Trace
Cake made from home recipe using enriched flour																
Boston cream pie with custard filling (1/12 of cake)	1 piece	69	35	210	3	6	34	46	70	.7	61	140	.09	.11	.8	Trace
Fruitcake, dark (1/30 of loaf)	1 slice	15	18	55	1	2	9	11	17	.4	74	20	.02	.02	.2	Trace
Pound (1/17 of loaf)	1 slice	33	16	160	2	10	16	6	24	.5	20	80	.05	.06	.4	0
Spongecake (1/12 of cake)	1 piece	66	32	195	5	4	36	20	74	1.1	57	300	.09	.14	.6	Trace
Cookies[27]																
Brownies with nuts, from home recipe	1 brownie	20	10	95	1	6	10	8	30	.4	38	40	.04	.03	.2	Trace
Chocolate chip	4 cookies	42	3	200	2	9	29	16	48	1.0	56	50	1.0	1.7	.9	Trace
Fig bars	4 bars	56	14	200	2	3	42	44	34	1.0	111	60	.04	.14	.9	Trace
Gingersnaps	4 cookies	28	3	90	2	2	22	20	13	1.7	129	20	.08	.06	.7	0
Macaroons[35]	2 cookies	38	4	180	2	9	25	10	32	.3	176	0	.02	.06	.2	0
Oatmeal with raisins	4 cookies	52	3	235	3	8	38	11	53	1.4	192	30	.15	.10	1.0	Trace
Sandwich type (chocolate or vanilla)	4 cookies	40	2	200	2	9	28	10	96	.7	15	0	.06	.10	.7	0
Crackers[28]																
Graham	2 crackers	14	6	55	1	1	10	6	21	.5	55	0	.02	.08	.5	0
Rye wafers, whole-grain	2 wafers	13	6	45	2	Trace	10	7	50	.5	78	0	.04	.03	.2	0
Saltines	4 crackers or 1 packet	11	4	50	1	1	8	2	10	.5	13	0	.05	.05	.4	0
Danish pastry (enriched flour) plain without fruit or nuts (piece, 4 1/4" diam. x 1")	1 pastry	65	22	275	5	15	30	33	71	1.2	73	200	.18	.19	1.7	Trace
Doughnut[27]																
Cake type, plain	1 doughnut	25	24	100	1	5	13	10	48	.4	23	20	.05	.05	.4	Trace
Yeast-leavened, glazed	1 doughnut	50	26	205	3	11	22	16	33	.6	34	25	.10	.10	.8	0
Macaroni, enriched, cooked	1 cup	130	64	190	7	1	39	14	85	1.4	103	0	.23	.13	1.8	0
Macaroni (enriched) and cheese from home recipe (served hot)	1 cup	200	58	430	17	22	40	362	322	1.8	240	860	.20	.40	1.8	Trace
Muffin[27]																
Blueberry	1 muffin	40	39	110	3	4	17	34	53	.6	46	90	.09	.10	.7	Trace
Bran	1 muffin	40	35	105	3	4	17	57	162	1.5	172	90	.07	.10	1.7	Trace
Corn (enriched degermed cornmeal and flour)	1 muffin	40	33	125	3	4	19	42	68	.7	54	120	.10	.10	.7	Trace
Noodles (egg), enriched, cooked	1 cup	160	71	200	7	2	37	16	94	1.4	70	110	.22	.13	1.9	0
Noodles, chow mein, canned	1 cup	45	1	220	6	11	26	–	–	.4	–	–	–	–	–	–
Pancake[28] (4" diam.)	1 cake	27	50	60	2	2	9	27	38	.4	33	30	.06	.07	.5	Trace
Pie[14] (9" diam.; 1/7 of pie)																
Apple	1 sector	135	48	345	3	15	51	11	30	.9	108	40	.15	.11	1.3	2
Banana cream	1 sector	130	54	285	6	12	40	86	107	1.0	264	330	.11	.22	1.0	1
Blueberry	1 sector	135	51	325	3	15	47	15	31	1.4	88	40	.15	.11	1.4	4
Cherry	1 sector	135	47	350	4	15	52	19	34	.9	142	590	.16	.12	1.4	Trace
Custard	1 sector	130	58	285	8	14	30	125	147	1.2	178	300	.11	.27	.8	0

APPENDIX TABLE. Nutritive Values of the Edible Part of Foods (*continued*)

Food, Approximate Measure, and Weight (in grams)		Water (%)	Food Energy (Cal)	Protein (g)	Fat (g)	Carbohydrate (g)	Calcium (mg)	Phosphorus (mg)	Iron (mg)	Potassium (mg)	Vitamin A Value (IU)	Thiamin (mg)	Riboflavin (mg)	Niacin (mg)	Ascorbic Acid (mg)
Grain Products (*continued*)															
Pie[14] (9" diam.; 1/7 of pie) (*continued*)	1 sector														
Lemon meringue		120	47	305	4	12	45	17	59	1.0	60	00	.09	.12	1.4	1
Mince		135	43	365	3	16	56	38	51	.9	240	Trace	.14	.12	1.4	1
Peach		135	48	345	3	14	52	14	39	1.2	201	990	.15	.14	2.0	4
Pecan		118	20	495	5	27	61	55	122	3.7	145	190	.26	.14	1.0	Trace
Pumpkin		130	59	275	5	15	32	66	90	1.0	208	3,210	.11	.18	1.0	Trace
Pizza (cheese), baked[14] (4¾" sector; 1/8 of 12" diam. pie)	1 sector	60	45	145	6	4	22	86	89	1.1	67	230	.16	.18	1.6	4
Popcorn popped																
Plain, large kernel	1 cup	6	4	25	1	Trace	5	1	17	.2	—	—	—	.01	.1	0
With oil (coconut) and salt added, large kernel		9	3	40	1	2	5	1	19	.2	—	—	—	.01	.2	0
Sugar coated		35	4	135	2	1	30	2	47	.5	—	—	—	.02	.4	0
Pretzels, made with enriched flour																
Dutch, twisted	1 pretzel	16	5	60	2	1	12	4	21	.2	21	0	.05	.04	.7	0
Thin, twisted	10 pretzels	60	5	235	6	3	46	13	79	.9	78	0	.20	.15	2.5	0
Stick	10 pretzels	3	5	10	Trace	Trace	2	1	4	Trace	4	0	.01	.01	.1	0
Rice, white, enriched																
Instant, ready-to-serve, hot	1 cup	165	73	180	4	Trace	40	5	31	1.3	—	0	.21	[36]	1.7	0
Long grain, cooked		205	73	225	4	Trace	50	21	57	1.8	57	0	.23	.02	2.1	0
Roll, enriched,[28] commercial	1 roll															
Brown-and-serve		26	27	85	2	2	14	20	23	.5	25	Trace	.10	.06	.9	Trace
Cloverleaf or pan		28	31	85	2	2	15	21	24	.5	27	Trace	.11	.07	.9	Trace
Frankfurter or hamburger		40	31	120	3	2	21	30	34	.8	38	Trace	.16	.10	1.3	Trace
Hard		50	25	155	5	2	30	24	46	1.2	49	Trace	.20	.12	1.7	Trace
Hoagie or submarine		135	31	390	12	4	75	58	115	3.0	122	Trace	.54	.32	4.5	Trace
Spaghetti, enriched, cooked	1 cup	130	64	190	7	1	39	14	85	1.4	103	0	.23	.13	1.8	0
Spaghetti (enriched) in tomato sauce with cheese, canned	1 cup	250	80	190	6	2	39	40	88	2.8	303	930	.35	.28	4.5	10
Spaghetti (enriched) with meat balls and tomato sauce, canned	1 cup	250	78	260	12	10	29	53	113	3.3	245	1,000	.15	.18	2.3	5
Toaster pastries	1 pastry	50	12	200	3	6	36	54[33]	67[33]	1.9	74[33]	500	.16	.17	2.1	33[33]
Waffle[27] (7" diam.)	1 waffle	75	41	210	7	7	28	85	130	1.3	109	250	.17	.23	1.4	Trace
Wheat flour																
All-purpose, enriched	1 cup	125	12	455	13	1	95	20	109	3.6	119	0	.80	.50	6.6	0
Whole-wheat, from hard wheats, stirred		120	12	400	16	2	85	49	446	4.0	444	0	.66	.14	5.2	0
Legumes (dry), Nuts, Seeds; Related Products																
Almonds, shelled, chopped	1 cup	130	5	775	24	70	25	304	655	6.1	749	0	.31	1.20	4.6	Trace
Beans, dry																
Common varieties as great northern, navy, and others																
Cooked, drained	1 cup	180	69	210	14	1	38	90	266	4.9	749	0	.25	.13	1.3	0

Food	Measure	Water (%)	Food energy (cal.)	Protein (g)	Fat (g)	Carbohydrate (g)	Calcium (mg)	Phosphorus (mg)	Iron (mg)	Potassium (mg)	Vitamin A (IU)	Thiamin (mg)	Riboflavin (mg)	Niacin (mg)	Ascorbic acid (mg)
Canned, solids and liquid, white with															
Frankfurters (sliced)	1 cup	71	365	19	18	32	94	303	4.8	668	330	.18	.15	3.3	Trace
Pork and tomato sauce	1 cup	71	310	16	7	48	138	235	4.6	536	330	.20	.08	1.5	5
Pork and sweet sauce	1 cup	66	385	16	12	54	161	291	5.9	—	—	.15	.10	1.3	—
Lima, cooked, drained	1 cup	64	260	16	1	49	55	293	5.9	1,163	—	.25	.11	1.3	—
Black-eyed peas, dry, cooked	1 cup	80	190	13	1	35	43	238	3.3	573	30	.40	.10	1.0	—
Cashews, roasted in oil	1 cup	5	785	24	64	41	53	522	5.3	650	140	.60	.35	2.5	—
Coconut meat, fresh, grated	1 cup	51	275	3	28	8	10	76	1.4	205	0	.04	.02	.4	2
Lentils, whole, cooked	1 cup	72	210	16	Trace	39	50	238	4.2	498	40	.14	.12	1.2	0
Peanuts, roasted in oil, salted	1 cup	2	840	37	72	27	107	577	3.0	971	—	.46	.19	24.8	0
Peanut butter	1 T.	2	95	4	8	3	9	61	.3	100	—	.02	.02	2.4	0
Peas, split, dry, cooked	1 cup	70	230	16	1	42	22	178	3.4	592	80	.30	.18	1.8	—
Pecans, chopped or pieces	1 cup	3	810	11	84	17	86	341	2.8	712	150	1.01	.15	1.1	2
Pumpkin and squash kernels, dry, hulled	1 cup	4	775	41	65	21	71	1,602	15.7	1,386	100	.34	.27	3.4	—
Sunflower seeds, dry, hulled	1 cup	5	810	35	69	29	174	1,214	10.3	1,334	70	2.84	.33	7.8	—
Walnuts, chopped	1 cup	3	785	26	74	19	Trace	713	7.5	575	380	.28	.14	.9	—
Sugars and Sweets															
Cake icing, boiled, white	1 cup	18	295	1	0	75	2	2	Trace	17	0	Trace	.03	Trace	0
Candy															
Caramels, plain or chocolate	1 oz.	8	115	1	3	22	42	35	.4	54	Trace	.01	.05	.1	Trace
Chocolate															
Milk, plain	1 oz.	8	115	1	3	22	42	35	.3	109	80	.02	.10	.1	Trace
Semisweet, small pieces (60/oz.)	1 cup or 6-oz. pkg.	1	860	7	61	97	51	255	4.4	553	30	.02	.14	.9	0
Chocolate-coated peanuts	1 oz.	1	160	5	12	11	33	84	.4	143	Trace	.10	.05	2.1	Trace
Fondant, uncoated (mints, candy corn, other)	1 oz.	8	105	Trace	1	25	4	2	.3	1	0	Trace	Trace	Trace	0
Fudge, chocolate, plain	1 oz.	8	115	1	3	21	22	24	.3	42	Trace	.01	.03	.1	Trace
Gum drops	1 oz.	12	100	Trace	Trace	25	2	Trace	.1	1	0	0	Trace	Trace	0
Hard	1 oz.	1	110	0	Trace	28	6	2	.5	1	0	0	0	0	0
Marshmallows	1 oz.	17	90	1	Trace	23	5	2	.5	2	0	0	Trace	Trace	0
Chocolate-flavored beverage powders (about 4 heaping t./oz.)															
With nonfat dry milk	1 oz.	2	100	5	1	20	167	155	.5	227	10	.04	.21	.2	1
Without milk	1 oz.	1	100	1	1	25	9	48	.6	142	—	.01	.03	.1	0
Honey, strained or extracted	1 T.	17	65	Trace	0	17	1	1	.1	11	0	Trace	.01	.1	Trace
Jams and preserves	1 T.	29	55	Trace	Trace	14	4	2	.2	18	Trace	Trace	.01	Trace	Trace
Jellies	1 T.	29	50	Trace	Trace	13	4	1	.3	14	Trace	Trace	.01	Trace	1
Syrup															
Chocolate-flavored syrup or topping	1 fl. oz. or 2 T.														
Thin type		32	90	1	1	24	6	35	.6	106	Trace	.01	.03	.2	0
Fudge type		25	125	2	5	20	48	60	.5	107	60	.02	.08	.2	Trace
Molasses cane	1 T.														
Light (first extraction)		24	50	—	—	13	33	9	.9	183	—	.01	.01	Trace	—
Blackstrap (third extraction)		24	45	—	—	11	137	17	3.2	585	—	.02	.04	.4	—
Sorghum	1 T.	23	55	—	—	14	35	5	2.6	—	—	.02	.02	Trace	—
Table blends, chiefly corn, light and dark	1 T.	24	60	0	0	15	9	3	.8	1	0	0	0	0	0

APPENDIX

APPENDIX TABLE. Nutritive Values of the Edible Part of Foods (*continued*)

Food, Approximate Measure, and Weight (in grams)	Water (%)	Food Energy (Cal)	Protein (g)	Fat (g)	Carbohydrate (g)	Calcium (mg)	Phosphorus (mg)	Iron (mg)	Potassium (mg)	Vitamin A Value (IU)	Thiamin (mg)	Riboflavin (mg)	Niacin (mg)	Ascorbic Acid (mg)
Sugars and Sweets (*continued*)														
Sugar														
Brown, pressed down 1 cup 220	2	820	0	0	212	187	42	7.5	757	0	.02	.07	.4	0
White														
Granulated 1 cup 200	1	770	0	0	199	0	0	.2	Trace	0	0	0	0	0
1 T. 12	1	45	0	0	12	0	0	Trace	Trace	0	0	0	0	0
1 packet 6	1	23	0	0	6	0	0	Trace	Trace	0	0	0	0	0
Powdered, sifted, spooned into cup 1 cup 100	1	385	0	0	100	0	0	.1	3	0	0	0	0	0
Vegetables and Vegetable Products														
Asparagus, green														
Cooked from raw, drained 4 spears 60	94	10	1	Trace	2	13	30	.4	110	540	.10	.11	.8	16
Canned 80	93	15	2	Trace	3	15	42	1.5	133	640	.05	.08	.6	12
Beans														
Lima, immature seeds, frozen, cooked, drained														
Thick-seeded types (Fordhooks) 170	74	170	10	Trace	32	34	153	2.9	724	390	.12	.09	1.7	29
Thin-seeded types (baby limas) 180	69	210	13	Trace	40	63	227	4.7	709	400	.16	.09	2.2	22
Snap														
Green														
Cooked from raw, drained 125	92	30	2	Trace	7	63	46	.8	189	680	.09	.11	.6	15
Canned, drained solids 135	92	30	2	Trace	7	61	34	2.0	128	630	.04	.07	.4	5
Yellow or wax														
Cooked from raw, drained 125	93	30	2	Trace	6	63	46	.8	189	290	.09	.11	.6	16
Canned, drained solids 135	92	30	2	Trace	7	61	34	2.0	128	140	.04	.07	.4	7
Bean sprouts (mung), cooked, drained 1 cup 125	91	35	4	Trace	7	21	60	1.1	195	30	.11	.13	.9	8
Beets, diced or sliced														
Cooked from raw, drained, peeled 1 cup 170	91	55	2	Trace	12	24	39	.9	354	30	.05	.07	.5	10
Canned, drained solids 1 cup 170	89	65	2	Trace	15	32	31	1.2	284	30	.02	.05	.2	5
Beet greens, leaves and stems, cooked, drained 1 cup 145	94	25	2	Trace	5	144	36	2.8	481	7,400	.10	.22	.4	22
Black-eyed peas, cooked, drained 1 cup 165	72	180	13	1	30	40	241	3.5	635	580	.50	.18	2.3	28
Broccoli, cooked, drained														
From raw 1 cup 155	91	40	5	Trace	7	136	96	1.2	414	3,880	.14	.31	1.2	140
From frozen 1 cup 185	92	50	5	1	9	100	104	1.3	392	4,810	.11	.22	.9	105
Brussels sprouts, cooked, drained														
From raw 1 cup 155	88	55	7	1	10	50	112	1.7	423	810	.12	.22	1.2	135
From frozen 155	89	50	5	Trace	10	33	95	1.2	457	880	.12	.16	.9	126
Cabbage, common varieties														
Raw 90	92	20	1	Trace	5	44	26	.4	210	120	.05	.05	.3	42
Cooked, drained 1 cup 145	94	30	2	Trace	6	64	29	.4	236	190	.06	.06	.4	48

Food	Approx. measure	Grams	Water (%)	Food energy (cal)	Protein (g)	Fat (g)	Carbohydrate (g)	Calcium (mg)	Phosphorus (mg)	Iron (mg)	Potassium (mg)	Vitamin A (IU)	Thiamin (mg)	Riboflavin (mg)	Niacin (mg)	Ascorbic acid (mg)
Carrots																
Raw	1 medium carrot	72	88	30	1	Trace	7	27	26	.5	246	7,930	.04	.04	.4	6
Cooked from raw, drained	1 cup	155	91	50	1	Trace	11	51	48	.9	344	16,280	.08	.08	.8	9
Cauliflower, cooked from raw, drained	1 cup	125	93	30	3	Trace	5	26	53	.9	258	80	.11	.10	.8	69
Celery, Pascal type, raw																
Stalk, large outer	1 stalk	40	94	5	Trace	Trace	2	16	11	.1	136	110	.01	.01	.1	4
Pieces, diced	1 cup	120	94	20	1	Trace	5	47	34	.4	409	320	.04	.04	.4	11
Collards, cooked from raw, drained	1 cup	190	90	65	7	1	10	357	99	1.5	498	14,820	.21	.38	2.3	144
Corn, sweet																
Cooked from raw, drained (ear, 5 x 1¾″)	1 ear	140[37]	74	70	2	1	16	2	69	.5	151	310[38]	.09	.08	1.1	7
Canned — Cream style	1 cup	256	76	210	5	2	51	8	143	1.5	248	840[38]	.08	.13	2.6	13
Whole kernel, vacuum pack		210	76	175	5	1	43	6	153	1.1	204	740[38]	.06	.13	2.3	11
Cucumber slices, ⅛″ thick, without peel	6½ large or 9 small pieces	28	96	5	Trace	Trace	1	5	5	.1	45	Trace	.01	.01	.1	3
Kale, cooked, drained	1 cup	110	88	45	5	1	7	206	64	1.8	243	9,130	.11	.20	1.8	102
Lettuce, raw																
Butterhead, as Boston types	1 head	220	95	25	2	Trace	4	57	42	3.3	430	1,580	.10	.10	.5	13
Crisphead, as iceberg	1 head	567	96	70	5	1	16	108	118	2.7	943	1,780	.32	.32	1.6	32
Looseleaf (bunching varieties as romaine or cos), chopped or shredded	1 cup	55	94	10	1	Trace	2	37	14	.8	145	1,050	.03	.04	.2	10
Mushrooms, raw, sliced or chopped	1 cup	70	90	20	2	Trace	3	4	81	.6	290	Trace	.07	.32	2.9	2
Okra pods, 3 x ⅝″ cooked	10 pods	106	91	30	2	Trace	6	98	43	.5	184	520	.14	.19	1.0	21
Onions																
Raw, chopped	1 cup	170	89	65	3	Trace	15	46	61	.9	267	Trace[39]	.05	.07	.3	17
Young green, bulb and white portion of top	6 onions	30	88	15	2	Trace	7	12	12	.2	69	Trace	.02	.01	.1	8
Parsley, raw, chopped	1 T.	4	85	Trace	Trace	Trace	Trace	7	2	.2	25	300	Trace	.01	Trace	6
Parsnips, cooked	1 cup	155	82	100	2	1	23	70	96	.9	587	50	.11	.12	.2	16
Peas, green, canned, drained solids	1 cup	170	77	150	8	1	29	44	129	3.2	163	1,170	.15	.10	1.4	14
Peppers, hot, red without seeds, dried (ground chili powder, added seasonings)	1 t.	2	9	5	Trace	Trace	1	5	4	.3	20	1,300	Trace	.02	.2	Trace
Peppers, sweet, raw, stem and seeds removed	1 pod	74	93	15	1	Trace	5	7	16	.5	157	310	.06	.06	.4	94
Potatoes, cooked																
Baked in skin, peeled	1 potato	156	75	145	4	Trace	33	14	101	1.1	782	Trace	.15	.07	2.7	31
Boiled in skin, peeled	1 potato	137	80	105	3	Trace	23	10	72	.8	556	Trace	.12	.05	2.0	22
French fried (strip, 2 x 3½″ long)	10 strips	50	45	135	2	7	18	8	56	.7	427	Trace	.07	.04	1.6	11
Hashed brown	1 cup	155	56	345	3	18	45	9	78	1.9	439	Trace	.11	.03	1.6	12
Mashed, prepared from — Raw, milk added	1 cup	210	83	135	4	1	27	50	103	.8	548	40	.17	.11	2.1	21
Raw, milk and butter added		210	80	195	4	9	26	50	101	.8	525	360	.17	.11	2.1	19
Dehydrated flakes; water, milk, butter, and salt added	1 cup	210	79	195	4	7	30	65	99	.6	601	270	.08	.08	1.9	11

APPENDIX TABLE. Nutritive Values of the Edible Part of Foods *(continued)*

Food, Approximate Measure, and Weight (in grams)	Weight (g)	Water (%)	Food Energy (Cal)	Protein (g)	Fat (g)	Carbohydrate (g)	Calcium (mg)	Phosphorus (mg)	Iron (mg)	Potassium (mg)	Vitamin A Value (IU)	Thiamin (mg)	Riboflavin (mg)	Niacin (mg)	Ascorbic Acid (mg)
Vegetables and Vegetable Products *(continued)*															
Potato chips — 10 chips	20	2	115	1	8	10	8	28	.4	226	Trace	.04	.01	1.0	3
Potato salad — 1 cup	250	76	250	7	7	41	80	160	1.5	798	350	.20	.18	2.8	28
Radishes — 4 radishes	18	95	5	Trace	Trace	1	5	6	.2	58	Trace	.01	.01	.1	5
Sauerkraut, canned — 1 cup	235	93	40	2	Trace	9	85	42	1.2	329	120	.07	.09	.5	33
Spinach															
Raw, chopped — 1 cup	55	91	15	2	Trace	2	51	28	1.7	259	4,460	.06	.11	.3	28
Cooked from raw, drained — 1 cup	180	92	40	5	1	6	167	68	4.0	583	14,580	.13	.25	.9	50
Squash, cooked															
Summer, diced, drained — 1 cup	210	96	30	2	Trace	7	53	53	.8	296	820	.11	.17	1.7	21
Winter, baked, mashed — 1 cup	205	81	130	4	1	32	57	98	1.6	945	8,610	.10	.27	1.4	27
Sweet potatoes															
Baked in skin, peeled — 1 potato	114	64	160	2	1	37	46	66	1.0	342	9,230	.10	.08	.8	25
Boiled in skin, peeled — 1 potato	151	71	170	3	1	40	48	71	1.1	367	11,940	.14	.09	.9	26
Candied — 1 piece	105	60	175	1	3	36	39	45	.9	200	6,620	.06	.04	.4	11
Tomatoes															
Raw (3/12-oz. pkg.) — 1 tomato	135	94	25	1	Trace	6	16	33	.6	300	1,110	.07	.05	.9	28[40]
Canned, solids, and liquid — 1 cup	241	94	50	2	Trace	10	14[41]	46	1.2	523	2,170	.12	.07	1.7	41
Tomato catsup — 1 T.	15	69	15	Trace	Trace	4	3	8	.1	54	210	.01	.01	.2	2
Tomato juice, canned — 1 cup	243	94	45	2	Trace	10	17	44	2.2	552	1,940	.12	.07	1.9	39
Turnips, cooked, diced — 1 cup	155	94	35	1	Trace	8	54	37	.6	291	Trace	.06	.08	.5	34
Turnip greens, cooked, drained — 1 cup	145	94	30	3	Trace	5	252	49	1.5	—	8,270	.15	.33	.7	68
Vegetables, mixed, frozen, cooked — 1 cup	182	83	115	6	1	24	46	115	2.4	348	9,010	.22	.13	2.0	15
Miscellaneous Items															
Barbecue sauce — 1 cup	250	81	230	4	17	20	53	50	2.0	435	900	.03	.03	.8	13
Beverages, alcoholic															
Beer — 12 fl. oz.	360	92	150	1	0	14	18	108	Trace	90	—	.01	.11	2.2	—
Gin, rum, vodka, whiskey — 1½ fl. oz. jigger															
80-proof	42	67	95	—	—	Trace	—	—	—	1	—	—	—	—	—
86-proof	42	64	105	—	—	Trace	—	—	—	1	—	—	—	—	—
90-proof	42	62	110	—	—	Trace	—	—	—	1	—	—	—	—	—
Wine — 3½ fl. oz. glass															
Dessert	103	77	140	Trace	—	8	8	—	—	77	—	.01	.02	.2	—
Table	102	86	85	Trace	—	4	9	10	.4	94	—	Trace	.01	.1	—
Beverages, carbonated, sweetened, nonalcoholic — 12 fl. oz.															
Carbonated water	366	92	115	0	0	29	—	—	—	—	0	0	0	0	0
Cola type	369	90	145	0	0	37	—	—	—	—	0	0	0	0	0
Fruit-flavored sodas and Tom Collins mixer	372	88	170	0	0	45	—	—	—	0	0	0	0	0	0
Ginger ale	366	92	115	0	0	29	—	—	—	0	0	0	0	0	0

Food	Approximate measure	Grams	Water (%)	Food energy (calories)	Protein (g)	Fat (g)	Carbohydrate (g)	Calcium (mg)	Iron (mg)	Vitamin A (IU)	Thiamin (mg)	Riboflavin (mg)	Niacin (mg)	Ascorbic acid (mg)
Root beer		370	90	150	0	0	39	—	—	0	0	0	0	0
Gelatin, dry	1 envelope	7	13	25	6	Trace	0	—	—	—	—	—	—	0
Gelatin dessert prepared with gelatine dessert powder and water	1 cup	240	84	140	4	0	34	—	—	—	—	—	—	0
Mustard, prepared, yellow	1 t. or individual serving pouch or cup	5	80	5	Trace	Trace	Trace	4	.1	—	—	—	—	0
Olives, pickled, canned: Green	4 medium, 3 extra large, or 2 giant	16	78	15	Trace	2	Trace	8	.2	40	—	—	—	—
Ripe, Mission	3 small or 2 large	10	73	15	Trace	2	Trace	9	.1	10	Trace	Trace	—	—
Pickles, cucumber: Dill, medium	1 pickle	65	93	5	Trace	Trace	1	17	.7	70	Trace	.01	Trace	4
Sweet, gherkin, small	1 pickle	15	61	20	Trace	Trace	5	2	.2	10	Trace	Trace	Trace	1
Relish, sweet, finely chopped	1 T.	15	63	20	Trace	Trace	5	3	.1	—	—	—	—	—
Popsicle, 3 fl. oz.	1 popsicle	95	80	70	0	0	18	0	—	0	0	0	0	0
Soup: Canned, condensed. Prepared with equal volume of milk: Cream of chicken	1 cup	245	85	180	7	10	15	172	.5	610	.05	.27	.7	2
Cream of mushroom	1 cup	245	83	215	7	14	16	191	.5	250	.05	.34	.7	1
Tomato	1 cup	250	84	175	7	7	23	168	.8	1,200	.10	.25	1.3	15
Prepared with equal volume of water: Bean with pork	1 cup	250	84	170	8	6	22	63	2.3	650	.13	.08	1.0	3
Beef broth, bouillon, consomme	1 cup	240	96	30	5	0	3	Trace	.5	Trace	Trace	.02	1.2	—
Beef noodle	1 cup	240	93	65	4	3	7	7	1.0	50	.05	.07	1.0	Trace
Clam chowder, Manhattan type (with tomatoes, without milk)	1 cup	245	92	80	2	3	12	34	1.0	880	.02	.02	1.0	—
Cream of chicken	1 cup	240	92	95	3	6	8	24	.5	410	.02	.05	.5	Trace
Cream of mushroom	1 cup	240	90	135	2	10	10	41	.5	70	.02	.12	.7	Trace
Minestrone	1 cup	245	90	105	5	3	14	37	1.0	2,350	.07	.05	1.0	—
Split pea	1 cup	245	85	145	9	3	21	29	1.5	440	.25	.15	1.5	1
Tomato	1 cup	245	91	90	2	2	16	15	.7	1,000	.05	.05	1.2	12
Vegetable beef	1 cup	245	92	80	5	2	10	12	.7	2,700	.05	.05	1.0	—
Vegetarian	1 cup	245	92	80	2	2	13	20	1.0	2,940	.05	.05	1.0	—
Dehydrated: Bouillon cube, 1/2"	1 cube	4	4	5	1	Trace	Trace	—	—	—	—	—	—	—
Mixes prepared with water: Chicken noodle	1 cup	240	95	55	2	1	8	7	.2	50	.07	.05	.5	Trace
Onion	1 cup	240	96	35	1	1	6	10	.2	Trace	Trace	Trace	Trace	Trace
Tomato vegetable with noodles	1 cup	240	93	65	1	1	12	7	.2	480	.05	.02	.5	2
Vinegar, cider	1 T.	15	94	Trace	0	0	1	1	.1	—	—	—	—	—
White sauce, medium, with enriched flour	1 cup	250	73	405	10	31	22	288	.5	1,150	.12	.43	.7	2
Yeast: Baker's, dry, active	1 pkg.	7	5	20	3	Trace	3	3	1.1	Trace	.16	.38	2.6	Trace
Brewer's, dry	1 T.	8	5	25	3	Trace	3	17[42]	1.4	Trace	1.25	.34	3.0	Trace

APPENDIX TABLE. Nutritive Values of the Edible Part of Foods (*continued*)

[1]Vitamin A value is largely from beta-carotene used for coloring.

[2]Applies to product without added vitamin A. With added vitamin A, value is 500 IU.

[3]Applies to product without added vitamin A.

[4]Applies to products that are made from thick shake mixes and do not contain added ice cream. Products made from milk shake mixes are higher in fat and usually contain added ice cream.

[5]Content of fat, vitamin A, and carbohydrate varies. Consult the label when precise values are needed for special diets.

[6]Applies to product made with milk containing no added vitamin A.

[7]Based on year-round average.

[8]Based on average vitamin A content of fortified margarine. Federal specifications for fortified margarine require a minimum of 15,000 IU of vitamin A per pound.

[9]Dipped in egg, milk or water, and breadcrumbs; fried in vegetable shortening.

[10]If bones are discarded, value for calcium will be greatly reduced.

[11]Dipped in egg, breadcrumbs, and flour or batter.

[12]Prepared with tuna, celery, salad dressing (mayonnaise type), pickle, onion, and egg.

[13]Outer layer of fat on the cut was removed to within approximately $\frac{1}{2}$ inch of the lean. Deposits of fat within the cut were not removed.

[14]Crust made with vegetable shortening and enriched flour.

[15]Value varies widely.

[16]About one-fourth of the outer layer of fat on the cut was removed. Deposits of fat within the cut were not removed.

[17]Vegetable shortening used.

[18]Also applies to pasteurized apple cider.

[19]Applies to product without added ascorbic acid. For value of product with added ascorbic acid, refer to label.

[20]Based on product with label claim of 100% of U.S. RDA in 6 fluid ounces.

[21]For white-fleshed varieties, value is about 20 IU per cup; for red-fleshed varieties, it is 1,080 IU.

[22]For products with added thiamin and riboflavin but without added ascorbic acid, values are 0.60 mg for thiamin, 0.80 mg for riboflavin, and trace for ascorbic acid. For products with only ascorbic acid added, value varies with the brand. Consult the label.

[23]Represents yellow-fleshed varieties. For white-fleshed varieties, value is 50 IU for one peach.

[24]Value represents products with added ascorbic acid. For products without added ascorbic acid, value is 103 mg per cup.

[25]Weight includes pits.

[26]Weight includes rind and seeds.

[27]Made with enriched flour and vegetable shortening.

[28]Made with vegetable shortening.

[29]Applies to product made with white cornmeal. With yellow cornmeal, value is 30 IU.

[30]Applies to white varieties. For yellow varieties, value is 150 IU.

[31]Applies to products that do not contain disodium phosphate. If disodium phosphate is an ingredient, value is 162 mg.

[32]Value may range from less than 1 mg to about 8 mg depending on the brand. Consult the label.

[33]Value varies with the brand. Consult the label.

[34]Applies to product with added ascorbic acid. Without added ascorbic acid, value is trace.

[35]Macaroons do not contain flour or shortening.

[36]Product may or may not be enriched with riboflavin. Consult the label.

[37]Weight includes cob. Without cob, weight is 77 g.

[38]Based on yellow varieties. For white varieties, value is trace.

[39]Based on white-fleshed varieties. For yellow-fleshed varieties, value is 70 IU.

[40]Based on year-round average. For tomatoes marketed from November through May, value is about 12 mg; from June through October, 32 mg.

[41]Applies to product without added calcium salts. Value for products with added calcium salts may be as much as 63 mg for whole tomatoes, 241 mg for cut forms.

[42]Value may vary from 6 to 60 mg.

NOTE: Dashes denote lack of reliable data for a constituent believed to be present in measurable amount.

SOURCE: Adapted from *Nutritive Value of Foods*, Home and Garden Bulletin No. 72, Agricultural Research Service, U.S. Department of Agriculture, revised April 1977.

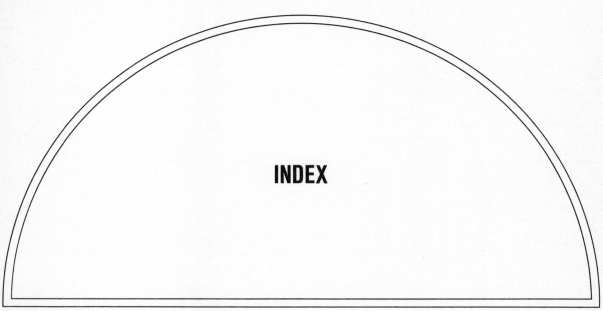

INDEX

ABOUT THE AUTHORS

Kristen McNutt majored in chemistry at Duke University and completed a master's degree at Columbia University Institute of Human Nutrition. She did nutrition research in a village outside Cairo, Egypt for a year and participated in the ICNND (Interdepartmental Committee on Nutrition for National Development) survey of Nigeria. Dave McNutt earned a bachelor's degree at Columbia University. He completed a master's degree in microbiology and a medical degree at Ohio State University, and interned at Tulane University.

The McNutts met at Vanderbilt University, where Dave was a resident in internal medicine and Kristen a Ph.D. candidate in biochemistry. After their marriage in 1969, they lived in San Francisco (he was training in hematology and immunology at UCSF and she did a fellowship in nutrition at UC Berkeley), Okinawa (he as an Air Force internist and she in clinical chemistry at the Army hospital), and Tucson (more Air Force medicine for Dave and

back to biochemistry research for Kristen). Next they worked for six months with the Hospital Ship HOPE in northeast Brazil.

Since 1973, the McNutts have resided in the Washington, D.C. area. Dave earned a master's in public health from Johns Hopkins University and became board certified in preventive medicine in 1975. He is currently Chief of Manpower Supply and Utilization with the Bureau of Health Manpower of DHEW. For four years Kristen was a research associate with the Nutrition Foundation. She is a member of the American Institute of Nutrition, the American Dietetic Association, and the Board of the Society for Nutrition Education. She was selected by FASEB (Federation of American Societies of Experimental Biology) as their 1977–78 Congressional science fellow and works on the staff of the Senate Committee on Agriculture, Nutrition, and Forestry.